Primary Care
for the PHYSICAL
THERAPIST

Examination and Triage

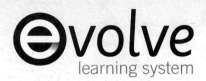
evolve
learning system

To access your Learning Resources, visit:

http://evolve.elsevier.com/ Boissonnault/primary

Evolve Student Learning Resources for Boissonnault: Primary Care for the Physical Therapist: Examination and Triage, Second edition, offers the following features:

- **Additional Resources**
  Printable versions of the appendices in chapters 4, 8, and 19.
- **Image Collection**
  These additional full color skin lesion figures supplement Chapter 10 in the textbook.
- **References**
  End of chapter References linked to Medline.
- **WebLinks**
  An exciting resource that lets you link to hundreds of websites carefully chosen to supplement the content of the textbook.

Evolve Instructor Resources for Boissonnault: Primary Care for the Physical Therapist: Examination and Triage, Second edition, offers the following features:

- **Image Collection**
  Search, view, and download the large selection of images from the textbook.
- **Exam Questions**
  Exam questions and answers for Section 2 of the book.
- **PowerPoint Slides**
  Teaching slides for Chapters 4 and 14.
- **PowerPoint Slides**
  Patient Case Studies with Questions for Chapters 6 to 9.
- **Test Bank**
  Exam questions and answers for Chapters 6 to 15.
- **Video**
  Video Simulations to supplement Chapters 5, 12, 13, and 20.
- **WebLinks**
  An exciting resource that lets you link to hundreds of websites carefully chosen to supplement the content of the textbook.

Primary Care
for the PHYSICAL THERAPIST

Examination and Triage

Second Edition

William G. Boissonnault, PT, DPT DHSc, FAAOMPT, FAPTA
Associate Professor
University of Wisconsin–Madison
Program in Physical Therapy
Madison, Wisconsin

ELSEVIER
SAUNDERS

3251 Riverport Lane
St. Louis, Missouri 63043

Boissonnault, William G.
  Primary care for the physical therapist : examination and triage / William G.
    Boissonnault. -- 2nd ed. p. ; cm.
  Rev. ed. of: Primary care for the physical therapist / [edited by] William G. Boissonnault. c2005
  Includes bibliographical references and index.
  ISBN 978-1-4160-6105-2 (hardcover : alk. paper) 1. Physical therapy--Practice. 2. Primary care (Medicine) 3. Physical diagnosis. 4. Triage (Medicine)
I. Primary care for the physical therapist. II. Title.
  [DNLM: 1. Physical Therapy Modalities. 2. Physical Examination. 3. Primary Health Care. 4. Triage. WB 460 B684p 2011]
  RM705.P756 2011
  615.8'2--dc22   2010019647

Vice President and Publisher: Linda Duncan
Executive Editor: Kathryn Falk
Senior Developmental Editor: Christie M. Hart
Publishing Services Manager: Catherine Jackson
Senior Project Manager: Mary Pohlman
Project Manager: Jennifer Boudreau
Book Designer: Paula Catalano

Printed in United States of America

Last digit is the print number: 9 8 7 6 5 4 3 2 1

To: Journeys driven by passion and understanding, and marked by discovery.

Contributors

Sandra Baatz, PT
Holy Family Memorial Medical Center
Manitowoc, Wisconsin

Janet R. Bezner, PT, PhD
Deputy Executive Director
American Physical Therapy Association
Alexandria, Virginia

Jill Schiff Boissonnault, PT, PhD, WCS
Assistant Professor
Program in Physical Therapy
University of Wisconsin–Madison;
Director
University of Wisconsin Hospitals and Clinics and
Meriter Hospital Orthopedic Physical Therapy Clinical
    Residency
Madison, Wisconsin

William G. Boissonnault, PT, DPT, DHSc, FAAOMPT, FAPTA
Associate Professor
Program in Physical Therapy
University of Wisconsin–Madison
Madison, Wisconsin

William P. Brookfield, RPh, MSc
Global Patient Safety Consultant
Eli Lilly and Company;
Adjunct Professor
College of Pharmacy
Butler University
Indianapolis, Indiana;
Adjunct Professor
School of Pharmaceutical Sciences
Purdue University
West Lafayette, Indiana;
Adjunct Professor
Krannert School of Physical Therapy
University of Indianapolis
Indianapolis, Indiana

Gail D. Deyle, PT, DSc, DPT, OCS, FAAOMPT
Associate Professor
Baylor University Graduate School;
Senior Faculty
US Army-Baylor University Doctoral Fellowship in
    Orthopaedic Manual Physical Therapy
Brooke Army Medical Center
San Antonio, Texas

Maureen (Reenie) Euhardy PT, MS, GCS
Doctor of Physical Therapy Program Admissions Advisor
University of Wisconsin–Madison
Madison, Wisconsin

Julie M. Fritz, PT, PhD, ATC
Associate Professor
Department of Physical Therapy
University of Utah
Salt Lake City, Utah

Matthew B. Garber, PT, DSc, OCS, FAAOMPT
Command Physical Therapist
US Army Special Operations Command
Fort Bragg, North Carolina;
Associate Professor
Rocky Mountain University of Health Professions
Provo, Utah;
Adjunct Faculty
Hardin-Simmons University
Abilene, Texas;
Adjunct Faculty
Shenandoah University
Winchester, Virginia

Joseph Godges, DPT
Coordinator
Clinical Education and Practice
OptimisCorp
Pacific Palisades, California;
Adjunct Associate Professor
Division of Biokinesiology and Physical Therapy
University of Southern California
Los Angeles, California

David G. Greathouse, PT, PhD, ECS, FAPTA
Director
Clinical Electrophysiology Services
Texas Physical Therapy Specialists
New Braunfels, Texas;
Adjunct Professor
US Army-Baylor University Doctoral Program in Physical Therapy
Fort Sam Houston, Texas

Kristine M. Hallisy, PT, MS, OCS, CMPT, CTI
Faculty Associate
Program in Physical Therapy
University of Wisconsin–Madison
Madison, Wisconsin

Michael P. Johnson, PT, PhD, OCS
Director of Clinical Leadership
Bayada Nurses, Skilled Visit Services
Moorestown, New Jersey

Connie J. Kittleson, PT, DPT
Adjunct Faculty
Program in Physical Therapy
Concordia University Wisconsin
Mequon, Wisconsin

Ronnie Leavitt, PhD, MPH, PT
Longmeadow, Pennsylvania

D. Michael McKeough, PT, EdD
Professor
Department of Physical Therapy
California State University–Sacramento
Sacramento, California

Rebecca G. Stephenson, PT, DPT, MS, WCS
Coordinator of Women's Health Physical Therapy
Brigham and Women's Hospital;
Adjunct Faculty
Massachusetts General Hospital Institute of Health Professions
Boston, Massachusetts

Steven H. Tepper, PT, PhD
President
Rehab Essentials, Inc.;
Freelance Professor
Monkton, Maryland

Kristin von Nieda, DPT, MEd
Associate Professor
Department of Physical Therapy
Arcadia University
Glenside, Pennsylvania

Sue Wenker, PT, MS, GCS
Faculty Associate
Program in Physical Therapy
Department of Orthopedics and Rehabilitation
University of Wisconsin–Madison
Madison, Wisconsin

Michael S. Wong, DPT, OCS, FAAOMPT
Associate Professor
Department of Physical Therapy
Azusa Pacific University
Azusa, California

Preface

As with the first edition of *Primary Care for the Physical Therapist: Examination and Triage,* this edition is written in the spirit of the American Physical Therapy Association's "Vision Statement for Physical Therapy 2020" (HOD 06-00-24-35):

By 2020, physical therapy will be provided by physical therapists who are doctors of physical therapy, recognized by consumers and other health care professionals as the practitioners of choice to whom consumers have direct access for the diagnosis of, interventions for, and prevention of impairments, functional limitations, and disabilities related to movement, function, and health.

Tremendous opportunities await physical therapist practitioners as the profession moves toward Vision 2020, including unlimited potential in the area of primary care. Primary care has been described by the Institute of Medicine (IOM) as "the provision of integrated, accessible health care services by clinicians who are accountable for addressing a large majority of personal health care needs, developing a sustained partnership with patients, and practicing within the context of family and community." The American Physical Therapy Association (APTA) has endorsed the concepts of primary care set forth by the IOM, noting that "primary care can encompass myriad needs that go well beyond the capabilities and competencies of individual caregivers and that require the involvement and interaction of varied practitioners." The 2002 APTA, *Interactive Guide to Physical Therapist Practice,* noted that "for acute musculoskeletal and neuromuscular conditions, triage and initial examination are appropriate physical therapist responsibilities, and for certain chronic conditions physical therapists should be recognized as principal providers of care within a collaborative Primary Care Team." Key words and phrases from these statements include examination, triage, principal providers of care for certain conditions, and collaborative team.

The APTA's collaborative team emphasis is an important message for those within and outside our profession. When I consider the delivery of primary care, I do not envision individuals (of any discipline), I picture a cohesive interdisciplinary health care delivery system. Such a cohesive system requires team building and communication skills, and a solid understanding of the various providers' backgrounds and potential roles. With the appropriate training, physical therapists can be active participants and leaders in the development of primary care delivery models, with training commensurate with the professional doctoral degree (DPT).

Since the publication of this textbook's first edition, signs of progress toward attaining the goals set by Vision 2020 are evident. More states have adopted direct access legislation, others have updated practice acts removing unnecessary patient access limitations, new publications have strengthened the evidence-based foundation for the goals of Vision 2020, and the public is becoming more aware of services provided by physical therapists and physical therapist assistants, and how these services can be accessed in a primary care environment. For decades, the only context of therapists working in the direct access model was the military model. In large part as a result of the success of physical therapists in the military, their performance, and reports of their experiences, the number of similar practice models in the public sector settings is increasing. Irrespective of how patients/clients access our services (primary care encompasses more than direct access to therapy services), the primary beneficiaries of this evolution of physical therapist practice are the patients and clients seeking our services.

The success stories associated with our changing practice and increased involvement in primary care are marked by themes of collaboration and interdependence. The adopted interdependence model of care delivery ensures that the consumer accesses the most appropriate practitioner in a timely fashion. Thus, a major focus of this edition is to promote the early recognition of patient warning signs (red flags) indicating that physician (or other provider) consultation is warranted. Considering the length of time that therapists tend to spend with patients and families and the rapport that can be established, combined with quality examination skills, the physical therapist is in a prime position to be a strong advocate for the health and wellness of those we serve. Effectively working interdependently with other health care providers in primary care settings is therefore an underlying theme of this text.

Despite the profession's progress toward achieving the goals of Vision 2020, there are many reminders that more work remains, which has helped create this second edition. Written for students, residents, fellows, and experienced clinicians, this new edition promotes a significant role in the primary care practice model for physical therapists, with major emphasis on the examination, triage, and interdisciplinary health care components related to the physical therapist's potential role. This text should complement other publications describing detailed regional examination and intervention approaches relevant to this model of health care delivery. Once again, an outstanding group of contributors has participated in this project. I am grateful for their commitment toward the completion of this text and for their overall passion and contributions to the growth of our profession. I have learned a great deal from their contributions. Through their efforts and feedback from readers over the past 5 years, preexisting chapters have been updated and expanded and new chapters have been added. These changes now reflect new evidence and the evolution of the physical therapist's practice. The book's original theme of examination, triage, and consultation has been broadened to include the healthy client. An excellent chapter has been added that provides a health and wellness perspective to therapists and the provision of primary care services. In addition, a concise presentation of screening for selected medical conditions that could warrant an urgent referral has been added (Chapter 20). Another new chapter expands the content related to the differential diagnosis of presenting complaints that therapists commonly encounter.

The book is divided into three sections: (1) Foundations, (2) Examination/Evaluation, and (3) Special Populations. Section One describes primary care models already in place, in which physical therapists are the entry point for selected patient populations (Chapter 1). The goals of these patient encounters include the following: (1) deciding whether certain imaging modalities are warranted to assist in the diagnostic process; (2) deciding whether a physician consultation is indicated; (3) determining whether a referral to a physical therapist certified clinical specialist is warranted; and (4) implementing a physical therapy plan of care, when appropriate. Considering that hypertension, diabetes mellitus, and low back pain are among the most frequently reported reasons for patient visits to a health care clinic, there are tremendous opportunities for physical therapists, not only as examiners and those who perform triage, but also as principal providers of care. Interestingly, much of the impetus for including physical therapists in the primary care models described in Chapter 1 has come from physician groups within the health care systems described. Chapter 2, "Evidence-Based Examination of Diagnostic Information," provides physical therapists with the tools necessary to practice in an evidence-based practice environment, with the focus on screening and diagnostic processes. Chapter 3, "Cultural Competence," provides essential information related to effective patient care in the ever-diversifying U.S. patient population. Chapter 4 discusses the importance of pharmacologic considerations for the physical therapist. Chapter 5, "The Patient Interview: The Science Behind the Art," details the art and science behind an effective patient-therapist interchange.

Section Two, Chapters 6 to 15—Examination/Evaluation—focuses on the physical therapist's examination and triage skills vital to a primary care environment. Central to these skills is the data evaluation process that leads to the differential diagnosis and establishment of the appropriate plan of care. An important part of the triage responsibilities is the recognition by physical therapists of those patients who need to be referred to other members of the primary care team, as well as determining which patients should be seen by a certified clinical specialist (physical therapist).

In an effort to promote efficient and effective practice, this section is organized in the same way that a physical therapist might collect patients' data; starting with the chief presenting complaint, "Patient what brings you here?", "How can I help you?" Chapters 6 (new chapter) and 7 present a differential diagnosis approach to common chief presenting complaints (e.g., back pain, joint pain dizziness). Conditions appropriate for therapists to manage are compared and contrasted to disorders that require physician involvement. Next, Chapter 8 discusses critical patient health history information (e.g., illnesses, medications, substance use, and family history). Effective and efficient means to collect the necessary patient data are presented, along with important follow-up questions and tests to help identify patient health care and wellness issues. Chapters 9 and 10 provide the basis for a detailed review of systems screening for health issues other than the chief presenting complaint. Chapter 10 makes a case for the physical examination beginning as soon as the therapist starts interacting with the patient. Chapters 11, 12, and 13 present physical examination screening including vital signs, and an upper and lower quadrant screening schematic. These important elements will help establish a baseline of general health status and guidance for where a more detailed examination needs to occur. Clinical medicine chapters are included that discuss the relevance of diagnostic imaging and laboratory tests and values to a therapist's clinical decision-making. Information in this Section should lead therapists to developing the appropriate plan of care for each individual patient/client.

Section Three, Special Populations, describes client groups (including the pediatric population, adolescents, obstetric patients, and geriatric patients), commonly served by physical therapists, with unique issues and challenges. Understanding the distinctive anatomic, physiologic, psychosocial, and pathologic factors associated with each group will help prepare the therapist to quickly establish an accurate and effective plan of care. Experts in the field present recommended examination modifications for these groups, with an overview of diseases and disorders commonly noted in these populations. Finally, this section presents potential practice niches in which physical therapists' involvement would greatly enhance the delivery of care.

The intent of this book is to complement therapists' knowledge and information from other texts and articles related to specific regional examination and intervention approaches. The information provided should facilitate the therapist's role in the primary care model as an active participant in shaping health care delivery in the United States and worldwide. The challenge that faces us is whether we can put the charges described in Vision 2020 into action, a challenge that must be met. I believe that maintaining the status quo of our practice is not a viable option. Two choices are available—either we regress back to the era when we were functioning more as aides, when we joined the ranks of supportive practitioners, or we become the decision makers. I am confident that you will agree that there is really only one option. "It's all about the patient/client" has been my mantra for years.

William G. Boissonnault, PT, DPT, DHSc, FAAOMPT, FAPTA

Acknowledgments

I am grateful to family, friends and colleagues for the ongoing support and encouragement-forever.

A special debt of gratitude goes to Giuseppe Plebani, Fisioterapista, Siena, Italy; whose vision of the level of practice physical therapists should aspire to, has opened international professional doors for me, and more importantly has led to a new-found friendship.

Last, a medal goes to Christie Hart, Senior Developmental Editor, of this edition and her colleagues at Elsevier for the perpetual patience and understanding throughout the project.

Contents

SECTION THREE   SPECIAL POPULATIONS

Primary Care: Physical Therapy Models

1

Michael P. Johnson, PT, PhD, OCS
Kristin von Nieda, DPT, MEd
David G. Greathouse, PT, PhD, ECS, FAPTA

Objectives

After reading this chapter, the reader will be able to:

1. Define primary and secondary health care.
2. Provide an overview of primary care from the perspective of physical therapists and physicians.
3. Describe examples of current physical therapy practice models that function within the realm of primary care.

Primary care, its definition, and the roles of various health professionals in the delivery of services has been evolving over the past 30 years. A definition of primary care was established by the World Health Organization (WHO) in 1978 through work at the International Conference on Primary Health Care.[30] Participants recognized that primary care includes the following:

1. A level of health service delivery that serves as the foundation of any health care system and "provides both the initial and the majority of health care services for a person or population."
2. An approach to health care practice that "addresses the main health problems in the community, providing promotive, preventive, curative and rehabilitative services accordingly."[30]

Physical therapy as commonly practiced has historically been considered a form of secondary health care rather than primary care. The WHO defines secondary health care as "consultative, short term, and disease oriented ... for the purpose of assisting the primary care practitioner."[30] Physical therapists (PTs) focus on function versus disease,[3] however, and identify themselves as autonomous practitioners of choice for patients with neuromusculoskeletal conditions (NMSCs), across a spectrum of well-being from prevention and health promotion to examination and intervention for individuals with functional limitations and disability.[2] An argument exists whether physical therapy can be a primary and a secondary health service.

Family physicians, general internists, and pediatricians provide most primary care medicine in the United States (Table 1-1). Primary care services are provided on a much smaller scale by a broad range of specialists, most notably obstetrician-gynecologists. In recent years, physician assistants (PAs) and nurse practitioners (NPs) have become important members of the primary care team, especially related to the management of general medical conditions. Primary care is distinguished by integration of care that encompasses three concepts: comprehensiveness, coordination, and continuity. As more health professionals participate in the delivery of services as part of primary care teams, the challenges of coordination and continuity become more paramount.

In 1996, the Institute of Medicine (IOM) defined primary care as "the provision of integrated, accessible health care services by clinicians who are accountable for addressing a large majority of personal health care needs, developing a sustained partnership with patients, and practicing in the context of family and community."[28] In the area of neuromusculoskeletal medicine, PTs have the capacity to function within the realm of primary care.

In their 2001 report titled "Crossing the Quality Chasm," which identified significant problems related to the delivery of quality care within the U.S. health system, the IOM recommended transitioning away from an autonomous physician model in health care delivery and moving toward a collaborative, multidisciplinary "team" model in which other clinicians also play a central role. Within this model, the "individual who serves as the (team) leader may not be ... associated with a particular discipline, such as medicine."[27] New opportunities exist for PTs to enhance their roles in the delivery of primary care services, in addition to their traditional roles of providing secondary health services.

The role of the PT in a primary care environment has been evolving rapidly. With specific expertise related to the management of patients with NMSCs, PTs are well positioned to contribute as key members and leaders of primary care teams. This is especially true given the prevalence of NMSCs among the U.S. population,[34,37,47,67,68] the number of primary care visits (20% to 30%) for neuromusculoskeletal complaints[65] (Figure 1-1), and the limited amount of education provided to internal and family

---

This chapter includes contributions by Ivan Matsui and Brian Murphy from the first edition of *Primary Care for the Physical Therapist, Examination and Triage.*

TABLE 1-1

Patient Visits to Physician Specialty

Physician Specialty and Professional Identity	No. Visits	%
All visits	901,954	100
PHYSICIAN SPECIALTY		
General and family practice	208,475	23.1
Internal medicine*	125,398	13.9
Pediatrics	122,344	13.6
Obstetrics and gynecology	69,436	7.7
Oncology	14,871	1.6
Ophthalmology	57,815	6.4
Orthopedic surgery	48,066	5.3
Dermatology	25,256	2.8
Psychiatry	25,150	2.8
General surgery	14,048	1.6
Urology	18,307	2
Cardiovascular disease	25,790	2.9
Otolaryngology	17,508	1.9
Neurology	12,532	1.4
All other specialties	116,958	13

*Includes only general internal medicine.

From U.S. Department of Health and Human Services, Public Health Service, Centers for Disease Control and Prevention, National Center for Health Statistics, 2006 (website). http://www.cdc.gov/nchs/data/nhsr/nhsr003.pdf.

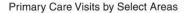
Primary Care Visits by Select Areas

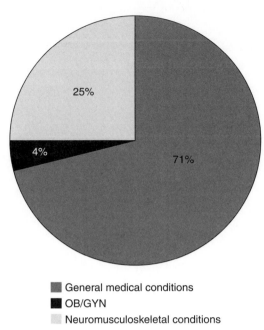

FIGURE 1-1 Primary care by selected condition areas. (From U.S. Department of Health and Human Services, National Center for Health Statistics, 2005.)

practice medical residents regarding the management of patients with NMSCs.[7] This chapter familiarizes PTs with the various providers and issues in primary care and helps PTs identify potential roles for themselves within multidisciplinary, interdependent models of primary care.

Modern Health Care in the United States

An awareness of the dynamics that have shaped the current health care system in the United States can help PTs appreciate the various demands placed on the primary care team. Beginning at the turn of the 19th century, with the advent of bacteriology and the focus on public health, physicians and hospitals began to play a dominant role in health care. Previously, most people were cared for at home by a family member or local healer.[56] As medical knowledge and technology improved, so did the quality of the care received by many Americans. As life expectancy and quality began to increase, there was a focus on policies that helped improve access to medical services. From the early 1930s to the mid-1960s, the following key events significantly shaped the U.S. health system: (1) the creation of health insurance that covered hospital (Blue Cross) and physician costs (Blue Shield) and was tied closely to employment as a benefit to attract workers during World War II when wage freezes were in effect, (2) an investment in research through the creation of the National Institutes of Health in 1930, and (3) widespread construction of hospitals resulting from the passage of the Hill-Burton Act in 1946. By 1965, the U.S. health care system could deliver high-quality care in hospitals and clinics in nearly every community across the United States.

With the passage of the Medicare and Medicaid Amendments to the Social Security Act (1965), the U.S. government guaranteed availability of health care services for elderly and poor individuals by ensuring payment for those services on a fee-for-service basis. Medicare and Medicaid were cornerstones of President Johnson's "great society." The Johnson administration envisioned subsequently offering similar programs to the entire population as a way of providing universal health care access. Health care expenditures for Medicare recipients increased dramatically, however, in the decade that followed. This rapid increase in health care costs put a halt to any plans to expand government-guaranteed health care coverage further and spawned several pieces of legislation that shaped later changes for health care delivery within the United States.[4]

In response to the rapid increase in health care costs in the private sector and Medicare, many strategies were used to contain costs, including the creation of peer review organizations, passage of the Health Maintenance Organization Act in 1973 (which led to the precipitous increase in managed care by the early 1990s), and the introduction of diagnosis-related groups (DRGs) as a method of prospective payment for inpatient services rendered to Medicare patients. The establishment of DRGs in 1984 resulted in the first reduction of use of Medicare services since the program's inception. Resource-based relative value scales (RBRVSs) were developed in 1989 to quantify outpatient Medicare services similar to the way DRGs were being used to define payment for inpatient services. RBRVSs were fully implemented in 1997.[23]

Although DRGs and RBRVSs were effective in controlling the increase in Medicare expenditures in the 1980s, health care expenditures for the remainder of the population continued to increase. Many federal administrations have attempted to reform health care primarily to control costs. The proliferation of health maintenance organizations (HMOs) in the 1990s charged the debate for health care reform in the United States. Many health care reformers at the time believed that the U.S. would follow the lead of most Western European nations and establish a national health care system. Despite the sense that reform was imminent, President Clinton's national health care reform initiative, the Health Security Act,[23] collapsed in 1994 under intense lobbying by the insurance and hospital industries and because of the sheer complexity of the task force's final recommendations.

With the demise of the Health Security Act, HMOs were aggressively promoted as the free market system's answer to controlling health care costs. The most common HMO model includes a physician gatekeeper. With this model, all services are provided directly by the patient's primary care provider or, if specialty services are required, authorized by the primary care provider. HMO plans assumed that requiring everyone to see a primary physician first would result in significant savings, because studies have consistently shown that patients with primary care physicians consume fewer services, have lower overall health care costs, and have better health outcomes than patients without primary care providers. Consumers developed a sense, however, that HMOs were limiting their access to care.

Double-digit increases in health care costs have again caused alarm in the business community and in the federal government. In 2009, there is a strong sense of impending health reform, and the Democratic administration under President Obama has pledged to overhaul the U.S. health care system. Primary care providers are watching closely to see how the most recent increases in health care costs will affect their role in the delivery of health care services in the near future.

Primary Care Providers in the United States

Family physicians, general internists, and pediatricians constitute the bulk of primary care physicians in the United States. PAs and NPs are increasingly being used to improve patient access to primary care services. Although all these groups are considered primary health care professionals, there are significant differences in training and patient populations served among groups.

Family physicians receive 3 years of training after graduation from medical school. The care of patients in an outpatient setting is the cornerstone of family practice residency training programs; the typical family physician spends 90% or more of his or her time in the outpatient setting. The first year of residency consists primarily of inpatient rotations of specialty services including, but not limited to, pediatrics, obstetrics/gynecology, surgery, adult medicine, emergency medicine, and intensive care. The family medicine resident maintains an outpatient continuity practice even during this first year of intensive inpatient training. During the second and third year of residency training, the amount of time spent in the outpatient setting increases. Further specialty training is received in various outpatient specialty clinics, such as otolaryngology, dermatology, urology, and rheumatology. A minimum of 1 month is spent concentrating on musculoskeletal conditions. This time may be spent with either an orthopedist or a sports medicine physician.

A heavy emphasis throughout the training is placed on the psychosocial model of medical care. This model emphasizes the influence the patient's social situation, family dynamics, and emotional well-being may have on his or her total health. All family medicine training facilities have full-time mental health specialists involved in the daily education and supervision of the residents. Family physicians potentially treat patients from "the cradle to the grave," although in reality many family physicians develop practices that are more limited in scope.

General internists also spend 3 years in postgraduate training. In contrast to family medicine residency training, the emphasis of general internal medicine is the caring for hospitalized patients such as patients with cardiac and medically intensive health problems. Outpatient services represent a small portion of the total time spent in the residency training programs. Little, if any, time is spent under the supervision of mental health educators, and there are no requirements for training with either orthopedists or sports medicine physicians to develop an understanding about musculoskeletal problems. On completion of their training, general internists tend to limit their practice to the care of adults, and many general internists do not provide women's health services. On completion of the residency training, internists generally spend as much, if not more, time caring for hospitalized patients as they do patients in the outpatient setting.

General pediatricians also spend 3 years in postgraduate training. Pediatric residents train in neonatal intensive care units, pediatric intensive care units, and general pediatric inpatient services. They also spend time in general and specialty pediatric outpatient clinics. The first year of most pediatric training programs is primarily spent in the hospital setting, with the subsequent 2 years more evenly split between the inpatient and outpatient settings. Pediatric training programs place great emphasis on childhood developmental stages. Recognition of congenital malformations, including orthopedic conditions, is part of formal pediatric training. Training in the care of musculoskeletal illness in older children is less formalized but has received greater emphasis in recent years. Pediatricians typically limit their scope of practice to patients younger than 18 years but can provide care for patients of any age.

An increasing number of other health professionals are delivering primary care services in the United States. NPs and PAs constitute the bulk of these professionals. PTs may also be considered primary care providers in states that authorize direct access to PTs. The focus, education, and training of these additional disciplines have important distinctions.

Enrollees in NP training programs are graduates of a registered nurse training program. The length and focus of an NP training program can vary dramatically depending on the focus of the particular program. Many NP training programs focus on a particular field of practice, such as geriatrics or pediatrics. A separate accrediting body determines the educational requirements for each of the areas of interest. Instructors within an NP training program are also typically nursing professionals and not physicians. NP programs award a Master of Science or a professional doctorate degree to their graduates. Each state has a defined certification process for NPs, which varies greatly from state to state. Depending on these regulations, NPs may function as independent practitioners or practice only under the direction of a physician supervisor. NPs have prescriptive authority in all states, but the level of supervision required varies. The local certification and review of NPs are functions of state boards of nursing, not local medical boards.

PAs were originally Army medics returning from the Vietnam War. These medics received an additional year of training to adapt what they had learned in the service and in the field to the needs of the civilian population. The training programs were expanded to include other individuals with prior health care experience, such as nurses or paramedics. Over time, PA programs grew in length and offered a broader level of health care training.

Although prior health care experience is encouraged for individuals applying to PA programs, most programs no longer require prior experience as a prerequisite for enrollment. Most programs are 2 years in length with 1 year spent in a classroom setting and 1 year involved in various inpatient and outpatient clinical experiences. In contrast to NP training programs, all PA training programs must meet the educational requirements established by a single national accrediting body. The organization is composed of PAs and representatives of various medical organizations. PA graduates are certified to practice after successfully completing an accredited training program and passing a national certification test. Graduates typically are awarded a Bachelor of Science or a professional Master of Science degree, but the certification process does not depend on the degree received. In contrast to NPs, PAs never practice as independent practitioners; rather they work solely in collaboration with a supervising physician. Each state sets the required level of physician supervision. Most states allow PAs prescriptive authority; however, as with NPs, the level of physician supervision varies. Supervising physicians are held liable for the scope of practice and the quality of care a PA renders. As such, medical oversight of PA practice is the responsibility of state medical boards. The type of patients seen by a PA depends on the supervising physician's expertise. PAs involved in primary care are typically supervised by family physicians, general internists, and emergency medicine physicians.

In the United States, PTs are required to receive a postgraduate degree. The minimum degree requirement is at the Master's level, but as of July 2009 approximately 95% of the PT programs are now at the doctoral level.[4] Program length varies, but is generally 3 to 4 years, and includes academic and clinical education. PT programs are accredited by the Commission on Accreditation in Physical Therapy Education, and content is required in basic sciences; behavioral sciences; and clinical sciences, including examination, intervention, medical screening, diagnostic imaging, clinical decision making, and pharmacology. Clinical education in specialty areas is not required, and PT students generally complete internships in inpatient settings and outpatient clinics, which may include rehabilitation centers, pediatric settings, skilled nursing facilities, sports medicine clinics, and women's health practices. PT graduates are eligible to apply for postgraduate residency programs and for specialty certification in eight areas of clinical practice: cardiovascular and pulmonary, clinical electrophysiologic, geriatric, neurologic, orthopedic, pediatric, sports, and women's health.

Role of Physical Therapy in Primary Care

Physicians, PAs, and NPs are clearly associated with the provision of primary care services in the United States. PTs can play an important role as primary care providers, as well. In jurisdictions with direct access to physical therapy services, patients are permitted to access PTs as the entry point into the health care system. The increasing practice demands for primary care physicians and the lack of time to meet the demands may have a negative effect on timely access to care. Often patients with soft tissue injuries are added to physicians' schedules as "walk ons" or "add ons," and there may be insufficient time to take a detailed history or conduct a thorough examination. Direct access to PTs as primary care providers for musculoskeletal problems may alleviate these demands by allowing more immediate and convenient access to heath care.

When NPs and PAs function as primary care providers for given patient populations, they consult with and refer to a physician or other provider when the medical problem is not within their scope of practice or expertise. The same is true for PTs functioning as primary care providers. Their roles include patient management, consultation, and referral.

Prevalence and Costs of Neuromusculoskeletal Conditions

NMSCs—injuries, disorders, and diseases of the musculoskeletal system—represent the most prevalent health problem in the United States.[34,37,46] The incidence of individuals reporting NMSCs increased 16% between 1996 and 2004, representing 76 million individuals. Of all mental and physical conditions, NMSCs have the largest estimated effect on disability.[41] Arthritis and other musculoskeletal conditions represent the most common chronic health problems that lead to activity limitation among working-age adults (18 to 64 years old).[46] The symptoms that lead to impaired activity (e.g., pain, weakness) have a greater effect on this population because these individuals are not only working but also often caring for children and aged parents.

In 2008, the expenditures for all medical care related to NMSCs (direct costs) totaled $510 billion (4.6% of gross domestic product).[60] An additional $339 billion of indirect costs were attributed primarily to lost wages. Overall health care costs are 50% greater for individuals with NMSCs compared with individuals without NMSCs,[67] and these costs are expected to increase as the U.S. population ages.[60] The sheer numbers of individuals with NMSCs and the costs associated with caring for them represent a significant challenge to primary care practice. A high level of expertise and attention is necessary to meet the goal of delivering safe, effective, timely, efficient, equitable, and patient-centered care[27] for individuals with NMSCs.

Primary Care Physician's Dilemma

Primary care medicine is particularly effective at managing nonmusculoskeletal problems, such as hypertension, diabetes, and asthma.[55] The treatment of NMSCs, traumatic and nontraumatic in origin, constitutes a major portion of the primary care physician's daily practice, however. Sprains and strains of the lower

TABLE 1-2

Delivery of Services to Patients with Musculoskeletal Conditions in the United States

Provider Type	Total Services Delivered (%)
Physical therapists	27
Family physicians	23
Chiropractors	23
Osteopathic physicians	15
Orthopedic surgeons	6
Other	6

Data from Karpman RR: Musculoskeletal disease in the United States: who provides the care? *Clin Orthop Relat Res* (385):52-56, 2001.

back are consistently in the top 20 diagnoses seen by primary care physicians; overall, musculoskeletal complaints are the second most common reason for consulting a physician and constitute 20% to 30% of all primary care visits[65] (see Figure 1-1).

Despite the volume of patients with NMSCs seen in the primary care setting by physicians, evidence suggests that medical education is lacking in the area of musculoskeletal medicine.[16,40,66] Graduates of family practice residency programs across the United States report low self-confidence in the physical examination, diagnosis, and treatment of NMSCs,[39] whereas PTs show an appropriate level of knowledge in screening and managing musculoskeletal disorders in the primary care setting.* Although various health professionals provide musculoskeletal care in the United States, PTs represent the greatest number of musculoskeletal care providers in the United States[58] (Table 1-2).

Efficiency

Most primary care physicians have no formal exposure to the practice of physical therapy during their training programs and have very little, if any, exposure to advancements that occur in the field. Despite a lack of formal training or continuing medical education in rehabilitation methods, primary care physicians are often expected to oversee the physical therapy services provided to their patients. Physicians often must function under significant restrictions regarding the services placed under their responsibility by insurance carriers. Few physicians provide detailed rehabilitation plans, but instead simply send a patient for "shoulder rehabilitation" or "treatment of ankle sprain." A referral may simply consist of the phrase "evaluate and treat," which provides the PT with an opportunity to suggest the most cost-effective approach to the patient's problem.

Many of the interventions provided by PTs, if applied during the acute or subacute phase of healing (i.e., 1 to 12 weeks), are likely to be more effective for decreasing pain and reducing the progression to chronic musculoskeletal dysfunction, particularly chronic back pain.[24,26,36,51] The long-term effects of failing to initiate timely intervention can result in significantly increased costs of care[35] and reduced quality of life for patients.[13] A more recent model for managing patients with low back pain showed

greater than 50% reduction in overall costs when PTs and primary care physicians were collaboratively involved in the initial triage of the patient (Figure 1-2).[17] In addition, a growing body of evidence lends credibility to the benefit of having PTs involved as key members of the primary care team in the role of neuromusculoskeletal experts.*

Primary Care Models in Physical Therapy

The use of PTs for screening and managing patients with musculoskeletal disorders in the primary care setting is widespread in other countries with universal health care systems† and within the U.S. military and Department of Veterans Affairs (VA) health systems.[45] PTs have been shown to have an appropriate level of knowledge in screening and managing patients with musculoskeletal disorders in the primary care setting.‡ The IOM has called for collaborative, multidisciplinary "team" models of care in which clinicians other than physicians also play a central role.[27] Johnson and Abrams, when considering physical therapy practice in the 21st century, noted that true, multidisciplinary practice will require "the collaboration and interdependence of all providers with a shared focus on efficient, accessible, quality patient care."[33] Opportunities exist for PTs to enhance their roles in the delivery of primary health care services as integral members of an interdependent health care team.

This section includes descriptions of four physical therapy primary care practice models. These models do not represent the entire current scope of such models, but they encompass four very different practice and health care environments: the military (U.S. Army), a large HMO structure (Kaiser Permanente), a large hospital system (VA), and a community hospital setting (Mercy Health System). The potential benefits from these proposed models of care are numerous and include the facilitation of (1) a more efficient use of health care resources because similar models show decreased unnecessary use of specialty orthopedic services[5,22]; (2) care being delivered in a more timely manner, potentially improving patient outcomes and limiting the burden of chronic illness§; and (3) interdisciplinary collaboration resulting in improved quality of care.[5,22,27]

An overview of these models provides PTs with a better understanding of the roles that they can play in the primary care arena. Ideally, the outcome would be the involvement of PTs in the creation of new primary care initiatives, with PTs taking a lead role.

United States Army Model

The mission of U.S. Army PTs is to provide physical therapy examination and intervention to correct or prevent physical impairments resulting from injury, disease, or preexisting problems.[18,19,44,45] Army PTs practice in direct access settings as nonphysician health care providers or in physician extender roles when performing primary care (i.e., evaluation and treatment) for patients with NMSCs.[18,19,44,45] In addition, Army PTs

---

*References 9, 12, 14, 22, 50, 63.

*References 5, 9, 12, 14, 22, 25, 38, 45, 50, 51, 53, 63.
†References 5, 14, 22, 25, 38, 45, 51, 53, 63.
‡References 9, 12, 14, 22, 50, 63.
§References 5, 14, 22, 38, 51, 53.

Paths to Recovery

As Virginia Mason streamlined its approach to back-pain treatment,
patients got in faster and employers and insurers saved money.

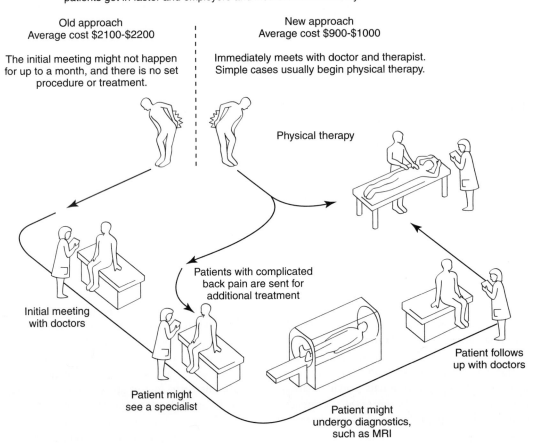

Old approach
Average cost $2100-$2200

The initial meeting might not happen
for up to a month, and there is no set
procedure or treatment.

New approach
Average cost $900-$1000

Immediately meets with doctor and therapist.
Simple cases usually begin physical therapy.

Physical therapy

Patients with complicated
back pain are sent for
additional treatment

Initial meeting
with doctors

Patient follows
up with doctors

Patient might
see a specialist

Patient might
undergo diagnostics,
such as MRI

FIGURE 1-2 Model of care from Virginia Mason Medical Center. *MRI,* magnetic resonance imaging. (From Furhmans V: Withdrawal treatment: a novel plan helps hospital wean itself off pricey tests—it cajoles insurer to pay a little more for cheaper therapies, *Wall Street Journal,* January 12, 2007.)

serve as technical advisors to commanders of troop units, providing guidance in the areas of physical fitness and wellness, physical training, and injury prevention. In the event of a mass casualty situation, Army physical therapy personnel assist in managing patients categorized through triage as "delayed" or "minor."[18,19,44,45]

HISTORICAL PERSPECTIVE. Before the Vietnam War, Army PTs had various wartime experiences but worked primarily in a prescriptive environment. Between 1962 and 1973, in support of the military mission in South Vietnam, Army PTs were assigned to Vietnam in response to a direct request for physical therapy services by hospital commanders.[18,19,48] The primary goals of physical therapy in Vietnam were the rehabilitation of patients who were capable of being returned to duty and basic rehabilitation procedures that would be continued at each evacuation stage for patients requiring evacuation out of the theater.[18,19]

During the Vietnam War, Army PTs took on extended roles in the management of the numerous patients with nonsurgical musculoskeletal problems who had to wait until physicians became available to evaluate and treat them.[18,19,21,45] The newly designated function for Army PTs was the early examination and intervention of patients with NMSCs in a direct access mode of health care delivery without physician referral.[18,19,21,45,61]

This new practice model led to positive outcomes, including decreased hospitalization, decreased patient waiting and treatment times, and facilitation of soldiers' rapid return to duty.[18,19,21,45] Since its implementation in the early 1970s, the use of Army PTs as primary care providers during military operations has been accepted by patients and practitioners, especially orthopedic surgeons. Presently, all other branches of the uniformed services, including Air Force, Navy, and Public Health Service, employ PTs as primary or direct access evaluators of NMSCs.[18,19,45]

PREPARATION FOR PRIMARY CARE PRACTICE. More recently, the roles of Army PTs have expanded to include planning and supervising physical therapy programs for patients accepted through patient self-referral or from a health professional in medical settings, the broader health care community, and the military field environment. Army PTs may obtain privileges as autonomous primary care providers through additional postgraduate training that allows them to examine, evaluate, and manage patients with emergent, acute, and chronic neuromusculoskeletal impairments, functional limitations, and disabilities.[44] Army PTs who opt for further training at an Army Medical Treatment Facility can serve in the direct access role for patients with NMSCs. They follow specific protocols before being credentialed to perform in their roles as primary care providers for the examination, evaluation, and treatment of patients with NMSCs.[18,19,45,49,52] Army PTs also attend a 1-week field readiness course, the Joint Operations Deployment Course, soon after entering active duty and before deployment overseas to prepare them better for their participation in the wartime environment.

NEUROMUSCULOSKELETAL EVALUATION

Triage Model. Traditionally, triage for patients with NMSCs consisted of an initial examination and diagnosis by a primary care physician, PA, or NP followed by a referral to an orthopedic surgeon, who then referred the patient for physical therapy services. The current triage practice for patients with NMSCs is entry-point "triage" by enlisted corps with skill levels consistent with those of nurse's aides or licensed practical nurses. The entry-level triage results in referrals to PTs for examination, evaluation, diagnosis, and treatment. PTs follow up with appropriate referral to orthopedic surgeons or other medical specialties as necessary.

Privileges. Army PTs have expanded privileges that include direct referral for appropriate imaging studies and the ability to restrict patients to quarters for 72 hours, to restrict work and training for 30 days, and to refer patients to all medical specialty clinics. In some medical treatment facilities, PTs are permitted to order certain analgesic and nonsteroidal anti-inflammatory medications.[18,19,45,49,52] They may obtain privileges as independent practitioners and physician extenders, evaluating, managing, and providing treatment to patients with emergent, acute, and chronic neuromusculoskeletal impairment, functional limitations, and disabilities.[52]

Army regulations specify formalized extensive training and privileging protocols for Army PTs to function in this role,[49,52] and they must be credentialed at the Army Medical Department where they practice. Army regulations also specify that a physician supervisor be assigned to PTs performing primary NMSC evaluations and that the physician be available for consultation in person or by telephone and, if absent, have an alternate.[49]

Outcome Studies. The peacetime use of Army PTs as the entry point for screening patients with neuromusculoskeletal disorders was first studied by James and Stuart in 1975.[32] Two Army hospitals and 2117 patients with low back pain participated, and two systems were compared. Data collected in a baseline phase under the prescriptive system were compared with data from a screening phase. The authors concluded that patients who went through the screening phase received more expeditious care, that radiographic examination was reduced by 50%, that job satisfaction increased, that patient acceptance was high, and that overall use of orthopedic physicians greatly improved. All of the 14 participating orthopedic surgeons believed that the program should be permanently adapted, with the exception of certain patient categories (e.g., pediatric patients younger than 12 years old).[32]

James and Abshier[31] assessed the neuromusculoskeletal evaluation program at Darnall Army Hospital, Fort Hood, Texas, in 1981. The study confirmed the program's efficiency, effectiveness, and acceptability in terms of PTs as primary care providers. PTs preferred the expanded role, and all preferred to include screening in their overall PT practice. The time required for neuromusculoskeletal evaluations by PTs was twice that for routine prescriptive visits. The typical neuromusculoskeletal evaluation took 30 to 45 minutes and was followed by direct PT intervention. Less than 4% of active duty patients screened by PTs required orthopedic consultation.[31]

More recently, Moore and colleagues[43] designed a study to ascertain whether direct access to physical therapy placed military health care beneficiaries at risk for adverse events related to their health care management. The findings from this preliminary study showed that patients in military health care facilities who are evaluated and managed by PTs with or without physician referral are at minimal risk for gross negligent care.[43]

Moore and colleagues[42] investigated clinical diagnostic accuracy for patients with musculoskeletal injuries referred for magnetic resonance imaging (MRI). They compared clinical diagnostic accuracy of PTs, orthopedic surgeons, and nonorthopedic providers at the Keller Army Community Hospital. There was no statistically significant difference between the clinical diagnostic accuracy of PTs and orthopedic surgeons for patients with musculoskeletal injuries, and the clinical diagnostic accuracy of PTs and orthopedic surgeons was significantly greater than that of nonorthopedic providers.[42]

The use of PTs as nonphysician primary care providers in the U.S. Army has been successful. The advantages of having PTs perform neuromusculoskeletal examination, evaluation, and treatment in their roles as nonphysician primary care providers include (1) prompt evaluation and treatment for patients with neuromusculoskeletal complaints; (2) promotion of quality health care; (3) decrease in sick call visits; (4) more appropriate use of physicians; and (5) more appropriate use of PT education, training, and experience.[6,11,18,19,45]

Kaiser Permanente Model

Another physical therapy model found in a primary care environment is currently being practiced within the largest nonmilitary setting in the United States, Kaiser Permanente. This practice model includes patient management responsibilities found in traditional physical therapy outpatient departments and involves a multitude of additional responsibilities. Despite the inherent challenges, the primary care setting that includes PTs affords significant service improvement for patients, professional growth opportunities for the PTs, growth for the physical therapy profession in line with the American Physical Therapy Association's Vision 2020, and a potential cost savings for health care organizations. Following is a description of the primary care model developed at Kaiser Permanente in Northern California, with key elements to consider when contemplating the inclusion of physical therapy services in other primary care settings.

Kaiser Permanente, the largest not-for-profit HMO in the United States, operates in nine states and the District of Columbia and serves 8.7 million members (6.3 million members are in California). The prepayment system used in today's HMOs was initiated by Sidney Garfield and Henry Kaiser for a health plan for workers and families at Kaiser-managed shipyards and steel mills. Kaiser Permanente became a federally qualified HMO in 1977. Physical therapy services have been integrated into primary care in some regions in the Kaiser Permanente system. One such region, the Northern California region, currently includes more than 3 million members.[30]

The medical practice model developed at Kaiser Permanente allows PTs to work in close proximity to other medical providers in shared clinic space with an integrated referral and medical record system. In addition to the physical layout, the philosophy of the organization provides support to its practitioners for making patient management decisions based on medical necessity and for medical management of the patients. The organization's mission includes goals of improved quality, accessibility, affordability, and patient satisfaction, but the health plan does not issue mandates regarding clinical care (e.g., number of visits, length of stay, limits on tests). The clinicians practice autonomously within the context of the organization's mission based on the medical needs of each patient.

In an increasingly competitive market, Kaiser Permanente decided to institute interdisciplinary teams as part of the primary care clinic. This move also addressed several goals of the organization:

• Increase quality of health care
• Increase patient satisfaction and accessibility to services
• Provide a more sustainable practice for physicians

Practitioners in the adult primary care (APC) clinic include physicians, NPs, medical assistants, health educators, behavioral medicine specialists, PTs, and in some cases pharmacists. Part of the impetus behind the APC redesign (Figure 1-3) at Kaiser Permanente came from a concern regarding the increasing practice and time demands on physicians in primary care. A consensus within the medical group that PTs possess the expertise to manage patients with musculoskeletal conditions and impairments led to a decision to include PTs on the APC team.[30] In 1997, after piloting physical therapy services in several primary care clinics for more than 2 years, PTs were placed in roughly half of the approximately 100 APC clinics located throughout the Northern California region. Table 1-3 provides a summary of the APC teams with integrated PTs. The need for PTs in the clinical model is supported further by the number of patients with musculoskeletal disorders, given that 20% to 25% of visits to the APC clinic were for patients with musculoskeletal disorders.

Referral processes and algorithms were developed that allowed appropriate triage by staff at the time of initial contact with the patient and facilitated more immediate access to the appropriate health provider within the APC clinic. Through this mechanism, patients have primary access to physical therapy services. In addition to this mechanism, a patient may access physical therapy services by referral from a physician at the time of the physician visit, by referral from the physician after review of the patient record, or by joint PT/physician consultation with the patient. Advantages of this system of triage and referral include earlier intervention for patients with higher acuity and more timely intervention for patients with identified recurrences or easily identified musculoskeletal problems.

As part of the primary care visit at the APC clinic, the PT is responsible for medical screening for red flags that would necessitate consultation with or referral to a physician; for consultation and discussion with the physician regarding the diagnoses and findings; for obtaining authorization from the physician; and for discussion with the physician about the need for specialty referrals or consultations, readiness for return to work, and other pertinent health issues. Not all PTs are prepared to work in the APC clinic, and Kaiser Permanente developed prerequisites and competencies to ensure readiness to practice in this model. A strong foundation in orthopedic PT is necessary, as well as at least 4 to 6 years of

TABLE 1-3		
Summary of Adult Primary Care Teams Including Physical Therapists		
Data Collected in First Quarter	**No. Teams with PTs**	**Total No. APC Teams**
1999	51	99
2000	65	99
2001	61	101
2002	56	101

APC, adult primary care; *PTs,* physical therapists.

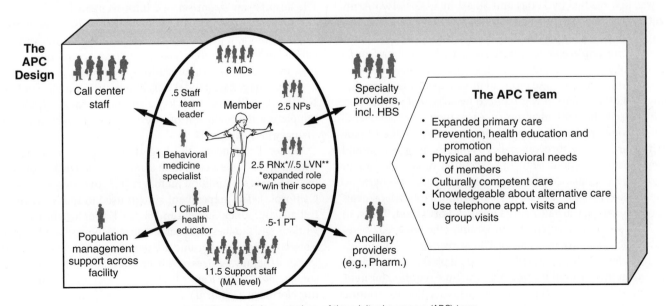

The APC Design

Call center staff

.5 Staff team leader

6 MDs

Member

2.5 NPs

Specialty providers, incl. HBS

1 Behavioral medicine specialist

2.5 RNx*//.5 LVN**
*expanded role
**w/in their scope

1 Clinical health educator

.5-1 PT

Population management support across facility

11.5 Support staff (MA level)

Ancillary providers (e.g., Pharm.)

The APC Team

• Expanded primary care
• Prevention, health education and promotion
• Physical and behavioral needs of members
• Culturally competent care
• Knowledgeable about alternative care
• Use telephone appt. visits and group visits

FIGURE 1-3 Various members of the adult primary care (APC) team.

outpatient orthopedic experience. PTs are required to participate in several mandated courses and to show competency in differential diagnosis, diagnostic imaging, pharmacology, laboratory values common in primary care, and acute musculoskeletal injuries. Kaiser Permanente supports PTs by providing clinical library modules for specific joints and by promoting a mentoring program within the system.

The Kaiser Permanente system supports primary care teams that include PTs. Within the team, the PT may function as a primary care provider, who is involved in direct care, referral, and consultation.

Department of Veterans Affairs Model

The VA runs the largest health care system in the United States with more than 1400 hospitals, clinics, and nursing homes. The VA system delivers health care services to more than 26.5 million living veterans. To address the needs of veterans comprehensively, the VA system uses primary care teams consisting of physicians, NPs, pharmacists, dietitians, and social workers. PTs became part of the primary care team more recently as experts in movement and exercise. They function on the team to identify and address impairments and dysfunction in the musculoskeletal, neuromuscular, cardiovascular/pulmonary, and integumentary systems of the body.

In February 2000, a group of PTs at the VA Salt Lake City Healthcare System began discussion on how to integrate physical therapy practice with primary care and used the U.S. Army model as a starting point. When looking at the applicability of this model to the VA population, it became apparent, however, that the role of a PT on an interdisciplinary primary care team was broader than neuromusculoskeletal care. PTs serving on the primary care team in the VA model assume responsibility for interventions directed at any and all systems that affect a patient's mobility, including the integumentary, musculoskeletal, neuromuscular, and cardiovascular/pulmonary systems.[3]

REQUIREMENTS FOR PHYSICAL THERAPISTS IN PRIMARY CARE. Similar to Kaiser Permanente, the VA system identified areas of competence that are required to work effectively with patients in a primary care model. These areas included not only differential diagnosis and orthopedic examination and evaluation, but also primary and secondary disease prevention and the effect of the four body systems on movement. Necessary skills in the affective domain included confidence, excellent communication abilities, a desire for personal and professional growth, and effective teaching abilities. These areas of competence are necessary to ensure consistent communication with the patient and all members of the primary care team, to assist in identifying and managing emerging health problems, and to risk-stratify patients for appropriate intervention. The VA developed a clinical internship program to mentor PT graduates to meet the identified areas of required competence. The goal is to prepare new graduates to work in the primary care model within the VA system.

Access to physical therapy services in the VA system occurs through three different mechanisms. PTs screen patients in the emergency department and function as consultants to determine whether there is a need for physical therapy services. If the patient is deemed appropriate for physical therapy, the physician generates a referral for physical therapy. Patients also access

physical therapy through the primary care clinic and through triage by a nurse. Whenever a mobility disorder is identified, an on-call PT is notified and functions as a consultant to identify specific needs related to mobility. Patents who are overweight or who wish to improve their general health are also eligible for primary interventions, such as therapeutic exercise and health promotion, delivered by a PT.

Mercy Model

In response to the prevalence of NMSCs in the local community and a need to address musculoskeletal education for internal medicine residents, one community hospital within the Mercy Health System of Southeastern Pennsylvania developed a model of education involving small group supervision and mentoring of physicians by PTs during the clinical care of patients with NMSCs. Previous recommendations have been made for the use of PTs as consultants and educators in relation to teaching medical residents how to initially examine and manage patients with NMSCs.[20,57,62] One specific goal for the clinic was to help manage the large population of patients seen in the hospital's primary care clinic who had long-standing chronic NMSCs and were dependent on pain medications.

The Musculoskeletal Consultation Clinic (MCC), which began in 2006, is located at Mercy Fitzgerald Hospital. It began as a monthly clinic, which expanded to occur bimonthly in the fall of 2008 because of an increasing need among patients and a growing interest in the clinic by local physicians. The MCC is staffed by five to six medical residents and a PT who mentors the residents and instructs them on the approach and examination of patients with NMSCs. Patients range in age from 22 to 90 years with most 50 to 60 years old. Back pain is the predominant condition, but there are also many patients with neck, shoulder, knee, foot, and hip pain. Included in this group are primarily patients with chronic conditions (>3 months in duration), although patients with acute or subacute symptoms are seen as well. Most patients are referred from the hospital's ambulatory medical clinic, which also serves as an educational site where medical residents practice other aspects of primary care medicine. The waiting time for patients to be seen in the MCC averages 1 to 2 weeks (Table 1-4).

Not all PTs are prepared to work in the MCC, and Mercy developed three guidelines to determine preparedness to serve in the role of a musculoskeletal consultant responsible for mentoring and training second-year and third-year internal medicine residents. These guidelines included (1) a strong foundation in orthopedic PT, which meant at least 3 to 5 years of outpatient orthopedic experience, and (2) demonstrated competency in differential diagnosis, diagnostic imaging, pharmacology, and laboratory values common in primary care and acute and chronic musculoskeletal injuries. This competency was often achieved among staff through the completion of a transitional DPT degree program. PTs who received their Board Certification in Orthopedic Physical Therapy (OCS) through the American Board of Physical Therapy Specialists[1] were deemed to have achieved expertise and competency. The final guideline was (3) an ability to work in a truly collaborative fashion with medical residents, while being an effective mentor and teacher.

TABLE 1-4

Mercy's Musculoskeletal Consultation Clinic: Descriptive Statistics*

Variable	Mean (Range)/%
Age (yr)	50 (22-90)
Gender	
Female	73%
Primary NMSC diagnosis	
Low back pain	55%
Neck pain	8%
Shoulder pain	9%
Knee pain	20%
Other	8%
Disease status	
Chronic (>3 mo)	93%
Acute	7%
Triage outcome (multiple referrals possible in same visit)	
Self-management (HEP)	44%
% of HEP to follow-up in MCC	(86%)
Physical therapy	53%
Occupational therapy	2%
Imaging	8%
Radiograph	7%
MRI	2%
Other (i.e., NCV testing)	1%
Physician specialty service	
Orthopedics	6%
Neurology	1%
Rheumatology	1%
Back to PCP	2%

*Scheduled appointments, $n = 336$; attended visits, $n = 150$; no show rate = 55%. *HEP*, home exercise program; *MCC*, Musculoskeletal Consultation Clinic; *MRI*, magnetic resonance imaging; *NCV*, nerve conduction velocity; *NMSC*, neuromusculoskeletal condition; *PCP*, primary care physician.

The MCC is open to provide patient care for a period of 3 hours. At the start of each clinic, a short 15- to 20-minute lecture/laboratory session occurs in which the PT instructs the medical resident in the cognitive and psychomotor components of a musculoskeletal screening examination. Each session covers examination related to one of the four most common body regions where patients experience NMSCs—low back, neck, shoulder, and knee. The residents rotate through the MCC once every 6 months (two rotations per month), so two topics are taught each month (one during each clinic session) for 6 months and then rotated to include the other two topic areas. Assigned readings from peer-reviewed articles related to the etiology, examination, and management of conditions in these areas are required for review by the residents before the teaching sessions. These four body areas are covered each year so that a medical resident is likely to receive education related to the low back, neck, shoulder, and knee twice during the final 2 years in the residency program. After the teaching session, time is available

for practice and discussion, then each medical resident is assigned a patient and expected to obtain a history and perform a focused physical examination. Every effort is made to ensure that residents have an opportunity to interact with patients whose diagnoses match the topic of the morning's teaching session.

After the initial examination, the resident presents the patient's case to the attending PT and fellow medical residents. The PT and residents discuss the patient and the features of the history and initial physical examination as needed. A working diagnosis is discussed, and recommendations for follow-up questions or examination procedures to be done by the residents are provided. After the medical resident has completed the initial history and physical examination, the attending PT and resident together meet with the patient. Most often, the PT performs some additional examination related to confirming the clinical diagnosis. A triage plan is developed and discussed with the patient. This plan often involves counseling; suggestions for lifestyle changes; recommendation for enhanced self-care with exercise instruction provided in the clinic (and follow-up appointments usually made within 2 to 4 weeks); and, as needed, referral for diagnostic testing (e.g., MRI, radiographs, nerve conduction velocity testing), medical specialists, or physical or occupational therapy services (Figure 1-4).

At each session, the medical residents have an opportunity to see many patients with different musculoskeletal conditions and to review some of the important pathophysiologic and clinical features of the patient's case. The residents observe the PT, then practice the physical examination maneuvers and evaluate findings that help confirm the musculoskeletal problem and subsequent course of action. Most residents who attend the MCC have very little training in the evaluation and treatment of patients with musculoskeletal problems and previously would often refer to the orthopedic surgeon because of their limited knowledge. The MCC has been important in helping medical residents develop skills to address more efficiently and effectively common NMSCs seen in an ambulatory primary care practice.

The MCC offers a new model to provide musculoskeletal education for medical residents, while delivering multidisciplinary care for patients with NMSCs. It is consistent with multidisciplinary, collaborative care models proposed by national[27] and international[29] organizations. The MCC offers a more efficient use of health care resources because specialty physician and imaging referrals occurred only 7% and 15% of the time, respectively. This efficiency is particularly important to note given that the patients served had a higher number of medical comorbidities and a greater burden of NMSC chronicity than the patients seen in a typical primary care practice. Referrals among patients for PT services were greater than 50%, however, which is a much higher referral rate than in previously described models.[22,38,51,53] These models focused on patients with acute injuries or were screened by PTs within an orthopedic specialty clinic, so it is difficult to compare whether the percentage of PT referrals for the MCC were excessive or appropriate for their population. Many of the referrals for physical therapy were provided only after an attempt at self-management was unsuccessful.

ASSESSMENT:

Patient presents with impairments above, which appear associated with:

• Capsular restriction • Connective tissue disorder • Localized inflammation • Peripheral nerve injury • Spinal disorder

Clinical examination findings are consistent with: _____

Recommendation: • Home exercise program   • Follow-up in _____ week(s)   • Referral to PT/OT

• Referral for physician consultation   • Imaging
    • Orthopedics   • Radiographs
    • Neurology   • MRI
    • Rheumatology   • Other _____

Consulting PT: _____

FIGURE 1-4 Triage assessment for the musculoskeletal consultation clinic. *MRI,* magnetic resonance imaging; *OT,* occupational therapist; *PT,* physical therapist.

Care was delivered in a timely manner, potentially improving patient outcomes and limiting the burden of chronic illness.* The interdisciplinary collaboration between the PT and the medical residents improved the quality of the patient care experience. The feedback from patients has been very positive related to the more holistic approach and a shorter wait time for expert consultation.

As a result of the success that has been seen at the MCC, there has been discussion and initial planning with physician leaders at the Philadelphia Department of Public Health regarding the implementation of a model using PTs as musculoskeletal consultants in the city's ambulatory health centers. Wait times for new appointments at city health centers can be 6 months,[8] and for a patient with an NMSC, it can take another 2 to 6 weeks to see an orthopedic physician. Many of the interventions provided by PTs, if applied in city health centers during the acute or subacute phase of healing (1 to 12 weeks), are likely to be much more effective for decreasing pain and reducing the progression to chronic musculoskeletal dysfunction, particularly chronic back pain.[24,26,36,51] Figures 1-5 and 1-6 graphically represent the model before and after the PTs are included as part of the primary care team. It is believed that such a model would help improve patient access, decrease costs for the Philadelphia Department of Public Health, and focus the management of patients with NMSCs on options, such as nonoperative interventions, prevention, wellness, and self-management, that would result in better long-term outcomes for the residents of Philadelphia.

Summary

At the beginning of this chapter, we introduced the reader to definitions of primary care. These definitions answered the following questions:

What is primary care?—a level of health service delivery that serves as the foundation of any health care system and "provides both the initial and the majority of health care services for a person or population."[30]

*References 5, 14, 22, 38, 51, 53.

How should primary care be delivered?—through integrated care, which is comprehensive, coordinated, and continuous.

Although the assumption is that physicians are the providers of primary care services, these definitions do not explicitly define "who" should and could provide primary care in the United States. As health care has evolved, primary care practice has expanded to include NPs and PAs. We are advocating that PTs can and are functioning within the role of primary care providers. The four models that have been described in this chapter provide clear and distinct examples of what the role of PTs in primary care can look like in practice.

Predicting how the coming years will affect the practice of physical therapy and medicine, and more specifically the role of PTs in primary care, is difficult. Continued increases in the cost of health care and a growing focus on quality have centered the attention of the United States on addressing major reform of the health care system. Dr. Carolyn Clancy, the Director for the Agency for Health, Research, and Quality, stated in testimony before the U.S. Senate Subcommittee on Health Care, Committee on Finance, that, "Simply put, health care quality is getting the right care to the right patient at the right time—every time."[64]

The health policy lexicon contains terms such as *value-based purchasing,*[59] *care coordination,*[10] *patient-centered medical home,*[54] and *accountable health care.*[15] These concepts and ideas, directed largely at the Medicare program, have grown out of the IOM's 2001 report titled "Crossing the Quality Chasm," which identified six aims for improving the quality of health care in the United States: care must be (1) safe, (2) effective, (3) timely, (4) efficient, (5) equitable, and (6) patient-centered.[27]

The achievement of high-quality health care that delivers the right care to the right patient at the right time and is in keeping with the six quality aims would be no small feat. When we understand the challenge and examine solutions, it becomes clear why the IOM recommended transitioning away from an autonomous physician model in health care delivery and moving toward a collaborative, multidisciplinary team model in which other clinicians also play a central role.[27] A coordinated team of clinicians, who are accountable for the value and the

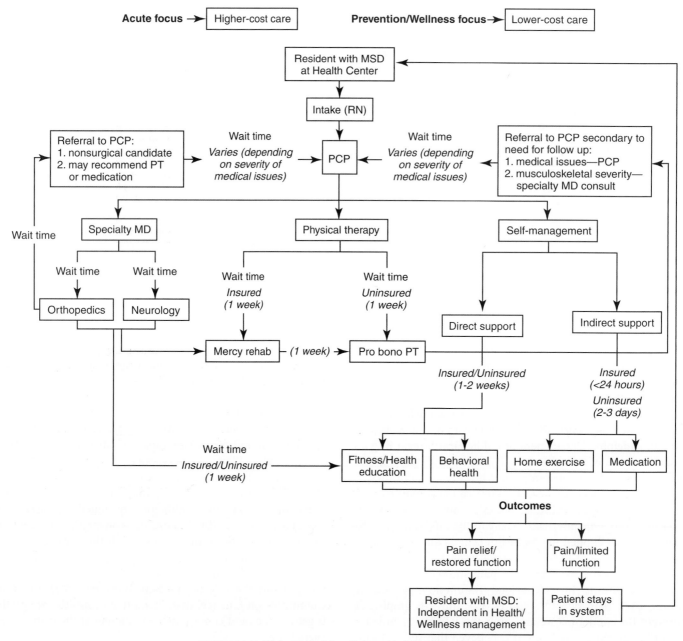

FIGURE 1-5 Original Patient Care Delivery Model and Flow Chart

volume of care they deliver, which is truly centered on what is best for the patient, is required to achieve high-quality health care for all Americans.

Primary care includes an approach to health care practice that "addresses the main health problems in the community, providing promotive, preventive, curative and rehabilitative services accordingly."[30] Within this definition and, more importantly, among the examples presented in this chapter, we see a clear role for PTs as members and leaders of multidisciplinary, interdependent health care teams. To this end, we would amend the IOM's definition of primary care to state "the provision of

integrated, accessible health care services by (teams) who are accountable for addressing a large majority of personal health care needs, developing a sustained partnership with patients, and practicing in the context of family and community."[28] In the area of neuromusculoskeletal medicine, and perhaps beyond, PTs have the capacity to function within the realm of primary care. The question that remains is whether we, as individual professionals and as a profession, will show the courage to *act*—not to "think" about, not to "ask" for, but to act—in a manner in which we are seen by patients and other health care professionals as essential members of the primary care team.

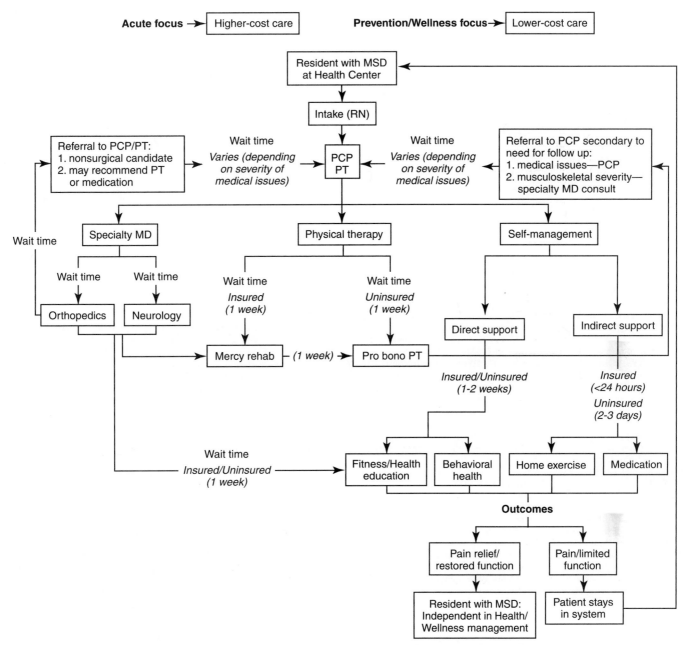

FIGURE 1-6 Established Patient Care Delivery Model with Physical Therapists as a Potential Entry-Point

REFERENCES

1. American Physical Therapy Association: About the American Board of Physical Therapy Specialties (website). http://www.apta.org/AM/Template.cfm?Section=Certification2&Template=/CM/ContentDisplay.cfm&CONTENTID=56659. Accessed August 4, 2009.

2. American Physical Therapy Association: APTA Vision Sentence for Physical Therapy 2020 and APTA Vision Statement for Physical Therapy 2020 (HOD 06-00-24-35).

3. American Physical Therapy Association. The guide to physical therapist practice. 2nd ed. Phys Ther 2001;81:9–746.

4. American Physical Therapy Association: Number of PT and PTA programs as of July 16, 2009 (website). http://www.apta.org/AM/Template.cfm?Section=Clear_Cache&TEMPLATE=/CM/ContentDisplay.cfm&CONTENTID=23652. Accessed August 4, 2009.

5. Belthur MV, Clegg J, Strange A. A physiotherapy specialist clinic in paediatric orthopaedics: is it effective? Postgrad Med J 2003;79:699–702.

6. Benson CJ, Schreck RC, Underwood FB, et al. The role of Army physical therapists as nonphysician health care providers who prescribe certain medications: observations and experiences. Phys Ther 1995;75:380–6.

7. Bernstein J, King T, Lawry GV. Musculoskeletal medicine educational reform in the Bone and Joint Decade. Arthritis Rheum 2007;57:1109–11.

8. Butkovitz A. Department of Public Health: assessment of pharmacy operations and impact of walk-in patients at district health centers. Philadelphia: Office of the Controller; 2008.

9. Byles S, Ling R. Orthopaedic out-patients: a fresh approach. Physiotherapy 1989;75:435–7.

10. Carmona RH. Evaluating care coordination among Medicare beneficiaries. JAMA 2009;301:2547–8; author reply 2548.

11. Childs JD, Whitman JM, Pugia ML, et al. Knowledge in managing musculoskeletal conditions and educational preparation of physical therapists in the uniformed services. Mil Med 2007;172:440–5.

12. Childs JD, Whitman JM, Sizer PS, et al. A description of physical therapists' knowledge in managing musculoskeletal conditions. BMC Musculoskelet Disord 2005;6:32.

13. Daffner SD, Hilibrand AS, Hanscom BS, et al. Impact of neck and arm pain on overall health status. Spine 2003;28:2030–5.

14. Daker-White G, Carr AJ, Harvey I, et al. A randomised controlled trial: shifting boundaries of doctors and physiotherapists in orthopaedic outpatient departments. J Epidemiol Community Health 1999;53:643–50.

15. Fisher ES, McClellan MB, Bertko J, et al. Fostering accountable health care: moving forward in Medicare. Health Aff (Millwood) 2009;28:w219–31.

16. Freedman KB, Bernstein J. Educational deficiencies in musculoskeletal medicine. J Bone Joint Surg Am 2002;84:604–8.

17. Furhmans V. Withdrawal treatment: a novel plan helps hospital wean itself off pricey tests—it cajoles insurer to pay a little more for cheaper therapies. Wall Street Journal January 12, 2007.

18. Greathouse DG, Schreck RC, Benson CJ. The United States Army physical therapy experience: evaluation and treatment of patients with neuromusculoskeletal disorders. J Orthop Sports Phys Ther 1994;19:261–6.

19. Greathouse DG, Sweeney JK, Hartwick AM. Physical therapy in a wartime environment. In: Dillingham TR, Belandres PV, editors. Military medicine: rehabilitation of the injured combatant. Washington, DC: Borden Institute (Walter Reed Army Medical Center); 1998. p. 19–30.

20. Hale LL, Schuch CP. Consultative and educational roles of a physical therapist in a family practice residency. Acad Med 1992;67:547–9.

21. Hartwick AM. Army Medical Specialist Corps 45th Anniversary Monograph. Washington, DC: Center of Military History, US Department of the Army; 1993.

22. Hattam P, Smeatham A. Evaluation of an orthopaedic screening service in primary care. Clin Perform Qual Health Care 1999;7:121–4.

23. Health Security Act, 1993. H.R. 1200; 103rd United States Congress. 1993-94.

24. Hemmila HM, Keinanen-Kiukaanniemi SM, Levoska S, et al. Long-term effectiveness of bone-setting, light exercise therapy, and physiotherapy for prolonged back pain: a randomized controlled trial. J Manipulative Physiol Ther 2002;25:99–104.

25. Hendriks EJ, Kerssens JJ, Nelson RM, et al. One-time physical therapist consultation in primary health care. Phys Ther 2003;83:918–31.

26. Hsieh CY, Adams AH, Tobis J, et al. Effectiveness of four conservative treatments for subacute low back pain: a randomized clinical trial. Spine 2002;27:1142–8.

27. Institute of Medicine. Crossing the quality chasm: a new health system for the 21st century. Washington, DC: Institute of Medicine; 2001.

28. Institute of Medicine. Primary care: America's health in a new era. Washington, DC: National Academy Press; 1996.

29. International classification of functioning, disability and health. Geneva: World Health Organization; 2001.

30. International Conference on Primary Health Care. Declaration of Alma-Ata. vol. 2009. Geneva: World Health Organization; 1978.

31. James JJ, Abshier JD. The primary evaluation of musculoskeletal disorders by the physical therapist. Mil Med 1981;146:496–9.

32. James JJ, Stuart RB. Expanded role for the physical therapist: screening musculoskeletal disorders. Phys Ther 1975;55:121–31.

33. Johnson MP, Abrams SL. Historical perspectives of autonomy within the medical profession: considerations for 21st century physical therapy practice. J Orthop Sports Phys Ther 2005;35:628–36.

34. Johnson MP, Metraux S. The prevalence of musculoskeletal conditions among the U.S. population: considerations for physical therapists. HPA Resource/HPA Journal 2009;9(2):J1–8.

35. Karpman RR. Musculoskeletal disease in the United States: who provides the care? Clin Orthop Rel Res 2001(385):52–6.

36. Korthals-de Bos IB, Hoving JL, van Tulder MW, et al. Cost effectiveness of physiotherapy, manual therapy, and general practitioner care for neck pain: economic evaluation alongside a randomised controlled trial. BMJ 2003;326:911.

37. Lubeck DP. The costs of musculoskeletal disease: health needs assessment and health economics. Best Pract Res Clin Rheumatol 2003;17:529–39.

38. Maddison P, Jones J, Breslin A, et al. Improved access and targeting of musculoskeletal services in northwest Wales: targeted early access to musculoskeletal services (TEAMS) programme. BMJ 2004;329:1325–7.

39. Matheny JM, Brinker MR, Elliott MN, et al. Confidence of graduating family practice residents in their management of musculoskeletal conditions. Am J Orthop 2000;29:945–52.

40. Matzkin E, Smith EL, Freccero D, et al. Adequacy of education in musculoskeletal medicine. J Bone Joint Surg Am 2005;87:310–4.

41. Merikangas KR, Ames M, Cui L, et al. The impact of comorbidity of mental and physical conditions on role disability in the US adult household population. Arch Gen Psychiatry 2007;64:1180–8.

42. Moore JH, Goss DL, Baxter RE, et al. Clinical diagnostic accuracy and magnetic resonance imaging of patients referred by physical therapists, orthopaedic surgeons, and nonorthopaedic providers. J Orthop Sports Phys Ther 2005;35:67–71.

43. Moore JH, McMillian DJ, Rosenthal MD, et al. Risk determination for patients with direct access to physical therapy in military health care facilities. J Orthop Sports Phys Ther 2005;35:674–8.

44. Moore JH: Evidence-based practice in US military physical therapy-sports medicine. From Garrison to Battlefield, Special Operations Medical Association Conference, Heidelberg, Germany, December 15, 2008.

45. Murphy BP, Greathouse D, Matsui I. Primary care physical therapy practice models. J Orthop Sports Phys Ther 2005;35:699–707.

46. National Center for Health Statistics. Health, United States, 2005: with chartbook on trends in the health of Americans. Hyattsville, MD: National Center for Health Statistics; 2005.

47. National Center for Health Statistics. Summary health statistics for U.S. adults: National Health Interview Survey, 2004. Hyattsville, MD: National Center for Health Statistics; 2006.

48. Neel S. Medical support of the US Army in Vietnam. Washington, DC: US Department of the Army; 1973.

49. Non-physician health care providers (Army Regulation 40-48). Washington, DC: US Department of the Army; 1992.

50. Overman SS, Larson JW, Dickstein DA, et al. Physical therapy care for low back pain: monitored program of first-contact nonphysician care. Phys Ther 1988;68:199–207.

51. Pinnington MA, Miller J, Stanley I. An evaluation of prompt access to physiotherapy in the management of low back pain in primary care. Fam Pract 2004;21:372–80.

52. Quality assurance administration (Army Regulation 40-68). Washington, DC: US Department of the Army; 1992.

53. Rymaszewski LA, Sharma S, McGill PE, et al. A team approach to musculoskeletal disorders. Ann R Coll Surg Engl 2005;87:174–80.

54. Sidorov JE. The patient-centered medical home for chronic illness: is it ready for prime time? Health Aff (Millwood) 2008;27:1231–4.

55. Starfield B, Shi L, Macinko J. Contribution of primary care to health systems and health. Milbank Q 2005;83:457–502.

56. Starr P. The social transformation of American medicine. New York: Basic Books; 1982.

57. Stirling J, Wood J, Lloyd J. An instructional module in musculoskeletal examination for residents incorporating physical therapists as patient-instructors and evaluators. Acad Med 1997;72:453–4.

58. Straus BN. Chronic pain of spinal origin: the costs of intervention. Spine 2002;27:2614–9; discussion 2620.

59. Tompkins CP, Higgins AR, Ritter GA. Measuring outcomes and efficiency in Medicare value-based purchasing. Health Aff (Millwood) 2009;28:w251–61.

60. United States Bone and Joint Decade. The burden of musculoskeletal diseases in the United States. Rosemont, IL: American Academy of Orthopedic Surgeons; 2008.

61. United States Department of the Army. DEPMEDS policies/guidelines and treatment briefs. Washington, DC: Defense Medical Standardization Board; 1992.

62. Vernec A, Shrier I. A teaching unit in primary care sports medicine for family medicine residents. Acad Med 2001;76:293–6.

63. Weale AE, Bannister GC. Who should see orthopaedic outpatients—physiotherapists or surgeons? Ann R Coll Surg Engl 1995;77:71–3.

64. What is health care quality and who decides? Statement of Carolyn Clancy before the Subcommittee on Health Care, Committee on Finance, U.S. Senate, March 18, 2009: Agency for Healthcare Research and Quality, Rockville, MD (website). http://www.ahrq.gov/news/test031809.htm. Accessed August 4, 2009.

65. Woolf AD, Pfleger B. Burden of major musculoskeletal conditions. Bull World Health Organ 2003;81:646–56.

66. Woolf AD, Walsh NE, Akesson K. Global core recommendations for a musculoskeletal undergraduate curriculum. Ann Rheum Dis 2004;63:517–24.

67. Yelin E, Herrndorf A, Trupin L, et al. A national study of Medical Care expenditures for musculoskeletal conditions: the impact of health insurance and managed care. Arthritis Rheum 2001;44:1160–9.

68. Yelin E. Cost of musculoskeletal diseases: impact of work disability and functional decline. J Rheumatol Suppl 2003;68:8–11.

Evidence-Based Examination of Diagnostic Information

Julie M. Fritz, PT, PhD, ATC

Objectives

After reading this chapter, the reader will be able to:

1. Describe the process physical therapists use to identify the most efficient and effective clinical diagnostic tests.
2. Describe the elements of a "best" clinical diagnostic test.
3. Provide an overview of evidence-based practice and diagnosis, including the rules to apply to judge the existing evidence.

The American Physical Therapy Association's *Guide to Physical Therapist Practice*[1] identifies five elements of patient management that must be integrated by physical therapists (PTs) to optimize the outcome of care (Box 2-1). The examination is the process of obtaining data from the patient. Evaluation requires the PT to make judgments based on of the data. The examination and evaluation lead to a diagnosis, or classification. Diagnosis has a preeminent role in the process of patient management because it represents the end result of the examination and evaluation process and is responsible for guiding the selection of interventions and establishing a prognosis.[21,22] Despite the importance of diagnosis, many clinicians are unaware of how to optimize the selection and interpretation of diagnostic tests and integrate this information into patient management decisions.

Selecting and Interpreting Diagnostic Tests: Reliability and Validity

Selecting the best diagnostic test for a particular clinical situation requires an understanding of the measurement properties of that test. This understanding requires consideration of the reliability and the validity of the diagnostic test. Although these two concepts are related, they describe distinct characteristics to consider when evaluating a diagnostic test. The concept of *reliability* describes the ability of a diagnostic test to produce the same result on repeated applications in which there has been no change in the condition being measured. *Validity* is concerned with the extent to which a diagnostic test measures what it intends to measure. Before proceeding to examine the validity of a diagnostic test, it is important to consider its reliability. If there is a large amount of error in the measurement of a particular diagnostic test, it is difficult to contend that this test would produce sufficiently valid results to be used in clinical practice. It is also important to consider, however, that all diagnostic tests would have some degree of error inherent in their measurement; careful consideration of the reliability of a diagnostic test is an important initial step in assessing its potential value in clinical practice.

Many diagnostic tests are measured on a nominal scale (i.e., they are either "positive" or "negative"). Perhaps the most apparent way to express the reliability of a diagnostic test measured in this way would be with the percentage of times two examiners agreed on the test result for the same patient, assuming his or her condition has not changed. If two different examiners evaluated the same 20 patients with neck pain, each examiner performed the neck distraction test with each patient, and both examiners agreed on the result in 19 of the 20 patients (95%), there would seem to be a high degree of interexaminer reliability for the neck distraction test.

The concern with focusing on percent agreement to express reliability for a diagnostic test measured using a nominal scale is that this approach does not account for the role of chance agreement between the examiners. If the neck distraction test were evaluated using 20 subjects without any neck pain, it would not be surprising that two examiners would agree on a judgment of "negative" in 20 of 20 subjects tested. In this example, the likelihood of agreement between examiners by chance would be high because all subjects would most likely have a negative test result because of their lack of any neck pain.

The preferred statistic to describe the reliability of a diagnostic test measured with a nominal scale is the $\varkappa$ statistic, which expresses the chance-corrected agreement.[34] In a study by Wainner and colleagues,[64] the neck distraction test was reported to have an interexaminer $\varkappa$ value of 0.88. Guides to evaluating $\varkappa$ statistics have described $\varkappa$ values greater than 0.75 as indicating excellent reliability; values 0.40 to 0.74, fair to good reliability; and values less than 0.40, poor reliability.[14] Although this guide may be helpful for examining the reliability of a diagnostic test, this guide is arbitrary. To determine the actual usefulness of a diagnostic test, one must consider measures of validity along with reliability. Reliability describes only the repeatability of a diagnostic test. A test could be highly reliable yet have little validity and no value in clinical decision making. A lack of reliability could be one explanation for poor validity results. In this instance, reducing measurement error could improve validity.

The validity of a diagnostic test examines whether the test actually measures what it is proposed to measure. An initial step in evaluating validity is to consider what a diagnostic test is intended to measure. The *Guide to Physical Therapist Practice*[1] describes diagnosis as having two aspects: (1) the process of evaluating data obtained from the examination and (2) the end result of that process. The process of evaluating diagnostic data requires the therapist to select and perform the necessary diagnostic tests for a particular patient and make the appropriate interpretation of the results. The second step, arriving at the end

BOX 2-1
Elements of Patient Management

Examination	Process of obtaining a history, performing relevant systems reviews, and selecting and administering specific tests and measures to obtain data
Evaluation	Dynamic process in which the PT makes clinical judgments based on data gathered during the examination
Diagnosis	Process and end result of evaluating information obtained from the examination, which the PT organizes into defined clusters, syndromes, or categories to help determine the most appropriate intervention strategies
Prognosis	Determination of level of optimal improvement that might be attained through intervention, and the amount of time required to reach that level
Intervention	Purposeful and skilled interaction of the PT with the patient and, if appropriate, with other individuals involved in the care of the patient using various physical therapy methods and techniques to produce changes in the condition that are consistent with the diagnosis and prognosis

PT, physical therapist.
From American Physical Therapy Association: The guide to physical therapist practice, ed 2, *Phys Ther* 81:9-746, 2001.

result, requires an integration of the results of all tests performed into a cluster, or classification, which directs the treatment. The classification may differ from the medical diagnosis because it is based on impairments and functional limitations assessed during the examination and not on pathologic origins.[8,30,55]

The need for developing classification systems within the profession of physical therapy has been emphasized to facilitate professional communication, improve the outcomes of care, and increase the power of clinical research.[50] Understanding the diagnostic process in physical therapy involves much more than simply memorizing a list of classification labels; it requires the PT to learn how to select the best tests to perform efficiently and effectively and how to integrate the results to arrive at a diagnostic decision.

One of the first steps in examining and interpreting diagnostic tests is to consider why the test is being performed. The tests used by PTs are performed for two basic purposes.[10,58] Some tests are performed to examine the status of an anatomic structure, exclude or include certain anatomic regions for further examination, or detect conditions for which physical therapy management would be inappropriate. These tests are often used as screening procedures and need to show diagnostic efficacy; they should have a high level of accuracy in distinguishing between individuals with or without the condition of interest. For example, a PT may use the anterior drawer test during the examination of a patient with knee pain in an attempt to assess the status of the anterior cruciate ligament. Another example is asking questions regarding unexplained weight loss or night pain in a patient with a musculoskeletal disorder to determine whether the patient's symptoms may be caused by a previously undiagnosed neoplasm. Tests designed for diagnostic efficacy are used to focus further examination and may be concerned with anatomic considerations instead of selecting specific treatment techniques.

The second reason PTs perform certain diagnostic tests is because the results, singularly or in combination with other findings, are believed to indicate that a particular type of

intervention would be most effective for the patient. Tests used in this manner form the foundation of classification systems and should show outcome efficacy. The observation of frontal plane displacement of the shoulders relative to the pelvis (i.e., lumbar lateral shift) in a patient with low back pain (LBP) is frequently cited as an important examination finding.[9,32,40,48] Several pathoanatomic hypotheses have been posited to explain the phenomenon, including disk herniation,[7,40] muscle spasm,[20] and segmental instability,[9] yet the precise condition resulting in a lateral shift is often unknown.[48] Despite this fact, the observation of a lateral shift is often an important diagnostic finding because it may indicate a specific intervention (e.g., correction of the lateral shift) that would be most useful in reducing pain and disability.[9,41]

One test may have the potential to serve diagnostic and classification purposes. The neck distraction test is commonly performed during the examination of patients with neck pain. The test is positive when manual distraction of the neck relieves the patient's symptoms. The distraction test has been described as a test for diagnosing cervical nerve root compression and has been shown to have some validity.[63,64] The test may also be used to select an intervention. A positive distraction test may be interpreted to indicate that the patient is likely to benefit from cervical traction.[43] Considering the purpose of a test is important for further consideration of the diagnostic process from an evidence-based perspective, because the purpose has significant implications for examining the evidence related to its usefulness in clinical practice.

Evidence-Based Practice and Diagnosis

Evidence-based practice can be defined as "the conscientious and judicious use of current best evidence in making decisions about the care of individual patients."[51] To practice in an evidence-based manner, the clinician must be able to determine what constitutes the "best" evidence. Developing proficiency at reading and interpreting the evidence in the literature related to diagnostic tests is an important skill for PTs who want to become efficient and skillful at clinical diagnosis. Many PTs are familiar with some of the principles for determining the best evidence when examining studies comparing different interventions. Most therapists understand that the best evidence in this area comes from randomized clinical trials with relatively long-term and complete follow-up periods among other criteria.[11,23,62] When one is seeking to determine the best evidence on diagnostic tests, the rules governing the evaluation of studies regarding treatment outcomes are no longer applicable.[52] Rules for judging evidence offered by a study of a diagnostic test have been described; however, these rules are not as familiar to most PTs.[3,26,37,44] These rules primarily apply to two important aspects of designing or interpreting a study of a diagnostic test: the study design and data analysis.

Judging the Evidence: Study Design

The optimal design for a study examining a diagnostic test is the one that most effectively reduces susceptibility to bias (a deviation of the results from the truth in a consistent direction).[17,26]

	Reference Standard Positive	**Reference Standard Negative**
Diagnostic test positive	True-positive results A	False-positive results B
Diagnostic test negative	False-negative results C	True-negative results D

FIGURE 2-1 Contingency table created by comparing the results of the diagnostic test and the reference standard.

The optimal design for examining a diagnostic test is "a prospective, blind comparison of the test and the reference test in a consecutive series of patients from a relevant clinical population."[37] In other words, a study investigating a diagnostic test should use a prospective design in which all subjects are evaluated by the diagnostic test and a reference standard representing the definitive, or best, criteria for the condition of interest. When the test is performed in this manner, the results and the reference standard can be summarized in a 2 × 2 table (Figure 2-1). Each subject fits into only one box in this table. The distribution of subjects into these different boxes is then used to determine the usefulness of the diagnostic test. Other aspects of the study design in addition to the basic layout are important for determining the strength of evidence offered by the study. These factors include the reference standard, the diagnostic test itself, and the patient population studied.

Reference Standard

When one is studying a diagnostic test, the test must be compared with a reference standard, or gold standard. The reference standard is the criterion that best defines the condition the test is attempting to detect.[27] Reference standards are not perfect but should offer the best approximation of the condition.[53] The selection and application of the reference standard are extremely important considerations in a study of a diagnostic test. If the reference standard cannot be accepted as the best method of determining whether the patient has the condition of interest, the study would be unable to provide meaningful information.[28] The reference standard must be consistent with the purpose of the test. If the test is primarily being used for diagnosing pathology in a certain anatomic structure, a reference standard related to pathoanatomy, such as a magnetic resonance image or radiograph, would likely be appropriate. If a test is being used to select an intervention, a reference standard related to pathoanatomy would be inappropriate. Because such tests are attempting to predict which patient would respond to a particular intervention, the reference standard needs to be related to the therapeutic outcome of the intervention.

A study investigating tests for carpal tunnel syndrome provides a good example of this distinction in reference standards.[6] One test that was examined in this study was Phalen's test. This test is typically used to diagnose compression of the median nerve in the carpal tunnel. The authors of the study also hypothesized that a positive Phalen's test result may be helpful in determining that a patient may respond to wrist splinting. To assess Phalen's test for both of these purposes, two different reference standards were needed—one to represent the pathoanatomic purpose of the test and the second to represent its role in selecting an intervention. The authors chose to use a nerve conduction velocity study as a pathoanatomic reference standard and the response of symptoms to 2 weeks of splinting as the intervention reference standard. This second reference standard permitted an examination of the usefulness of Phalen's test in determining whether splinting should be performed, regardless of its ability to help diagnose pathology in the median nerve.

The results of a study that uses a reference standard reflecting one purpose cannot be generalized to other possible uses of the test. Spurling's test is typically described as a test for cervical radiculopathy.[60] One study that examined the validity of Spurling's test compared the results against a reference standard of subject-reported neck pain present during the week preceding the examination.[56] By using this reference standard, the authors conceptualized the tests as essentially screening procedures designed to distinguish between individuals with or without a recent history of neck pain. This is not the reason why most PTs perform Spurling's test during an examination. PTs typically use the test to help determine whether a cervical nerve root lesion is present. PTs may use the results of Spurling's test to make an intervention decision. Some PTs may consider a positive Spurling's test result an indication to perform cervical traction.[43] A reference standard of self-reported neck pain makes the results difficult to interpret because it is inconsistent with what Spurling's test is used for.

Examining the reference standard and ensuring its consistency with the purpose of the test are essential for evaluating diagnostic test studies. Although most studies in the literature use pathoanatomic reference standards, PTs are often concerned with issues related to classification and outcome efficacy. If the reference standard is inappropriate for the purpose of the test, the study would not provide useful results.

Other factors related to the reference standard are important to consider. The reference standard must be consistently applied to all subjects in the study. A study of screening examinations was performed by nurses with goniometry to detect cerebral palsy in preterm infants.[47] Infants with a high suspicion of cerebral palsy were referred to a neurologist whose evaluation served as the reference standard; a less rigorous reference standard consisting of chart reviews was used for the remaining subjects.[47] The adequacy of chart reviews for diagnosing cerebral palsy with the same accuracy as a clinical examination leaves this study susceptible to bias, which can lead to an overestimation of the diagnostic value of a test.[37,49]

In addition, the reference standard should be judged by an individual who is unaware of, or blinded to, the diagnostic test results and the overall clinical presentation of the subject. If blinding is not maintained, judgments of the reference standard may be influenced by expectations based on knowledge of the test results.[19] Review bias occurs in situations when either the reference standard or the diagnostic test is judged by an individual with knowledge of the other result.[48] In a study by Lauder and associates,[35] various clinical diagnostic tests were compared against a reference standard of electrodiagnostic testing to determine their utility in diagnosing lumbar radiculopathy. In the study, it is unclear whether the individual performing the diagnostic tests was aware of the results of the electrodiagnostic studies. If the examiner was aware of the electrodiagnostic test results, this knowledge could have influenced the judgment of the diagnostic test results.

Diagnostic Tests

The diagnostic tests being studied must be described in sufficient detail to allow the reader to understand and replicate the procedures. The actual physical performance of the test also needs to be described, because the same test may be performed differently by different examiners. A study's results can be generalized to the test only as it was performed in the study. Levangie[36] examined the diagnostic usefulness of pelvic asymmetry for detecting the presence of LBP among subjects referred to physical therapy. If asked how to test for the presence of pelvic asymmetry, most PTs would probably describe the palpation of certain bony landmarks, with the patient standing or sitting. In this study, however, pelvic asymmetry was determined by using a pelvic inclinometer to assess iliac crest height. It cannot be assumed that determination of pelvic asymmetry with palpation would yield similar results.

Description of the diagnostic test should cover physical performance and the criteria defining positive and negative results. Many tests commonly used by PTs have variable or unclear grading criteria. Determining the presence of centralization in patients with LBP is an example. What constitutes a positive finding of centralization varies. Some authors use definitions strictly based on movement of symptoms from distal to proximal.[16,40] Others have defined centralization to include diminishment of pain during testing.[31] Such disagreements point out the need to clarify how positive and negative results are defined within a particular study. Grading the diagnostic test is also susceptible to review bias if the individual judging the test is aware of the results on the reference standard. If this blinding is not maintained, the usefulness of the test is likely to be overestimated, possibly to a large degree.[37]

Study Population

The subjects of a diagnostic test study are an important consideration. The subjects should be similar to patients to whom a PT would consider applying the test in clinical practice. Some subjects in the study would end up having the condition of interest, whereas others would not. Subjects who do have the condition should reflect a continuum of severity from mild to severe.[28] Subjects who do not have the condition should have similar symptoms.[25] Many studies include some healthy subjects. Any diagnostic test would look more useful than it really is when it is used to distinguish between healthy individuals and subjects with severe conditions.[37] Spectrum bias occurs when study subjects are not representative of the population in whom the test is typically applied in practice.[37] Spectrum bias can profoundly affect the results of a study. The best way to avoid spectrum bias is to use a prospective design in which a consecutive group of subjects from a clinical setting is studied.[3]

Comparing the study by Burke and colleagues[6] with another study examining the value of Phalen's test for diagnosing carpal tunnel syndrome illustrates the concern over spectrum bias. A study by Gellman and coworkers[18] also compared Phalen's test against a reference standard of nerve conduction velocity. The only substantial difference between the two studies was the subjects. All the subjects in the study by Burke and colleagues[6] had symptoms consistent with carpal tunnel syndrome. The study by Gellman and coworkers[18] involved subjects with symptoms consistent with carpal tunnel syndrome but also included a group of 50 hands that were asymptomatic. Inclusion of hands without symptoms creates a spectrum bias. The results of this study showed much greater diagnostic accuracy for Phalen's test than the study relatively free from spectrum bias.

Using the Data: Analysis

The basic layout of the results from a study of a diagnostic test is shown in Figure 2-1. The result for each subject fits into only one of the four categories based on a comparison of the results of the diagnostic test and the reference standard. The defining characteristics of the four categories are as follows:

- True-positive (*A*) subjects are positive on the reference standard and the diagnostic test.
- False-positive (*B*) subjects are negative on the reference standard but positive on the diagnostic test.
- False-negative (*C*) subjects are positive on the reference standard but negative on the diagnostic test.
- True-negative (*D*) subjects are negative on the reference standard and the diagnostic test.

Several statistics can be calculated from this layout that are useful for understanding the value of a diagnostic test [19] (Table 2-1).

TABLE 2-1

Statistics Commonly Used in Studies of Diagnostic Tests

Statistic	Formula	Description
Positive predictive value	$a/(a + b)$	Given a positive test result, the probability that the individual has the condition
Negative predictive value	$d/(c + d)$	Given a negative test result, the probability that the individual does not have the condition
Sensitivity	$a/(a + c)$	Given that the individual has the condition, the probability that the test will be positive
Specificity	$d/(b + d)$	Given that the individual does not have the condition, the probability that the test will be negative
Positive LR	sensitivity/ (1 − specificity)	Given a positive test result, the increase in odds favoring the condition
Negative LR	(1 − sensitivity)/ specificity	Given a negative test result, the decrease in odds favoring the condition

LR, likelihood ratio.

Sensitivity, Specificity, and Predictive Values

Sensitivity and specificity values are calculated vertically from the 2 × 2 table and represent the proportion of correct diagnostic test results among individuals with and without the condition. *Sensitivity* (or true-positive rate) is the proportion of true-positive subjects among all subjects who have the condition of interest. *Specificity* (or true-negative rate) is the proportion of true-negative subjects among all subjects without the condition.[53]

Predictive values are calculated horizontally from the table and represent the proportion of subjects with a positive or negative diagnostic test result that are correct results. The *positive predictive value* is the proportion of true-positive subjects among all subjects with a positive diagnostic test. The *negative predictive value* is the proportion of true-negative subjects among all subjects with a negative diagnostic test.[21] The predictive values are generally of less value in interpreting the usefulness of a test because they depend highly on the prevalence of the condition of interest in the study population. Positive predictive values are lower and negative predictive values are higher in study populations with a low prevalence of the condition. If prevalence is high, the trends reverse.[25] Sensitivity and specificity values remain fairly consistent across different prevalence levels[53] and are preferred over predictive values.

Sensitivity and specificity values provide useful information for interpreting diagnostic tests. A test with high sensitivity has few false-negative results. High test sensitivity attests to the value of a negative test result.[54,57] In other words, if a test has high sensitivity, few false-negative results would be found, and the examiner can have some level of trust that the negative result actually represents the absence of the condition. Sackett and colleagues[53] have advocated the acronym *SnNout* (if sensitivity is high, a negative result is useful for ruling out the condition). High sensitivity indicates that a test is useful for excluding, or ruling out, a condition when it is negative but does not address the value of a positive test. A diagnostic test with high specificity has few false-positive results and speaks to the value of a positive test result.[54,57] The acronym advocated is *SpPin* (if specificity is high, a positive result is useful for ruling in the condition).[53]

Few diagnostic tests have high sensitivity and high specificity. Knowledge of sensitivity and specificity of a diagnostic test can improve clinical decision making by helping clinicians weigh the value of positive and negative results. A study examining history and physical examination findings in predicting rotator cuff tears in older patients provides an illustration.[38] Numerous diagnostic tests were compared against a reference standard of shoulder arthrogram. No test had high levels of sensitivity and specificity (Table 2-2). A painful arc during passive elevation of the arm was the most sensitive, and limited external rotation passive range of motion to less than 70 degrees was the most specific.[38] The high sensitivity (97.5%) of the presence of a painful arc indicates that this finding is useful for ruling out a rotator cuff tear; however, the low specificity (9.9%) indicates that a positive painful arc has little meaning. Few false-negative results are found when testing for a painful arc, and it would be unlikely that the patient actually has a rotator cuff tear if a painful arc is not present. Conversely, limited external rotation was highly specific (83.6%), indicating that a positive test is useful for confirming a rotator cuff tear. The sensitivity of limited external rotation was poor (19%), indicating a lack of value for a negative test result.

Likelihood Ratios

Sensitivity and specificity values provide helpful information; however, they do not provide a complete picture. The actual performance of a diagnostic test is related to sensitivity and specificity values and depends on the pretest probability that the condition is present. Useful tests should produce large shifts in probability when the result of the test is known.[12,33,39] Sensitivity and specificity values cannot quantify shifts in the probability given a certain test result. The best statistics for quantifying shifts in probability, based on the results of a diagnostic test, are likelihood ratios (LRs).[5,29] LRs combine sensitivity and specificity values into a value that can be used to quantify shifts in probability when the diagnostic test result is known.[59] The positive LR is calculated as sensitivity/(1 − specificity) and indicates the increase in odds favoring the condition given a positive test result. The negative LR is calculated as (1 − sensitivity)/specificity and indicates the change in odds favoring the condition given a negative test result.[26] An LR value of 1 indicates the test result does nothing to change the odds favoring the condition, whereas an LR value greater than 1 increases the odds of the condition, and an LR value of less than 1 diminishes the odds of the condition. Table 2-3 provides a guide for interpreting the strength of an LR.[29]

A diagnostic test with a large positive LR (e.g., >5) indicates that the shift in odds favoring the condition would be relatively

---

TABLE 2-2
Diagnostic Efficacy of Clinical Tests for Detecting Rotator Cuff Tears

Diagnostic Test	Sensitivity	Specificity	Positive LR	Negative LR
Presence of night pain	87.7	19.7	1.09	0.62
Presence of supraspinatus atrophy	55.6	72.9	2.05	0.61
Shoulder elevation PROM <170 degrees	30.2	78.1	1.38	0.89
Shoulder external rotation PROM <70 degrees	19	83.6	1.16	0.97
Neer impingement sign	97.2	9	1.07	0.31
Weakness with external rotation strength test	75.9	57.3	1.78	0.75
Painful arc during elevation PROM	97.5	9.9	1.08	0.25

LR, likelihood ratio; *PROM,* passive range of motion.
Modified from Litaker D, Pioro M, El Bilbeisi H, et al: Returning to the bedside: using the history and physical examination to identify rotator cuff tears, *J Am Geriatr Soc* 48:1633-1637, 2000.

TABLE 2-3

Guide to Interpretation of Likelihood Ratio (LR) Values

Positive LR	Negative LR	Interpretation
>10	<0.10	Generate large, often conclusive shifts in probability
5-10	0.1-0.2	Generate moderate shifts in probability
2-5	0.2-0.5	Generate small, but sometimes important, shifts in probability
1-2	0.5-1	Alter probability to a small, and rarely important, degree

Data from Jaeschke R, Guyatt GH, Sackett DL: Users' guides to the medical literature, III: how to use an article about a diagnostic test, B: what are the results and will they help me in caring for my patients? *JAMA* 271:703-707, 1994.

large when the diagnostic test is positive. It is desirable for a test to have a large positive LR value. In general, diagnostic tests with high levels of specificity also have large positive LR values because both attest to the usefulness of the positive test result. The negative LR value indicates the change in odds *favoring* the condition given a negative diagnostic test result. Because a negative test result is supposed to reduce the odds that a condition is present, it is desirable for a test to have a small (e.g., <0.20) negative LR value. A small negative LR indicates a diagnostic test that is useful for ruling out a condition when the result is negative. Tests with high sensitivity values generally have small negative LR values.

Examining the tests for rotator cuff tears discussed earlier provides an example of the importance of combining sensitivity and specificity values (see Table 2-2). The most sensitive test was a painful arc (97.5%), and this test also had the smallest negative LR. The most specific test was external rotation range of motion (83.6%); however, positive LR value was greater for the presence of supraspinatus atrophy (1.78 versus 2.05). This is because the sensitivity value for the finding of supraspinatus atrophy was much better than the sensitivity for external rotation range of motion limitation.

Using the Data: Interpretation

The diagnostic process requires PTs to think in terms of probability and revision of probabilities. Before performing a diagnostic test, a PT would have some idea of the likelihood that the patient being evaluated has the condition of interest. Although this probability is rarely articulated or quantified in the PT's mind, all clinicians develop at least a sense that certain conditions are more likely, and others less likely, for certain patients. The condition of interest in the therapist's mind may be related to pathology or pathoanatomy: For instance, is it likely that this patient has a cervical disk lesion that is causing arm pain? The condition of interest being considered by the PT may involve treatment decision making: Would this patient's arm pain be relieved with traction treatments?

The PT also has some threshold level of certainty, at which point he or she would be "sure enough" and ready to act.[39,45] This threshold is typically not quantified, but there is some amount of assurance that any PT must reach before an action is taken

with the patient. The threshold is a factor of the costs associated with making an incorrect decision versus the benefits of being correct.[4,46] A high threshold of certainty would be required if the question involved ruling out metastatic disease in the lung as a source of arm pain. If a PT had any lingering doubts about such a diagnosis, it would be incumbent to refer the patient for further diagnostic workup before pursuing physical therapy.

If the question concerned the application of a treatment with minimal cost and low potential for risk, such as mechanical cervical traction, the threshold for action would be lower. A PT would likely be willing to initiate traction treatment if he or she is fairly certain the patient may benefit and if there is not greater certainty that the patient would benefit from an alternative treatment. LRs provide the information needed to select the diagnostic test or tests that would most efficiently move the PT from the uncertainty associated with the pretest probability to a posttest probability that crosses a threshold for action.

The probability that a patient has a particular condition before performing the diagnostic test can come from sources other than the clinical experience and expertise of the examiner. Other sources of pretest probabilities include epidemiologic data on prevalence rates for certain conditions, the prevalence of the condition in studies examining diagnostic test properties, clinical databases, and information already obtained on the patient from the examination.[4] Whatever the source of the pretest probability, LR values quantify the direction and magnitude of change in the pretest probability based on the diagnostic test result.[27] To illustrate the process, consider the case of a 37-year-old man with a 1-week history of LBP and right buttock pain that does not extend below the knee. The question is one related to treatment decision making: "Is this patient likely to respond to a manipulation intervention?"

What is a reasonable pretest probability that this patient would respond to manipulation? Based on a randomized trial showing that many patients with LBP respond to manipulation[24,42] and clinical experience, the probability may be fairly high, perhaps 60%. What information should be gathered to alter this probability? To answer this question, a study examined the usefulness of various diagnostic tests against a reference standard of success with manipulation (defined as a 50% decrease in self-reported disability occurring over two treatment sessions).[15] The results of this study (Table 2-4) show that the best test would be asking the patient how long the symptoms have been present (positive LR = 4.4 for ≤15 days). Factors from the history commonly prove more useful than factors from the physical examination.

If the test is positive (i.e., duration of symptoms is <16 days), what should the new probability of success with manipulation be? Two methods can be used to make this determination. The simpler but less precise method uses a nomogram (Figure 2-2).[13] A straight edge is anchored along the left side at the point representing the pretest probability. The straight edge is aligned with the appropriate LR value (4.4 in this example), and the line is extended through the right side of the nomogram. The point of intersection on the right side indicates the posttest probability.[52] In this example, if the duration of the patient's symptoms was less than 16 days, the posttest probability of success with manipulation seems to be approximately 83%. The posttest probability

TABLE 2-4

Diagnostic Usefulness of Signs and Symptoms for Determining Whether a Patient with Low Back Pain Would Respond to a Manipulation Technique

Test	Sensitivity	Specificity	Positive LR	Negative LR
FACTORS FROM HISTORY				
Duration of symptoms ≤15 days	0.56	0.87	4.4	0.51
Symptom distribution not distal to the knee	0.88	0.36	1.4	0.33
Episodes of LBP not becoming more frequent	0.75	0.44	1.3	0.59
FACTORS FROM PHYSICAL EXAMINATION				
Hypomobility with prone spring testing in at least one lumbar segment	0.97	0.23	1.3	0.13
Hip internal rotation PROM >35 degrees in at least one hip	0.50	0.85	3.3	0.59
No peripheralization during lumbar standing AROM	0.84	0.33	1.3	0.48

AROM, active range of motion; *LBP*, low back pain; *LR*, likelihood ratio; *PROM*, passive range of motion.
Adapted from Flynn T, Fritz J, Whitman J, et al: A clinical prediction rule for classifying patients with low back pain who demonstrate short term improvement with spinal manipulation, *Spine* 27:2835-2843, 2002.

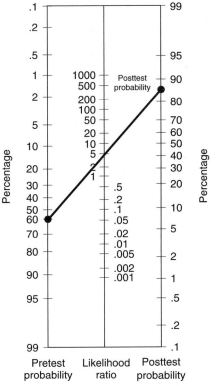

FIGURE 2-2 Nomogram for estimating posttest probability of a diagnosis. (From Fagan TJ: Nomogram for Bayes's theorem, *N Engl J Med* 293:257, 1975.)

BOX 2-2

Calculation of Posttest Probability

Step 1: Convert pretest probability to pretest odds:

$$\text{Pretest odds} = \frac{\text{Pretest probability}}{1 - \text{Pretest probability}}$$

Step 2: Multiply pretest odds by LR value:

$$\text{Pretest odds} \times \text{LR} = \text{Posttest odds}$$

Step 3: Convert posttest odds to posttest probability:

$$\frac{\text{Posttest odds}}{\text{Posttest odds} + 1} = \text{Posttest probability}$$

LR, likelihood ratio.

can be quantified with greater precision by using a calculation process described by Sackett and colleagues[53] and outlined in Box 2-2.

By using these calculations, the pretest probability of 60% would correspond to pretest odds of 1.5:1. Multiplying this by the LR value of 4.4, the posttest odds would be 6.6:1. Converting this back to probability results in a posttest probability of 87%. Examples such as this highlight the importance of attending to the most important examination findings for clinical decision making. If the examiner had instead focused on the lack of symptoms distal to the knee as confirming evidence that this patient was likely to benefit from manipulation, the actual

posttest probability would increase to only a 68% probability of success. Without knowledge of the relative unimportance of this finding, the PT might overinterpret the finding.

If the pretest probability were lower, the PT may instead want to seek a finding that would confirm that the patient does not need manipulation but instead would benefit more from another type of intervention.[7] Consider if the patient told the PT that for previous episodes of LBP, treatment with spinal manipulation had been unsuccessful. In this case, the therapist would likely believe the pretest probability of success with a manipulation technique to be much lower, perhaps only 15%. In this circumstance, the finding that the current duration of symptoms was less than 16 days would increase the probability of success to only 44%. The PT may be better served to use the test with the smallest negative LR value because if this finding is negative, it is likely that the posttest probability would be small enough to exclude manipulation as a treatment option and move on to other considerations. The test with the smallest negative LR value was prone posterior-to-anterior spring testing over the spinous processes in the lumbar spine (see Table 2-4). If this testing did not reveal any hypomobility, the posttest probability of success with manipulation would be only 2%.

It is common within the process of clinical decision making to seek to rule out, or reduce the likelihood of, a condition instead of ruling in. This is typically the situation with screening procedures, where the goal is to exclude a diagnosis adequately and move on to alternative diagnostic hypotheses. Consider a 25-year-old man who had an inversion ankle sprain while playing basketball the previous evening. He was able to finish playing the game but experienced substantial swelling within a few hours after finishing. No radiographs have been taken, and before initiating treatment, the PT wants to rule out the possibility of a fracture. What is the pretest probability of a fracture in this individual? It is likely low, perhaps 5%.

The Ottawa Ankle Rules,[61] a well-validated decision-making aid for determining whether a patient requires radiographs after an acute trauma, can be applied to determine whether this patient should be referred for radiographs before treatment. The Ottawa Ankle Rules are positive if either one of two findings is present: (1) the inability to bear weight immediately and at the time of examination or (2) bony tenderness at the navicular, base of the fifth metatarsal, or distal end of the medial or lateral malleolus.[61] If neither of these findings is present, the patient is negative for the Ottawa Ankle Rules. What is the patient's posttest probability of a fracture? Because the patient is negative for the Ottawa Ankle Rules, the negative LR is the appropriate statistic to use. A systematic review of studies reported a pooled negative LR of 0.08 for the Ottawa Ankle Rules.[2] Using the procedures outlined previously, this negative LR would reduce the posttest probability of a fracture to 0.4%, which may be sufficient to permit continuing treatment without referral for radiographs.

Summary

LRs provide the most powerful tool for quantifying the importance of a particular test within the diagnostic process. Because LR values can be calculated for positive and negative results, the importance of positive and negative test results can be examined independently. This examination is important because few tests provide useful information in both capacities, and understanding the relative strength of evidence provided by a negative or a positive test result helps refine interpretation of the diagnostic test. Understanding the information contained in statistics, such as sensitivity, specificity, and LRs, can assist PTs in improving their diagnostic and decision-making skills. Developing these skills is paramount for PTs working in primary care settings.

REFERENCES

1. American Physical Therapy Association. The guide to physical therapist practice, 2nd ed. Phys Ther 2001;81:9–746.
2. Bachmann LM, Kolb E, Koller MT, et al. Accuracy of Ottawa ankle rules to exclude fractures of the ankle and mid-foot: systematic review. BMJ 2003;326:417–9.
3. Begg CB. Methodologic standards for diagnostic test assessment studies. J Gen Intern Med 1988;3:518–20.
4. Bernstein J. Decision analysis. J Bone Joint Surg 1997;79A:1404–14.
5. Boyko EJ. Ruling out or ruling in disease with the most sensitive or specific diagnostic test. Med Decis Making 1994;14:175–9.
6. Burke DT, Burke MA, Bell R, et al. Subjective swelling: a new sign for carpal tunnel syndrome. Am J Phys Med Rehabil 1999;78:504–8.
7. Charnley J. Orthopaedic signs in the diagnosis of disc protrusion. Lancet 1951;1:186–92.
8. Delitto A, Snyder-Mackler L. The diagnostic process: examples in orthopedic physical therapy. Phys Ther 1994;75:203–11.
9. Delitto A, Erhard RE, Bowling RW. A treatment-based classification approach to low back syndrome: identifying and staging patients for conservative management. Phys Ther 1995;75:470–89.
10. Deyo RA, Haselkorn J, Hoffman R, et al. Designing studies of diagnostic tests for low back pain or radiculopathy. Spine 1994;19(suppl):2057s–63s.
11. Dickersin K, Scherer R, Lefebvre C. Identifying relevant studies for systematic reviews. BMJ 1994;309:1286–91.
12. Dujardin B, Van den Ende J, Van Gompel A, et al. Likelihood ratios: a real improvement for clinical decision making? Eur J Epidemiol 1994;10:29–36.
13. Fagan TJ. Nomogram for Bayes's theorem. N Engl J Med 1975;293:257.
14. Fleiss JL. Statistical methods for rates and proportions. 2nd ed. New York: John Wiley; 1981.
15. Flynn T, Fritz J, Whitman J, et al. A clinical prediction rule for classifying patients with low back pain who demonstrate short term improvement with spinal manipulation. Spine 2002;27:2835–43.
16. Fritz JM, Delitto A, Vignovic M, et al. Inter-rater reliability of judgments of the centralization phenomenon and status change during movement testing in patients with low back pain. Arch Phys Med Rehabil 2000;81:57–61.
17. Geddes JR, Harrison PJ. Closing the gap between research and practice. Br J Psychiatry 1997;171:220–5.
18. Gellman H, Gelberman RH, Tan AM, et al. Carpal tunnel syndrome: an evaluation of the provocative diagnostic tests. J Bone Joint Surg 1986;68A:735–7.
19. Greenhalgh T. How to read a paper: papers that report diagnostic or screening tests. BMJ 1997;315:540–3.
20. Grieve GP. Treating backache: a topical comment. Physiotherapy 1983;69:316.
21. Griner PF, Mayewski RJ, Mushlin AI, et al. Selection and interpretation of diagnostic tests and procedures: principles and applications. Ann Intern Med 1981;94:557–92.
22. Guccione AA. Physical therapy diagnosis and the relationship between impairments and function. Phys Ther 1991;71:499–504.
23. Guyatt GH, Sackett DL, Cook DJ. Users' guide to the medical literature, II: how to use an article about therapy or prevention, A: are the results of the study valid? JAMA 1993;270:2598–601.
24. Hadler NM, Curtis P, Gillings DB, et al. A benefit of spinal manipulation as an adjunctive therapy for acute low-back pain: a stratified controlled study. Spine 1987;12:703–5.
25. Hagen MD. Test characteristics: how good is that test? Med Decis Making 1995;22:213–33.
26. Irwig L, Tosteson ANA, Gatsonis C, et al. Guidelines for meta-analyses evaluating diagnostic tests. Ann Intern Med 1994;120:667–76.
27. Jaeschke RZ, Meade MO, Guyatt GH, et al. How to use diagnostic test articles in the intensive care unit: diagnosing weanability using f/Vt. Crit Care Med 1997;25:1514–21.
28. Jaeschke R, Guyatt G, Sackett DL. Users' guides to the medical literature, III: how to use an article about a diagnostic test, A: are the results of the study valid? JAMA 1994;271:389–91.
29. Jaeschke R, Guyatt GH, Sackett DL. Users' guides to the medical literature, III: how to use an article about a diagnostic test, B: what are the results and will they help me in caring for my patients? JAMA 1994;271:703–7.
30. Jette AM. Diagnosis and classification by physical therapists: a special communication. Phys Ther 1989;69:967–9.
31. Karas R, McIntosh G, Hall H, et al. The relationship between nonorganic signs and centralization of symptoms in the prediction of return to work for patients with low back pain. Phys Ther 1997;77:354–60.
32. Khuffash B, Porter RW. Cross leg pain and trunk list. Spine 1989;14:602–3.
33. Kortelainen P, Puranen J, Koivisto E, et al. Symptoms and signs of sciatica and their relation to the localization of the lumbar disc herniation. Spine 1985;10:88–92.
34. Landis RJ, Koch GG. The measurement of observer agreement for categorical data. Biometrics 1977;33:159–74.
35. Lauder T, Dillingham R, Andary M, et al. Effect of history and exam in predicting electrodiagnostic outcome among patients with suspected lumbosacral radiculopathy. Am J Phys Med Rehabil 2000;79:60–8.
36. Levangie PK. The association between static pelvic asymmetry and low back pain. Spine 1999;24:1234–41.
37. Lijmer JG, Mol BW, Heisterkamp S, et al. Empirical evidence of design-related bias in studies of diagnostic tests. JAMA 1999;282:1061–6.
38. Likater D, Pioro M, El Bilbeisi H, et al. Returning to the bedside: using the history and physical examination to identify rotator cuff tears. J Am Geriatr Soc 2000;48:1633–40.
39. Lurie JD, Sox HC. Principles of medical decision making: spine update. Spine 1999;24:493–8.
40. McKenzie RA. The lumbar spine: mechanical diagnosis and therapy. Waianae, NZ: Spinal Publications; 1989.
41. McKenzie RA. Manual correction of sciatic scoliosis. N Z Med J 1972;76:194–9.
42. Meade TW, Dyer S, Browne W, et al. Randomised comparison of chiropractic and hospital outpatient management for low back pain: results from extended follow up. BMJ 1995;311:349–51.

43. Moeti P, Marchetti G. Clinical outcome from mechanical intermittent cervical traction for the treatment of cervical radiculopathy: a case series. J Orthop Sports Phys Ther 2001;31:207–13.

44. Mulrow CD, Linn WD, Gaul MK, et al. Assessing quality of diagnostic test evaluation. J Gen Intern Med 1989;4:288–95.

45. Pauker SG, Kassirer JP. The threshold approach to clinical decision making. N Engl J Med 1980;302:1109–17.

46. Pauker SG, Kassirer JP. Therapeutic decision-making: a cost benefit analysis. N Engl J Med 1975;293:229–34.

47. Pinto-Martin JA, Torre C, Zhao H. Nurse screening of low-birth-weight infants for cerebral palsy using goniometry. Nurs Res 1997;46:284–7.

48. Porter RW, Miller CG. Back pain and trunk list. Spine 1986;11:596–600.

49. Reid MC, Lachs MS, Feinstein AR. Use of methodological standards in diagnostic test research: getting better but still not good. JAMA 1995;274:645–51.

50. Rose SJ. Physical therapy diagnosis: role and function. Phys Ther 1989;69:535–7.

51. Sackett DL, Richardson WS. Evidence based medicine: what it is and what it isn't. BMJ 1996;312:71–2.

52. Sackett DL, Wennberg JE. Choosing the best research design for each question: it's time to stop squabbling over the "best" methods. BMJ 1997;315:1636.

53. Sackett DL, Haynes RB, Guyatt GH, et al. Clinical epidemiology: a basic science for clinical medicine. 2nd ed. Boston: Little, Brown; 1992.

54. Sackett DL. A primer on the precision and accuracy of the clinical examination. JAMA 1992;267:2638–44.

55. Sahrmann SA. Diagnosis by the physical therapist—a prerequisite for treatment. Phys Ther 1988;68:1703–6.

56. Sandmark H, Nisell R. Validity of five common manual neck pain provoking tests. Scand J Rehab Med 1995;27:131–6.

57. Schulzer M. Diagnostic tests: a statistical review. Muscle Nerve 1994;17:815–9.

58. Schwartz JS. Evaluating diagnostic tests—what needs to be done? J Gen Intern Med 1986;1:266–76.

59. Simel DL, Samsa GP, Matchar DB. Likelihood ratios with confidence: sample size estimation for diagnostic test results. J Clin Epidemiol 1991;44:763–70.

60. Spurling RG, Scoville WB. Lateral rupture of the cervical intervertebral discs: a common cause of shoulder and arm pain. Surg Gynecol Obstet 1944;78:350–8.

61. Stiell IG, Greenberg GH, McKnight RD, et al. Decision rules for the use of radiography in acute ankle injuries: refinement and prospective validation. JAMA 1993;269:1127–32.

62. van Tulder MW, Assendelft WJ, Koes BW, et al. Method guidelines for systematic reviews in the Cochrane Collaboration back review group for spinal disorders. Spine 1997;22:2323–30.

63. Viikari-Juntura E, Porras M, Laasonen EM. Validity of clinical tests in the diagnosis of root compression in cervical disc disease. Spine 1989;14:253–7.

64. Wainner RM, Fritz JM, Irrgang JJ, et al. Reliability and diagnostic accuracy of the clinical examination and patient self-report measures for cervical radiculopathy. Spine 2003;28:52–62.

Cultural Competence: An Essential Element of Primary Health Care

3

Ronnie Leavitt, PhD, MPH, PT

Objectives

After reading this chapter, the reader will be able to:

1. Describe the concept of and the variables associated with a culturally competent practitioner.
2. Describe cultural considerations associated with treating a diverse population.
3. Provide specific strategies associated with a culturally competent organization and practitioner.

In today's world, human diversity is the norm rather than the exception. Patients seeking care in the health care system are likely to look, think, and act, at least in some ways, differently from the health care professional. People have a wide range of ethnic identifications, religions, material realities, beliefs, and behaviors that lead to rich diversity and cultural complexity. Each patient and each physical therapist (PT) is a unique individual.

This book addresses the needs of the PT outpatient practitioner in a primary care environment. The concept of primary health care is especially appropriate for the wide range of physical impairments likely to be seen in an outpatient setting. By definition, primary health care by a PT presumes practice to meet the needs of a patient within the context of the individual patient, family, community, and broader cultural milieu. There is increasing interest in the need to provide health care in a more effective and efficient way to maximize limited resources and meet an ever-expanding array of health concerns. We want to do our job well; we do not want to be ineffective or waste precious resources.

This chapter facilitates the process by which PTs can become culturally competent in a primary health care setting. The goal of cultural competence, as is the goal of competence in any area, is to maximize the potential for a successful interaction between the clinician and patient. Today, rehabilitation practitioners, organizations, and systems need to be culturally competent.

Cultural competence is a set of behaviors, attitudes, and policies that come together on a continuum to enable a system, agency, or individual to function effectively in transcultural interactions.[17] Cultural competence is an essential element for physical therapy outpatient practitioners to facilitate effective and efficient examination, diagnosis, and development of a plan of care. Developing rapport, collecting and synthesizing patient data, recognizing personal functional concerns, and developing treatment suggestions for a particular patient require cultural competence.

Understanding the concept of culture is key to understanding cultural competence. Lynch and Hanson[44] described culture as the framework that guides and binds life practices. This definition is in contrast to a rigidly prescribed set of behaviors or characteristics. Individuals do not inherit a culture biologically; they learn it. People may share cultural tendencies and pass them among generations. Cultural frameworks are constantly evolving, however, and many factors, such as ethnic identification, socioeconomic status, migration history, gender, age, and religion, have a profound effect on one's cultural way of life. Based on these variables, individuals may be members of several subcultures, or smaller units within a larger culture. One's culture is closely interrelated to cultural value systems, health beliefs and behaviors, and communication styles. These variables are particularly relevant to the PT working in a cross-cultural environment, such as an outpatient orthopedic setting.

A culturally competent practitioner must do the following:

- *Acknowledge the immense influence of culture.* It is essential to understand that each of us is immersed in our own culture, with its associated beliefs, attitudes, and behaviors that guide our personal and professional interactions. Human nature is such that we all tend to be ethnocentric, however—believing that our own cultural way of life is the norm, the standard by which all others are judged. What we forget is that the next person, from another culture, is also ethnocentric. The relevance of this self-awareness, or lack of it, is especially crucial when PTs are working with patients who are different from themselves. It is not merely the "other" who has a unique culture, but each of us.

- *Assess cross-cultural relations* and be vigilant toward the dynamics that result from cultural differences. With cross-cultural interaction comes the possibility of misjudging the other's intentions and actions. Each party to an interaction brings to the encounter a specific set of experiences and styles. One must be vigilant to minimize misperception, misinterpretation, and misjudgment.

- *Expand one's cultural knowledge* and institutionalize it so that it can be accessed and incorporated into the delivery of services. We must attempt to seek out sociocultural information about the individual patient, which helps us have a better understanding of how to perform an interview or history—what to ask, how to ask—and how to modify treatment interventions appropriately based on a person's cultural reality. It is impossible, and unnecessary, to learn all there is to know about all cultural subgroups, but clinicians must be aware of the ethnographic information related to the local community and relevant beliefs and behaviors of their patients and the patients' families.

- *Adapt to diversity.* PTs need to develop culturally sensitive examination and treatment techniques that allow a patient to be culturally comfortable. The clinic should be adapted to create a better fit between the needs of the individuals requiring services and the providers meeting their needs.

It is important to remember what cultural competence is *not*. It is not abandoning your own culture and becoming a member of another culture by taking on their attitudes, values, and behaviors.

Developing cultural competence is a lifelong process, and all PTs are not equally culturally competent. Cross and colleagues[17] described at least six possibilities along a continuum of cultural competence ranging from cultural destructiveness to cultural proficiency. Many PTs today are moving from stage 3 to 4:

- *Cultural blindness (stage 3)* presumes an unbiased philosophy and that all people are the same. Facility policy and practices do not recognize the need for culturally specific approaches to solve problems.
- *Cultural "precompetence" (stage 4)* moves toward the more positive end of the continuum. Here PTs recognize weaknesses in the system or their personal cultural knowledge base and explore alternatives. There is a commitment to responding appropriately to differences.
- *Cultural competence (stage 5) and cultural proficiency (stage 6), the last stage,* are where one recognizes the need to conduct research, disseminate the results, and develop new approaches that might increase culturally competent practice.

Campinha-Bacote[10] suggested five factors that contribute to a culturally competent model of care:

- *Having cultural desire:* The motivation of the health care professional to "want to" engage in the process of becoming culturally competent (as opposed to "have to").
- *Developing cultural awareness (cultural sensitivity):* Becoming aware of and minimizing cultural biases.
- *Increasing cultural knowledge:* Understanding the theoretic and conceptual frameworks for others' worldviews and some of the details influencing daily life.
- *Developing cultural skills:* How we assess and treat individuals appropriately.
- *Experiencing cultural encounters:* Exposure to people from different cultures and an opportunity to work with them toward achieving shared goals.

This chapter focuses primarily on the second factor of PTs increasing their knowledge base so that cultural awareness and skill development can be facilitated. A cultural encounter is bound to occur in all work environments. Examples are derived from a variety of cultures and patient populations, emphasizing those cultures PTs are more likely to come into contact with by virtue of national demographic trends or working in an outpatient orthopedic practice setting.

TERMINOLOGY AND DEMOGRAPHICS

Terminology identifying individuals and groups of people is often controversial. From a sociocultural perspective, the term *ethnicity* is a better label than *race*. Ethnic identification is classified by common traits or customs. It is based on one's identity as belonging to a distinct behavioral or ideational group with presumed shared cultural heritage. Ethnicity may be based on color, religion, one's own or ancestor's place of origin, language, or geographic territory. Race, a concept historically used to divide the world into three biologic species, is an increasingly meaningless concept.

Broad categories are often a necessity for expedience but fail to represent subgroups and the presence of *intracultural*

diversity and individuality. The category *Asian* encompasses at least 18 subgroups, and *Hispanic* or *Latino* encompasses more than 20 subgroups. There are more than 500 American Indian tribal groups in the United States. *Black* may refer to African Americans, Jamaicans, Nigerians, or other Africans. There is also an enormous variety of individuality among white cultures. The term *Euro-American* encompasses people whose ancestors come from many European nations, including England, Italy, Greece, and Poland. Considerable individual differences exist within each of the aforementioned groups—that is, not all people from Mexico are the same. Assessment of the culture and of each patient as an individual is crucial. The phrase *people of color* is often the preferred terminology used in the United States today for nonwhite individuals. According to census data, this combined group of people will become the majority over the next generations, and they will require rehabilitation services.[40]

In 2000, approximately 75% of the population of the United States was white; 12.5%, black or African American; 12.5%, Hispanic/Latino; 1%, American Indian or Alaska native; 3.7%, Asian, Native Hawaiian, or other Pacific Islander; 2.4%, identified as two or more ethnic groups; and 5.5%, identified as other. Between 1980 and 1990, the total U.S. population increased 9.8%, but the rate of growth varied widely: The Asian/Pacific Island population growth was 107.8%; Hispanic/Latino, 53%; American Indian, 37.9%; black, 13.2%; and white, 6%.[61,62] Between 1990 and 2000, this population trend continued. During that time, there was a tremendous influx of immigrants from South and Central America and Asia, and this trend is expected to continue.[22]

Understanding the 2000 census is complicated by the fact that, although seen as necessary by many, there were 63 possible ethnic categories from which to choose (to accommodate individuals who identify themselves in ways that are different from the afore-mentioned classifications or as multiracial) instead of the previously used 5 categories. Still, the trends are clear, and the raw percentages speak for themselves.

Statistics from the 2008 census[63] show a continuation of the aforementioned trends. The Hispanic population, showing the fastest rate of growth, has grown to 15.1% of the U.S. population (45.5 million people) and is the largest "minority" group. Blacks are reported to be 13.9% (40.7 million); Asians, 5.04% (15.2 million); American Indian/Alaska natives, 1.49% (4.5 million); and Pacific Islanders, 0.33% (1 million). The population of whites (non-Hispanic) totaled 66% (199.1 million), a decrease from the 75% reported in 2000. The greatest number of immigrants coming to the United States are Mexican. In addition, birth rates are generally higher for Hispanics, especially Puerto Ricans.[61,62]

By 2050, based on immigration patterns and fertility rates, it has been projected that white, non-Hispanic Americans will represent approximately 53% of the total population, showing a continued downward trend. Hispanic Americans will account for 24%; African Americans, 15%; and Asian/Pacific Island Americans, 9%.[66] Previous estimations have been revised, however. The 2008 estimate is that whites will no longer be in the majority by 2042—8 years ahead of the earlier predictions.

Also relevant to the practice of outpatient physical therapy is the great increase in the population older than 65 years expected during the next decades. The relative increase is expected to be greatest for people of color.

An additional consideration is the substantial disparity between the number of individuals from particular ethnic groups enrolled in health professional schools and their representation in the society as a whole. The American Physical Therapy Association estimates that approximately 10% to 12% of their members are people of color.[3] Although moving in the right direction, the profession of physical therapy remains "diversity challenged." It is essential to realize that, yes, it is best if professionals are proportionately represented within the treatment setting, but it is equally important for *all* PTs, no matter what their own ethnic background, to be culturally competent. In addition, the didactic and clinical educational materials we have historically learned from are generally presented from a Western medical model/Eurocentric point of view with regard to disability, health, and illness. All this contributes to a less-than-ideal delivery of professional service to people from diverse backgrounds and can result in a cultural clash and conflicting expectations between patient and PT.

A strong word of caution is in order. Broad categories as used in the previous paragraphs are practical for descriptive purposes, but they can perpetuate culturally biased racial or ethnic stereotyping and prejudices; this is not the intent. Rather, the intent is to incorporate knowledge about the patient population, considering the extensive cultural landscape in which they live and their individual characteristics, to recognize *interethnic* and *intraethnic* diversity. In an orthopedic outpatient setting, generalization about an ethnic group is as inappropriate as generalizing about a frozen shoulder or torn knee ligament. In addition, if a patient came in with an unfamiliar diagnosis, you would obtain information about the problem. Similarly, it is appropriate to obtain information about the patient's cultural ways of life.

CULTURAL CONSIDERATIONS WHEN TREATING A DIVERSE PATIENT POPULATION: DEVELOPING CULTURAL COMPETENCE

To facilitate the process of becoming culturally competent in physical therapy practice, especially in the primary health care setting, PTs must, in essence, perform a medical ethnography. *Ethnography* is the work of describing a culture with the aim of understanding another way of life from the native point of view. The ethnographer seeks to learn from a culture; be taught by the population; and discover the insider's, or emic, point of view rather than the outsider's, or etic, point of view.[59] This chapter introduces several variables that must be considered during the process of ethnography. Assessing each of these domains is crucial so that the examination and treatment interventions may be appropriately modified based on an individual's cultural reality. The following subheadings never stand alone. Each is intertwined with the others.

This brief introduction to several variables should not be used to stereotype individuals but can be used as a starting point from which to assess further how PTs and patients may view the world from different vantage points. PTs need to sense patterns and variations without overgeneralizing. Diversity and

contradictions abound among populations. Improving one's understanding of the many subcultures encountered in practice requires greater research of individual ethnic groups and different geographic regions. Further emphasis needs to be placed on the difficult task of parsing out the relative influence of biologic/genetic factors from socioeconomic factors and from cultural lifestyle habits.

Socioeconomic Status

Socioeconomic status may be the most relevant variable affecting someone's worldview. Poverty is not randomly distributed throughout the population. Rather, it is strongly related to race or ethnicity, sex, and age. In the United States, approximately 20% of African American families and 17% of Hispanic families live in poverty compared with 9.5% of Asian and Pacific Islander and 8.7% of white families.[67] Although urban poverty is more visible, rural residents are more likely to be poor than urban residents and because of their isolation have less access to needed services and programs.[24,32] In 2007, individuals with disabilities also had an increased rate of poverty at 30.4% compared with 10.5% of individuals without disabilities.[64]

Although most poverty in the United States is categorized as relative (i.e., people are able to afford basic necessities but are unable to maintain an average standard of living), it is commonly known that individuals who live in poverty have more health problems than individuals with higher incomes. Many frequently cited obstacles to maintaining health are associated with poverty, such as poor housing (or even homelessness) and environmental conditions, inadequate nutrition, harmful lifestyle habits, and lack of access to transportation and child care services. Poverty is known to influence the use of and interaction with the health care system and the outcomes associated with health care.[14,52]

Specifically in an outpatient setting, hours of operation and available means of transportation if a patient does not have a car should be assessed. Hourly workers may not have the flexibility to take off from work during the typical workday, and public transportation may be less available at certain times. Can you assume that your patient has electricity or running water at home? Can resistive weights be bought, or do you need to be creative by filling a bag with rocks or cans of food? Availability of resources should not be assumed.

PTs should keep in mind the possibility of domestic violence. Although not just a problem among low-income individuals, it is nevertheless an issue often associated with the stresses of poverty. PTs working in a primary care environment need to be familiar with the signs and symptoms of abuse and helpful resources related to domestic violence. PTs might be the first ones to notice indications that abuse is present. Sensitivity to these socioeconomic and cultural issues can be tricky. How do you inquire without being insulting or taking away the patient's pride? Level of skill development can be especially important in this area.

The patient's health insurance status and the effect of federal policy on Medicare and Medicaid are important to the primary health care outpatient practitioner. The changing economic and political landscape of the early 21st century is likely to affect low-income and less acculturated people of color disproportionately because of their considerable reliance on these programs. The ethnic group most likely to be completely uninsured is the Hispanic population (more than one third of the population). Recent immigrants are also less likely to be insured.[46,60]

Racism

Although a detailed discussion of the effects of racism is beyond the scope of this chapter, PTs must be cognizant of the marked effect of racism on health status and health care interactions.[14,56,57] The collective experience of African Americans includes the Tuskegee syphilis study, sterilization initiatives, and sickle cell screening abuses, which have led to distrust of the medical profession by many black Americans.[7] There is a large body of evidence to suggest that health disparities are often partly related to racism. According to research by Schneider and colleagues,[55] after adjustment for potential confounding factors, black Medicare beneficiaries enrolled in managed care plans were less likely than whites to receive eye examinations, beta-blocker medication after myocardial infarction, and follow-up after hospitalization for mental illness.

Degree of Acculturation

Acculturation is a process through which individuals in subcultures adopt traits of the larger, or normative, culture. Individuals range from being highly assimilated (in which the boundaries between the old and new culture are erased) to bicultural to highly traditional (in which values and behaviors are similar to those found in the country of origin). The degree to which individuals acculturate to the mainstream North American culture (heretofore the white, Anglo-Saxon, Protestant culture) is influenced by such things as age, level of education, number of years in a new country, and socioeconomic status and affects a person's health status and interaction with the health care system.

The PT should be aware of the patient's migration history as a means to initiate an assessment of degree of acculturation. Vietnamese who arrived in the United States during the mid-1970s were primarily well-educated, upper class, Christian individuals escaping a repressive political regime. In contrast, during the 1980s, Vietnamese immigrants were more likely to be escaping economic and political deprivation, and they had fewer economic resources, different and more considerable health problems, and a more marginalized social support system. A look at the migration history for the Cuban American population reveals a similar distinction between the first and second waves of immigrants.[30]

Predictive of more traditional beliefs and behaviors are emigration from a rural area, frequent returns to the country of origin, limited formal education, poor English language skills, low socioeconomic status, recent immigration to the United States or immigration at an older age, and housing segregation. Typical ways to measure the degree of acculturation are based on the language used within the home, the language of preferred media sources, and who makes up a primary support system.[30] Although the PT might not formally measure a patient's acculturation status, a primary care PT can ask questions of the patient that would give a better understanding of the patient's degree of assimilation.

INCIDENCE AND PREVALENCE OF DISEASE AND DISABILITY. A primary care orthopedic physical therapy practice setting is likely to treat patients with a range of diagnoses, impairments, and functional disabilities. Disease and disability are not randomly distributed among humans. Many factors, including race, ethnicity, socioeconomic status, geography, and migration history, play a role in determining the incidence and prevalence of disease and disability. Discovering the determinants of disease— that is, risk factors that relate to the development and cause of the condition—is a major aspect of epidemiologic work. Broadly speaking, risk factors can be related to inherited characteristics, environmental factors, or personal behavior and lifestyle.[8,35,49,57]

In the United States, people of color have many more health problems than the white population.* They are also more likely to report poor health and more restricted activity than white people. Women are especially disadvantaged and report greater limitation in activities of daily living. People of color have a lower life expectancy, higher infant mortality rates, and higher morbidity and mortality rates for a wide range of diseases. Cardiovascular disease, hypertension, and strokes disproportionately affect African Americans.[11,39,70] The death rate for individuals having a stroke is 52 per 100,000 for African American men and 39.9 per 100,000 for African American women (97.7% higher than white American men and 77.3% higher than white American women).[47] Approximately 85% of elderly Hispanics have one or more chronic diseases, such as diabetes (especially among Mexican Americans), arthritis, and depression, resulting in greater rates of morbidity and mortality. Chronic liver disease and acquired immunodeficiency syndrome (AIDS) are far more prevalent among blacks and Hispanics.[53,65-71]

The incidence of non–insulin-dependent diabetes mellitus (type 2) has shown an alarming increase in recent years, especially among young and old American Indian, African American, and Hispanic populations. Family history, genetics, obesity, and age are key risk factors. An example of the interaction of genetic and lifestyle variables is the implication of the so-called thrifty gene theory as it relates to Mexican American and American Indian diabetics. When particular tribes were seminomadic, they frequently subsisted on a feast-or-famine diet. The tribes genetically developed an ability to metabolize their food efficiently. Today, when food is more abundant and likely to be high in fat and calories, and when exercise is less a part of daily living, a higher rate of obesity and diabetes occurs. Individuals with more Indian admixture are more inclined to insulin resistance and the inability to break down glucose in the blood. On the positive side, some American Indians have the benefit of a gene that causes their blood glucose levels to respond to moderate exercise more quickly than others.[12,30,50,63,72]

Representative studies evaluating health disparities within physical therapy per se from the perspective of access, referral patterns, prevention, interventions, and outcomes are sparse but increasing. Allen and coworkers[1] found that African American women were significantly less likely to receive a referral or to enroll in cardiac rehabilitation, even though there are greater levels of functional disability and higher rates of morbidity and

---

*References 2, 14, 27, 39, 54, 56, 68.

mortality among people of color with cardiac disease. In a study evaluating knee replacement outcomes, Lin and Kaplan[43] suggested that black individuals might be referred for surgery later in their disease process, negatively influencing their outcome.

Healthy People 2010, a guiding document for the U.S. Public Health Service, has as one of its three major goals the elimination of disparity between people of color and the white population.[61,69] PTs working in a cross-cultural environment need to be knowledgeable about the variables affecting the incidence and prevalence of orthopedic and medical conditions so that they can be better prepared to treat these conditions, answer patient and family questions concerning the condition, and develop special preventive and educational programs targeted to patients in need.

Comparative Value Orientations

In contrast to material culture, or the more easily observed and understood parts of culture (e.g., clothing, food, music, forms of greeting, ceremonial rites of passage), nonmaterial culture is more difficult to assess. Sometimes similarities in the material culture obscure profound differences in the nonmaterial culture that are relevant to the therapist-patient interaction. These value orientations are as important, or even more important, for the PT to pay attention to.

Many observers have identified recurrent themes and patterns in cultures (Table 3-1). These cultural elements may be the core of one's *worldview,* or values people live by. Typically, cultures that have been most heavily influenced by Euro-American values match those cultural characteristics listed in the left column of Table 3-1, whereas cultures influenced by Latin or Hispanic, Asian, Middle Eastern, or African values fit the characteristics listed on the right. Worldview can be heavily influenced, however, by personality traits and socioeconomic and acculturation status. In addition, people do not fit into a rigid category; some may fall at the far end of one dichotomous scale, in the middle, or at the other end.

If forced to choose one contrasting element for these two columns, it might be an individualist society versus a collectivist society. These adjectives symbolize general social organization and relationships and can be linked to many of the other values listed. There are innumerable ways in which these characteristics can influence the therapeutic encounter. Euro-American values emphasize the importance of the individual and the ability of each person to affect his or her future through hard work. In this type of cultural orientation, time and nature are commodities to be used profitably, and the success—or lack of success—of each person is credited to that individual. Professionals with this type of cultural value system would emphasize the autonomy and personal responsibility of their patients and expect them to work hard while in therapy. Desires and expectations would be clearly stated in a direct manner.

In contrast, patients may have a cultural value system that emphasizes the importance of the group over the individual. In the Hispanic culture, possibly the most significant value is that of *familismo.* Consistent with a collectivist society, the emphasis is on family commitment and responsibility. The welfare and honor of the family are preeminent concerns. The father is typically the final arbiter of decision making. The mother is central

TABLE 3-1	
Comparative Value Orientations	
Euro-American	**Cross-Cultural Comparison**
Individualism/privacy	Collectivism/group welfare
Personal control over environment	Fate
Time dominates	Human interaction dominates
Precise time reckoning	Loose time reckoning
Future orientation	Past orientation
Doing (working, achieving)	Being (personal qualities)
Human equality	Hierarchy/rank/status
Self-help	Birthright inheritance
Competition	Cooperation
Informality	Formality
Directness/openness/honesty	Indirectness/ritual/"face"
Practicality/efficiency	Idealism/theory
Materialism	Spiritualism
Values youth	Values elders
Relative equality of sexes	Relative inequality of sexes

Adapted from Ferraro G: *The cultural dimension of international business,* 2nd ed, Englewood Cliffs, NJ, 1994, Prentice-Hall; and Lynch E, Hanson M: *Developing cross-cultural competence,* Baltimore, 1998, Paul Brookes.

within the household and is responsible for childrearing and cultural and social stability.[53] Kinship bonds across generations are common. A patient may arrive at the clinic with several family members and think there is little point to working too hard because he or she will be cared for by the family. Another common belief is that much of what happens to people—including disability—is predetermined by fate. For both of you to save face, Hispanic patients might act politely and be accommodating when in fact they may not understand your instructions or know that your goals and theirs are not in sync. Other cultural values associated with the Hispanic culture include *personalismo* (friendliness), *simpatia* (kindness, avoid conflict; sympathy), and *fatalismo* (fatalism).

Core cultural values associated with African Americans include community and connection to ancestors and history, religion and spiritualism, oral expressiveness, commitment to family, and intuition and experience.[8] Core cultural values of Asian individuals are associated with the teachings of Buddhism, Taoism, and Confucianism. Harmony between and among humans and nature is critical.[58]

Perhaps the most difficult cultural differences to overcome in an outpatient orthopedic clinic, especially for North Americans, relates to pace of life and notion of time.[29] The different views on the importance of an appointment time can have profound psychologic and business impact. *Monochronism* is the view that events happen in chronologic order, work tasks and socialization are separate, and adherence to schedules is important. Euro-Americans are monochronic: They are action oriented and are often unforgiving about such things as missed appointments and a casual approach to punctuality, "red tape," bureaucratic delays, and the sense that time is an unimportant concept.

Polychronism is the view that events can happen concurrently and that fixed schedules are insignificant. The focus is on a more personal interaction, with less concern toward completion of the task at hand. With Hispanic patients as an example, there is the value for *personalismo,* or a more humanistic approach. The attention to a work orientation and the acquisition of material goods may not be present among individuals who more highly value a relaxed, human relationship–oriented lifestyle. Imagine the potential for misunderstanding if a Cuban patient arrives late for an appointment and expects the PT to chat for a few minutes about nontherapeutic issues, such as the well-being of his family, and the PT, already annoyed about her schedule being interrupted, immediately launches into a discussion about how to do exercises. In a rehabilitation setting, even the development of group exercise programs may be influenced by comparative value systems. For example, does the patient value competition or cooperation?

The role and status of medical personnel may be different depending on cultural orientation. A patient from a Middle Eastern culture would more naturally defer to the health professional, who is considered an authority figure worthy of high esteem. An interactive conversation about health options is less likely to occur.

Comparative value systems may affect behaviors around a particular age group of patients. There may be particular expectations of Asian American adolescents that are different from those of a typical Euro-American adolescent. In contrast to how young children are obliged and indulged, older children are expected to be well disciplined and to take on some adult roles. An older, adolescent sibling may be expected to accept personal sacrifice and assume child care for young children in the extended family, while maintaining a strong academic record. A sense of duty or obligation to the family may be pronounced, and this is learned through proper role modeling. If there is misbehavior by a younger sibling, an older sibling might be rebuked for not setting a good example. High expectations may be a source of stress. Adolescents are likely to be recipients of a parenting style that is controlling, restrictive, and protective; this may lead to distancing behaviors or distrust of outsiders. Discussions about sensitive topics such as sexuality may be avoided, and the willingness to discuss personal issues related to treatment can be minimal.[44]

Similarly, special considerations may be necessary when working with elder or terminal patients that reflect a particular worldview. Widespread respect for elders is prevalent among many ethnic groups. Signs of respect may include use of the terms "Ma'am" or "Sir" or asking for tales of wisdom. Although the orthopedic primary care PT is not typically faced with discussions regarding end-of-life decisions, this is still a possible topic of conversation, especially with family members. In Asian and Hispanic cultures, disclosure of a terminal disease may take away any hope that the patient may have. Family members have a strong obligation to protect loved ones from emotional distress.

Elder adults are likely to have variations in attitudes toward advance directives. Chinese elders may be less likely to write something down because they honor the spoken word. In actuality, Chinese elders commonly do not discuss the likelihood of death at all because it is believed to be a bad omen. The Navajo feel similarly. Negative thoughts would be in conflict with the concept of *hozho,* which involves goodness, harmony, and positive attitude. Japanese elders place great faith in family and professional relationships, and it is less likely that individual decision making would be a norm. Children, particularly the oldest son, feel the duty to maintain a parent's life. For the Navajo as well, major decisions are collaborative, and family and tribespeople would have input into any advance health directives.[7]

African Americans who have been socioeconomically marginalized tend to be more likely to desire life-sustaining treatment and are less likely to desire or receive hospice care. In contrast, white people are more likely to feel empowered and in control, which may account for their greater willingness to forgo life-sustaining treatment.[7] Finally, considering an individual's value system may influence whether accepting a gift from a patient or his or her family is ethically appropriate. In many cultures, it would be a great insult to refuse a gift; a person's pride may be at stake.

Communication

Communication, language, cultural value orientations, and culture overall are intertwined and inseparable. Communication is another exceptionally important variable when working cross-culturally or seeking to understand one's cultural value system and explanatory model. In addition to the problems encountered when the provider and patient do not speak the same language, obvious and subtle differences in the interactive styles of the individuals exist. Verbal communication in individualistic societies is associated with direct, "low-context" communication. It is expected that someone will get right to the point, and it is assumed that surrounding context is unnecessary for interpretation. Rather, what is heard in the verbal message is what is being communicated. The notion of privacy is important, and questions of a more personal nature might be considered off-limits.

In contrast, an individual from a collectivist culture may speak indirectly, in a more circular fashion, always keeping in mind the need for everyone to "save face." The Hispanic culture relies more on *indirectas.* Communication is more high context, or sensitive to situational and contextual features. There is a more spiral logic, more indirect verbal negotiation, and subtle nonverbal nuances. The notion of privacy is less pervasive, but this must take into account the idea of not embarrassing someone or causing either party to "lose face." The focus is more on human relationships. Individuals are especially more reluctant to express negative feelings and unlikely to share concerns about taking medication ordered by a physician or ask questions that may be perceived as stupid.[9]

Another difference in verbal communication is the amount of "wait time," or pace of conversation. American Indians typically have a slower pace of conversation, which requires waiting until the individual has finished speaking before interrupting or asking questions. Euro-Americans are typically uncomfortable with silence. Wait time is also increased if patients need to translate the words into their own language in their minds before responding.[38] In some cultures, many people may speak at once.

Many nonverbal, observable differences exist in communication style among different cultural groups. As much as 93% of the total meaning of an encounter is communicated by nonverbal factors.[46] Differences occur regarding eye contact, facial expression, body movement, comfortable distance zones, and overall formality. The PT may believe a patient is acting disinterested if eye contact is not direct, yet the patient may believe it is impolite to look directly at someone perceived as the authority figure. A white PT may firmly shake the hand of an American Indian or traditional Asian patient on introduction and may presume this is an appropriate, friendly, polite gesture. The patient may consider this aggressive or hostile because he or she is more used to a subtle, soft, nonthreatening handshake.

What is the preferred distance zone for the patient? How close does the patient like to stand when speaking with the PT? It is wise for the PT to observe a patient's response when the PT stands closer or further away during a general conversation. During a treatment session, does a person of the opposite sex seem more uncomfortable than one might expect? The PT should observe how individuals from a different culture act with each other compared with how they act with the PT. Touch can provide reassurance and kindness, or it can be a discomfort and annoyance. Gender and age are important variables influencing distance zones.

A PT who is educating a patient about a diagnosis or a home program must also recognize that methods of teaching and learning differ among cultures. Knowledge transmission in Euro-American cultures often relies on taking notes and studying written texts and intense discussions with a great deal of interaction between the PT and patient. Other cultures rely more on a straight lecture format with few questions and little discussion. Still other cultural groups, such as African Americans, rely almost entirely on oral training and demonstration. A written list of exercises, even with diagrams, may not be as effective as "hearing and feeling" such exercises. Typically, family members should be included in a discussion about a home program and prevention of further problems.[42,44]

It is ideal for the PT and patient to speak the same language, but it is often not possible. PTs should learn at least a few key words in the patient's language, but realize there are often differences in dialects and accents between and within countries. More typically, family (often children) or friends act as translators; although this may be the only available alternative, it is fraught with problems. The PT must be aware that the untrained third party may be interpreting the information before passing it on to the PT, or there may be topics that are inappropriate to discuss with the translator because they are more personal or sensitive in nature (e.g., family planning, spousal abuse, terminal illness). Interpretation requires knowledge of medical terminology, a good memory, ability to concentrate, and ability to know how and when to edit messages so that the true meaning of the interpretation can be accurately transmitted. If possible, a professional translator should be used. A professional interpreter is likely to be bicultural and have a good grasp of the medical and cultural nuances.

Any written materials should be translated in grammatically correct, simple language with appropriate, meaningful vocabulary so that they may be used for their intended purpose and be culturally relevant to the patient. Materials always should be translated back into the original language to verify accuracy.

Because language barriers are such a significant and prevalent obstacle to good health care, the Office of Civil Rights within the U.S. Department of Health and Human Services has developed policies for individuals with limited English proficiency. These include assistance options appropriate to each facility's needs. Massachusetts is the first state to require the services of competent interpreters for individuals with limited English proficiency, and more states are expected to follow suit.[16]

The key question is how best to develop rapport with patients to enhance the likelihood of the patient and the PT being satisfied with an encounter. Understanding a range of verbal and nonverbal communication styles and the ability to interpret an interaction properly and engage in good communication minimize barriers that may otherwise exist.

Health Beliefs and Behaviors

Historically, the available models for the provision of care have generally relied on the values and belief systems of the "majority"—the white, middle-class person. These models have been culturally insensitive by denying the realities of non-Western systems of thinking. Although it is recognized that biomedicine and its professionals have a lot to offer, there is an increased awareness of the limitations of a system based solely on a biologic understanding of the human being. In the pluralistic medical systems that exist throughout the world, a range of health care beliefs and behaviors and practitioners is present.

When working in a multicultural environment, PTs must make an effort to understand how people in different cultures and social groups explain the causes of ill health, the types of treatment they believe in, and to whom they turn if they do get ill. One process of medical ethnography through which local health care systems are analyzed was developed by Kleinman, a psychiatrist and medical anthropologist.[35] Specifically, Kleinman developed the theory of an *explanatory model* (EM) to analyze such things as patterns of belief about the causes of illness, decisions about how to respond to specific episodes of sickness, and actions taken to effect a change: "EMs are the notions about an episode of sickness and its treatment that are employed by all those engaged in the clinical process. The study of patient and family EMs tells us how they make sense of given episodes of illness, and how they choose and evaluate particular treatments."[35]

Open-ended questions should be used to allow patients to explain and expand on their situations based on their own perceptions of a particular illness or condition. The therapist can ask the patient questions such as the following:

"What do you call your problem?"
"What do you think caused your problem?"
"What are the greatest problems your illness has caused for you?"
"What do you fear most about the consequences of this illness?"
"What are the most important results you hope to get from your treatment?"

Kleinman's EM is considered an internal, clinical view of the patient's cultural health care system. Because the EM is recognized to depend on many variables—such as societal attitudes toward the sick and disabled, the degree to which the disabled are stigmatized, the material realities of the environment, and the adaptation mechanisms that are available—it is necessary to analyze EMs in a concrete setting.

Presumably, for individuals with a disease or disability and their families, there are specific medical care systems and EMs that account for the beliefs about the impairment and the cultural patterns of behaviors relating to diagnosis and treatment. Although PTs need to focus on the patient EM, it is essential to explore and understand that practitioners also have an EM and operate within their own distinct culture. To enhance the relationship between interacting parties and to affect the outcome of an interaction positively, the culture of the patient and the practitioner must be taken into account. Patients and their families cannot always completely comply with the practitioner EM, and the health professional cannot always accept the patient EM.

Much variation exists in culturally perceived causes of chronic illness or disability.[25-28,35] Patients may have a naturalistic or supernatural belief system. One naturalistic explanation by a Jamaican mother of a child was "jaundice at birth and she premature. The hospital didn't have the facilities for the jaundice, to burn it out, so the jaundice damage her."[41] A different mother, when asked why she believed her child had a disability, answered "like how I have the children fast, and the food me eat. Maybe I did need more nutritious food …. Me had a problem with me big daughter … sent her to buy shoes and she run away with a guy and she never come back until long after the baby born. I was very worried." In actuality, this child had Down syndrome, so the explanation is not scientifically feasible.[41]

Although scientific rationales may exist, traditional beliefs are in some patients' cultural backgrounds and may be brought to the forefront during times of stress or uncertainty. In some instances, individuals believe that disability is a form of punishment. A person may have sinned or violated a taboo, either in this life or a previous life, causing the wrath of God or a source of wickedness. Throughout much of the world, there is belief in the evil eye. In general, the concept implies that an evil spell has been put on a person, which causes the individual to fall ill. The motive is usually envy. As quoted by Mardiros[45] in an article about disability in Mexico, one informant stated, "Before we were married my husband had a lot of women. One of them asked this lady to put a hex on us. She's a bruja [sorcerer or witch]. Because of her we always had bad luck. People are so mean these days …."

Alternatively, in some cultures, an imbalance of elements, or humors, may be responsible for the ailment. In the Asian Indian Ayurvedic system, health is equated with balance. Similarly, traditional Chinese medicine requires a balance of *yin* and *yang*. The Navajo believe that their health depends on harmony with family, community, self, and nature; they do not have the concept of communicable disease. The Navajo language does not have a word for *germ*.[7] In some communities, importance is placed on a balance of hot and cold. These mutually complementary forces are required to be in harmony with nature.

Treatment for a disease or disability is also culture specific, although intraethnic variation abounds. Indigenous healers, or practitioners of traditional medicine, are prevalent in every society. The *espiritismos* may be the preferred source of care for Puerto Ricans. *Espiritismo* involves the belief in the importance of the spiritual world, and "do unto others as you would have them do unto you" is considered the highest ethical principle. The *espiritista*, usually a female medium, helps patients with physical and emotional problems by connecting with good spirits and exorcising evil spirits.[47] The *curanderos* may be preferred for Mexican Americans; the singer, for Navajo; the voodoo priest,

for Haitians; and the herbalist, for Chinese. For Laotian Hmong, the *shaman* may use herbal concoctions and animal sacrifice.[21] For Jamaicans, the *obeah* may use blood, feathers, parrots' beak, grave dirt, egg shell, and medicinal herbs to treat a person with a disability.[41] For American Indians, "talking circles," where stories are shared, are used to show the interconnectedness of life, the cycle of life and death, and the balance required for good health. They may be used to educate about preventive and treatment measures so that the notion of fatalism can be replaced with the idea of control over one's health.[50]

Primary health care PTs today should be especially tuned into the use of complementary and alternative medical therapies (CAM). Seminal work has been done by Eisenberg and colleagues,[18,19] who published the first national survey describing the use of CAM (i.e., defined as health care and medical practices that are not currently an integral part of conventional medicine). The first report stated that approximately one third of adults in the United States had used at least one CAM during the last year. A follow-up survey in 1997 concluded that 42% of the population used CAM.[19] More recently, the U.S. National Health Interview Survey concluded that greater than one third of adults used CAM during the preceding year.[4] When the definition of CAM was expanded to include prayer, the percentage increased to 62%. CAM includes mind-body interventions (hypnosis or prayer), biologic-based interventions (herbal therapies and dietary supplements), manipulative and body-based interventions (massage, manipulation), and energy therapies (focusing on the role of energy sources within the body). For individuals with non-Western belief systems, these types of intervention may be the norm, and it is the Western biomedical model that can be complementary and alternative.

There are two theoretic explanations for why ritual healing practices may be successful. One is neurobiologic. There is increasing evidence that endorphins may play a role in diminishing pain. These neurochemicals produced by the brain may be released by psychologic experiences. Alternatively, the placebo effect may help the body to heal itself. A placebo may be word or action, not just a pharmaceutical substance. By engaging the patient's mind and emotions, the healer may aid physiologic repair.[47]

Traditional practices may also influence the response of a patient to a suggested Western medical protocol. Many Vietnamese believe that Western medicine is designed to suit the body size of Westerners. The quantity prescribed may be seen as inappropriate for the typical Vietnamese, who is much smaller than the typical American.[37] Likewise, many Hispanic and Asian people classify substances as hot or cold. These categorizations affect the patient's decision regarding what medicines to use and foods to eat.

A practitioner working in the area of women's health might want to know that there may be special considerations associated with childbirth. Within the traditional Asian culture, a woman who is pregnant or has recently given birth may have a diet with selected hot or cold foods. During the first trimester of pregnancy, a woman may eat "hot" foods, such as eggs, meat, black pepper, or ginger. In the second trimester, she eats "cold" foods, such as squash, fruits, bean curd, sugar, and herbal tea. During the last trimester, when she is in a "hot period," "hot" foods or medicines are strictly limited. During the entire pregnancy, shellfish, lamb, and rabbit are forbidden. Immediately postpartum, during the "cold" period, there is a specific taboo against some "cold" foods. Different Asian cultures prepare special dishes to assist with the involution of the uterus, chase the "bad blood" away, and regulate menstrual flow. In the Cambodian culture, a postpartum mother may be placed on a slatted bed with a heat source under the bed. The practice is referred to as "mother roasting," and it is meant to replace the heat lost during childbirth. Going out doors, drinking cold water, washing the hair, and taking a shower are not advised.[13]

Clinicians should not assume that the father will take part in labor and delivery. Although the presence of the father is common among Euro-Americans, in many cultures childbirth is not a "family" matter, but a job for the woman and her female support system. Social roles are separate, and other female family members or women trained specifically to assist with childbearing and child care are deemed more appropriate.[13]

The use of an alternative treatment is often the source of misunderstanding and conflict. Asian practices used to draw evil from the body, such as coin rubbing—in which a coin is rubbed on the skin until a raised red mark appears—or cupping—when a heated glass is placed on the body to create a vacuum, causing the skin to become raised and red—may be perceived as harmful to a child by a Western practitioner. The traditional Hmong harbor superstitions toward American health practitioners. Some Hmong believe that surgeons cut out body parts of the deceased to sell them as food or eat them themselves.[21]

When using typical Western physical therapy treatment procedures, it is necessary to consider the appropriateness of that treatment within the context of the patient's culture. In many Asian cultures, people usually squat rather than sit, necessitating greater range of motion even at the expense of stability. In addition, eating with hands or chopsticks may require different movement patterns and range than those typically used by Westerners.

Especially relevant to PTs working with patients who have a wide range of orthopedic impairments is the notion that pain means different things to people from various ethnic groups and that their response to pain is guided by cultural rules. Research on the psychosocial and behavioral aspects of pain has found a significant relationship between ethnic variation and perception of pain intensity and the responses to pain.

In his famous study comparing different white populations, including Jewish, Italian, Irish, and "old" or "Yankee" Americans, Zborowski[74] determined that in some groups it was permissible to complain about pain, whereas other groups were expected to report pain in a dispassionate manner. Members of some groups wanted immediate relief of pain with painkillers, whereas others worried more about the long-term implications of pain and did not want medications for fear that pharmacologic treatment would mask a more serious problem. Societal rules also promote gender or age differences regarding pain tolerance, but these are not cultural universals.

During the late 1990s, Bates and Edwards[6] completed a similar study to determine patient meanings and explanations associated with pain. American-born white (mostly Protestant), Hispanic, Irish, Italian, French Canadian, and Polish people, all

of whom were outpatients in a Massachusetts pain treatment facility, were studied. Variation in ethnic identity and locus of control style was consistently associated with differences in pain intensity and response. The Hispanic group showed the highest pain expressiveness, the greatest interference with work and social activities, and the highest degree of emotional and psychologic stress. The Italian group was second in each of these categories, and either the Polish or "old" American group was the lowest in each category. The notion of interethnic group variation was supported.

Nevertheless, intragroup variation analysis shows within-group differences based on generation and degree of heritage consistency. More recent immigrants or first-generation American-born individuals, who have high degrees of heritage consistency and who believe that they have a strong support system, report less severe responses to pain. The notion of intraethnic variation is supported as well.

Looking more closely at one particular group, Santana and Santana[53] cited a 1995 study by Villarruel, who identified the ways in which Mexican Americans experience pain. Beliefs about pain include (1) pain is an accepted and expected part of life, (2) pain does not negate one's responsibilities and duties, (3) pain is predetermined by the gods, (4) pain is a consequence of immoral behavior, (5) pain should be endured with a stoic attitude, and (6) pain may best be alleviated by maintaining balance. PTs need to contemplate the meaning of pain for an individual patient.

A study comparing normative pain responses among college students in the United States and India found that students in India were less accepting of overt pain expression than students in the United States. Female students believed that overt pain expression was more appropriate than male students. Indian men had the highest pain tolerance. Reported pain intensity predicted 28% of the variance in pain tolerance, and beliefs predicted another 5%.[48] (For more information on pain and culture, see *Culture, Health and Illness,* by Cecil Helman[29a] and *Pain as Human Experience: An Anthropological Perspective,* edited by Good et al[27a].)

PTs serving as primary health care practitioners would also benefit from knowledge about their patients' dietary practices. In addition to nutritional value, there is profound social and cultural meaning in food. Specific foods for the African American community are identified as "soul food." These may be unhealthy from a nutritional perspective, but significant to an individual, representing a rich cultural history and memories. It is unlikely that an individual would completely alter his or her eating habits on the PT's suggestion to eat more healthfully. Finding a compromise is likely the best solution.

Practices that can appear in pregnant African American women are pica (eating inedible substances such as laundry starch) and geophagy ("earth eating"). Eating clay or dirt is a practice brought from Africa during slavery and was presumed beneficial to the mother and unborn child. Red clay is rich in iron. In more recent times, because working on a farm is less common, laundry starch may be substituted.[58]

Health beliefs and behaviors that are closely intertwined with comparative value systems relate to the role that religion plays in one's EM. Religious beliefs and customs may affect the acceptance and the administration of more orthodox rehabilitation-related practices. This may be an area in which the PT has difficulty accepting someone else's moral and ethical viewpoint and actions. A common point of conflict is the willingness of a practitioner to accept the refusal of a Jehovah's Witness to allow a medical intervention if it involves the need for a blood transfusion. Another common frustration occurs when patients have strong faith in the ability of their supreme spiritual being (e.g., God, Allah, Brahma) to cure them, avoiding any other treatments. It may be less than ideal from a PT's perspective if a Lubavitcher orthodox Jew turns to a *rebbe* for healing prayers or an African American to a "tent meeting." From the Mexican study, in which the respondents were Roman Catholic, "the most commonly reported cultural prescription was prayer through which children were given spiritually to either the patron saint or the Lady of Guadeloupe. Through the fulfillment of vows and pilgrimages, by offering the child to God, cutting off one's hair, ceasing drinking, becoming dedicated to the child and family, the child would be ensured a perpetual place next to God."[45]

A fascinating domain unlikely to be familiar to the PT is that of culture-bound syndromes, sometimes referred to as folk illnesses. These culture-specific syndromes exist in most cultures and are associated with unique beliefs about the cause of an illness and specific prescribed treatments. *Susto* is the most studied culture-bound psychosomatic illness within Hispanic cultures. *Susto,* or "shock," refers to a magical fright or soul loss, which happens when a frightening event causes the soul to leave the body. Symptoms include sleepiness, loss of appetite, insomnia, and generalized depression and are considered body metaphors for psychologic distress. Other culture-bound syndromes within the Hispanic community include *emphacho* (stomachaches, diarrhea, vomiting, and fever are symptoms of having eaten an inappropriate food, which is said to "stick" to the stomach lining), *envidia* (set off when a person is envious of another), and *mal aire* (bad air caused by an evil wind, with symptoms similar to those of a cold or flu).[47,51]

A culture-bound syndrome from the Haitian culture is "arrested pregnancy syndrome," in which a woman who is expected to be carrying a child and feels as though she is pregnant actually is not. It is often associated with infertility in a culture that highly values the ability to have children.[15] Anorexia nervosa, a psychologic disorder with which most PTs are familiar, is considered a North American culture–bound syndrome.[5]

It is expected that most people, to varying degrees, intertwine modern or Western medicine with indigenous or folk medicine. People are more likely to partake in indigenous practices if they are less acculturated, poorer, and more rural based. Family and a hierarchy of lay healers are often the first line of defense. Practical matters, such as cost, seriousness of illness, and availability of practitioners, often determine the use of traditional practices. This results in medical pluralism, or the existence and use of many different health care alternatives within societies.[20,73]

The PT should learn as much as possible about the relevant traditional practitioners in his or her community. Most patients do not report the use of CAM to their health provider, so the PT must ask the right questions.[7] To learn more, the PT can ask the patient to bring him or her to a session with a traditional healer or take him or her to the local *botanica* (store for herbal remedies and religious items in a Hispanic community). The PT should be concerned only if the traditional healer prescribes an unhealthy, dangerous remedy. Why not think in terms of multiple treatment options—each serving its own purpose? The best scenario, in theory, involves the PT serving as a "culture broker" between the patient, the traditional healers, and the mainstream health care system. Expanded information on particular cultural group beliefs and behaviors can be accessed from the resources listed in the Suggested Readings.

More Practical Strategies to Facilitate Cultural Competence

The information in this chapter provides the PT with knowledge to enhance cultural competence. The following additional practical strategies are offered to support a climate in which multiculturalism is the norm. Multiculturalism encompasses cultures that differ in age, color, ethnicity, sex, national origin, political ideology, race, religion, and sexual orientation and includes the presence and participation of individuals with disabilities and individuals from differing socioeconomic backgrounds. As an organization, practice, or individual becomes multicultural, cultural competence is imperative.

ORGANIZATIONAL POLICY CONSIDERATIONS

- Does the mission statement of the organization have a commitment to cultural competence?
- Does the budget and the strategic plans of the organization show a commitment to culturally competent practice?
- Does the organizational leadership set a good example with regard to their approach to a diverse range of client cultural ways of life?
- Does the organization know the community demographic data, needs, health care practices, and barriers to care?
- Is the organization committed to cultural competence training for health care personnel?
- Has the organization become aware of, and abided by, the state, federal, and professional organization standards requiring cultural competence?*
- Does the organization work to build culturally appropriate resource networks?

HUMAN AND PERSONNEL CONSIDERATIONS

- What is the ethnic background of the staff and the board of directors? Is there a commitment to a diverse workforce? Is there an effort to hire people who speak the same languages as the patients or staff who are bicultural?

---

*For example, to ensure that the health care system better responds to the needs of an increasingly diverse patient population, the U.S. Department of Health and Human Services Office of Minority Health has developed national standards for culturally and linguistically appropriate services. The 14 standards are organized by themes: culturally competent care (standards 1 to 3), language access services (4 to 7), and organizational supports for cultural competence (8 to 14). Although these standards are intended to be inclusive of all cultures, they are particularly designed to assist in the elimination of racial and ethnic health disparities in the United States by making the health care environment more inviting to the groups that historically have experienced unequal access to health services.[16] Specific ways to put culturally and linguistically appropriate services into action are found in the document. Standard 2 states that diversity is a necessary but insufficient condition to achieve a culturally competent organization. The notion of a diverse staff includes all personnel from maintenance to administrative to medical professionals. The use of proactive incentives, mentoring programs, staff education, and training all are given forethought to avoid the need for resolution of conflict.

- If you drew an organizational chart, what would it look like? Who is in a position of power? Who is at the bottom of the hierarchy?
- Who is the "face to the wider world" for the organization? Who represents the organization?
- Are the employee benefits meeting the needs of individuals with unique circumstances?
- Is there a commitment to ongoing discussion and training on issues of cultural competence on the staff/board level?
- Has the organization established collegial and collaborative relationships with other relevant community groups to improve the health status of patients?
- Are there clear recruitment and retention/affirmative action goals for the organization? Does everyone in the organization understand the meaning of affirmative action and know these goals?
- Do the white people in the organization value working in a diverse setting? How is this evident?
- Is there a safe forum for people to learn how they may have unknowingly excluded or slighted their colleagues?
- Has anyone ever been rewarded in any way for their efforts to become culturally competent? Has anyone in the organization ever been penalized in any way for their inappropriate behavior?
- Is there a specific survey to assess patient and staff satisfaction with the facility and personnel?

ENVIRONMENTAL CONSIDERATIONS

- What images decorate the space?
- What magazines are placed in public meeting spaces or in the waiting area? Are publications in more than one language? Do pictures in the literature look like the people who frequent the facility?
- Are the signs around the workplace in more than one language?
- What types of foods are served at group gatherings?
- Does the organization follow the Christian calendar? Do people of a different religious faith have the option to observe their holidays?
- Who considers the "fun" days (e.g., group picnics, parties, dinners) fun?
- Is the workplace fully wheelchair accessible?
- Is public transportation available to the practice?
- Are the workplace hours of operation conducive to meeting the needs of the clients?

MOVING FROM CONCERN TO ACTION: PERSONAL INVENTORY

- Have I consciously thought about my own cultural identity and come to realize how much it is a part of who I am? Does my name have a relationship to my ancestors' ethnic identity? What belongings in my home are meaningful to me and why? Do my preferences regarding food, music, and clothes give an indication of who I am? Do I have health beliefs and behaviors that have been passed down to me from my ancestors?
- Have I spent some time reflecting on my own childhood and upbringing and analyzing where, how, and when I was receiving cultural, ethnocentric, and racist messages?
- Have I spent some time recently looking at my own attitudes and behaviors as an adult to determine how I am contributing to or combating ethnocentrism? Do I recognize that I may be prejudiced and may stereotype even if it is unconscious?
- Have I intentionally and aggressively sought to educate myself on other cultural ways of life and on issues of bias and racism by talking with others, viewing films and videos, finding reading material, attending lectures, or joining a study group?
- Have I evaluated my use of language, light and dark imagery, and other terms or phrases that might be degrading or hurtful to others? Do I make comments or jokes about cultural groups?
- Have I grown in my awareness of subliminal messages in television programs, advertising, and news coverage?
- Have I supported political candidates or contributed financially to an agency, fund, or program that actively confronts the problems of inequality and discrimination or enhances my patients' likelihood of receiving more culturally competent health care?
- Have I worked directly or indirectly to dispel misconceptions, stereotypes, prejudices, and other adverse feelings that members of one group have against members of another group? Have I openly disagreed with an insensitive comment, joke, reference, or action among those around me?
- Have I taken the initiative in dispelling prejudices, stereotypes, and misunderstandings among staff and discouraging or preventing patterns of informal discrimination, segregation, or exclusion of individuals?
- Do I listen with an open mind to staff members of other groups, even if their communications are initially disturbing or divergent from my own thinking? Do I welcome constructive feedback from others about how I relate to people from different cultures?

MOVING FROM CONCERN TO ACTION: PROFESSIONAL INVENTORY

- Have I asked my patients appropriate questions about their culture and way of life and let them know I have a lot to learn?
- Have I made the necessary adaptations to ensure that my patient and I are able to communicate effectively?
- Have I recognized that my patients may be from a different socioeconomic class than I am? Have I considered a sliding scale for fees? Do I assume my patient has the same comforts and capabilities for a home program as I might? Do I recognize the need to minimize potential barriers to service for my patients?
- Have I considered doing research that includes people of diverse backgrounds to enable the profession of physical therapy to become more culturally proficient? Have I considered the need for assessment tools that address culture-specific functional tasks such as squatting or eating with chopsticks?
- Have I made overtures toward traditional healers to collaborate and increase my understanding of their ideas and ways?
- Does my clinic conduct inspire patients to respect one another and be open and honest in their communications with others and me?
- Have I adapted my physical therapy examination and intervention to reflect my patient's culture and desires?
- Have I worked toward aiding my patients to navigate the health care system as needed?

Culture Shock

When working cross-culturally, *culture shock* can be experienced. This term describes the more pronounced reactions to the psychologic disorientation most people have when immersed in a culture markedly different from their own. Culture shock is a cyclic phenomenon in which one moves through four basic phases of adjustment: excitement in a new environment, withdrawal and hostility, adjustment and appreciation of differences, and adaptation.[36]

In a sense, culture shock is an occupational hazard of cross-cultural immersion. There are no easy remedies, but there are some things the PT can do to help lessen its effect. Admitting one's ethnocentrism and understanding one's own culture are the first steps. In addition, the PT should continue to learn about the particular cultures with which he or she works. The PT should ask questions and be astute in observations. The PT should have realistic expectations of himself or herself and others and remember that problems and challenges are inevitable.

What personal characteristics are likely to foster a more successful cross-cultural encounter? High on the list are a sense of adventure, patience, flexibility, tolerance for ambiguity and difference, a sense of humor, and cultural sensitivity. Ironically, many successful professionals have some of the characteristics that are not conducive to working cross-culturally. That is, they are task-oriented, overachievers, and fearful of failure. It is important to acknowledge that, although almost all PTs are likely to work with patients who are culturally different from themselves, not all are equally suitable for working cross-culturally.

SUMMARY

In the 21st century, national population patterns will continue to shift, and practitioners will increasingly be required to share and practice their knowledge and skills in less familiar multicultural settings. The challenges to delivering effective and humanistic care will become even greater than they are today. The obstacles to achieving the goal of cultural competence should not be underestimated. Yet competency in recognizing bias, prejudice, discrimination, and one's own discomfort when faced with difference and using cultural resources and overcoming cultural barriers can be learned. PTs must be cognizant of useful strategies to minimize existing barriers between individuals from different cultural contexts and seek ways to make therapeutic goals and the patients' or families' goals compatible rather than conflicting. An understanding of the macrolevel and microlevel sociocultural variables in the health care setting and an individual patient's worldview should lead to an improved clinical encounter. Health professionals increasingly understand that health care interaction that incorporates negotiation and preservation of cultural health-related beliefs and practices is likely to increase treatment adherence and self-efficacy for both parties.[33] As Ibrahim[31] proposed, "Each individual in a professional-consumer dyad [should] be viewed as a unique 'cultural entity' with an emphasis on the individual's 'subjective reality' or worldview …. [This] can lead to professional-consumer cultural matching."

In essence, the "culture of rehabilitation" needs to change and adapt in response to the environment and conditions present in a particular time and place. So it is that the PT is increasingly becoming skilled as a primary health care practitioner. The path of intercultural learning to cultural proficiency takes a long time and conscious effort. The challenge of embracing diversity and differences, reshaping practice protocols, redefining research priorities, and developing the most appropriate service models and public policy to benefit the patient must be faced.

REFERENCES

1. Allen J, Scott L, Stewart K, et al. Disparities in women's referral to and enrollment in outpatient cardiac rehabilitation. J Gen Intern Med 2004;19:747–53.
2. American Cancer Society: Cancer facts and figures 2008 (website). http://www.cancer.org/downloads/STT/2008CAFFfinalsecured.pdf. Accessed August 6, 2009.
3. APTA Office of Minority and International Affairs. APTA minority membership statistics. Washington, DC: American Physical Therapy Association; 2008.
4. Barnes P, Powell-Griner E, McFann K, et al. Complementary and alternative medicine use among adults: United States, 2002. Advance data from vital and health statistics, no. 3443. Hyattsville, MD: National Center for Health Statistics; 2004.
5. Basch P. Textbook of international health. Oxford: Oxford University Press; 1999.
6. Bates M, Edwards WT. Ethnic variations in the chronic pain experience. In: Brown P, editor. Understanding and applying medical anthropology. Mountain View, CA: Mayfield Publishing; 1998.
7. Berger J. Culture and ethnicity in clinical care. Arch Intern Med 1998;158:2085–90.
8. Braithwaite R, Taylor S, editors. Health issues in the black community. San Francisco: Jossey Bass; 2001.
9. Brice A, Campbell L. Cross-cultural communication. In: Leavitt R, editor. Cross-cultural rehabilitation: An international perspective. Philadelphia: Saunders; 1999.
10. Campinha-Bacote J. The process of cultural competence in the delivery of healthcare services: a culturally competent model of care. Wyoming, OH: Transcultural C.A.R.E Associates; 2003.
11. Centers for Disease Control and Prevention (CDC): Chronic disease prevention and health promotion (website). 2008. http://www.cdc.gov/nccdphp. Accessed August 6, 2009.
12. Centers for Disease Control and Prevention (CDC): National diabetes fact sheet: United States 2007 (website). 2008. http://www.cdc.gov/diabetes/pubs/pdf/ndfs_2007.pdf. Accessed August 6, 2009.
13. Chan S. Families with Asian roots. In: Lynch E, Hanson M, editors. Developing cross-cultural competence. Baltimore: Paul Brookes; 1998.
14. Collins K, Hughes D, Doty M, et al. Diverse communities, common concerns: assessing health care quality for minority Americans. New York: The Commonwealth Fund; 2002.
15. Coreil J, Barnes-Josiah D, Augustin A, et al. Arrested pregnancy syndrome in Haiti: findings from a national survey. Med Anthropol Q 1996;10:424–36.
16. Closing the gap. Washington, DC: Office of Minority Health and Science, U.S. Department of Health and Human Services; February/March 2001.
17. Cross TL, Bazron BJ, Dennis KW, et al. Towards a culturally competent system of care vol. 1. Washington, DC: National Technical Assistance Center for Children's Mental Health, Georgetown University; 1989.
18. Eisenberg D, Kessler R, Foster C. Unconventional medicine in the United States. N Engl J Med 1993;328:246–52.
19. Eisenberg D, Davis R, Ettner S, et al. Trends in alternative medicine use in the United States. JAMA 1990-1997;280(18):1569–77.
20. Fabrega H. Disease and social behavior: an interdisciplinary perspective. Cambridge, MA: MIT Press; 1974.
21. Fadiman A. The spirit catches you and you fall down: a Hmong child, and her American doctors, and the collision of two cultures. New York: Farrar, Straus & Giroux; 1997.
22. Federal Register (vol. 65, no. 247, pp 80865-80879), Washington, DC: December 22, 2000, Office of Minority Health, Public Health Service, U.S. Department of Health and Human Services.
23. Ferraro G. The cultural dimension of international business. 2nd ed. Englewood Cliffs, NJ: Prentice-Hall; 1994.
24. Fisher M. Rural residents: cause or effect from poverty. Perspectives on Poverty, Policy, and Place 2007;4:2–5.

25. Foster G. Disease etiologies in non-Western medical systems. Am Anthropologist 1976;78:773–82.

26. Galanti GA. Caring for patients from different cultures. Philadelphia: University of Pennsylvania Press; 1991.

27. Gamble V, Stone D. U.S. policy on health inequities: the interplay of politics and research. J Health Politics Policy Law 2006;31:93–126.

27a. Good MJ, Brodwin PE, Good BJ, Kleinman A, editors. Pain as human experience: an anthropological perspective. Berkley (CA): University of California press; 1994.

28. Groce N, Zola I. Multiculturalism, chronic illness, and disability. Pediatrics 1993;91:1048–55.

29. Hall ET. The dance of life. New York: Doubleday; 1983.

29a. Helman C. Cuture, health and illness. 4th ed. Oxford: Butterworth-Heinemann; 2000.

30. Huff R, Kline M. Promoting health in multicultural populations: a handbook for practitioners. Thousand Oaks, CA: Sage Publishing; 1999.

31. Ibrahim F. Multicultural influences on rehabilitation training and services: the shift to valuing non-dominant cultures. In: Karan O, Greenspan S, editors. Community rehabilitation services for people with disabilities. Boston: Butterworth-Heinemann; 1995, p. 187–205.

32. Institute for Research on Poverty: Who is poor? (website). http://irp.wisc.edu/faqs/faq3.htm. Accessed August 6, 2009.

33. Kavanagh K, Absalom K, Beil W, et al. Connecting and becoming culturally competent: a Lakota example. Adv Nurs Sci 1991;21:9–31.

34. Kleinman A. Patients and healers in the context of culture. Berkeley, CA: University of California Press; 1980.

35. Knutson L, Leavitt R, Sarton B. Race, ethnicity and other factors influencing children's health and disability: implications for pediatric physical therapists. Pediatr Phys Ther 1995;7:175–83.

36. Kohls R. Survival kit for overseas living. Chicago: Intercultural Press; 1979.

37. Ladinsky JL, Volk ND, Robinson M. The influence of traditional medicine in shaping medical care practices in Vietnam today. Soc Sci Med 1987;25:1105–10.

38. Ladyshewsky R. Cross-cultural supervision of students. In: Leavitt R, editor. Cross-cultural rehabilitation: an international perspective. Philadelphia: Saunders; 1999.

39. La Veist T. Minority populations and health: an introduction to health disparities in the United States. San Francisco: Jossey-Bass; 2005.

40. Leavitt R, editor. Cross-cultural rehabilitation: an international perspective. Philadelphia: Saunders; 1999.

41. Leavitt R. Disability and rehabilitation in rural Jamaica: an ethnographic study. Madison, NJ: Fairleigh Dickinson University Press; 1992.

42. Levitt S. The collaborative learning approach in community based rehabilitation. In: Leavitt R, editor. Cross-cultural rehabilitation: an international perspective. Philadelphia: Saunders; 1999.

43. Lin J, Kaplan R. Multivariate analysis of the factors affecting duration of acute inpatient rehabilitation after hip knee arthroplasty. Am J Phys Med Rehab 2004;83:344–52.

44. Lynch E, Hanson M. Developing cross-cultural competence. Baltimore: Paul Brookes; 1998.

45. Mardiros M. Conception of childhood disability among Mexican-American parents. Med Anthropol 1989;12:55–68.

46. Mehrabian A. Silent messages. Belmont, CA: Wadsworth; 1971.

47. Nakamura R. Health in America: a multicultural perspective. Upper Saddle River, NJ: Allyn & Bacon; 1999.

48. Nayak S. Cultural and gender effects in pain beliefs and the prediction of pain beliefs and the prediction of pain. Cross-Cultural Research 2000;34:135–51.

49. Paul T, Thorburn M. Epidemiological considerations in the assessment of disability. In: Leavitt R, editor. Cross-cultural rehabilitation: an international perspective. Philadelphia: Saunders; 1999.

50. Pember M. The Ho-Chunk way, The Washington Post, Health section, April 9, 2002.

51. Rebhun LA. Swallowing frogs: anger and illness in Northeast Brazil. Med Anthropol Q 1994;8:360–82.

52. Reviere R, Hylton K. Poverty and health: an international overview. In: Leavitt R, editor. Cross-cultural rehabilitation: an international perspective. Philadelphia: Saunders; 1999.

53. Santana S, Santana F. An introduction to Mexican culture for rehabilitation service providers. Buffalo, NY: Center for International Rehabilitation Research Information and Exchange (CIRRIE); 2001.

54. Satcher D, Pamies R. Multicultural medicine and health disparities. New York: McGraw-Hill; 2006.

55. Schneider E, Zaslavsky A, Epstein A. Racial disparity in the quality of care for enrollees in Medicare managed care. JAMA 2002;287:1288–94.

56. Smedley B, Stith A, Nelson A, editors. Committees on understanding and eliminating racial and ethnic disparities in health care. Washington, DC: Institute of Medicine; March 2002.

57. Smey J. Understanding racial prejudice, discrimination and racism and their influence on health care delivery. In: Leavitt R, editor. Cross-cultural rehabilitation: an international perspective. Philadelphia: Saunders; 1999.

58. Spector R. Cultural diversity in health and illness. East Norwalk, CT: Appleton & Lange; 1996.

59. Spradley J. The ethnographic interview. New York: Holt, Rinehart & Winston; 1979.

60. UCLA Center for Health Policy and Kaiser Family Foundation. Racial and ethnic disparities in access to health insurance and health care. Los Angeles: UCLA Center for Health Policy and Kaiser Family Foundation; 2000.

61. United States Bureau of the Census. Current population reports. Washington, DC: U.S. Bureau of the Census; 2000.

62. United States Bureau of the Census. Current population reports. Washington, DC: U.S. Bureau of the Census; 1990.

63. U.S. Census Bureau: US Hispanic population surpasses 45 million: now 15 percent of total, US Census Bureau News, May 1, 2008 (website). http://www.census.gov/Press-Release/www/releases/archives/population/011910.html. Accessed August 6, 2009.

64. U.S. Census Bureau: Table 3: Poverty status of people, by age, race, and Hispanic origin: 1959 to 2006 (website). 2008. http://www.census.gov/hhes/www/poverty/histpov/hstpov3.html. Accessed August 6, 2009.

65. U.S. Census Bureau: Annual Statistical Abstract: Table 176: Estimated numbers of persons living with acquired immunodeficiency syndrome (AIDS) by year and selected characteristics: 2000-2005 (website). 2008. http://www.census.gov/prod/2007pubs/08abstract/health.pdf. [SG11] Accessed August 6, 2009.

66. United States Department of Commerce. Population projections of the United States by age, sex, race, and Hispanic origin, 1995 to 2050. Washington, DC: U.S. Bureau of the Census; February 1996.

67. USDHHS: Prior HHS poverty guidelines and Federal Register references (website). http://aspe.hhs.gov/poverty/figures-fed-reg.shtml. Accessed May 13, 2008.

68. United States Department of Health and Human Services. Report of the secretary's task force on black and minority health. Washington, DC: USDHHS; October 1998.

69. United States Department of Health and Human Services. Office of Disease Prevention and Health Promotion: Healthy People 2010. Washington, DC: USDHHS; 1998.

70. United States Department of Health and Human Services: Healthy People 2010 (website). 2008. http://www.healthypeople.gov/default.htm. Accessed August 6, 2009.

71. Villa VM, Torres-Gil FM. The health of elderly Latinos. In: Aguirre-Molina M, Molina C, Zambrana R, editors. Health issues in the Latino community. Washington, DC: Jossey-Bass; 2001.

72. Wasson S. Treatment of the Native American population. Orthop Phys Ther Clin North Am 1999;8:215–23.

73. Young J, Garro L. Variations in the choice of treatment in two Mexican communities. Soc Sci Med 1982;16:1453–65.

74. Zborowski M. Cultural components in responses to pain. J Soc Issues 1952;8:16–30.

SUGGESTED READINGS

Particular Ethnic Groups

Braithwaite R, Taylor S, editors. Health issues in the black community. San Francisco: Jossey-Bass; 2001.

Fadiman A. The spirit catches you and you fall down: a Hmong child and her American doctors, and the collision of two cultures. New York: Farrar, Straus & Giroux; 1997.

Galanti GA. Caring for patients from different cultures. Philadelphia: University of Pennsylvania Press; 1991.

Huff R, Kline M. Promoting health in multicultural populations: a handbook for practitioners. Thousand Oaks, CA: Sage Publishing; 1999.

Lattanzi J, Purnell L. Developing cultural competence in physical therapy practice. Philadelphia: Davis; 2006.

Leavitt R, editor. Cross-cultural rehabilitation: an international perspective. Philadelphia: Saunders; 1999.

Leavitt R. Disability and rehabilitation in rural Jamaica: an ethnographic study. Madison, NJ: Fairleigh Dickinson University Press; 1992.

Lynch E, Hanson M. Developing cross-cultural competence. Baltimore: Paul Brookes; 1998.

Nakamura R. Health in America: a multicultural perspective. Upper Saddle River, NJ: Allyn & Bacon; 1999.

Royeen M, Crabtree J. Culture in rehabilitation: from competency to proficiency. Upper Saddle River, NJ: Pearson Education Inc; 2006.

Satcher D, Rubens P. Multicultural medicine and health disparities. New York: McGraw-Hill; 2006.

Spector R. Cultural diversity in health and illness. East Norwalk, CT: Appleton & Lange; 1996.

Web Resources

American Physical Therapy Association: Tips to increase cultural competency (website). http://www.apta.org/AM/Template.cfm?Section=Cultural_Comp etence1&Template=/TaggedPage/TaggedPageDisplay.cfm&TPLID=48&Con tentID=20219.

Center for International Rehabilitation Research Information & Exchange. http://cirrie.buffalo.edu/mseries.html.

The Commonwealth Fund's 2001 health care quality survey report (website). http://www.commonwealthfund.org/.

U.S. Department of Health and Human Services Office of Minority Health. http://www.omhrc.gov.

U.S. Department of Health and Human Services Health Resources and Services Administration. http://www.hrsa.gov/culturalcompetence/indicators/.

Pharmacologic Considerations for the Physical Therapist

William P. Brookfield, RPh, MSc

Objectives

After reading this chapter, the reader will be able to:

1. Describe the principles of pharmacokinetics as they apply to the general patient population and to elderly patients.
2. Explain the principles of pharmacodynamics, including the role of receptors and the modes of action of drugs as they apply to the learning of pharmacology.
3. Apply the principles of patient screening to the subject of pharmacovigilance.
4. Describe clinical considerations of commonly prescribed medications germane to physical therapy practice.
5. Identify valuable clinical sources of drug information.

The role of the pharmacist as a member of the health care team is evolving. The standard academic training (Doctor of Pharmacy degree) now encompasses a 6-year program, with 1 year of clinical rotations included in the educational process. This training includes emphasis on clinical decision making and has produced many pharmacists with improved clinical skills. As a result of this academic evolution, the role of the practicing pharmacist is in transition. The educational experience has produced a practitioner with the ability to monitor drug therapy effectively for side effects and suggest drug therapy to physicians and nurse practitioners.

The physician community has not yet widely accepted the pharmacist as a prescriber of drugs. In the future, categories of drugs that fall somewhere between prescription-only and over-the-counter (OTC) may be prescribed directly by the pharmacist. The future may bring numerous circumstances in which the physical therapist (PT) and the clinical pharmacist can interact to improve the care of the patient.

PTs work with patients who are taking medications in virtually every health care setting. Medications are being administered to a large percentage of physical therapy outpatients, and polypharmacy may be pronounced in some. Medication use in many situations has a significant effect on the health of the patient and may alter the clinical presentation or course of treatment. The PT must have a working knowledge of pharmacology to help the patient, physician, and pharmacist in the management of disease. This knowledge allows the PT to participate fully in a collaborative medical model within a primary care environment.

Understanding how drugs work and mastering the vast amount of information about drugs are seemingly insurmountable tasks. When the health care practitioner learns pharmacology by regurgitating isolated facts, he or she has great difficulty applying the information in a practical manner to improve patient care. Only when the teacher and the student understand and practice certain principles can the student learn pharmacology and be able to apply it to the treatment of a patient. Some key tips in the study and presentation of pharmacology are presented in Box 4-1.

The presenter of pharmacology information must be able to give the student of pharmacology some guidance to ease the anxiety that often accompanies learning pharmacology. This chapter provides a framework that allows the reader to apply the knowledge that he or she has gained to foster safe and effective patient care, while avoiding rote memorization of information. In addition, the PT can learn to apply this knowledge to communicate effectively with pharmacists and physicians.

Pharmacokinetics

Pharmacokinetics should be considered "what the body does to the drug"; this definition can help the PT keep information about the term in perspective. Pharmacokinetics incorporates all aspects of the transport of a drug to its target site and subsequent removal of the drug and its metabolites from the body. Pharmacokinetics has four primary divisions: absorption at the site of administration, distribution within the body to the tissues, metabolism of the drug to more active or inactive forms, and excretion of the drug and its metabolites.[4,9,18]

Absorption

Absorption is the process by which drugs are made available to the body fluids that distribute the drugs to organ systems.[4,9,18] A key term within any discussion of absorption is *bioavailability*. Bioavailability is the study and measurement of the completeness of absorption. It is the most important concept within the study of absorption within pharmacokinetics. The two primary factors associated with drug absorption and ultimately bioavailability are the route of administration and the dosage formulation. Primary routes of administration include oral, sublingual, buccal, transdermal, inhalation, subcutaneous, intramuscular, intravenous, rectal, and topical. Examples of drugs and their primary routes of administration are aspirin (oral), nitroglycerin (sublingual), insulin (subcutaneous), meperidine (intramuscular), and hydrocortisone (topical). These examples should help the reader appreciate the variety of choices available for administration of a drug.

This discussion focuses primarily on the oral route of administration because this route is the most common mode of drug delivery. Some drugs cannot be administered orally because of degradation by intestinal enzymes (proteases). Insulin is an example of such a drug; the insulin product undergoes complete degradation and is not absorbed. For any drug to be effective after oral administration, it must be absorbed through the intestinal epithelium and enter the blood vessels of the intestinal tract. The drug is carried directly to the liver by the hepatic portal system before it reaches the systemic circulation.

Tips in the Study and Presentation of Pharmacology

- Focus on principles relevant to health care professionals in their everyday practice.
- Concepts or principles applied to a particular class of drugs vary little, if any, among drugs within the class. In the study of pharmacology, a person *cannot* learn everything about all available drugs.
- Knowledge of pharmacology allows one to bring *systematic* order to drug-related information.
- Therapeutic responses vary widely among different drugs.

If a drug has properties that allow the liver to metabolize it rapidly, little, if any, actually enters the systemic circulation. The liver extraction is called the *first-pass effect* and may render an orally administered drug ineffective. An example of such a drug and its pharmacokinetic application is lidocaine. Lidocaine is not available in an oral formulation but is available in topical, subcutaneous, and intravenous forms because of the 100% first-pass effect of the molecule.

Many other molecules exhibit partial first-pass effects and require oral doses that may be significantly larger than doses needed for parenteral (injectable) dosing. An example of a partial first-pass effect can be observed with the beta-receptor blocker propranolol. Propranolol intravenous dosing is 1 to 3 mg, whereas the oral route requires 10 to 80 mg to produce a similar pharmacologic response.

Changes in the formulation may significantly change absorption properties. The first-pass effect can be altered in some situations by changes in the oral formulation. *Timed-release* or *sustained-release* formulations are designed to produce slow, uniform dissolution of the drug and allow more drug to reach the systemic circulation. An example of a timed-release medication is nifedipine (Procardia XL and Adalat CC).

Enteric-coated or *delayed-release* formulations may be used with orally administered medications to alter absorption. If a medication is prone to acidic degradation in the stomach, it may be helpful to give the medication an outer coat of a chemical that resists acid. The outer-coat chemical dissolves in the alkaline environment of the intestine, and the actual drug may be released effectively from the intestinal location and produce a pharmacologic response. An example of a medication with such a formulation is omeprazole (Prilosec). The granules within the capsule are enteric-coated. Enteric coating (delayed release) of a medication also is used when the medication may be irritating to the stomach to avoid this gastrointestinal side effect. This formulation allows the stomach-irritating drug to be released in the intestine rather than in the stomach. Many aspirin formulations are enteric-coated to minimize stomach irritation.

Distribution

The second division of pharmacokinetics is distribution, the movement or transport of a drug to the site of action.[4,9,18] Distribution of a drug to the different tissues depends on blood flow. The transportation phase of distribution in the blood is facilitated by the binding of a percentage of the drug molecules to serum protein. The primary protein that binds drug molecules is serum albumin. The "free" drug or "unbound" molecules are the portion that can penetrate capillary walls to reach the site of action. The "bound" drug cannot exert any pharmacologic action.

A problem sometimes may arise when two or more drugs compete for the same binding site. This competition may create higher levels of "free" drug or unbound drug for one of the competing molecules. The anticoagulant warfarin can potentially compete for protein binding sites with ibuprofen. The nonsteroidal anti-inflammatory drug (NSAID) ibuprofen has a much greater affinity for serum albumin than warfarin does. If a patient taking warfarin starts taking ibuprofen, the anti-inflammatory drug may "bump" the warfarin off the albumin, resulting in higher concentrations of warfarin as *free drug* now available to act on the body. The concentration of warfarin may reach toxic levels, putting the patient in danger. The PT may be the practitioner who discovers that the patient has recently started taking ibuprofen for a minor musculoskeletal symptom.

Despite adequate blood flow, all drugs do not gain access to all areas of the body (e.g., the central nervous system [CNS]). When a drug reaches the plasma, it must cross several barriers before it can reach its final site of action. For any drug to have effects in the CNS, it must be able to cross the *blood-brain barrier*. A drug may enter the cerebral circulation yet be unable to enter the cells of the brain. The blood-brain barrier is a "tight" barrier that does not allow the molecules to "squeeze" through or diffuse through the barrier.

The blood-brain barrier was originally postulated from experiments in which dyes were injected into the systemic circulation but were found not to reach the cells of the brain. Later work has shown that, although there is such a barrier, it is not an absolute barrier. A more appropriate term may be the *blood-brain sieve*.

Many drugs that easily penetrate other body organs do not appreciably enter the brain. A practical application of this concept for the PT is a comparison of the safety profiles of morphine and ibuprofen. Morphine is prone to cause vivid dreams (nightmares) and hallucinations, whereas ibuprofen does not have these issues in its safety profile. This is because morphine readily crosses the blood-brain barrier while acting on the CNS, but ibuprofen does not. An important question to ask about a medication is the drug's propensity to cross the blood-brain barrier. The drug's blood-brain barrier profile is information that may assist in the prediction of whether an undesired CNS effect is drug-induced or induced by the disease state.

Lipid-soluble drugs are more likely to penetrate the blood-brain barrier than other drugs because they pass through the cell membrane instead of "squeezing through the openings." In addition, lipid-soluble drugs may be stored in adipose tissue, which acts as a drug repository. This storage has the potential to cause a lower plasma concentration but a longer duration of action. Storage in fatty tissue is of concern in obese patients, in patients who have an absolute increase in adipose tissue, and in elderly patients when the ratio of body fat to lean body weight increases although the body weight remains the same.

Finally, an important term in distribution is *bioavailability,* just as it was in the absorption phase. Bioavailability from the distribution aspect is defined as the amount of drug that reaches its target of action, and it may be affected by protein binding, gastrointestinal absorption, adipose tissue storage, metabolism to other products, and elimination.

Metabolism

Metabolism is the process of transforming drugs into more water-soluble compounds so that they can be excreted by the kidneys.[4,9,18] Metabolism occurs primarily within the liver, although other organs, such as the kidneys and cardiovascular system, may be involved. Most drugs are not excreted unchanged by the body but undergo a biotransformation after they enter the body. Metabolism usually changes active drugs to inactive metabolites. A few drugs are not active, however, until transformed by the liver to an active metabolite. Most drugs are detoxified in the liver, but in some circumstances, metabolites may be more toxic than the parent compound. An example is the seizure potential of meperidine compared with its metabolite normeperidine. Normeperidine has a threefold greater seizure potential than meperidine and has increased toxicity regarding seizures.

Many drugs are metabolized by the microsomal mixed-function oxidase enzyme system in the liver. Most microsomal enzyme reactions degrade a drug to more water-soluble end products, which are excreted by the kidneys. The cytochrome P-450 enzyme system is the most clinically important system of microsomal enzymes in the liver. Many clinically important drug interactions involve the cytochrome enzyme system. The enzymes are inducible by drugs that may stimulate the metabolism of another drug. Carbamazepine (Tegretol) has the ability to stimulate or induce numerous enzymes. This induction may increase the metabolism of drugs such as olanzapine (Zyprexa). In addition, some drugs may reduce the metabolism of another drug, resulting in a plasma level of the drug that is higher than normal. An example of the latter is the elevated levels of terfenadine (Seldane) caused by concomitant administration of erythromycin, leading to ventricular arrhythmias and ultimately withdrawal from the market. The coadministration of terfenadine and erythromycin did not allow the terfenadine to be fully metabolized to a less toxic metabolite.

Some drugs are secreted with the bile into the intestinal tract and can be either reabsorbed or excreted with the feces. When a drug is reabsorbed by this mechanism involving the intestinal tract and given a second chance to exert its effect, it is considered to have undergone enterohepatic circulation. This process affects only a few drugs but may have some clinical significance. The presence of liver disease may interfere with the metabolism of a drug so that repeated dosing may result in the development of elevated serum levels that may prove toxic to the body. The PT should be aware of the patient's liver function and understand the primary route of excretion for the drugs being taken.

Excretion

Excretion of drugs or their metabolites is carried out in the kidney by two processes, glomerular filtration and tubular secretion.[4,9,18] Glomerular filtration is the process in which drugs are filtered through the glomerulus and then carried through the tubule into the urine. A drug may be reabsorbed to some extent, depending on the lipid solubility of the drug and pH of the urine, whereas others are not reabsorbed and are eliminated in the urine. The other process of elimination or excretion is the

active secretion of the drug by the tubule into the urine. Drugs also may be excreted in fluids other than urine, including milk, saliva, sweat, and feces. The preceding discussion of metabolism mentioned biliary secretion; this process places drugs in the feces for elimination.

The health care professional must recognize that a patient with reduced kidney function may have problems eliminating certain drugs that are excreted primarily unchanged in the urine. Elderly patients and patients with renal disease fit the category of reduced kidney function. Drugs that depend entirely on the kidney for elimination have the highest risk for adverse reactions in geriatric patients. The elimination aspect of pharmacokinetics is the most clinically significant in alterations of drug response and issues of adverse events or side effects.

The health care professional should be able to estimate the patient's ability to avoid problems with drugs that are excreted by the renal system. One method for estimating the glomerular filtration rate of any patient is the Cockcroft and Gault formula. The formula generates an estimate of the creatinine clearance for a given patient. Creatinine clearance measures the elimination capabilities of the patient. The larger the creatinine clearance value in milliliters per minute, the greater the ability of the patient to avoid problems with a drug that uses renal excretion. The Cockcroft and Gault formula and key facts are presented in Box 4-2.

The normal value for creatinine clearance would be 90 to 120 mL/min, with the female value toward the lower end of the range. A male patient would have a normal creatinine clearance toward the high end of the range. The lower the number, the more compromised the creatinine clearance and degree of change in the handling of renally excreted drugs.

Drug Half-Life

In any discussion of pharmacokinetics and elimination, one must understand the concept of drug half-life.[4,9,18] *Elimination half-life* and the *biologic half-life* are two terms that one should understand. The elimination half-life is defined in all books that discuss pharmacokinetics, but for some drugs it is less practical than the biologic half-life when working with patients.

The elimination half-life of a drug is the time in which the concentration of the drug in the plasma decreases to one half of its original amount. The elimination half-life describes a drug's rate of disappearance from the body, whether by metabolism, excretion, or a combination of both. The half-life usually is measured in hours, but for some drugs the half-life is measured in days, and for others in minutes or even seconds. In contrasting the cardiac drugs amiodarone, propranolol, and adenosine, one

Pharmacokinetics in Geriatric Patients

Pharmacokinetic Functions	Alterations in Geriatric Patients	Clinical Consequences
A—Absorption	Decreased gastrointestinal tract motility. Slower gastric emptying. Increased gastric pH.	Bloating after eating more common. Medication effects may be altered. Less important than **M** and **E**.
D—Distribution	Decreased cardiac output. Increased body fat. Decreased lean body mass.	Less important than **M** and **E** to drug action changes. Cardiac output change when accompanied by decreased renal and liver blood flow can be important.
M—Metabolism	Decreased liver mass. Decreased liver enzyme activity. Decreased liver blood flow.	Liver enzyme changes (reduced activity) can increase intensity of drug action.
E—Excretion	Decreased kidney blood flow. Decreased glomerular filtration rate.	Change in renal function is most important pharmacokinetic factor resulting in adverse drug reactions.

can appreciate the great variation in half-life. The elimination half-life for amiodarone is 26 to 107 days because the drug is very lipid-soluble, the elimination half-life for propranolol is 3 to 4 hours, and the elimination half-life for adenosine is 10 seconds.

The half-life of a drug is useful information when determining the amount of time the drug would remain in the body and potentially exert a pharmacologic effect. In addition, this information helps determine how often a drug should be administered to the patient.

The biologic half-life of the drug is the time in which the duration of action decreases to one half of its original duration. This half-life refers to the time of the drug's response, rather than the plasma concentration. Several drugs have durations of action that are longer than the plasma levels indicate. This difference may result from interactions of the drug with its receptor that may initiate activity that continues even without the presence of the drug. With some drugs, the biologic half-life may be more clinically useful than the elimination half-life.

The half-life information can be applied to discussions about the loading dose of a drug, the therapeutic range of a drug, and the steady-state level of a drug. One must understand the concept of *steady state* because this term is used in many articles that discuss drug therapy. Steady-state plasma levels are more important in understanding and interpreting long-term drug therapy rather than short-term drug therapy. Drugs tend to accumulate in the body if given on a regular schedule until the amount eliminated is equal to the amount administered. When this happens, the steady-state level is reached.

At the steady-state level, plasma concentrations oscillate around the mean plasma concentration. The concentration varies between the peak plasma level after administration of the drug and the minimum plasma level just before the next administered dose. If a drug has been administered on a regular basis, the steady-state level usually is reached after five half-lives of the drug have passed. Some authors also call the steady-state level the *plateau level*.

When the patient stops taking the drug, five half-lives usually must pass before the drug is considered no longer to have the ability to affect the patient's system. This information is important to the PT because when investigating a patient's use of medication, asking the question, "Have you recently stopped taking any medications?" is very important. A drug with a long half-life stopped only a couple of days ago may account for the presence of symptoms or complications noted by the PT.

Another important consideration in drug response is patient compliance. A patient who is noncompliant may not be allowing the drug to reach steady state. The patient's level of compliance with medications also may indicate his or her compliance with a home exercise program or modifications of body mechanics with daily activities.

Key facts about pharmacokinetics and geriatric patients are presented in Box 4-3. The examples in this box illustrate some of the challenges of determining proper dosing for elderly patients. See Chapter 18 for further discussion of polypharmacy and elderly patients.

Pharmacodynamics

The pharmacodynamic principles are the heart of pharmacology. The PT should think of *pharmacodynamics* as "what the drug does to the body," that is, the study of the mechanisms and action created by drugs.[4,9,18]

The study of pharmacodynamics includes four areas that the PT should understand: the general mode of action, including secondary modes of action; the indications for use; the safety profile; and rehabilitation considerations. Pharmacodynamics involve the biochemical and physiologic effects of a drug. The site of action of a drug may be a specific organ system, or the drug may cause a more generalized body effect. In general, drugs act by forming a bond, usually reversible, with some cellular constituent (receptor).

Most drugs act on a specific receptor. For a drug to have an action in the body, the drug must bind to a receptor to a sufficient degree to create a pharmacologic response. A *receptor* is defined as a specific macromolecule that recognizes the drug. The receptor may be on the cell membrane or inside the cell. *Affinity* describes the degree of attraction or binding power a given drug has for the receptor. Some degree of affinity must be inherent in the drug for it to bind to a receptor.

A drug that binds to a receptor and produces an action is called an *agonist*. An agonist is a drug with affinity that can elicit a pharmacologic response. A drug that binds to a receptor and does not produce an action is called an *antagonist* or blocker. An example of the concepts of agonist activity and antagonist activity is seen in histamine-antihistamine interaction. Diphenhydramine (Benadryl) is an antihistamine that blocks the histamine-1 (H_1) receptor site by binding to the receptor. This binding prevents histamine from binding to the receptor and creating responses such as itching of the skin. The drug diphenhydramine has affinity for the histamine receptor (binds to the receptor) and displays antagonist activity in that the histamine cannot exert a physiologic change (increased itching). *Partial agonist* drugs are drugs that bind with a receptor but cannot produce maximal response compared with the agonist.

Potency and Efficacy

Two confusing terms associated with pharmacodynamics are *potency* and *efficacy*. Potency describes the dose of a drug required to produce a given effect relative to a standard. This information is usually unimportant clinically. Efficacy is the capacity to stimulate or produce an effect for a given occupied receptor. Efficacy in everyday terms describes how well the drug works or the maximum response to a drug. This information is clinically important. The word *potency* can mislead one into believing that because a drug is more potent, it is more effective. An illustration of this difference is the use of morphine and meperidine (Demerol) in treating pain. If morphine, 10 mg, and meperidine, 75 mg, both alleviate the pain of a patient, one can state that morphine is more potent (10 mg versus 75 mg for meperidine); however, both drugs may display equal efficacy.

Tolerance

Pharmacodynamics may involve the development of *tolerance* to a given drug. The pharmacologic effect of tolerance has developed with a given drug when increasing amounts (more milligrams) are required to produce the same effect or when the same dose on repeated occasions produces lower responses. Tolerance may occur with some drugs but not with others. Narcotic analgesics are a class of drugs that are well known to exhibit tolerance because increasing doses are required to produce the same effect. The other aspect of *tolerance* is classified as *tachyphylaxis*. Tachyphylaxis is considered a rapidly developing tolerance and may be seen after only a few administrations of some drugs. Nasal decongestants for allergic rhinitis have been associated with tachyphylaxis.

Autonomic Nervous System and Pharmacodynamics

An extremely important concept in the understanding of pharmacodynamics for the PT is the autonomic nervous system. The discussion of receptor activity along with agonist and antagonist properties strongly affects one's ability to understand pharmacologic responses of the autonomic nervous system. Terminology regarding the autonomic nervous system and the subsequent pharmacologic changes should be reviewed. The PT must understand the following terms to study pharmacodynamics:

- Parasympathetic (cholinergic) subdivision
- Sympathetic (adrenergic) subdivision
- Parasympathomimetic drug (cholinergic agonist or stimulant)
- Parasympatholytic drug (cholinergic antagonist) (anticholinergic)
- Sympathomimetic drug (adrenergic agonist or stimulant)
- Sympatholytic drug (adrenergic antagonist or blocker)
- Alpha blocker (specialized adrenergic antagonist)
- Beta blocker (specialized adrenergic antagonist)

- Beta$_1$-blocking properties only (cardioselective adrenergic antagonist)
- Beta$_1$-blocking plus beta$_2$-blocking properties (nonselective adrenergic antagonist)
- Beta$_2$-agonist properties (bronchoselective adrenergic agonist)
- Beta$_2$-agonist plus beta$_1$-agonist properties (nonselective beta-receptor agonist)

Some examples of prototype drugs within the aforementioned therapeutic categories may help the PT understand pharmacology better. In the study of pharmacology, it is always helpful to apply focused rote memorization to the indications for use and safety profiles of a prototype drug within each major mode-of-action category. This approach offers a more systematic way to learn pharmacology across the wide array of available drugs. Examples of such drugs follow:

- Parasympathomimetic drug: bethanechol (Urecholine) or pilocarpine
- Parasympatholytic drug: atropine or ipratropium (Atrovent)
- Sympathomimetic drug: epinephrine (Adrenalin)
- Sympatholytic drug: must determine alpha-receptor or beta-receptor antagonist
- Alpha antagonist: prazosin (Minipress) or terazosin (Hytrin)
- Alpha agonist: norepinephrine (Levophed) or phenylephrine (Neo-Synephrine)
- Combined beta$_1$ and beta$_2$ antagonist: propranolol (Inderal)
- Beta$_1$ antagonist: atenolol (Tenormin) or metoprolol (Lopressor)
- Beta$_2$ agonist: albuterol (Ventolin)
- Combined beta$_2$ and beta$_1$ agonist: isoproterenol (Isuprel)

The concept of alpha receptors and beta receptors is associated with the sympathetic subdivision of the autonomic nervous system only.

An understanding of the primary changes that occur with agonist and antagonist activity within these two subdivisions of the autonomic nervous system is extremely useful in learning pharmacology. One should master some key pharmacologic responses within each subdivision. This key information is provided in the following section.

Parasympathetic (Cholinergic) Subdivision: Selected Pharmacologic Responses

Tables 4-1 and 4-2 describe the clinically important aspects of the cholinergic subdivision of the autonomic nervous system. As can be seen from these tables, these pharmacologic changes are *daily functional aspects* and typically are not life-threatening aspects, as can be the case with adrenergic pharmacologic changes. The mnemonic *SLUD* is helpful in learning the parasympathetic (cholinergic) actions (see Table 4-1).

Changes in the urinary bladder are an example of how the tables might be used. Urinary incontinence and benign prostatic hypertrophy are common problems in some patient groups. One can develop an understanding of drug-induced bladder function changes regarding urinary flow by reviewing the parasympathetic and sympathetic nervous systems. Table 4-2 displays the detrusor muscle surrounding the urinary bladder as innervated by the parasympathetic system. Drugs that are parasympathetic agonists promote the flow of urine. Any drug that is a

TABLE 4-1

Possible Cholinergic Responses: SLUD Acronym

	Pharmacologic Response	Parasympathetic (Cholinergic) Stimulation	Cholinergic Blockade (Anticholinergic Activity)
S	Salivation	Increased saliva/drooling	Xerostomia (dry mouth)
L	Lacrimation	Increased tearing/watery eyes	Dry eyes/blurred vision/loss of power of accommodation
U	Urination	Increased genitourinary motility (urine flow increased)	Retention of urine
D	Defecation	Increased gastrointestinal motility (diarrhea)	Constipation

TABLE 4-2

Cholinergic Actions

Pharmacologic Response	Parasympathetic (Cholinergic) Stimulation	Cholinergic Blockade (Anticholinergic Activity)
Detrusor muscle around urinary bladder	Muscle contraction (increase in urine output)	Muscle relaxation (decrease in urine output)
Pupil size	Miosis (pupil constriction)	Mydriasis (pupil dilation)
Lungs (bronchioles)	Bronchoconstriction	Bronchodilation (slow dilation)
Heart rate (chronotropic)	Decrease in heart rate (bradycardia)	Increase in heart rate (tachycardia)

parasympathetic antagonist would tend to cause retention of urine, however. A male patient with benign prostatic hyperplasia may notice an exacerbation of urinary retention when taking drugs with parasympathetic antagonist properties. The PT must review drug therapy regimens for any and all medications with parasympathetic antagonistic (anticholinergic) actions.

Autonomic Nervous System Sympathetic (Adrenergic) Subdivision: Selected Pharmacologic Responses

Table 4-3 describes important clinical pharmacologic parameters of the receptor site that has the ultimate control on the given pharmacologic parameter. Several of the adrenergic responses are critical to the cardiovascular system, and alterations can be *life-threatening*.

Pharmacodynamic Considerations in Elderly Patients

- *Orthostatic (postural) hypotension*: Orthostatic (postural) hypotension in an elderly patient may be aggravated by some drug therapy. Any drug that has the ability to deplete vascular volume, or has vasodilating activity, or has sympatholytic (adrenergic blocking) activity is prone to cause clinically significant orthostatic hypotension.
- *Confusion and mental fuzziness*: Elderly patients are vulnerable to increased response to agents that have parasympatholytic (anticholinergic) effects. An aging patient has increased sensitivity of the CNS resulting from decreased cerebral blood flow (20% decreased by the aging process).
- *Mobility alteration (prone to falls and gait disturbance)*: Elderly patients are profoundly affected by drugs that cause sedation, reduce coordination, and cause tremors. In addition to the previously mentioned effects, their mobility may be affected by orthostatic hypotension and confusion and mental fuzziness.

- *Extrapyramidal effects*: Elderly patients are more prone to the complex of side effects called *extrapyramidal symptoms* resulting from a decrease in the activity of dopamine in the CNS. This decrease is due in part to a decreased production of dopamine in elderly patients. Altered levels of CNS dopamine change the frequency and intensity of extrapyramidal effects when medications that block dopamine receptors, such as the neuroleptics, are given.

Extrapyramidal symptoms include akathisia, parkinsonism-like symptoms (e.g., tremor, cogwheel rigidity), dystonia, and dyskinesia. Tardive dyskinesia also is included in the broad category of extrapyramidal symptoms. These symptoms may be very prominent in any patient taking antipsychotic medications but can be especially troublesome in an elderly patient. An imbalance between the neurotransmitters of acetylcholine and dopamine is the basis for the development of extrapyramidal symptoms. This imbalance is focused toward the CNS rather than the autonomic nervous system.

In the study of pharmacology, one must not only understand the autonomic nervous system but also have a basic understanding of serotonin and dopamine as neurotransmitters. Antipsychotic drugs (neuroleptics) have multiple modes of action that are used for therapeutic indications and that can produce side effects. Table 4-4 can help the PT learn the pharmacologic profile of drugs for mental disease.

All drugs classified as antipsychotics used to treat schizophrenic symptoms are classified as neuroleptics.[11] Some medications used as ancillary medications in the treatment of schizophrenia may work by other modes of action. Neuroleptics have differing blockade properties and intensities of blockade. The ideal neuroleptic would have strong blockade of the $5HT_{2a}$ receptor and moderate blockade of the D_2 receptor along with no blockade of the H_1, cholinergic, or alpha receptors (no side effects). Such an agent does not exist. Moderate blockade at the D_2 receptor allows control of schizophrenic symptoms and minimal extrapyramidal side effects. Extrapyramidal side effects occur with strong blockade of the D_2 receptor.

In the area of pharmacodynamics, an ideal drug would produce only one effect (desired therapeutic effect), but this is not reality. In addition to the desired action, drugs have undesired effects called *side effects*. Side effects are responses other than the intended medical effect. *Side effects often are an extension of the known pharmacologic activity of the drug.* Many side effects of medications affect the mobility of geriatric patients.[2,3,17] Table 4-5 presents a few of the many categories of medications that can have a clinically significant effect on geriatric patients.

In addition to mobility issues in elderly patients, medications with anticholinergic activity (cholinergic antagonist) may

TABLE 4-3

Adrenergic Responses with Receptor Site

Pharmacologic Parameter	Alpha-Receptor Stimulation	Beta₁-Receptor Stimulation	Beta₂-Receptor Stimulation	Dopamine Receptor Stimulation (Non-CNS Receptors)
Heart rate (chronotropic)		Increase in heart rate (positive chronotropic)		
Heart contractility (pumping force) (inotropic)		Increase in pumping force of heart (positive inotropic)		
Peripheral vasculature*	Vasoconstriction		Vasodilation	
Renal vasculature	Vasoconstriction			Vasodilation
Lungs (bronchioles)			Bronchodilation	
Uterine smooth muscle			Relaxation (reduced contractions)	
Urinary bladder internal sphincter muscle tone	Contraction (closure of bladder outlet)			Non-CNS dopamine

Note: The lack of a comment in any box in this table does not imply that the receptor has no effect on the parameter, *only that the primary influence resides with the receptor that has the comment in the box.*
*Although alpha and beta₂ responses affect the peripheral vasculature parameter, the alpha influence is the stronger of the two. In the normal condition, homeostasis is maintained with input from both aspects.
CNS, central nervous system.

TABLE 4-4

Neuroleptic Receptor Blockade and Resulting Pharmacodynamics

Receptor Type	Pharmacologic Changes from Blockade	Comments
Dopamine (D₂)	Treatment of schizophrenic positive symptoms. Production of extrapyramidal side effects. Increase in prolactin blood levels.	Prolactin level increase can lead to breast swelling and tenderness and galactorrhea
Serotonin (5HT₂ₐ)	Treatment of schizophrenic negative symptoms.	Action seen with some newer neuroleptics that may block serotonin
Serotonin (5HT₂c)	Anxiolytic properties. Increase in food intake (weight gain).	Reduction of anxiety prompts use in anxiety states and in treating panic attacks
Histamine (H₁)	Sedation. Weight gain.	Blockade of histamine is a secondary effect and leads to side effects
Cholinergic	Peripheral anticholinergic effects (SLUD): dry mouth, blurred vision, retention of urine, and constipation. CNS anticholinergic effects: confusion, delirium, and cognitive deficits.	CNS effects may mimic schizophrenic symptoms and may not be readily recognized as drug-induced side effects
Alpha-adrenergic (alpha receptors)	Orthostatic (postural) hypotension. Syncope from blood pressure changes. Nasal congestion. Priapism.	Most troublesome is hypotension resulting from vasodilation, leading to falls

CNS, central nervous system.

cause confusion and mentation difficulties. Many therapeutic categories contain drugs that may create undesired anticholinergic effects in geriatric patients. Anticholinergic effects include mental confusion and hallucinations. Box 4-4 lists some therapeutic categories that have these anticholinergic properties.[2,3,17] To review the study of pharmacodynamics, see the key facts in Box 4-5.

Pharmacovigilance

Pharmacovigilance is the practice of monitoring the safety of a drug therapy regimen. In addition, it can be defined as "watchfulness in guarding the safety of drugs," and through this function the PT can offer meaningful input as part of a health care team. Adverse events (side effects) caused by drug therapy are best monitored by the individuals who spend the most time with the patient. The physician in many cases does not spend sufficient quality time with the patient to perform good pharmacovigilance. The PT can apply knowledge of pharmacokinetics and pharmacodynamics toward the application of pharmacovigilance and use the examination tools described in Sections Two and Three of the book to screen the patient for such events. See Chapters 6 through 9 for detailed explanations of how to screen patients for medication use and adverse reactions.

The key to understanding pharmacovigilance is to remember that drugs do not do just one thing. Drugs display the desired effect, if they have efficacy, but also display undesired effects. Side effects can be divided into two categories: *predictable* and *unpredictable reactions.*

Predictable side effects constitute 80% of all drug reactions and in most situations are an extension of the known pharmacology of the compound. Another explanation of a predictable side

TABLE 4-5
Adverse Drug Reactions Affecting Mobility in Elderly Patients

Drug Category	Adverse Reactions	Comments
Tricyclic antidepressants (e.g., amitriptyline [Elavil])	Postural hypotension, tremors, sedation, arrhythmias	May lead to syncope and balance difficulty. Cardiac rhythm changes may cause dizziness and mobility problems.
Benzodiazepines (e.g., diazepam [Valium], alprazolam [Xanax], lorazepam [Ativan])	Sedation, weakness, decreased coordination, confusion	Prone to cause oversedation and morning balance problems. Many hypnotics are in this class, such as flurazepam (Dalmane) and temazepam (Restoril).
Sedative hypnotics (e.g., secobarbital [Seconal], zolpidem [Ambien])	Sedation, weakness, decreased coordination, confusion	May lead to falls. Prone to cause morning hangover.
Antihypertensives, alpha-receptor blockers (e.g., prazosin [Minipress], terazosin [Hytrin], doxazosin [Cardura])	Orthostatic (postural) hypotension	May cause significant problems with syncope and lead to falls. Not all classes of drugs for hypertension are prone to postural hypotension.
Narcotic analgesics (e.g., morphine or Vicodin)	Sedation, reduced coordination, confusion	May contribute to clouded thinking and balance problems.
Beta-receptor blockers (e.g., propranolol [Inderal], atenolol [Tenormin])	Reduced ability to respond to workload changes	May lead to weakness and lethargy because of blunting of homeostasis mechanisms. Heart rate and cardiac output may not respond to workload change number.
Antipsychotics or neuroleptics (e.g., haloperidol [Haldol], risperidone [Risperdal], olanzapine [Zyprexa], fluphenazine [Prolixin])	Orthostatic hypotension, sedation, extrapyramidal effects	Significant number of movement disorders and fainting spells. Extrapyramidal effects may take the form of tremors, abnormal gait, or muscle rigidity.

BOX 4-4
Drugs with Potential to Cause Confusion in Elderly Patients

Medication Category	Examples
Antispasmodics	Dicyclomine (Bentyl), hyoscyamine (Levsin)
Antiparkinsonism	Benztropine (Cogentin), trihexyphenidyl (Artane)
Antihistamines	Diphenhydramine (Benadryl), chlorpheniramine
Antidepressants	Amitriptyline (Elavil), imipramine (Tofranil)
Antiarrhythmics	Quinidine, disopyramide (Norpace), procainamide
Antipsychotics (neuroleptics)	Risperidone (Risperdal), haloperidol (Haldol), aripiprazole (Abilify), quetiapine (Seroquel)
Selected hypnotics	Hydroxyzine (Vistaril)
Over-the-counter medications	Antidiarrheals such as loperamide (Imodium), sleep aids such as doxylamine (Unisom), cold remedies such as Contac

BOX 4-5
Key Concepts in the Study of Pharmacodynamics

- An agonist drug displays affinity and activity at the receptor.
- An antagonist drug displays only affinity and no activity at the receptor.
- Drug efficacy is important clinically, whereas drug potency is not important clinically.
- Most pharmacologic responses (desired and undesired) can be predicted when one knows the mechanism of action of the drug (pharmacodynamic activity).

drug (reduction of heart rate). This type of side effect may be dose-related or the result of comorbidities of a given patient. The dose of the metoprolol may have been excessive for the patient, or the dose may have been low, but this patient might have had a history of myocardial infarction and altered cardiac activity.

The second category of side effects is unpredictable reactions. Unpredictable side effects may be subdivided into idiosyncratic and allergic reactions. An *idiosyncratic reaction* is an unusual or unexpected reaction that cannot be explained by the pharmacology of the drug. An example of this type of reaction is a patient who becomes hyperexcitable and hyperactive on a sedating drug such as phenobarbital. *Allergic reactions* also are examples of unpredictable side effects caused by medication. These reactions constitute only approximately 8% of all side effects and are not related to the pharmacologic profile of the drug. The allergic reaction is unlikely to be dose-related and normally is not reproducible across many different patients. The reaction is reproducible only in the individual who experienced the reaction.

The PT also should understand the term *anaphylactic reaction*. An anaphylactic reaction is considered an unpredictable side effect and is an allergic reaction that may occur quickly and is manifested with the symptoms of bronchospasm, hypotension, shock, and potentially death.

A final concept in pharmacovigilance is *drug interaction*. A drug interaction is an adverse event involving the interplay between two or more drugs. In addition, an interaction may occur between a drug and herbal preparations. The more drugs or herbal preparations in a therapeutic regimen, the greater the propensity for drug interactions, and the greater the need for pharmacovigilance. The most important contributor to drug interactions is polypharmacy. Polypharmacy is common because many patients have multiple disease states in addition to communication problems. Many clinicians have prescribed drugs over the telephone rather than performing an examination in the office. Unrecognized side effects may be treated with more

effect is an increased intensity of a predictable action of the drug. For a key example of a predictable side effect, consider the use of metoprolol (Lopressor) to treat hypertension. Metoprolol is a beta-receptor antagonist drug that reduces blood pressure and heart rate. When metoprolol excessively reduces the heart rate (bradycardia), the patient may experience dizziness, lack of energy, and even fainting spells. The bradycardia would be an increased or unexpected intensity of a predictable action of the drugs. The clinician may view an elderly patient as having problems that are disease-state driven rather than medication driven (side effects). Clinicians often are more thorough in investigating patient symptoms in younger patients than in elderly patients. Indifference to the finer points of medication management seems to contribute to drug interactions.

By strict definition, a drug interaction does not have to be adverse, but the common use of the term implies an adverse event. An example of a drug interaction that is not adverse is the use of levodopa and carbidopa in Sinemet to treat Parkinson's disease. The carbidopa creates more efficient use of levodopa and increases the ability of levodopa to penetrate the blood-brain barrier. Most drug interactions do involve adverse events, however, and should be closely monitored.

Drugs may interact through pharmacokinetic and pharmacodynamic mechanisms. An extremely important key to predicting drug interactions is the ability to recognize underlying liver or renal disease in the patient. The PT should constantly ask the important question, "Is the drug necessary?" This question alone can prevent drug interactions or at least uncover problems early in a drug regimen.

Often drugs are released on the market while the patient care team has limited knowledge about its safety profile. From the perspective of the pharmaceutical manufacturers, clinical trials are performed to establish efficacy (to determine whether the drug works), and the development of a safety profile is only a secondary goal in most cases. The patient in clinical trials typically is not treated for a sufficiently long enough time to guarantee the detection of all the adverse effects of the study medication. In addition, the adverse effects may be rare, delayed, or a result of interactions with other drugs. Clinical trials may not have allowed the drug to be tested in a particular subgroup of patients who may be very vulnerable to the pharmacologic actions of the drug. Caregivers who spend the most time with patients must monitor these drugs after they enter the market.

Pharmacovigilance also has an increasingly important role in the risk/benefit assessment of drugs. The risk/benefit assessment continues regardless of whether the drug is new to the market or has been on the market for years. The efficacy and the safety of a drug are of equal importance, and the PT can provide information on both. The focus of the caregiver regarding pharmacovigilance should be on the safety concerns or hazards of a drug, however, rather than on its benefits. An example of a hazard is the case of the antihistamine terfenadine (Seldane). The safety concern with terfenadine was not discovered until the drug was on the market for more than 10 years. The disturbances in cardiac rhythm created by terfenadine resulted from a drug interaction that was not detected in clinical trials or in the early marketing stages of the drug. The discipline of pharmacovigilance requires the PT to ask constantly whether the patient's symptom or problem is drug related or disease-state related. Box 4-6 lists some key concepts in understanding pharmacovigilance.

Over-the-Counter Medications

The PT, in examining drug regimens, must never overlook the influence of OTC medications. The patient often does not consider OTC drugs to be important information to pass along to

---

BOX 4-6

Key Concepts in Understanding of Pharmacovigilance

- Drug safety is monitored by watching over therapeutic regimens.
- Most side effects are increased intensity of a predictable action of the drug.
- The more drugs (polypharmacy), the greater the need for pharmacovigilance.
- Listen to the patient's symptoms and weigh the risk/benefit ratio of every drug.
- Use of over-the-counter medication must be investigated with direct questions.
- Use of herbal preparations should be investigated after over-the-counter medication questioning.

---

the health care professional. The patient often assumes the OTC drug is safe and devoid of side effects. The patient may believe that an OTC drug would not have been approved as an OTC medication by the U.S. Food and Drug Administration (FDA) unless it was completely safe. Aspirin and oral contraceptives are only two of the many drugs that many patients do not list when questioned about their medication. The PT must ask direct questions and incorporate any mentioned medications into the evaluation plan.

The PT should apply the principles of pharmacovigilance and must incorporate knowledge of OTC medications into the screening plan. Many OTC medications began as prescription-only drugs and are not without safety issues. NSAIDs, such as naproxen (Aleve), and histamine-2 receptor antagonists, such as cimetidine (Tagamet), are two of the many therapeutic categories that now appear in the OTC list of medications. The PT must not overlook OTC medications in the patient's drug regimen.

Herbal Preparations

The PT should not overlook the potential influence of herbal preparations. Numerous herbal users and promoters and sellers of herbs (herbalists) do not consider herbal preparations to be medications. If patients do not consider herbal preparations to be a medication, they may omit this information during medication questioning. Herbal preparations should always be included in any medication screening process because of the potential for side effects and drug-herb interactions leading to altered pharmacologic responses. Herbals include any "natural" or "traditional" remedies and are sometimes called *herbal medications*. The terminology of herbal medication may be inaccurate and misleading, however. [8] Many herbal preparations are suggested for use based on their "adaptogenic" properties; they may help the body return to a normal state by resisting stress but may completely lack any medicinal effects. Sometimes clinicians involved in patient care refer to herbs as herbal medicine, which may convey an unintended meaning, and it may not be appropriate to term herbs as herbal medications. The more appropriate term would seem to be *herbal preparations*.

Herbal preparations are classically considered to be a subset of alternative medical therapies.[6] These therapies are interventions that are neither taught in medical schools nor generally available in U.S. hospitals. For regulatory purposes, herbal preparations are recognized through the FDA as a dietary supplement. This classification seems to suggest the FDA sees herbal preparations as nutrients with a nondrug status rather than as medications. Although the FDA does not classify these preparations as

TABLE 4-6
Commonly Used Herbal Preparations

Herbal Preparation	Also Known as	Indications (Uses)	Side Effects
Garlic	*Allium sativum*	Infections, hypertension, colic, cancer	Contact dermatitis, gastroenteritis, nausea, vomiting, herb interactions with antiplatelet drugs and anticoagulant drugs
Ginkgo	*Ginkgo biloba*	Alzheimer's disease, peripheral vascular disease	Relatively safe but has potential drug-herb interactions with antiplatelet drugs leading to bleeding
Echinacea	*Echinacea purpurea, Echinacea angustifolia*	Cold and flu symptom management	Allergic reactions
Saw palmetto	*Serenoa repens*	Benign prostatic hypertrophy/hyperplasia	Mode of action is as 5α-reductase inhibitor; considered a safe remedy in appropriate doses
Ginseng	*Panax ginseng*	Respiratory illness, gastrointestinal disorders, impotence, stress and fatigue	Hypertension, nervousness, sleep problems, morning diarrhea, interaction with warfarin (Coumadin)
St. John's wort	*Hypericum perforatum*	Depression	Photosensitivity reactions, drug interactions with medications metabolized by CYP3A4
Black cohosh	*Cimicifuga racemosa*	Premenstrual syndrome and perimenopausal symptoms, arthritis, mild sedative	Seems safe in appropriate doses
Valerian	*Valeriana officinalis*	Anxiety and sleep aid	Interaction with sedative-hypnotic medications
Kava kava	*Piper methysticum*	Sleep aid, stress reliever, muscle relaxant	Ataxia, hair loss, loss of appetite, dry/yellow discoloration of skin, liver injury
Soy	*Glycine max*	Menopausal symptoms	Contains isoflavones: concern about breast cancer development with high level of isoflavones

medications, they often are used by the public with the intent of preventing illness or treating medical illness. On several occasions, the FDA has urged manufacturers to stop producing dietary supplements containing unsafe products. The study of herbal preparations is challenging because standardized nomenclature is lacking, and there is diversity in the naming conventions (common names, proprietary names, and botanical names), increasing confusion. A result is difficulty in accurately classifying herbal preparations, limiting the effective study.

Herbal preparations and other dietary supplements are no longer sold only in health food stores but are readily available in many grocery stores, drug stores, and mail order companies. Factors supporting high usage of herbal preparations include lower cost, ease of purchasing compared with prescription-only medication, dissatisfaction with conventional therapy, and a general perception by some that herbals are somehow better and safer.[6] Information has appeared over the last 5 years concerning the potential dangers of herbals, however. Information regarding the dangers of using ephedra and kava preparations along with a lack of efficacy for preparations such as ginkgo and St. John's wort has created negative publicity for herbals and reduced their usage.

Herbal preparations may be beneficial in the treatment of certain medical conditions, however; some pharmacologic ingredients in the preparations may provide a potential benefit. Saw palmetto is an herbal preparation with efficacy suggested to be similar to finasteride (Proscar) in the treatment of benign prostatic hyperplasia. In addition, glucosamine and chondroitin may be useful in the treatment of osteoarthritis. Some Chinese herbal preparations may be effective in the treatment of irritable bowel syndrome. Based on preliminary studies, herbal preparations have systematic flaws, however, limiting their external validity.[10] Additional scientific evidence is required to prove the effectiveness of herbal preparations by current scientific standards. There has been an initiative through the National Center for Complementary and Alternative Medicine (NCCAM) at the National Institutes of Health to support research in complementary and alternative medicines.[15] The NCCAM has stimulated and developed research to increase the understanding regarding efficacy and safety of herbal preparations.

Currently, herbal preparations can be marketed without any evidence of testing for efficacy or safety. Occasionally, health claims for herbal preparations have been made without approval from the FDA. The Dietary Supplement Health and Education Act (DSHEA) passed in 1994 gave some guidance to the FDA regarding new products classified as dietary supplements. Most dietary supplements were in use before 1994, however, and most have not been subject to premarket safety evaluations. After marketing, if the FDA determines a manufactured dietary supplement is unsafe, the FDA may take action ranging from warning the public to an extreme action such as the ban of a product from the marketplace. In November 2004, the FDA announced it intends to change its strategy and will work with other agencies to make safety more evidence-based and begin making stronger decisions regarding dietary supplements. The FDA has elucidated that herbal preparations carry potential for various toxic manifestations. Table 4-6 presents commonly used, top-selling herbal preparations and their corresponding uses and side effects.

Many herbal preparations are pharmacologically active and have the potential for toxic effects.[7,13,16] Health care professionals including the PT should be aware that these preparations are generally poorly studied, and scientific evidence of efficacy and safety is often lacking. PTs should always include questions about herbal preparations in any patient history and not assume other health care professionals have screened the patient. A patient who does not view the herbal preparation as an OTC drug may not volunteer the information.

Clinical Considerations of Selected Drug Classes for the Physical Therapist

A list of selected therapeutic categories and their corresponding clinical considerations is provided in Appendix 4-1 at the end of this chapter. The considerations noted are associated with commonly prescribed drugs.

Reference Sources for Drug Information

A vast array of information on drugs and the therapeutic application of drugs is available. With the wide use of various computer programs and the Internet, one can find a great deal of information that was unavailable to the health care professional in past years. All pharmacologists and physicians must consult the literature for drug information. This section discusses some of the most-consulted sources of drug information known to the PT and some valuable sources not readily known.

The *Physicians' Desk Reference* (PDR) is a drug information source that nurses and physicians often consult. This reference is published once a year in the spring and contains information provided by the manufacturers of drugs (pharmaceutical industry). The information is the same as that found in the package insert or package circular approved by the FDA.

The PDR has some major limitations that the PT should keep in mind. Older, established medications may not be included in the current PDR because the pharmaceutical industry uses the PDR as a method of promoting newer drugs. Aspirin is not discussed in the current PDR. Generic products also are not discussed in the PDR. The generic drug fluoxetine is not addressed in the current PDR, although the brand name Prozac can be found.

The PDR is tremendously selective in its product information. Many PTs are surprised to learn that the pharmacologist rarely, if ever, consults the PDR for drug information. The pharmacologist may consult the PDR to help identify a product by looking in the section that contains pictures of dosage formulations.

Many other sources of useful drug information are available to the PT in addition to the PDR. One excellent resource is *Mosby's Drug Consult 2004,* a traditional textbook reference that also contains a CD-ROM.[14] It provides information on pharmacology, indications for use, available dosage formulations, dosing recommendations, and adverse reactions. The four sections include keyword and international brand indices; complete drug information; monographs on the 50 most commonly used herbal drugs and supplements; and appendices containing comparative drug tables, additional information, and supplier profiles. *Mosby's Drug Consult* lists all medications alphabetically by generic name. The trade name is listed in a shaded summary text box immediately after the generic drug entry name. The detailed information for each drug follows.

In addition, the PT should readily consult with the pharmacist on hand when facing important medication-related clinical questions. See the References for other valuable resources for drug information.[1,5,12]

Use of Basic Pharmacology in Screening Drug Regimens: A Patient Case

The following case provides the reader with a significant number of decisions or considerations in regards to a drug regimen.

A 74-year-old man with a history of peptic ulcer disease, type 2 diabetes (15 years' duration), peripheral neuropathy, moderate autonomic neuropathy, and anxiety states including some agitation was recently diagnosed with hypertension and started on terazosin (Hytrin). The medication has been administered for 2 weeks. In addition, the patient has complained of joint stiffness and was started on naproxen (Naprosyn) therapy. The patient, who lives alone, also has had trouble sleeping and began taking an OTC antihistamine (diphenhydramine) for sleep on the recommendation of a friend. The patient's complete drug regimen includes the following eight medications:

- Omeprazole (Prilosec), 20 mg daily
- Amitriptyline, 50 mg at bedtime increased from 25 mg at bedtime 7 days ago
- Fludrocortisone, 0.1 mg daily
- Haloperidol, 2 mg three times daily
- Benztropine (Cogentin), 1 mg twice daily
- Naproxen (Naprosyn), 500 mg two times daily
- Terazosin (Hytrin), 2 mg at bedtime
- OTC antihistamine diphenhydramine (Benadryl), 25 mg at bedtime

The patient recently fell at home; severely straining his lower back, and now is being seen twice each week in the physical therapy outpatient department at the local hospital. The goal of physical therapy is to assist the patient in his ability to ambulate and generally to speed his recovery from the fall. The PT has observed the patient has attention and memory problems and has had difficulty finding the treatment areas on some days. The patient also has shown speech difficulties with increased tendencies to ramble in his conversation since starting therapy. In addition, the patient has had difficulties with urination and has complained of dizziness.

Assessing the Effect of a Patient's Drug Therapy Regimen

All regimens should be assessed for the number of medications with the potential for CNS influence and autonomic nervous system responses. Any elderly patient should be assessed for the presence of medications that might contribute to dizziness, balance problems, or confusion.

The chief examination findings of concern for the above-described patient include dizziness, urinary retention, confusion, and balance problems. Considerations should be: Is he taking medications that have anticholinergic properties? Are there medications present with sympathetic nervous system influences (alpha and beta receptor)? Applying information provided earlier in the chapter reveals the following:

- Anticholinergic properties can be found with haloperidol, benztropine, diphenhydramine, and amitriptyline.
  - Anticholinergic influences can lead to confusion and urinary retention.
- Alpha blockade properties can be found with terazosin and haloperidol.

- Alpha blockade properties can lead to vasodilation, followed by orthostatic hypotension, followed by dizziness.
- Other considerations include renal function and the influence of drugs such as naproxen.
- Disease-state considerations include diabetes and the presence of autonomic neuropathy leading to orthostatic hypotension, and why fludrocortisone is used in the drug regimen.

It would seem many of the patient's clinical issues might be associated with his current drug therapy. The PT should apply critical thinking in regard to patient evaluation and could present opportunities for improvement to the patient and to the attending physician.

Summary

The medical team, including the physician, pharmacist, nurse, dietitian, respiratory therapist, and PT, has a responsibility to monitor patients' drug therapies. The primary goal in screening drug regimens is measuring general efficacy of a drug regimen and noting any adverse events (side effects) associated with the regimen. For a given drug, there is no single dose of a drug treatment that is optimal for *all* patients. An optimal dose should provide efficacy and be devoid of toxicity (no side effects) or at least have minimal toxicity.

An understanding of pharmacology and drug regimens and applying basic pharmacologic principles allows PTs to meet their responsibility. The training or awareness of the practicing physician is not always adequate for the task of pharmacovigilance. Not all prescribers could possibly become experts in the evaluation of the causal relationship between a drug and an adverse clinical event. Assessing the role of a drug is only one aspect of the classic medical diagnostic process, which includes a differential diagnosis and an etiologic diagnosis. The etiologic diagnosis, as far as drugs are concerned, is based on evidence for or against a temporal relationship (the timing of the event) and on the elimination of other principal non–drug-related causes of the observed event. The PT traditionally has not been considered an important source of information about adverse clinical events associated with medication use and has not been assigned the role of identifying patients at risk for an adverse event. By working closely with pharmacists, nurses, and physicians, however, PTs can improve patient care and educate others about the important role they can play. Understanding terms presented in Appendix 4-2 will facilitate therapist communication with other providers.

REFERENCES

1. American Society of Health-System Pharmacists. ASHP drug information. Bethesda, MD: American Society of Heath-System Pharmacists; 2004.
2. Applegate WB, Blass JP, Williams TF. Instruments for the functional assessment of older patients. N Engl J Med 1990;322:107–214.
3. Brawn LA, Castleden CM. Adverse drug reactions: an overview of special considerations in the management of the elderly patient. Drug Saf 1990;5:421–35.
4. Ciccone CD. Pharmacology in rehabilitation. 4th ed. Philadelphia: Davis; 2007.
5. Drug Facts and Comparisons, St Louis, Facts and Comparisons (website). www.drugfacts.com. Accessed August 6, 2009.
6. Eisenberg DM, Davis RB, Ettner SL. Trends in alternative medicine use in the United States, 1990-1997: results of a follow-up national survey. JAMA 1998;280:1569–75.
7. Fugh-Berman A. Herb-drug interactions. Lancet 2000;355:134–8.
8. Gilroy CM, Steiner JF, Byers T, et al. Echinacea and truth in labeling. Arch Intern Med 2003;163:699–704.
9. Gilman AG, Rall TW, Nies AS, editors. The pharmacological basis of therapeutics. 10th ed. New York: Pergamon Press; 2000.
10. Haller CA, Anderson IB, Kim SY, et al. An evaluation of selected herbal reference texts and comparison to published reports of adverse herbal events. Adverse Drug React Toxicol 2002;21:143–50.
11. Keltner NL, Folks DG. Psychotropic drugs. 4th ed. St Louis: Mosby; 2001.
12. Lacy CF, Armstrong LL, Goldman MP, et al. Drug information handbook. 12th ed. Hudson, OH: Lexi-Comp; 2004.
13. Miller LG. Herbal medicinal: selected clinical considerations focusing on known or potential drug-herb interactions. Arch Intern Med 2000;158:2200–11.
14. Mosby's Drug Consult 2004. St Louis: Mosby; 2004.
15. National Center for Complementary and Alternative Medicine: Clinical trials (website). http://nccam.nih.gov/research/clinicaltrials. Accessed August 6, 2009.
16. O'Hara MA, Kiefer D, Farrell K, et al. A review of 12 commonly used medicinal herbs. Arch Fam Med 1998;7:523–36.
17. Peters NL. Antimuscarinic side effects of medications in the elderly. Arch Intern Med 1989;149:2414–20.
18. Pratt WB, Taylor P, editors. Principles of drug action: the basis of pharmacology. 4th ed. New York: Churchill Livingstone; 1995.
19. Thomson Corporation (website). www.micromedex.com. Accessed August 15, 2009.
20. Wilt TJ, Ishani A, Stark G. Saw palmetto extracts for treatment of benign prostatic hyperplasia. JAMA 1998;280:1604–9.

Appendix **4-1** Clinical Considerations of Pharmacologic Agents in Rehabilitation Patients

Therapeutic Category	Clinical Considerations	Drug Examples
Sedative-hypnotic/ antianxiety drugs (anxiolytics)	Prevalence of use is high. Tension and anxiety are significant in some patient populations, and these agents may be required to treat these symptoms to assist in rehabilitation. The rationale of these agents can backfire if the drug produces significant sedative effects or morning hangover. Some types of rehabilitation are best accomplished through scheduling the dose of the drug at least 2 hours before or after rehabilitation efforts	*Benzodiazepines*: diazepam (Valium), alprazolam (Xanax), lorazepam (Ativan), flurazepam (Dalmane), temazepam (Restoril). *Barbiturates*: secobarbital (Seconal), pentobarbital (Nembutal). *Miscellaneous*: buspirone (BuSpar), zolpidem (Ambien)
Antidepressants/ antimanic drugs	May make patient more optimistic and improve therapy potential. Patient may become more interested in rehabilitation. Certain side effects can be troubling during physical therapy treatments. Tricyclic antidepressants can produce orthostatic hypotension, causing syncope and subsequent injury from falls. Sedation, lethargy, and muscle weakness may occur	*Tricyclic agents*: amitriptyline (Elavil), imipramine (Tofranil), desipramine (Norpramin), nortriptyline (Aventyl). *SSRIs*: fluoxetine (Prozac), paroxetine (Paxil), sertraline (Zoloft). *Antimanic*: Lithium
Antipsychotics (neuroleptic drugs)	These drugs tend to "normalize" patient behavior. Withdrawn patient becomes more active. Agitated patient becomes calmer and more relaxed. These drugs cause sedation and anticholinergic side effects. Guard against orthostatic hypotension. Major side effects are EPS. PT always should be alert for motor involvement manifested as balance changes, involuntary movements, and other motor dysfunction	Chlorpromazine (Thorazine), fluphenazine (Prolixin), trifluoperazine (Stelazine), perphenazine (Trilafon), prochlorperazine (Compazine), thioridazine (Mellaril), haloperidol (Haldol), clozapine (Clozaril), olanzapine (Zyprexa), risperidone (Risperdal). Some antiemetics are in this category of neuroleptics, such as droperidol (Inapsine). The promotility drug metoclopramide (Reglan) may cause some EPS
Anticonvulsants (antiepileptic agents)	PT should be aware of any patient with a history of seizure disorder. Common side effects of headache, dizziness, sedation, and gastrointestinal disturbances may be bothersome during rehabilitation. Cerebellar side effects such as ataxia are the most important to monitor and may impair rehabilitation ability. All of these drugs have therapeutic serum levels (look for toxic levels). Many of these drugs often are used as mood stabilizers with antipsychotics	Phenobarbital, primidone (Mysoline), phenytoin (Dilantin), carbamazepine (Tegretol), valproic acid (Depakote), gabapentin (Neurontin), lamotrigine (Lamictal)
Antiparkinsonism drugs	PT should coordinate therapy sessions with peak effect of the drug. In a patient taking levodopa, the peak usually occurs 1 hour after a dose. Optimal therapy sessions can be achieved by scheduling after the breakfast dose of levodopa (may find maximal drug effect and lower fatigue levels in the patient). PT should monitor blood pressure in patients because most are prone to hypotension. Dizziness with positional changes sometimes produces falls	*Levodopa*: Sinemet. *Anticholinergic agents*: benztropine (Cogentin), trihexyphenidyl (Artane), procyclidine (Kemadrin), biperiden (Akineton). *Dopamine agonists*: pergolide (Permax), bromocriptine (Parlodel), pramipexole (Mirapex), ropinirole (Requip). *Miscellaneous*: selegiline (Eldepryl), amantadine (Symmetrel)
Skeletal muscle relaxants	By reducing muscle tone in spasticity, these drugs may allow more effective passive range of motion and stretching activities. General muscle weakness may occur with some drugs, such as dantrolene. Patients' ability to support themselves during ambulation may be impeded by the drug, which causes overall muscle weakness. PT should be aware of drug choices and work closely with patient	Dantrolene (Dantrium), baclofen (Lioresal), cyclobenzaprine (Flexeril), diazepam (Valium), carisoprodol (Soma)

Appendix 4-1 Clinical Considerations of Pharmacologic Agents in Rehabilitation Patients—cont'd

Therapeutic Category	Clinical Considerations	Drug Examples
Analgesics: opiates	Side effects of sedation and gastrointestinal upset may be particularly troublesome. Relief of pain may have a positive effect on rehabilitation. Drugs may tend to blunt the respiratory response to exercise. Respiratory depression usually does not occur unless preceded by mental alteration. Recognize mental change. Overall blunting effect is a descending response, and diaphragm changes usually follow mental changes	Morphine, oxycodone (Percocet and Percodan), hydrocodone (Vicodin), hydromorphone (Dilaudid), meperidine (Demerol), fentanyl (Duragesic), pentazocine (Talwin), buprenorphine (Buprenex), nalbuphine (Nubain)
Analgesics: NSAIDs	Aspirin and other NSAIDs are among the most common medications used by patients in rehabilitation. Side effects usually do not interfere with physical therapy. Gastrointestinal symptoms are the most common problems, but renal symptoms are the most critical issue. Renal problems with an increasing potassium level may put the patient at risk for severe problems. The patient often asks questions about the use of Tylenol versus aspirin; be able to explain the differences	*Salicylate NSAIDs*: aspirin and others. *Nonsalicylate NSAIDs*: ibuprofen, naproxen, sulindac, ketoprofen, tolmetin, indomethacin. *COX-2 inhibitors*: rofecoxib (Vioxx), celecoxib (Celebrex), valdecoxib (Bextra)
Antihypertensive drugs	These common medications produce a diverse set of side effects. Be aware of orthostatic hypotension. Activities that produce widespread vasodilation, such as whirlpools, should be used with caution with patients taking vasodilator drugs. Exercise tolerance may be impaired when beta blockers are used; myocardium does not respond as strongly to sympathetic influences. Be aware of coughing problems when patient is using ACE inhibitor medications	*Beta blockers*: propranolol (Inderal), metoprolol (Lopressor), atenolol (Tenormin). *ACE inhibitors*: captopril (Capoten), lisinopril (Zestril), enalapril (Vasotec), ramipril (Altace). *Calcium channel blockers*: nifedipine (Procardia), diltiazem (Cardizem), verapamil (Isoptin), isradipine (DynaCirc), hydralazine (Apresoline), minoxidil (Loniten). *Alpha blockers*: doxazosin (Cardura), terazosin (Hytrin), prazosin (Minipress)
Antianginal drugs	Activities in rehabilitation increase myocardial oxygen demand with subsequent anginal pain. If patient uses sublingual nitroglycerin, have patient bring drug to rehabilitation. Beta blockers may slow heart rate and reduce myocardial contractility in some situations. Nitrates and calcium channel blockers produce peripheral vasodilation. Heat and exercise may be additive to the drug's effect, resulting in syncope	*Nitrates*: nitroglycerin, isosorbide dinitrate (Isordil), isosorbide mononitrate (Ismo). *Beta blockers*: see above. *Calcium channel blockers*: see above. Dipyridamole (Persantine)
Antiarrhythmic drugs	These drugs may produce side effects that can affect rehabilitation. These drugs usually do not alter exercise parameters such as heart rate or blood pressure. PT should monitor for faintness and dizziness because these may be signs of a rhythm disturbance	Quinidine, procainamide (Procan SR), disopyramide (Norpace), lidocaine, mexiletine (Mexitil), flecainide (Tambocor), propafenone (Rythmol), digoxin (Lanoxin), adenosine (Adenocard)
Anticoagulants	Primary outpatient agent is warfarin (Coumadin). PT should be aware of increased tendency to bleed. Any situation that involves open wounds should be handled with caution. Be aware of all antiplatelet drugs that may increase bleeding tendency	Warfarin (Coumadin). Heparin. Low-molecular-weight heparins, including enoxaparin (Lovenox). *Antiplatelet drugs*: aspirin, dipyridamole (Persantine), ticlopidine (Ticlid)
Antibiotics	PT should be aware of gastrointestinal side effects with antibiotics and recognize diarrhea, nausea, vomiting, and gastrointestinal cramping. Some antibiotics increase sensitivity to ultraviolet light (ciprofloxacin [Cipro]) and make the patient more prone to burns	Sulfa: sulfamethoxazole/trimethoprim (Bactrim). Quinolones: ciprofloxacin (Cipro), ofloxacin (Floxin), tetracycline (Sumycin), doxycycline (Vibramycin), demeclocycline (Declomycin)

ACE, angiotensin-converting enzyme; *COX-2,* cyclooxygenase 2; *EPS,* extrapyramidal symptoms; *NSAIDs,* nonsteroidal anti-inflammatory drugs; *SSRIs,* selective serotonin reuptake inhibitors.

Appendix **4-2 Glossary**

Affinity—Amount of attraction or binding power a given drug has for its receptor site. Some degree of attraction must be inherent in the drug for it to bind to a receptor.

Agonist—Drug with affinity that can elicit a pharmacologic response. The pharmacologic action generally is stimulation, but inhibition also may be the action.

Antagonist—Drug with affinity (binds to receptor) but that does not produce an inherent action.

Bioavailability—Measure of the completeness of absorption combined with a measure of the amount of drug that reaches the target organ.

Biologic half-life ($t_{1/2}$)—Time in which the pharmacologic response decreases to one half of its original effect.

Blood-brain barrier—Sieve through which a drug must pass from the cerebral circulation into the brain cells to exert a pharmacologic effect in the central nervous system.

Efficacy—Capacity to produce an effect for a given occupied receptor. The term describes how well a drug works or the maximum response to a drug.

Elimination half-life ($t_{1/2}$)—Time in which the plasma concentration of a drug decreases to one half of its original amount.

First-pass effect—Rapid extraction and metabolism of a drug by the liver, blocking all of the drug or greatly minimizing the amount of drug available in the systemic circulation.

Pharmacology—Study of the action of any chemical on a living system. The methodology of the field relies heavily on physiology and biochemistry.

Pharmacotherapeutics—Study of the use of drugs in the treatment, prevention, and diagnosis of disease. This aspect of pharmacology correlates pharmacodynamics with the pathophysiology of the clinical issue and applies principles of rigorous patient monitoring.

Pharmacovigilance—Monitoring of the safety profile (side effects) of medications to protect the patient. It applies the aspect of watchfulness in protecting the patient's safety from untoward conditions with the use of medications.

Potency—Amount of drug required to produce a given effect relative to a standard. The amount of drug usually is not important clinically.

Steady-state level—Condition in which the amount of drug eliminated is equal to the amount administered, and the plasma levels oscillate around the mean. This is one of the goals of drug therapy for the clinician.

Tachyphylaxis—Rapidly developing tolerance that prevents the desired pharmacologic effect from being achieved. Rebound congestion that occurs with a nasal decongestant is an example.

Tolerance—Clinical situation in which increasing amounts of drug are required to produce the same pharmacologic effect, or the situation in which the same dose of the drug on repeated occasions produces a less intense pharmacologic effect.

The Patient Interview: The Science Behind the Art

Matthew B. Garber, PT, DSc, OCS, FAAOMPT
William G. Boissonnault, PT, DPT, DHSc, FAAOMPT

Objectives

After reading this chapter, the reader will be able to:

1. Identify potential impediments to an effective and efficient patient interview.
2. Describe the elements of the patient-centered interview.
3. Describe strategies, including setting the environment and nonverbal and verbal communication skills, physical therapists can use to enhance the interview process.
4. Provide an overview of strategies designed to enhance the interview process of patients with hearing deficits, patients who are angry or combative, and patients who are depressed.

We have been given two ears and but a single mouth in order that we may hear more and talk less.

Zeno of Citium

Physical therapy management for patients with neuromusculoskeletal conditions without a physician referral is now a reality in most states. With direct access comes a heightened awareness of the obligation to all patients of providing a comprehensive, evidence-based examination to diagnose accurately the spectrum of conditions likely to respond to physical therapy interventions, while promptly recognizing conditions that require referral to other medical providers. The patient interview is a crucial element of this process.

Most of the essential diagnostic information arises from the patient interview.[17,23,72] Despite the recognized importance of this core clinical skill, many health care providers perform inadequate patient interviews. Platt and McMath[60] observed more than 300 clinical interviews by physicians and found five primary areas of deficiency: (1) interviews with low therapeutic content; (2) inattention to primary data (symptoms); (3) a high control style; (4) an incomplete database, usually omitting patient-centered data and active problems other than the present illness; and (5) thoughtless interviews in which the physician fails to formulate a needed working hypothesis.

The typical length of a physician visit, including the physical examination, ranges from 3 to 74 minutes[64,65,67] the average visit lasts 15 to 21 minutes.[47,65,67,69,81] In primary care, the average consultation times for family physicians, internists, and pediatricians are 13 minutes, 19 minutes, and 13 minutes, respectively.[65] In an informal survey of Army physical therapy clinics, Garber[21] found the average length of a new patient visit was 35 minutes, whereas the average follow-up visit was 23 minutes. In two unrelated studies, researchers found that only 23% to 28% of patients are able to complete their opening statement of concerns before being interrupted or redirected.[9,47] In one study, only one patient was able to complete his entire opening statement.[47] Patients are interrupted by the physician an average of 18 to 23 seconds into the interview—typically after only one initial concern is stated.[9,47] This finding is important because if given the opportunity, patients typically express an average of three concerns per visit, and the first concern is not always the primary complaint.[47,87] After being interrupted, patients may not mention the information again.[62]

Interrupting the patient may hinder the amount and quality of pertinent data gained through the interview.[62] Physicians typically take control of the interview after interrupting and use more closed-ended questions for the remainder of the interview.[9] Patients allowed to complete their initial statements take only 6 seconds longer than patients who are interrupted.[47] The average time for a patient to disclose main concerns fully is 32 to 90 seconds, with a maximum of approximately 2 minutes.[9,47] An average of 21 interruptions occur in a typical primary care visit.[62] Patients bring up new problems not previously mentioned—commonly referred to as the "Oh, by the way ..." concerns—during the closing moments of approximately 20% of patient visits.[47,87]

Most studies have focused on the physician-patient relationship, but physical therapists (PTs) are not exempt from these same inadequacies. These data should make PTs reflect on their own interview styles and relationships with patients. Positive communication characteristics noted during patient-physician encounters are also valued by patients working with PTs. Beattie and colleagues[5] reported a strong association between patient satisfaction and the perceived quality of patient-PT interactions. In particular, PTs spending adequate time with the patient, exhibiting strong listening and communication skills, and offering clear explanations of treatments were desirable qualities.

One can question, "How much time is adequate," and "How long is this initial visit going to last?" When comparing "no-claims" physicians with physicians who had suits filed against them, the average length of patient encounter time difference was only 3 minutes. The difference in length of visits had an independent effect in predicting the physicians' claim statuses.[41] These results support the notion that quality, and not amount, of time alone is key for a positive encounter. Most of the aforementioned physician studies were performed in primary care settings. For PTs working in primary care environments, the challenges faced should be similar.

Considering the importance of the patient interview as described in the current medical literature, why are health care providers so poor at this core clinical skill? Why is so little time devoted to teaching the skills associated with performing an effective interview? Given the time constraints common in clinical practice, how can PTs gather these data accurately, efficiently, and in adequate detail and still have time to complete the physical examination, provide an intervention, and educate the patient?

The primary objective of this chapter is to provide PTs and students with the communication, technical, and clinical decision-making skills associated with the interview process. The development of these skills results in the PT (1) developing an accurate clinical hypothesis; (2) developing an examination and intervention approach to meet the individual's cultural, communication, anatomic, and physiologic needs and abilities; (3) recognizing patient symptoms and signs that necessitate communication with other health care providers; and (4) participating in the decision-making process regarding the selection of appropriate diagnostic testing. Excellent communication skills are a vital foundation for all these aspects of patient care. The end result is the PT providing high-quality patient care and assuming a valuable role on an interdisciplinary health care team.

Communication: Overview of the Medical Literature

I know that you believe you understand what you think I said, but I am not sure you realize that what you heard is not what I meant.

Anonymous

In the medical professions, clinicians need to use effective and sharply honed communication skills routinely. These critical skills are taught in medical school and entry-level allied health training programs, yet are rarely emphasized.[54,57,72] To make a correct diagnosis and to establish an effective intervention, PTs must have the communication skills that allow them to comprehend completely important details of the patient's problem. Proficiency in communication skills is necessary to collect important patient data efficiently and effectively, provide exercise instruction, explain the diagnosis and prognosis, and teach the details of a treatment program to a patient. Patience and repeated hard work, humility, clarity, and self-criticism all are required to acquire highly effective communication skills.[13,45]

Increased public dissatisfaction with the medical professions is related to deficiencies in clinical communication. Studies in many countries have confirmed that serious communication problems are common in clinical practice. These findings led Simpson and coworkers[72] to conclude that there is a "clear and urgent need" for teaching core clinical communication skills to medical students and that this training should be continued in the postgraduate setting and continuing medical education courses. Similarly, PTs could benefit from communication skills training at all levels of their professional and postprofessional education. In 1987, Singleton[73] called for an increased emphasis on written and oral communication skills in physical therapy curricular offerings when direct access was approved in North Carolina. Malpractice claims could possibly increase against PTs as they take on more responsibility for patient management in primary care. PTs working in primary care must develop excellent communication skills to try to defuse potentially disgruntled patients.

Clinicians need to understand the many complexities surrounding effective communication. Successful communication can be difficult to achieve. Wright and Hopkins[90] found that physicians, PTs, and patients disagree about the definition of commonly used medical terms. Physicians and patients showed poor agreement on more than 40% of the words included in a questionnaire. PTs and patients showed poor agreement for the terms *numbness, ligaments, lumbar, back,* and *sciatic nerve.* What may be even more alarming is that physicians and PTs could not agree on 30% of these commonly used medical terms. Among words with fair to poor agreement were *arthritis, back, weakness of the arm, swelling of a joint,* and *sciatic nerve.* It is a travesty that physicians and PTs cannot agree on the definition of *back.* Similar results were found in a study performed by neurologists.[29] Perhaps this is one reason Waddell[84] called low back pain "a twentieth century medical disaster."

In a comprehensive review of patient-physician communication, Roter and associates[69] found that many different types of communication are used throughout the interview process. They grouped these communication patterns into broad categories of communication process variables: information-giving, information-seeking, partnership-building, social conversation (positive talk), and negative talk. These same authors found that patients provide 40% of the talk in the visit and physicians contribute approximately 60%.[69]

Roter and associates[68] later identified many distinct communication patterns in primary care visits. Patients and physicians prefer different styles.[69] The "narrowly biomedical" pattern occurred in 32% of visits. Closed-ended medical questions and primarily biomedical talk characterize this pattern. An "expanded biomedical" pattern, similar to the narrow biomedical pattern, but including moderate levels of psychosocial discussion, constituted 33% of visits. The "biopsychosocial" pattern contained a balance of biomedical and psychosocial topics. This pattern constituted 20% of the visits. High levels of psychosocial interaction characterized "psychosocial" visits. The "consumerist" pattern primarily consisted of patient questions and physician information-giving. The psychosocial and consumerist patterns each constituted 8% of the visits. Physician satisfaction was lowest in the narrowly biomedical pattern and highest in the consumerist pattern, whereas patients preferred the psychosocial pattern.

Jensen and colleagues[33,34] provided observations on novice and expert PTs. Clinical experts spend considerable time with patients in hands-on care, seeking information and evaluating and educating the patient. Expert clinicians enter the lives of their patients, listen well, detect confusion, seek clarification, and know when they are being understood—they are patient-centered. Although novice PTs tend to be more procedural and mechanical when dealing with patients, experts are more responsive, listen intently, and build on what the patient says.

Similar to expert PTs, Marvel and coworkers[48] found that exemplary family physicians with excellent communication skills involve patients more in the medical interview, offer more emotional support, and use a more biopsychosocial approach to patient care. Community physicians serving as control subjects focused more on the biomedical model. The exemplary physicians used no more time per patient than the control subjects.

In addition to communicating with patients, PTs need to develop expertise in communicating with physicians and insurance companies.[20] In a study of communication between physicians and PTs, Hulme and coworkers[32] found that PTs desire more accessibility to and communication with physicians, whereas physicians want brief communication with clear objective data provided by the PT. They found that PTs prefer a more autonomous practice in which the physician recognizes the PT's expertise. Physicians want to communicate with PTs who have high levels of expertise, yet they generally do not facilitate PT autonomy.[32] The idiosyncratic attitudes of physicians and PTs toward communication, combined with the lack of agreement on definitions of common medical terms,[90] make this one area of communication that still needs to be fostered. This is especially true if PTs are to be successful practitioners in a primary care setting.

More recent surveys have revealed that disruptive behavior, including the use of intimidation by health care professionals, is common.[10] Although most research on disruptive behavior centers on physicians and nurses, it is also prevalent in other professions, including physical therapy.[63] Unprofessional behavior has been shown to have negative effects on patient and family satisfaction and patient outcomes and can impede communication, relationship building, and the transfer of information between providers.[64] Health care providers perceived as disrespectful or condescending have also been linked to a higher malpractice risk.[30,31,78] PTs should use reflective clinical practice not only to assess their direct patient care skills but also their attitude toward patients and other members of the health care team. It is never appropriate to speak negatively about other providers in front of patients or to create a disruptive work atmosphere.

Another important aspect of communication relates to patient education and compliance. Increased compliance may occur if the PT is able to communicate effectively with patients.[85] A PT who speaks highly of all members of the health professions helps assure patients that they are being cared for by a team of cooperative and knowledgeable providers. PTs need to portray a level of confidence when interacting with patients, never giving the impression of incompetence. This confidence includes showing a willingness to explore multiple health issues or make an appropriate referral when indicated. In addition to confidence, the communicator should provide information in a friendly, sympathetic, and concerned manner, which increases the likelihood of compliance.[85] People remember best what they are told first. They remember what they believe is important and what has been repeated to them.[85] Providing patients with the most important information first, stressing how important it is, using short words and sentences, repeating key points frequently, and providing specific information may improve compliance.[85] For instance, "Do your exercises regularly" is likely not as effective as telling the patient to do "three 30-second repetitions of each stretch once per day." Determining patients' preferred learning style promotes the most effective manner to educate patients.

Health care professionals often undervalue or forget the potency of good communication skills.[50] Limiting communication with patients because of managed care, capitation, and other work pressures could lead to longer recovery times for patients simply because of gaps or errors in patient data collection.[50] Becoming a skilled communicator with patients, physicians,

and insurers, among others, should be a high priority for any PT desiring to work in a primary care arena.

Listening: An Active Process

> Listening is itself, of course, an art: that is where it differs from merely hearing. Hearing is passive; listening is active. Hearing is voluntary; listening demands attention. Hearing is natural; listening is an acquired discipline.[45]

The average person spends approximately 45% of his or her waking hours involved in listening activities, but with an efficiency of 25%.[12] Being a good listener—picking up new lines of thought or inquiry from verbal and nonverbal cues—is vital to the success of the examination and intervention.[52] Grieve[26] stated that PTs are "in danger of overlooking the simple (psychological) potency of giving patients a good hearing, listening attentively, giving them the benefit of the doubt." This inability to examine fully in a patient-centered format, according to Grieve, "may lead to unnecessary mischief." Many authors have reported on the therapeutic effect of the patient interview.[12,17,79]

Listening attentively and allowing patients to provide their perspective regarding their health has many potential benefits. The PT may learn something important about the patient's personality, background, and values, leading to a better understanding of the patient's problem. This attentive listening may make the patient listen more attentively to the PT, which improves rapport through more effective communication.[13,61]

Listening becomes effective only when what is said is also heard and understood.[61,85] Hearing connotes attention to sounds and perhaps the interpretation of their literal meanings, whereas listening requires that the listener grasp the true meaning of what is communicated through verbal and nonverbal cues.[12] Effective listening is hindered by numerous factors, including (1) the listener being unwilling to listen, (2) the listener attending only to what he or she wishes to hear (i.e., selective listening), (3) the listener's thoughts wandering, and (4) language differences leading to perceptual differences between the listener and the speaker. Controlling these factors is a major determinant of good listening.[13]

Although the content of verbal communication is important, other factors influence interpretation of what is said. Tone of voice, inflection, and facial expressions affect how a verbal message is perceived.[34]

Several authors have also found that patients commonly offer verbal and nonverbal clues that frequently go unrecognized by physicians.[37,40,81] This lack of recognition has been attributed to the physician being "off in differential-land"[37] rather than focusing on the patient's psychosocial needs. In contrast to commonly held beliefs, visits in which physicians took the time to use active listening and responded to these clues were shorter than visits in which clues were missed.[40]

Setting the Environment

A patient-friendly environment promotes more active and comfortable participation in the examination process. Patients are often asked important but very personal questions; a more comfortable and trusting environment may enable patient willingness to share this information. In addition, any action that assists patients to be accurate historians enhances accurate and timely decision making by the PT. Ideally, the patient interview should be conducted in a room or area with minimal noise and as few distractions as possible. PTs can control the frequency of interruptions when the patient visit begins, allowing for contact of an urgent nature only. What constitutes urgent contact should be clearly communicated to receptionists and other support staff. Clinic areas equipped with most commonly used instruments (e.g., reflex hammers, goniometers, tape measures) and stocked with adequate linens minimizes the number of PT forays to find necessary items. Rooms with bright lights and clutter inhibit good eye contact[15] and should be avoided. Patients should be offered the choice of where to sit (or lie down) so that they can remain comfortable and the desirable level of eye contact can be established.[15] Allowing patients to remain in their clothing during the interview when possible protects modesty and enhances comfort when the room temperature may not be ideal. A patient-friendly environment enhances patients' initial impressions of the upcoming encounter. Similar effect can be imparted with nonverbal interaction between the PT and the patient.

Nonverbal Communication

Looking (observing) is itself a skill: that is where it differs from merely seeing. Seeing is passive; looking is active. Seeing is natural; looking is an acquired discipline.[45]

Of equal importance to listening and verbal communication skills is nonverbal communication. The exchange of verbal messages during the medical encounter may not correlate with nonverbal communication.[83] The effect of nonverbal signals is usually stronger, quicker, and more direct than the effect of verbal signals.[45] Nonverbal communication is a subconscious reflex action and can be expected to be more genuine.[45] Verbal communication is discontinuous, with periods of silence, whereas body language, facial expressions, and other nonverbal mannerisms are continuous—even when we are not conscious of them.[83]

Skillful understanding of nonverbal communication is similar to active listening. It involves conscious effort and discipline. Many messages are conveyed through nonverbal communication. Pain may be expressed by a grimace or wince on the patient's face. Direct eye contact, nodding of the head in agreement, and facing the patient during the interview may convey sincerity and acknowledgment of the patient's problem. Sensitivity to cultural influences regarding nonverbal communication is important; what may be considered to be a desirable strategy (e.g., eye contact) may not be for all people. Chapter 3 provides multiple examples of cultural considerations and communication.

Despite the perceived importance of nonverbal communication, this topic has received much less systematic research by health professionals than verbal communication. Thornquist[83] reviewed videos of 30 interviews from PTs in three different practice settings. Patients were more likely to look down during

the greeting, and PTs tended to decide on the spatial relationship between the patient and PT. PTs occasionally writing notes had a distancing effect by decreasing eye contact and turning away from the patient. Manual PTs were especially good at active listening, eye contact, posture, and limited writing; this indicates interest, approachability, and attentiveness.[83] In addition, manual PTs made active use of their hands throughout the interaction, remained physically close to the patient, and adapted their tempo and rhythm to match the patient, creating interaction. Thornquist[83] concluded that this behavior communicated a sense of caring and acknowledgment that can create an atmosphere of confidence. This confidence, in addition to credibility of the communicator, is an important aspect of effective communication.[85]

Patient-Centered Interview

To know what kind of person has a disease is as essential as to know what kind of a disease a person has.[77]

A growing body of literature shows that good interpersonal skills of health care providers result in increased patient satisfaction,[70,75] improved patient outcome,[64,67] increased provider satisfaction,[4,43,69,74,76,80] improved efficiency,[19,79] decreased patient anxiety,[64] and decreased malpractice claims.[41] Despite complaints by many health care providers that interviews that attend to the patient's feelings, ideas, and values take longer, there is clear evidence that these interviews take the same or less time as the biomedical interview.[19,40,47]

Most complaints about health care providers are not associated with clinical competency problems but with communication problems.[63,71] Most malpractice allegations against physicians arise from problems in communication.[66] The difference between sued and never-sued physicians is not explained by negligence, quality of care, or poor documentation. Patients and families are more likely to sue if they believe the physician is not caring or compassionate.[39] Beckman and associates[8] found that 70% of malpractice depositions were attributed to communication problems between the patient and the physician. Primary care physicians who use active listening, use more statements of orientation, laugh and use humor, and facilitate patient input are less likely to have malpractice claims than other physicians.[41] How health care providers communicate with patients—through tone of voice, demeanor, and empathy—is perhaps more important than the context of the message.[41,46,50]

Although asking for patient input and inquiring about feelings makes sense, this is done in less than 50% of patient visits.[17,18] Many health care providers find it difficult to go beyond the disease-centered or biomedical model of patient care. Others simply do not have the training to investigate adequately the patient's feelings, values, or ideas, leading to interviews focusing only on the patient's disease or diagnosis. Some providers wish to focus more on the patient but simply "don't know what to say."[58,60] The patient-centered interview is one method of addressing the patient as a person by incorporating biopsychosocial concepts and encouraging more patient participation during the medical encounter in addition to diagnosing and treating the patient's disorder.[8] The patient-centered interview provides a mechanism for the health care provider to develop a more effective relationship with patients and to ensure that patients are understood and valued[60]; a process that starts with a brief, general discussion of what is about to occur during the initial visit, and confirmation that this is what the patient was expecting, can set the stage for meaningful verbal interchange.

Within this model are six interactive components[73]: (1) exploring the patient's disease/diagnosis and its effect on his or her life, (2) understanding the whole person, (3) finding common ground regarding intervention or management, (4) advocating prevention and health promotion, (5) enhancing the patient-provider relationship, and (6) providing realistic expectations. Within this framework, the provider must also explore the dimensions of the illness experience,[60] including the following:

1. Who is the patient (patient profile)? This consists of information on the patient's hobbies, interests, and professional and personal life.

2. What does the patient want from the provider (patient's goals)? It is important to know whether the patient wants advice on diagnosis and prognosis, desires only a home exercise program, or expects a full return to prior level of activity. Depending on the scenario, it is important to determine whether the patient has realistic expectations based on the nature, stage, and history of the disorder.

3. How does the patient experience illness (functional limitations)? It is important to know how the patient deals with being sick; how he or she responds to symptoms and changes in function; and how the patient's family, coworkers, and social network deal with illness or disability.

4. What are the patient's perceptions about the disorder? It is important to ask for the patient's opinion about what the source of the symptoms is and what he or she thinks about the diagnosis, prognosis, or intervention.

5. What are the patient's feelings about the disorder? It is important to note whether the patient is sad, depressed, optimistic, or motivated.

In addition to strong evidence that the patient-centered interview improves outcomes and patient and provider satisfaction, and decreases malpractice claims, there is evidence that these communication skills can be taught and learned by medical students, PT students, and practicing clinicians.* This evidence dispels the theory that communication skills and good listening are character traits rather than acquired skills.[17] Clinical experience alone does not improve communication skills.[66]

Interview Process

A health care provider who cannot take a good history, and a patient who cannot provide one, are at risk of giving and receiving poor care.

Author unknown

The patient history provides 80% of the information needed to determine the source of symptoms.[23] The goals of obtaining

---

BOX 5-1

SINSS: Operational Definitions and Guidelines

Severity: This term describes the clinician's assessment of the intensity of the patient's symptoms as they relate to a functional activity. PTs may consider the patient's perception of the severity and their assessment of the severity.

Irritability: This term describes the clinician's assessment of the ease with which the symptoms can be provoked or stirred up. It has three components: (1) the amount of activity needed to trigger the patient's symptoms, (2) the severity of the symptoms provoked, and (3) what activity and the amount of time before the patient's symptoms subside (duration).

Nature of the complaint: This term describes the clinician's assessment of the following:

1. Hypotheses of the structures (if appropriate), syndrome/classification, or pathoanatomic structures or syndromes responsible for producing the pain (e.g., nerve root, disk, inflammatory component, lumbar dysfunction versus sacroiliac joint dysfunction)

2. Anything about the problem or overall condition that may warrant caution with the objective examination (e.g., trauma, whiplash)

3. The character of the presenting patient or the problem: consider the psychologic, personality, ethnic, and socioeconomic factors or the patient's pain tolerance

Stage of pathology: This term describes the clinician's assessment of the stage in which the disorder is presenting (acute, subacute, chronic, acute on chronic). It involves a time frame from onset, which depends on the pathoanatomic nature of the problem and phase of tissue healing (e.g., fracture versus soft tissue). Stage may be obtained from the past and present history. A chronic symptom pattern with episodic acute aggravation of symptoms is common.

Stability: This term describes the progression of the patient's symptoms over time (the current episode or of all episodes over time). Is the problem getting better, getting worse, or staying the same?

Adapted from *Orthopaedic manual physical therapy: a description of advanced clinical practice,* Biloxi, MS, 1998, American Academy of Orthopaedic Manual Physical Therapists.

---

the patient history include establishing rapport, identifying any barriers to communication, identifying the patient's preferred learning style, and establishing the patient's goals for physical therapy. In addition, the PT can use this information to assist in determining the severity, irritability, nature, stage, and stability of the patient's condition[45] (Box 5-1). The history enables the PT to establish an early hypothesis regarding the source of the patient's symptoms, plan an appropriate physical examination, and establish a baseline of symptoms and functional level to measure changes subsequent to any interventions. Formation of an early hypothesis is a characteristic that distinguishes expert clinicians from novice clinicians.[33,34]

Verbal skills are vital during the patient interview. Starting with open-ended questions and then "funneling" to closed-ended questions that require a "yes" or "no" response to clarify information is recommended (Table 5-1). Open-ended questions allow patients to elaborate on details surrounding their primary concerns, whereas closed-ended questions provide more limited information. Closed-ended questions should come later in the interview. Also important is avoiding the use of biased questions that lead the patient to give the answer the PT wants to hear.[44] Instead of asking, "Did the treatment make you feel better?," it may be more effective to ask "How did the treatment make you feel?" or "Did the treatment make you any worse?" If the patient truly does feel better, the clinician may have more confidence in the patient's response with answers to the latter two questions.

TABLE 5-1

Open-Ended versus Closed-Ended Questions

Open-Ended Questions	Closed-Ended Questions
What makes your pain worse?	Does bending increase your pain?
What happens to your pain at night?	Does the pain worsen at night?
How did you feel after our last visit?	Were you any better after our last visit?
Can you describe the pain for me?	Is the pain dull or sharp?
How do you feel on waking?	Are you still or sore on waking?

Other effective verbal communication strategies include asking only one question at a time, speaking slowly and deliberately, and keeping questions brief. These strategies prevent the patient from getting confused and help the patient answer questions more accurately.[45] Periodically restating or summarizing what the patient has reported can also be beneficial, especially when the clinician is about to change topics or categories of questions. Using the patient's own words whenever possible can facilitate this process.[45] Simple sentences free of medical jargon are also helpful in preventing patient confusion.[45] Asking the patient to "flex" or "extend" the arm, or referring to patient's "signs and symptoms" should be avoided. Likewise, the PT should avoid using medical jargon for diagnosis. Terms such as *subacromial* or *retropatellar* typically do not have meaning to patients. Instead, the PT should use common terms, such as "under your shoulder" or "behind your kneecap."

Using the patient's line of thought, or paralleling the patient's mental processes, may also be helpful. In doing so, the PT is more likely to get an accurate picture of the patient's symptoms and how they are affecting his or her life.[45] Assumptions should be avoided, and any misunderstanding that does occur should be blamed first on the PT's inability to communicate effectively.[45] Physicians have been found most often to attribute communication problems to the patient rather than their own limitations.[43] Attributing frustration to patient characteristics alone may interfere with building a trusting relationship necessary for an optimal patient-provider relationship.[43]

Instead of blaming the patient for the miscommunication, the PT should rephrase the question instead. "I'm sorry, I wasn't very clear with that question. What I meant was …" is a good way to clarify without blaming the patient. These moments of misunderstanding and clarification are excellent opportunities for the PT to use self-evaluation and reflection to improve verbal skills. Reflecting on various aspects of clinical practice is another characteristic of expert clinicians.[31,34] Periodic self-assessment of the entire examination process, including the interview, with videotapes and audiotapes is a useful tool to critique one's ability to conduct an examination.

Throughout the patient interview, remembering that each question has a specific purpose that assists in early hypothesis formation and differential diagnosis is important. With each question, PTs must know what they want to know and why, what is the best way to word the question, what possible answers the patient may provide, and how the answer may influence future questions.[44]

Ethics, Empathy, and Humanism

> I have not been critical of the quality of services you deliver; I have been critical of the quality of their delivery.[82]

The complexities of clinical practice coupled with the spectrum of patient needs and personalities pose significant challenges for the PT. With changes in Medicare, capitation, health maintenance organizations, and managed care, clinical practice continues to be even more complex. As a result, clinicians can easily lose sight of the humanistic side of clinical practice. With advanced technology, clinicians often focus more on the pathoanatomic components of patients rather than the patients themselves. Many of us have caught ourselves referring to "the ACL reconstruction patient" or "the fibromyalgia patient" rather than "Mr. Jones, the plumber with three children who is unable to return to work 6 months after an ACL reconstruction."

Clinicians often shift from the human experience of illness or disability to various technologic facts about the disorder.[2] Clinicians sometimes have difficulty understanding human suffering that cannot be explained by specific anatomic or physiologic conditions. To help bridge this gap between the patient's experience with illness or functional limitations and the health care provider's focus on the most appropriate anatomic diagnosis, we need to have a paradigm that incorporates a more complete understanding of the human predicament.[2] We must reconcile scientific understanding with human understanding, using one to guide the other.[2] Although active listening, good eye contact, and open-ended questions are examples of strategies to incorporate empathy and humanism into the patient encounter, we must also be willing to venture beyond this to recognize and understand fully the concerns of the patient.[51] To make the humanistic aspect of patient care a habit, it is important to identify the multiple health issues present during a patient visit, reflect on possible conflicts, and support the patient's perspective.[51]

The foundation of humanistic patient care is understanding that each patient visit consists of three perspectives: the provider, the patient, and the patient's family.[51] Providers must learn to reflect and think critically about their own behavior and skills. True behavioral change occurs only when reflecting on new experiences and changing the structure of our own knowledge.[49] This reflective practice is also one of the characteristics of clinical expertise in physical therapy practice identified by Jensen and colleagues.[33] Finally, the provider must choose altruism— supporting the patient's perspective, even if it conflicts with the provider's own agenda.[51]

Similar to patient-centered interviewing skills, empathy and humanism can also be learned.[59,65,81] This process involves recognizing when the patient is expressing strong feelings or emotions, allowing the patient to express these feelings, acknowledging that these feelings make sense, and offering assistance.[59] Often, complicated and frustrating patient encounters can become productive interactions for the patient and the provider by pausing—doing nothing other than listening to the patient rather than feeling compelled to "do something."[14,59] Several words and phrases have been identified that build empathy, enabling the provider to connect with the patient (Box 5-2).[14] "Will you tell

---

BOX 5-2
Words that Build Empathy

QUERIES
Would you tell me more about that?
What has this been like for you?
Is there anything else?
Hmm ...

CLARIFICATIONS
Let me see if I have this right.
I want to make sure I understand you.
Am I hearing this right?
You let me know if I'm off track, OK?

RESPONSES
That sounds tough.
I imagine you might feel ...
I can see that you are ...
That's very good. You should feel good about that.

Adapted from Coulehan JL, Platt FW, Egener B, et al: "Let me see if I have this right ...": words that help build empathy, *Ann Intern Med* 135:221-227, 2001.

---

me more about that," "Is there anything else," and "Let me see if I have this right ..." all are useful in practicing clinical empathy.[14]

Ethical practice is a hallmark of the physical therapy profession. If patients or other health care providers perceive, through verbal and nonverbal communication, the personal values and attributes of the PT as deficient, it is likely to have a negative effect on the patient visit. PTs must use conduct that is decent, modest, sensitive, honest, sincere, benevolent, empathetic, courteous, and capable.[22]

Communication Challenges

Cultural differences, gender-related issues, and sensory impairments must be considered during any patient interaction. Female physicians have been found to conduct longer medical visits than male physicians (22.9 minutes versus 20.3 minutes), with approximately 40% more discussion occurring during the patient interview.[68] Patients of female physicians talk 58% more than patients of male physicians.[68] Female physicians engage in more positive talk, partnership-building, question-asking, and information-giving.[68] Based on these statistics, Roter and colleagues[68] concluded that female physicians might be more patient-centered in their interviewing than their male counterparts.

White patients tend to receive more information and more positive talk than African Americans or Hispanics.[69] Working class patients are less likely to question the health care provider than patients from higher social classes.[69] Although these differences in content were noted, there was no difference in overall length of visits by race,[69] and no differences in outcomes have been reported.

Language barriers and other sources of communication barriers must also be considered.[35] Effective communication may be hindered in patients with hearing loss, difficulty reading or seeing, social anxiety disorders, and other cultural issues. The patient is not the barrier, and either the patient or the provider

with these impairments has to develop strategies to be an effective communicator. Sometimes it is unclear whether language is the barrier or whether cultural practices prevent clear understanding between the patient and PT.[13] Understanding and respecting any cultural differences that may exist because of ethnic, social, and religious beliefs of the patient is important (see Chapter 3). Likewise, knowing one's own cultural values and biases is helpful because these attitudes can influence communication with patients and potentially affect outcome.[15,42,45] Developing a familiarity with the cultural values, health beliefs, and illness behaviors of the ethnic and religious groups commonly served in one's clinical practice may help improve communication.[14] Having health screening forms and patient outcome measures translated into several languages may also assist with gathering pertinent information (see Chapter 8).

Patients with Hearing Deficits

For the purposes of this discussion, it is assumed that the patient's hearing deficit does not warrant a physician consultation (see Chapter 10 for a discussion of how to determine whether hearing loss should be reported to the physician). Interviewing patients with hearing disturbances has unique challenges for the PT. The PT's history-taking goals described earlier are no different for these patients, but the PT needs to make adjustments for the interview to be judged a success by the patient and the PT. The following discussion presents strategies for interviewing patients with partial hearing and patients who are deaf.[11,16]

Finding a quiet area for the interview is paramount when working with a patient who is hearing-impaired, because excessive background noise can interfere with communication. Patients with hearing aids should be wearing them, and if glasses are necessary for clear vision, they should be worn as well. For the patient to read lips, the PT should be sitting in a well-lit area and positioned directly facing the patient. An exception to the recommendation of directly facing the patient is if the patient has unilateral hearing loss, in which case the PT should sit more toward the patient's "hearing side." Sitting 3 to 6 feet from the patient is recommended as the ideal distance to facilitate the communication process.[16] To facilitate continued visual facial contact, the PT should avoid covering his or her mouth while speaking and should avoid speaking to the patient while looking away to write down patient responses. Looking away to write down patient responses can also lead to the PT's voice "trailing off."

Speaking deliberately and in a relatively low-pitched voice can also aid communication. Presbycusis, hearing loss associated with aging, is the most common cause of hearing deficits in elderly adults and in most cases begins with a reduced capacity to hear higher frequencies.[27,91] To compensate for the patient's hearing impairment, PTs may be prone to speak very loudly, but yelling is not recommended. Speaking at a slightly louder than normal volume is more appropriate, and not allowing the voice to trail off at the end of sentences or questions is important. Gestures and demonstrations are important strategies designed to reinforce the verbal communication. In certain situations, handwritten questions and answers may be necessary (although they are time-consuming) to ensure accurate collection of data. Written questionnaires can facilitate the efficiency of collecting these data (see Chapter 8 for an example). Beyond the history-taking process, any oral instructions for these patients should be complemented with written instructions to ensure safe and accurate patient follow-through.

For patients who are deaf, the PT should determine the patient's preferred mode of communication. If lip reading is the choice, the aforementioned strategies are appropriate. If using sign language is the patient's preference, and the PT does not have this skill, working with an interpreter is appropriate.[11] Most importantly, the interpreter should have specific qualifications, including familiarity with medical concepts and terminology. A general rule to follow is that the interpreter should not be a family member or a child. Before starting the patient interview, the interpreter should be oriented to how the examination will proceed, and time should be provided for the interpreter and the patient to establish some rapport. The PT should pose all questions directly to the patient, keeping them short and simple and avoiding highly technical jargon. Verifying mutual understanding by periodically asking the patient to restate what has been discussed is important to ensure obtaining accurate information. Last, to avoid frustration on the part of the PT, it is important to understand that these visits take longer than usual and to make plans accordingly.

Patients Who Are Angry

Clinicians periodically encounter a patient who seems angry. How the clinician reacts and responds to such a patient determines whether the rehabilitation visit is productive or not, and whether the situation escalates into a hostile situation. Recognizing that the patient may be angry is the first step toward resolving the situation. For some patients, the anger is obvious—expressed verbally with direct statements that reflect unreasonable demands, annoyance, and resentment—and may be a part of an outburst. Other patients may express their anger in a more subtle fashion, such as with statements marked with sarcasm, cynicism, or negativism. Actions that are potentially self-destructive, such as noncompliance with recommended treatment, may also represent angry behavior. Finally, for some patients, nonverbal manifestations may be the initial cues that something is awry. A patient who is angry often has clenched fists or jaw, a pronounced frown on the face, or lips tightly compressed, and their gestures may be abrupt or jerky in nature.[3,86] When the PT recognizes that anger may be an issue, confirming that observation with the patient and determining why he or she is angry are the next important steps.

If the PT is uncertain but suspects that the patient may be angry, simply asking whether the patient is upset or angry about something is appropriate. If the patient asks why the question is being asked, the PT should describe the observations that led to the inquiry. If the angry behavior is overt, simply stating the obvious is appropriate: "You appear to be upset today, Mr. Jones; are you?" In either scenario, when the manifestations associated with the anger are subtle or obvious, the PT needs to inquire about the reason for the anger.

Potential reasons for a patient's anger are numerous and many times legitimate: adverse life events, a response to the suffering and disability associated with the patient's illness, or the sense of being helpless or mistreated within the health care system. Other possible reasons for anger include the patient waiting for an unacceptable period of time because the PT is behind schedule, the patient being treated in an inconsiderate or insensitive manner by the PT or other staff, or the patient's behavior reflecting that of the PT who seems to be angry.[11] When the source of anger is identified, the clinician can begin exploring the issues and formulating a specific plan.

The clinician should not react to any of the patient's comments with hostility or come across as being judgmental. Maintaining a calm voice and relaxed posture and making it clear that one is there to work with the patient can help prevent the situation from escalating. Actively engaging the patient in addressing the identified issues and possible solutions, and *not* focusing on the patient's behavior, can also facilitate a constructive resolution.[86] Displaying this empathetic attitude does not mean that the PT agrees with the patient's sentiments, but it is essential for an open and frank professional discussion to occur. If the anger is present during multiple patient visits, communication with the patient's physician is warranted. Persistent anger may be a manifestation of an organic or psychologic disorder, including chemical dependency or withdrawal.[1,3]

Finally, to protect the PT and the patient, the PT must be vigilant for signs of potential violence on the patient's part. The following are behavioral clues suggesting potential violent behavior[38]:

- Patient tensely moving to the edge of the chair
- Patient tensely gripping the arm rests
- Loud, forceful speech
- Restless agitation, pacing, and inability to sit still

In addition to staying calm, as described earlier, showing respect, maintaining eye contact, listening attentively, maintaining a safe distance from the patient, and avoiding any physical contact can help begin to defuse the situation. Trying to redirect the patient away from the factors contributing to the agitation and appealing to the patient to work with the PT toward identifying goals and solutions may also help.[86] In addition to these strategies, each facility should have operational procedures established in the event of a hostile interaction. These procedures should be reviewed as frequently as procedures associated with fire or violent weather.

Depressed Patients

A patient who is depressed may present the PT with multiple challenges during the interview. Impaired concentration is often a manifestation of depression[1] and can result in some patients being "poor historians." Strict adherence to the strategies outlined earlier in this chapter may facilitate the transfer of information from the patient to the PT, but short, delayed, and vague responses to questions can lead to frustration on the part of the PT. This frustration, if unchecked, impairs the communication process further. To complete an adequate examination within the usual time constraints, the PT may need to prioritize the interview questions even more than usual. Focusing on questions designed to assist in the planning of the physical examination should be emphasized initially. When the physical examination begins, the PT can continue to ask questions to collect additional information geared toward treatment planning and developing a prognosis. Ultimately in this scenario, the PT's clinical decision making may be directed primarily by the physical examination findings and much less so by the data collected during the history.

Beyond the examination process, the impaired concentration can affect the patient's ability to follow through with home instructions. For these patients, it is not a matter of purposely disregarding the PT's advice; the depression interferes with their ability to follow seemingly simple (from the PT's perspective) instructions. The PT should prioritize the exercises and the postural or ergonomic instructions to avoid overloading the patient. Providing written materials that are clear and concise may also facilitate compliance, but sometimes it may be necessary to recruit a caregiver or family member to assist with the home program.

Awareness that impaired concentration is a manifestation of this disease, just as chest pain can be a manifestation of ischemic heart disease, may keep this communication challenge in perspective. An understanding of how the impaired concentration can affect the rehabilitation process may help minimize frustration on the part of the PT. This awareness should direct the PT to use strategies designed to promote follow-through other than just scolding the patient for not doing the exercises. Last, contacting the attending physician or clinical psychologist for suggestions of strategies may be necessary.

Another potential challenge when working with patients who are depressed is that the depressed behavior or affect may be so intense that a productive visit is prohibitive. Counseling strategies (cognitive, behavioral, and interpersonal therapies) as summarized by Brody and colleagues[12] can be adapted and used by the PT to help salvage the visit of a patient with mild to moderate major depression. First, simply acknowledging that the patient seems to be depressed or feeling down, by saying "You appear to be having a rough day today," or "You appear to be down in the dumps today," may open the door to a constructive conversation. Exploring the potential reasons for the patient's condition occurs next. Sometimes stating the obvious is necessary: "Two weeks ago you were completely independent, but the fall and hip fracture have rendered you reliant on others for most of your daily care." Pointing out that these feelings are common in individuals who have had such a loss may help patients recognize that their predicament is not a result of failure or shortcomings on their part.

This communication portrays empathy and acknowledgment that you are aware of their feelings, and in some sense these statements give the patient permission to feel as they do. Discussing the short-term rehabilitation goals with the patient, and clearly describing the plan of how they will be attained, is very important. The thought of how much the patient needs to overcome to return to the preinjury level of function can seem insurmountable, leading to despondency, or the patient may have unrealistic expectations. This can be an equally important conversation to have with family members and caregivers to promote appropriate support for the patient.

Finally, suicide is a potential risk in patients who are depressed, as evidenced by the estimate that 15% of patients with a major depressive disorder commit suicide.[1] The expression of hopelessness is considered a risk factor for suicide in patients with major depression.[6,7,44,89] Statements such as, "I am not sure how much longer I can stand this," or "I am not sure this therapy is going to help," may be expressions of this sentiment. Follow-up questions related to the expression of hopelessness are important to determine the depth of the patient's despair. If the patient seems to have truly given up, the question, "Have things gotten so bad that you are considering harming yourself or taking your life?" is appropriate. If the answer is affirmative, the PT should follow with questions regarding the patient's plan and the availability of resources to carry out the plan. Avoiding the topic with a patient is an inappropriate action, and many patients with suicidal ideation are relieved to be asked about their intentions.[89] When this information is collected, implementing the facility's standing "suicidal patient procedure" is appropriate. Practitioners should not avoid asking patients whether they have had thoughts of hurting themselves or taking their lives in the fear of suggesting the idea of suicide to the patient.[88] Acknowledging suicidal ideation must occur first for proper management to occur. Chapter 20 further describes screening for conditions such as depression and suicidal ideation.

Summary

> A painstaking exercise in discernment and a grasp of small detail are infinitely worthwhile because in time they provide a grasp of musculoskeletal problem behavior which no other exercise in education can give.
>
> **G.P. Grieve, on the patient interview**

Communication between health care providers and patients is more than just an art. The concepts of patient-centered care, empathy, and humanism are not simply acquired skills. These skills can be taught, learned, and retained by aspiring health care providers and experienced clinicians. Specific training in psychosocial medicine improves patient and provider satisfaction, patient outcomes, and diagnostic efficiency and decreases malpractice claims. Despite the pressures and time constraints of managed care, patient-centered interviews require no more time to complete than purely biomedical examinations. In light of this convincing evidence, clinicians should strive to improve their communication skills and remember that the patient is the focus of clinical practice. Without the patient, we would not have a mechanism to learn, grow, and reflect on why we chose a career in the health sciences.

The late Geoff Maitland was one of the most highly skilled communicators in physical therapy practice. He "is prepared to visit carefully and thoughtfully that subjective world of [his] patients to ensure that [he] really does approximate [his] way of thinking to that of the patient."[25,45] Maitland "enters a close, point-to-point, moment-to-moment feedback loop" with his patients.[25,45] This is the essence of patient-centered care. Many health care providers remain inadequate at this core clinical skill. The age of paternalistic medicine has passed. Patients hold clinicians accountable for their attitudes, as well as their actions. As a result, clinicians, educators, and students must place more emphasis on this often-neglected science behind the art of clinical practice.

REFERENCES

1. American Psychiatric Association. Diagnostic and statistical manual of mental disorders. 4th ed. Washington, DC: American Psychiatric Association; 1994.
2. Baron RJ. An introduction to medical phenomenology: I can't hear you while I'm listening. Ann Intern Med 1985;103:606–11.
3. Barsky AJ. Approach to the angry patient. In: Goroll AH, Mulley AG, editors. Primary care medicine. Philadelphia: Lippincott Williams & Wilkins; 2000. p. 1187–8.
4. Bates AS, Harris LE, Tierney WM, et al. Dimensions and correlates of physician work satisfaction in a Midwestern city. Med Care 1998;36:610–17.
5. Beattie PF, Pinto MB, Nelson MK, et al. Patient satisfaction with outpatient physical therapy: instrument validation. Phys Ther 2002;82:557–64.
6. Beck AT, Steer RA, Kovacs M, et al. Hopelessness and eventual suicide: a 10 year prospective study of patients hospitalized with suicidal ideation. Am J Psychiatry 1985;142:559–63.
7. Beck AT, Brown G, Berchick RJ, et al. Relationship between hopelessness and ultimate suicide: a replication with psychiatric outpatients. Am J Psychiatry 1990;147:190–5.
8. Beckman HB, Markakis KM, Suchman AL, et al. The doctor-plaintiff relationship: lessons from plaintiff depositions. Arch Intern Med 1994;154:1365–70.
9. Beckman HB, Frankel RM. The effect of physician behavior on the collection of data. Ann Intern Med 1984;101:692–6.
10. Behaviors that undermine a culture of safety. Sentinel Event Alert 40 July, 2008.
11. Bickley LS. Bates' guide to physical examination and history taking. 7th ed. Philadelphia: Lippincott; 1999.
12. Brody DS, Thompson TL, Larson DB, et al. Strategies for counseling depressed patients by primary care physicians. J Gen Intern Med 1994;9:569–75.
13. Conine TA. Listening in the helping relationship. Phys Ther 1976;56:159–62.
14. Coulehan JL, Platt FW, Egener B, et al. "Let me see if I have this right …": words that help build empathy. Ann Intern Med 2001;135:221–7.
15. Croft JJ. Interviewing in physical therapy. Phys Ther 1980;60:1033–6.
16. Dwyer B. Detecting hearing loss and improving communication in elderly persons. In Focus on geriatric care and rehabilitation. Rockville, MD: Aspen Publishers; 1987. p. 6.
17. Duffy DF. Dialogue: a core clinical skill. Ann Intern Med 1998;128:139–41.
18. Epstein RM. The science of patient-centered care. J Fam Pract 2000;49:805–7.
19. Evans BJ, Stanley RO, Mestrovic R, et al. Effects of communication skills training on students' diagnostic efficiency. Med Educ 1991;25:517–26.
20. Farrell JP. In search of clinical excellence. J Orthop Sports Phys Ther 1996;24:115–21.
21. Garber MB: Informal survey (unpublished data), March 2001.
22. Gartland G. Essentials of ethics in clinical practice: a communications perspective. Physiother Canada 1987;39:179–82.
23. Goodman CC, Snyder TE. Differential diagnosis in physical therapy. 3rd ed. Philadelphia: WB Saunders; 2009.
24. Gordon JH, Walerstein SJ, Pollack S. The advanced clinical skills program in medical interviewing: a block curriculum for residents in medicine. Int J Psychiatry Med 1996;26:411–29.
25. Graham J. Communication. In Maitland's vertebral manipulation. 6th ed. London: Butterworth-Heinemann; 2001. p. 21–2.
26. Grieve GP. Mobilization of the spine. 5th ed. London: Churchill Livingstone; 1991.
27. Gulya AJ. Evaluation of hearing loss. In: Goroll AH, Mulley AG, editors. Primary care medicine. Philadelphia: Lippincott Williams & Wilkins; 2000. p. 1108–12.
28. Haber RJ, Lingard LA. Learning oral presentation skills: a rhetorical analysis with pedagogical and professional implications. J Gen Intern Med 2001;16:308–14.
29. Hawkes CM. Communicating with the patient in an example drawn from neurology. Br J Med Educ 1974;8:57–63.
30. Hickson GB, Federspiel CF, Pichert JW, et al. Patient complaints and malpractice risk. JAMA 2002;287:2951–7.
31. Hickson GB, Federspiel CF, Blackford J. Patient complaints and malpractice risk in a regional healthcare center. South Med J 2007;100:791–6.
32. Hulme JB, Bach BW, Lewis JW. Communication between physicians and physical therapists. Phys Ther 1988;68:26–31.
33. Jensen GM, Gwyer J, Hack LM, et al. Expertise in physical therapy practice. London: Butterworth-Heinemann; 1999.
34. Jensen GM, Shepard KF, Hack LM. The novice versus the experienced clinician: insights into the work of the physical therapist. Phys Ther 1990;70:314–23.
35. Joint Commission on Accreditation of Hospitals and Organizations handbook. Chicago: Joint Commission on Accreditation of Hospitals and Organizations; 2001.
36. Ladyshewsky R, Gotjamanos E. Communication skill development in health professional education: the use of standardised patients in combination with a peer assessment strategy. J Allied Health 1997;26:177–86.
37. Lang F, Floyd MR, Beine KL. Clues to patients' explanations and concerns about their illnesses: a call for active listening. Arch Fam Med 2000;9:222–7.
38. Leonard J, Harbst T. Medical emergencies in physical therapy. In: Boissonnault WG, editor. Examination in physical therapy practice: screening for medical disease. 2nd ed. New York: Churchill Livingstone; 1995. p. 358–60.
39. Levin MF, Riley EJ. Effectiveness of teaching interviewing and communication skills to physiotherapy students. Physiother Canada 1984;36:190–4.
40. Levinson WL, Bhat RG, Lamb J. A study of patient clues and physician responses in primary care and surgical settings. JAMA 2000;284:1021–7.
41. Levinson W, Roter DL, Mullooly JP, et al. Physician-patient communication: the relationship with malpractice claims among primary care physicians and surgeons. JAMA 1997;277:553–9.
42. Levinson W, Roter D. Physicians' psychosocial beliefs correlate with their patient communication skills. J Gen Intern Med 1995;10:375–9.
43. Levinson W, Stiles WB, Inui TS, et al. Physician frustration in communicating with patients. Med Care 1993;31:285–95.
44. Lewinsohn PM, Rohde P, Seeley JR. Adolescent suicidal ideation and attempts: prevalence, risk factors, and clinical implications. Clin Psychol Sci Pract 1996;3:25–46.
45. Maitland G, Hengeveld E, Banks K, et al. Maitland's vertebral manipulation. 6th ed. London: Butterworth-Heinemann; 2001. p. 23-36.
46. Maitland GD. Peripheral manipulation. 3rd ed. London: Butterworth-Heinemann; 1991.
47. Marvel MK, Epstein RM, Flowers K, et al. Soliciting the patient's agenda: have we improved? JAMA 1999;281:283–7.
48. Marvel MK, Doherty WJ, Weiner E. Medical interviewing by exemplary physicians. J Fam Pract 1998;47:343–8.
49. Maxwell M, Dickson DA, Saunders C. An evaluation of communication skills training for physiotherapy students. Medical Teacher 1991;13:333–8.
50. May WF. Listening carefully. Second Opinion 1994;20:47–9.
51. Miller SZ, Schmidt HJ. The habit of humanism: a framework for making humanistic care a reflexive clinical skill. Acad Med 1999;74:800–3.
52. Moore A, Jull G. The art of listening. Manual Therapy 2001;6:129.
53. Novack DH, Volk G, Drossman DA, et al. Medical interviewing and interpersonal skills teaching in US medical schools: progress, problems, and promise. JAMA 1993;269:2101–5.
54. Novack DH, Dube C, Goldstein MG. Teaching medical interviewing: a basic course on interviewing and the physician-patient relationship. Arch Intern Med 1992;152:1814–20.
55. Oh J, Segal R, Gordon J, et al. Retention and use of patient-centered interviewing skills after intensive training. Acad Med 2001;76:647–50.
56. Orthopaedic manual physical therapy: a description of advanced clinical practice. Biloxi, MS: American Academy of Orthopaedic Manual Physical Therapists; 1998.
57. Payton OD. Effects of instruction in basic communication skills on physical therapists and physical therapy students. Phys Ther 2001;63:1292–7.
58. Platt FW, Gaspar DL, Coulehan JL, et al. "Tell me about yourself": the patient-centered interview. Ann Intern Med 2001;134:1079–85.
59. Platt FW, Keller VF. Empathic communication: a teachable and learnable skill. J Gen Intern Med 1994;9:222–6.
60. Platt FW, McMath JC. Clinical hypocompetence: the interview. Ann Intern Med 1979;91:898–902.
61. Ramsden EL. Interpersonal communication in physical therapy. Phys Ther 1968;48:1130–2.
62. Realini T, Kalet A, Sparling J. Interruption in the medical interaction. Arch Fam Med 1995;4:1028–33.
63. Richards T. Chasms in communication. BMJ 1990;301:1407–8.
64. Rosenstein AH, O'Daniel M. Disruptive behavior and clinical outcomes: perceptions of nurses and physicians. Am J Nurs 2005;105:54–64.
65. Rosenstein AH, O'Daniel M. A survey of the impact of disruptive behaviors and communication defects in patient safety. Jt Comm J Qual Patient Saf 2008;34:464–71.
66. Roter DL, Stewart M, Putnam SM, et al. Communication patterns of primary care physicians. JAMA 1997;277:350–6.
67. Roter DL, Hall JA, Kern DE, et al. Improving physicians' interviewing skills and reducing patients' emotional distress: a randomized clinical trial. Arch Intern Med 1995;155:1877–84.
68. Roter D, Lipkin M, Korsgaardt A. Sex differences in patients' and physicians' communication during primary care medical visits. Med Care 1991;29:1083–93.

69. Roter DL, Hall JA, Katz NR. Patient-physician communication: a descriptive summary of the literature. Patient Educ Couns 1988;12:99–119.

70. Rubin FL, Judd MM, Conine TA. Empathy: can it be learned and retained? Phys Ther 1977;57:644–7.

71. Shapiro RS, Simpson DE, Lawrence SL, et al. A survey of sued and nonsued physicians and suing parents. Arch Intern Med 1989;149:2190–6.

72. Simpson M, Buckman R, Stewart M, et al. Doctor-patient communication: the Toronto consensus statement. BMJ 1991;303:1385–7.

73. Singleton MC. Independent practice—on the horns of a dilemma: a special communication. Phys Ther 1987;67:54–7.

74. Smith RC, Lyles JS, Mettler J, et al. The effectiveness of intensive training for residents in interviewing: a randomized, controlled clinical trial. Ann Intern Med 1998;128:118–26.

75. Smith RC, Lyles JS, Mettler JA, et al. A strategy for improving patient satisfaction by the intensive training of residents in psychosocial medicine: a controlled, randomized study. Acad Med 1995;70:729–32.

76. Smith RC, Osborn G, Hoppe RB, et al. Efficacy of a one-month training block in psychosocial medicine for residents: a controlled study. J Gen Intern Med 1991;6:535–53.

77. Smyth FS. The place of the humanities and social sciences in the education of physicians. J Med Educ 1962;37:495–9.

78. Stelfox HT, Gandhi T, Orav E, et al. The relation of patient satisfaction with complaints against physicians, risk management episodes, and malpractice lawsuits. Am J Med 2005;118:1126–33.

79. Stewart M, Brown JB, Donner A, et al. The impact of patient-centered care on outcomes. J Fam Pract 2000;49:796–804.

80. Stewart MA. Effective physician-patient communication and health outcomes: a review. Can Med Assoc J 1995;152:1423–33.

81. Suchman AL, Markakis K, Beckman HB, et al. A model of empathic communication in the medical interview. JAMA 1997;277:678–82.

82. Swartz F. The rehabilitation process: a view from inside. Rehabil Lit 1970;3:203–4.

83. Thornquist E. Body communication is a continuous process: the first encounter between patient and physiotherapist. Scand J Prim Health Care 1991;9:191–6.

84. Waddell G. The back pain revolution. London: Churchill Livingstone; 1998.

85. Wagstaff GF. A small dose of commonsense—communication, persuasion and physiotherapy. Physiother Canada 1982;68:327–9.

86. Welk F. Managing the hostile patient. PT Magazine 2000;8:68–70.

87. White J, Levinson W, Roter D. "Oh by the way …": the closing moments of the medical visit. J Gen Intern Med 1994;9:24–8.

88. Whooley MA, Simon GE. Managing depression in medical outpatients. N Engl J Med 2000;3443:1942–50.

89. Worthington JJ, Rauch SL. Approach to the patient with depression. In: Goroll AH, Mulley AG, editors. Primary care medicine. Philadelphia: Lippincott Williams & Wilkins; 2000. p. 1157–62.

90. Wright V, Hopkins R. What the patient means: a study from rheumatology. Physiotherapy 1978;64:146–7.

91. Zeeger LJ. The effects of sensory changes in older persons. J Neurosci Nurs 1986;18:325–32.

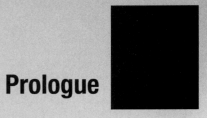

Prologue

William G. Boissonnault, PT, DPT, DHSc, FAAOMPT

Chapters 6 through 15 of Section Two present a recommended patient examination scheme; the author encourages the learner to read these chapters in order the first time through the text. The 10 chapters, each representing an important patient data category, are sequenced in accordance with an actual initial patient visit. These chapters also contain suggested tools, such as patient self-report questionnaires, that promote efficient data collection and allow for a smooth examination flow from one patient category to the next.

Figure 1 presents a flow chart illustrating patient data categories to be addressed in a recommended sequence during an initial visit. Sequencing the examination in such a manner allows for a more efficient collection of patient data and a more effective clinical decision-making process concerning the following:

- Deciding what questions to include or exclude as one progresses through the patient history
- Deciding what physical examination tests and measures to include or exclude
- Choosing interventions to be initiated during the first visit
- Determining whether a patient referral or consultation is needed

Access to patient demographic and social and health history information (see Chapter 8) before the start of the patient/family interview is very helpful to promote efficiency and effectiveness during the patient interview. In an inpatient setting, the patient medical record can be read before the interview, whereas in an outpatient setting, physician notes, a completed patient health history self-report form, or both could be read. This information is useful in determining the detail and depth of patient medical screening, establishing potential safety precautions for subsequent examination and intervention procedures, and formulating diagnoses and prognoses.

When the interview begins, the initial focus should be on what has precipitated the physical therapy visit. The emphasis differs depending on the nature of the visit—pain, neurologic complaints, or both that are interfering with function (see Chapters 6 and 7) or an interest in health and wellness issues (see Chapter 19). When this part of the interview is completed, investigating relevant health history (see Chapter 8) and screening for symptoms unrelated to the chief presenting complaint (review of systems) occurs (see Chapter 9). Finally, in terms of the patient interview process, the concept that the physical examination begins during the history portion of the examination is an important one. In terms of general observation, the physical examination begins as soon as the physical therapist (PT) makes visual contact with the patient and continues throughout the patient interview (see Chapter 10). This element of the physical examination includes a general assessment of posture, skin, and neurologic status.

Review medical history/Patient profile
↓
History/Interview begins
↓
Presenting complaints/Functional limitations
↓
Review relevant medical history
↓
Review of systems
(general health)
↓
Review of systems
(specific systems)
↓

| Cardiovascular Pulmonary Gastrointestinal Urogenital | Psychologic Endocrine | Nervous system Integumentary (Physical examination begins) |

Physical Examination
↓

| Vital signs Height/weight | Upper/lower quarter Screening examinations | Systems review |

Evaluation of data (ongoing throughout above process)
↓

| Treat | Treat and refer | Refer only |

FIGURE 1 Examination/evaluation.

Chapters 11, 12, and 13 cover the physical examination proper, including elements appropriate for all patients and other elements to be included based on patient history information and initial physical examination findings. Chapter 11 covers topics appropriate for all patients, including vital signs and patient height and weight. Chapters 12 and 13 describe an upper and lower quarter screening examination scheme. Finally, as presented in Chapters 14 and 15, diagnostic imaging and laboratory values represent patient information that may be critical to the PT's decision making, including knowing when to refer patients for such testing.

Symptom Investigation, Part I: Chief Complaint by Body Region

6

Joseph Godges, DPT
Michael S. Wong, DPT, OCS FAAOMPT
William G. Boissonnault, PT, DPT, DHSc, FAAOMPT

Objectives

After reading this chapter, the reader will be able to:

1. Describe the types of patient data that fall under the category of symptom investigation, including the information that constitutes a red flag requiring physician contact.
2. Summarize symptoms and signs associated with medical disorders that may result in patient pain syndromes common to physical therapy practice.
3. Describe medical screening questionnaires and incorporate them into an examination scheme for patients with common pain syndromes.

Many individuals seek physical therapy services for chief complaints of lower back, shoulder, or knee pain.[12,29,53] Many of these patients assume the symptoms are related to a sprain, strain, poor posture, or arthritic condition. For some of these patients, however, the symptoms are related to a more serious medical condition. Low back pain may be related to cancer, infection, visceral disease, or fractures. Jarvik and Deyo[50] estimated that, of patients with low back pain presenting to ambulatory primary care clinics, 4% have symptoms associated with an osteoporosis-related fracture; 1% to 2%, with a traumatic fracture including spondylolisthesis/spondylolysis; 2%, with visceral disease; 0.7%, with cancer; and 0.5%, with infection.

These estimates of disease-related back pain highlight the initial primary objective of the examination process: deciding whether (1) physical therapist (PT) intervention is appropriate; (2) consultation with another health care provider is required along with PT intervention; or (3) PT intervention is not indicated, and the patient needs to be managed by another provider.[25] A detailed description of the back pain is often the point in the examination at which the PT's suspicion of a potentially serious etiology of symptoms is first raised. This suspicion is based on an atypical description of symptoms provided by the patient, often described as a nonmechanical pain presentation. Does the patient provide a story of how and when the symptoms began, and how they change (or do not) with postures and movements—as the region is being mechanically loaded and unloaded—that makes sense based on the PT's understanding of basic and clinical sciences and the PT's clinical experiences?

The detailed symptom investigation includes subcategories of symptom location and description, onset (history) of symptoms, and behavior or pattern of symptoms. The location and description of symptoms should alert the PT to other possible "pain generators" (e.g., ischemic heart disease manifesting as shoulder pain or mid-back pain). The PT must know what diseases could produce local pain or referred pain in a region so that he

or she can screen for other symptoms or signs associated with these conditions. The follow-up questions related to when and how the back pain began, how the pain fluctuates over a 24-hour period, and what makes the pain better or worse are critical to the screening process. The assumption is that most impairment-driven conditions (mechanical pain patterns) manifest with pain onset marked by macrotrauma or microtrauma (repetitive overuse) and consistently vary based on time of day and associated activities, with assumption of specific postures, and during movements and functional activities that load and unload the involved body region.

This chapter provides the medical screening principles associated with investigating patients' chief presenting symptoms based on location of symptoms. Various causes of pain in specific body regions (low back; pelvis, hip, and thigh; knee, leg, ankle, and foot; thorax; cervical spine and shoulder; head and face; and elbow, wrist, and hand) are presented, providing PTs with a list of diseases to "think about" as they examine patients. The remainder of the examination will, it is hoped, allow the PT to state with confidence, "I am not worried about heart or lung disorders causing the shoulder pain," or maybe, "I need to worry about such conditions," with subsequent physician contact. Recognizing important history and physical examination information common to these disorders is a key step in this differential diagnosis process. To assist the reader, summary tables and self-report medical screening questionnaires for each of the seven body regions are presented as quick clinical reference guides.

Part of the discussion in this chapter includes knowing what follow-up questions to ask related to potential red flag findings. Night pain (pain that wakes a patient from sleep) is considered a red flag and has been linked to serious pathology, such as cancer, infection, ischemic heart disease, and peptic ulcer disease—all conditions that require physician examination and management. Yet some authors have associated night pain with degenerative joint disease, especially of the lumbar spine, hip, and knee joints, and others have noted that night pain occurs in a large proportion of patients who apparently do not have a serious disease. So, when is night pain a red flag, suggestive of a potentially life-threatening disorder? Can the clinician determine the seriousness of this symptom with further questioning after the patient reveals the night pain?

The goal of the screening process is early recognition of the need for a physician referral, speeding up the diagnosis of systemic and other pathologic processes. The more timely the diagnosis, the greater chance of minimizing morbidity and mortality. The most common symptom associated with back pain and cancer is simply a dull ache, with an average of 9 months passing between when the ache begins and the tumor diagnosis is made.[80] In this case, the PT has contributed to the diagnosis being made by the physician.[14]

Symptom Investigation

Location of Symptoms

To help document symptoms, the authors recommend using a body diagram for noting the exact location of symptoms and describing symptoms, including pain quality (e.g., ache, burning, shooting), paresthesia, numbness, and weakness. The questioning should start with the patient's chief presenting complaint, the symptoms that are most interfering with function: "What brings you here today," or "I understand you are having some trouble with your knee—is that what brings you here today?" Depending on the patient's response to these open-ended questions, follow-up questions can provide the detail needed to proceed through the rest of the examination. Examples of follow-up questions regarding symptom location include the following:

- Do the chief complaint symptoms move or spread up, down, or around you?
- Can you rate the symptom intensity on a 0-to-10 scale—when you are feeling your best, your worst, and an average?
- Do you have symptoms anywhere else?

Figure 6-1 shows the patient presented with low lumbar and right buttock pain (dull ache). After reporting these symptoms, the patient stated, "That is all of the symptoms I have."

The next follow-up question is: "So you don't experience any pain, pins and needles, weakness, or numbness down the backs of your legs; on the bottoms of your feet; up the front of your body, including the pelvis, stomach, chest, neck, or face; or between your shoulder blades, and you don't experience any headaches?" Noting where the patient *does not* have symptoms

(the check marks on the body diagram) is just as important as documenting where the patient does experience symptoms. Patients may not volunteer that they have abdominal pain or facial pain. Their rationale may be, "Why does the PT need to know if my stomach hurts? I am here for my low back pain," or "My physician takes care of my stomach problem, not my PT." One reason disease-related symptoms may be missed is that the patient has such severe or intense symptoms in one area that he or she pays little attention to a mild ache that was present before the injury. This aching may not be limiting function at all, and it is perceived as not being a big deal. That ache may or may not be associated with the chief presenting complaint and may be the initial manifestation of a more serious disorder. Asymptomatic areas should be noted on the body diagram with a check mark or some other notation, as shown in Figure 6-1.

Pain from visceral structures typically would be thought to be located in the anterior chest wall or abdominal regions, but numerous viscera are located in the retroperitoneal region of the trunk. These structures include portions of the duodenum, ascending and descending colon, abdominal aorta, pancreas, and kidneys, and if these structures are diseased, back pain, rather than abdominal pain, may be manifested. Ischemic heart disease may manifest in the classic middle-aged male pattern noted in Figure 6-2, but cardiac pain may also be noted in the epigastric, interscapular, right shoulder, throat, jaw, or tooth regions. There is considerable "overlap" between pain location patterns associated with visceral disorders and common musculoskeletal disorders (Table 6-1; see Figure 6-2). In addition, many pain-generating diseases simply manifest as a dull ache, stiffness, or mild to moderate soreness in their early or middle stages; these also are very common conditions for many patient populations that respond to physical therapy interventions.

Although the symptom location helps differentiate diseases from impairments only occasionally, these patient data do play an important role in the medical screening process. Knowledge of potential pain patterns associated with viscera can guide the PT in selecting the organ systems to screen with questions related to review of systems (see Chapter 9). Finally, knowing the pain patterns associated with various diseases helps the PT know which disorders should be suspected as he or she performs the examination. The tables in this chapter are designed to provide such information.

The investigation of symptoms also includes the patient's description of the symptoms. Patients use more than one descriptor for their back pain, including ache and stiffness, or aching, and sharp soreness. The PT must assess each descriptor independently of the others, including the onset and pattern of symptoms. Hearing a similar pattern (aggravating and alleviating factors) for each of the descriptors would lead the PT to believe all three symptoms are related to the same lesion, but hearing different symptom fluctuation patterns should lead the PT to consider the back pain might have more than one source.

Certain descriptors are unusual for musculoskeletal impairment disorders, as follows[9,40,68,89]:

- Vascular disorders—throbbing, pounding, pulsating
- Neurologic disorders—sharp, lancinating, shocking, burning
- Visceral disorders—aching, squeezing, gnawing, burning, cramping

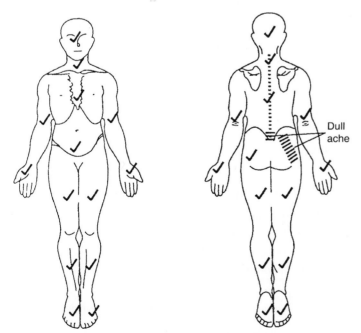

Dull ache

FIGURE 6-1 Body diagram used to illustrate symptomatic and asymptomatic body regions. (From Boissonnault WG: *Examination in physical therapy practice: screening for medical disease*, 2nd ed, New York, 1995, Churchill Livingstone, p 5.)

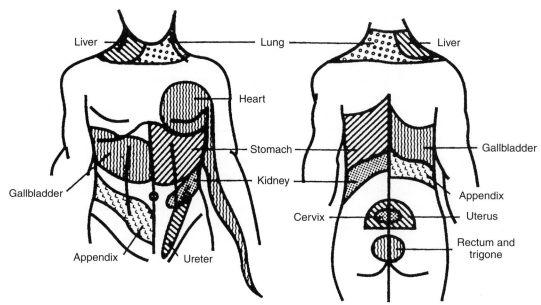

FIGURE 6-2 Possible local and referred pain patterns of visceral structures. (From Boissonnault WG: *Examination in physical therapy practice: screening for medical disease,* 2nd ed, New York, 1995, Churchill Livingstone, p 6.)

TABLE 6-1
Visceral Local and Referred Pain Patterns

Structure	Segmental Innervation	Possible Areas of Pain Location
PELVIC ORGANS		
Uterus including uterine ligaments	T1-L1, S2-S4	Lumbosacral junction, sacral, thoracolumbar
Ovaries	T10-T11	Lower abdominal, sacral
Testes	T10-T11	Lower abdominal, sacral
RETROPERITONEAL REGION		
Kidney	T10-L1	Thoracolumbar junction (ipsilateral), middle lumbar, lower abdominal, upper abdominal
Ureter	T11-L2, S2-S4	Groin, medial/proximal thigh, upper abdominal, suprapubic, thoracolumbar, iliac crest
Urinary bladder	T11-L2, S2-S4	Sacral apex, suprapubic, thoracolumbar
Prostate gland	T11-L1, S2-S4	Sacral, perineal, testes, thoracolumbar
DIGESTIVE SYSTEM ORGANS		
Esophagus	T4-T6	Substernal and upper abdominal
Stomach	T6-T10	Upper abdominal, middle and lower thoracic spine
Small intestine	T7-T10	Middle thoracic spine
Pancreas	T10	Upper abdominal, lower thoracic spine, upper lumbar spine
Gallbladder	T7-T9	Right upper abdominal, central and right-sided middle and lower thoracic spine, right scapula
Liver	T7-T9	Right middle and lower thoracic spine, right cervical spine
Common bile duct	T8-T10	Upper abdominal, middle thoracic spine
Large intestine	T11-L1	Lower abdominal, middle lumbar spine, buttock
Sigmoid colon	T11-T12	Upper sacral, suprapubic, left lower quadrant of abdomen
CARDIOPULMONARY SYSTEM		
Heart	T1-T5	Cervical anterior, jaw, teeth, upper thorax, epigastric, left upper extremity, right shoulder and upper extremity
Lungs and bronchi	T5-T6	Ipsilateral thoracic spine, chest wall, cervical (diaphragm involved)
Diaphragm (central portion)	C3-C5	Cervical spine

Adapted from Boissonnault W, Bass C: Pathological origins of trunk and neck pain: parts I, II, III, *J Orthop Sports Phys Ther* 12:191-221, 1990.

Hollow viscus pain may come in waves—called *colicky pain*. Often associated with organ distention or smooth muscle spasm, the pain builds to a crescendo and then may slowly recede. Terms commonly used in medical literature for such conditions include *biliary* or *renal colic* depending on which structures are involved. Gastroenteritis, constipation, menstruation, gallbladder disease, and ureteral obstruction all have been implicated in causing colicky pain experienced in the abdominal or back areas.[73]

If the peritoneum is involved, the pain tends to be more intense and severe—more easily localized by the patient, With peritoneum involvement, coughing and movements can be very painful, and patients choose to lie very still.[9,40] As noted earlier, visceral pain may be noted on the posterior aspect of the trunk and pelvis depending on anatomic location of the structure and pain referral patterns. Critical to pain assessment is patients noting associated symptoms indicative of organ involvement and systemic disorders. Chapter 9 presents detailed material regarding review of systems and key symptoms that may assist in interpreting pain complaints. Although some descriptors are unusual for musculoskeletal conditions, other diseases manifest with pain complaints frequently heard from patients commonly seen by PTs. Slipman and colleagues[80] noted that a dull ache is the most common pain complaint associated with cancer. Many patients seen by PTs present with a dull diffuse ache. As with location of symptoms, symptom descriptors alone often do not provide enough information on which to base a referral.

Symptom History

For many patients, the current episode of symptoms is not the first episode, but the most relevant information for this initial visit is investigating the most recent injury or flare-up. If the patient is asked, "When did your symptoms begin?," the reply may be "20 years ago," and after a 5-minute discussion of the incident 20 years past, the PT might conclude that he or she has learned nothing that influences today's clinical decision making. To promote practice efficiency, the discussion should be started with the current or most recent episode, working backward chronologically.

Impairment-related symptoms typically are associated with a traumatic incident, an accident, repetitive overuse, or sustained postural strains. These events may include lifting an object, falling, or taking an extended car ride or plane trip, or the patient may report shoulder or back pain after a day of heavy yard work. Many patients cannot relate the onset of their symptoms to any particular incident or accident, however. Careful questioning by the PT reveals a likely cause, such as the patient beginning to run after not running for 3 months, being promoted to an administrative position that requires sitting for 8 hours per day, or beginning gardening or yard work after a winter of inactivity. If the onset of symptoms is truly insidious, if new symptoms occur insidiously during the course of treatment, or if resolved symptoms return for no apparent mechanical reason, the PT should be concerned about the underlying nature of the condition.[105]

Comparing and contrasting current and past events can reveal important information. One way pain-generating diseases may "slip through" the health care system occurs when a patient with chronic neck pain has a new episode. In the patient's

mind, this is the "usual" neck pain, and if a PT already has seen this patient a few times for neck pain, the PT may make the same assumption. These assumptions may lead the patient to fail to report a unique finding about his or her current episode, and may cause the PT to skip steps in the examination process. In the past, the flare-ups might have always been associated with prolonged travel or time at a computer, but neither travel nor computer time is associated with this episode. An overview of symptom onset and the 24-hour report would quickly reveal a story that is or is not consistent with previous episodes. For the initial visit, starting with the current or recent onset consistently provides the PT with information relevant to critical decision making. Discerning how the current complaints may be consistent with the complaints of the past is important, but requesting, "Tell me when this all started," can lead to a long, unproductive discussion.

Behavior and Pattern of Symptoms

The patient report of symptom site and intensity changes over a defined time period produces information vital to the medical screening process. The PT should ask questions regarding the following:

- The relationship symptoms have to rest, activities, time of day (morning, midday, evening, or night) and positions and postures
- The constancy, frequency, and duration of symptoms, including fluctuations in intensity[65]

For many patients with neuromusculoskeletal disorders, a description of how symptoms do or do not change over a 24-hour period is adequate. For patients with disorders such as multiple sclerosis, stroke, or head injury, the time frame may be 3 to 6 months.

In addition to insidious onset of symptoms, reports of unexpected or atypical behavior of symptoms may be the initial clue that raises the suspicion of a serious underlying condition. Symptoms associated with impairments or movement disorders typically fluctuate as the mechanical loads on the body increase or decrease with time of day, onset or cessation of specific activities, and assumption or avoidance of certain postures. This expected symptom behavior pattern fits many patients seeking physical therapy services, with or without a pathoanatomic etiology of symptoms. In a study of pain profiles for patients with low back pain, Boissonnault and DiFabio[13] found no difference in the time of day pain was most intense, movements and postures that altered symptoms, or frequency of night pain in patients with disk pathology (degeneration, internal disruption, herniation, or bulging) versus patients with no pathoanatomic findings on magnetic resonance imaging (MRI) or computed tomography (CT) scans. If the symptom pattern reveals no consistent pattern, the PT should begin questioning whether physical therapy intervention is warranted. This inconsistent symptom pattern should alert the PT to screen specific body systems later in the examination (see Chapter 9).

The fact that symptoms do vary in intensity or are intermittent does not rule out the presence of serious medical disorders. If a patient's thoracic spine pain is the result of a duodenal ulcer, gastrointestinal system activity may alter the symptoms. The ulcer symptoms probably would be reduced shortly after the patient eats because the food acts as a buffer, and a few hours after eating, the pain would return or intensify. Most patients probably would not make the connection between eating and pain level; the patient may attribute the symptoms to certain activities or to working at a computer for many hours. Careful questioning about the change of symptoms over a 24-hour period may reveal inconsistencies that catch the clinician's attention.

Finally, an inconsistent pattern of change in symptom intensity is not the only warning sign that may be discovered during questioning regarding behavior of symptoms. Symptoms that move from one body location to another for no apparent mechanical reason are also an atypical report for many patients seeking physical therapy services. A patient may note right shoulder and wrist pain during the initial visit, and at the second visit report right and left shoulder and left elbow and wrist pain. This patient cannot describe any reason why the apparently new pains have started. Primary neurologic, endocrine, or rheumatic disorders or adverse drug reactions may account for a symptom pattern such as this (see Chapters 7 and 9).

The investigation of symptom behavior over a defined time includes questions about night pain. Night pain (pain that wakes someone from sleep) has been associated with serious diseases such as cancer and infection.* One cannot assume serious disease is not present in patients not experiencing night pain, however. Slipman and colleagues[80] reported that approximately 50% of patients with musculoskeletal tumors experienced night pain. Many studies also describe night pain as being associated with degenerative joint disease, especially of the lumbar, hip, and knee regions.† In addition, a significant percentage of patients with low back pain reported night pain with no evidence of serious disease. So, when is night pain a red flag? When night pain is reported, follow-up questions should include the following:

- How many nights per week?
- Is there a consistent time when you wake up?
- How does the intensity of the night pain compare with the pain experienced at other times of the day?
- What do you have to do to fall back asleep?

Boissonnault and DiFabio[13] noted that 53% of patients with a complaint of back pain reported night pain. Only one patient of this group stated that the night pain was more intense than the pain in the morning, midday, or evening, and almost 80% stated that they simply had to change position in bed to fall back to sleep. This pattern would be expected for a patient with nonacute low back pain. The practitioner would assume that the lumbar area would be mechanically loaded to a greater degree, and more painful, when the patient was physically active. In addition, many patients with low back pain start the night sleeping supine with a pillow under the knees or side-lying with a pillow between the legs to support the lumbar region but wake up with the pillows on the floor and lying halfway onto their stomach. Low back discomfort wakes these patients up, but they fall back to sleep with minimal effort after the pillows are back in place. More concern would be warranted if the night pain was the patient's most intense pain, and if it took more than minimal

effort to fall back to sleep (nonpositional night pain and non-acute conditions). Based on the current evidence, one must conclude that the presence of night pain as the sole red flag has little diagnostic value but must be considered in context of the other examination findings.

The symptom investigation often is the step that first alerts the PT to the possible need for a patient referral. Careful questioning reveals a pattern of symptoms that is unusual for patients with impairment-driven conditions. Using a body diagram to document the location of symptoms and a description of the symptoms can save documentation time for the PT. A well-organized sequence of questions allows a patient to give an accurate history of his or her reasons for seeking medical care:

- In which area are symptoms most interfering with functions or daily activities?
- Describe the symptoms (e.g., ache, pins and needles).
- Do these symptoms spread to any other body regions or parts?
- Can you rate the intensity of the symptoms on a 0-to-10 scale—at best, at worst, and on average?
- Was there a recent injury or flare-up? If so, when?
- If not, can you explain why these symptoms may have begun?
- Are the symptoms constant, or do they come and go?
- What makes the symptoms worse or better?
- Do the symptoms wake you up at night?
- Have you had any previous episodes similar to this?
- Do you have symptoms anywhere else? (If the answer is yes, repeat the previous questions.)

Regional Pain Patterns and Associated Diseases and Disorders

Low Back Pain

Consider a 55-year-old patient with a recent history of insidious low back pain who is being examined by a PT. In the waiting room, the patient was given four forms to fill out: one outcome measure (Modified Oswestry Low Back Pain Disability Questionnaire),[37] one prognosticating tool (Fear-Avoidance Beliefs Questionnaire [FABQ][39]), a typical medical history intake form, and a body region–specific red flag screening form. The modified Oswestry score was 44%, and the key red flag finding here was that the patient marked, "The pain is moderate and does not vary much." The modified Oswestry score indicates severe disability, which is uncommon especially when pain is occurring with no clear precipitating factors, again raising suspicion in the clinician's mind that something other than typical musculoskeletal back pain should be screened for. The FABQ scores were 6 for physical activity scale and 4 for the work scale. With typical back pain, a more recent study[39] suggests that elevated FABQ work scale scores greater than 20 would have indicated a two to five times higher likelihood of showing no improvement at 6 months (poor prognosis).

In this patient's case, the low FABQ scores indicate to the clinician that work beliefs play a minimal role in this patient's overall pain schema, and FABQ work scale scores of less than 5 also indicate that this patient is three times more likely to experience improvement at 6 months, which is contrary to this patient's course of symptom progression, which is staying the

---

*References 1, 8, 10, 77, 95, 98.
†References 1, 32, 35, 51, 55, 79.

same or getting worse. These tools lead the clinician to consider other potentially nonmusculoskeletal sources for the pain. Four serious conditions that may manifest as low back pain are tumors, spinal infections, vertebral fracture, and cauda equina syndrome.[10] As this patient is describing the pain and activity limitations, he reports that his pain has not resolved with rest or anti-inflammatory medications over the past 6 weeks. The PT recalls that lack of improvement for a patient older than 50 years with acute low back pain is a red flag, increasing the index of suspicion that the patient's low back pain is caused by a tumor rather than by a less serious musculoskeletal disorder such as a lumbar or sacroiliac ligament sprain.[28]

This patient's reported lack of improvement leads the PT to verify the patient's age and ask whether the patient has a history of cancer or has experienced recent, unexplained weight loss. Evidence supporting the value of these inquiries is found in a study by Deyo and Diehl[27] on patients with low back pain who had cancer. Deyo and Diehl[27] reported that of the 13 patients whose low back pain was caused by cancer (out of a total subject pool of 1975 patients with low back pain), all 13 were older than 50 years of age, had a history of cancer, had experienced unexplained weight loss, or had failed to improve with conservative therapy. The PT asks the 55-year-old patient the following questions to increase or decrease the index of suspicion that this patient's low back pain is caused by cancer:

- Do you have a history of cancer? If so, what type of cancer (e.g., lung, breast, prostate)?
- Have you recently lost weight, even though you have *not* been attempting to eat less or exercise more? If so, how much?

The patient responds "no" to each question. Next, the PT considers three other serious pathologies that may cause low back pain. One of these conditions is a back-related infection, such as spinal osteomyelitis.[97] The red flags that raise suspicion of osteomyelitis as a cause of the low back pain all are factors that put the patient at risk for spinal infection. These factors are current or recent bacterial infection (e.g., urinary tract or skin infections), intravenous drug use or abuse, and concurrent suppression of the patient's immune system. The PT asks the following questions to increase or decrease the index of suspicion that this patient's low back pain is caused by a back-related infection:

- Have you recently had a fever?
- Have you recently taken antibiotics or other medicines for an infection?
- Have you been diagnosed with an immunosuppressive disorder?
- Does your pain ease when you rest in a comfortable position?

Again, the patient responds "no" to all of the above-listed questions. Negative responses to the first three questions reduce the suspicion that this patient has a back-related infection. A negative response to the fourth question suggests, however, that the patient's low back pain is *not* due to a musculoskeletal disorder because pain related to musculoskeletal disorders typically is eased when the patient rests in a comfortable position.

To rule out the likelihood of spinal fracture as a cause of this patient's low back pain, the patient is asked whether any trauma to the spine triggered the onset of pain. In addition, the PT asks whether the patient has any history of osteoporosis because minor strains or falls may produce an unsuspected spinal fracture

in an individual with osteoporosis. The PT also asks whether the patient has a history of other disorders that increase the risk of decreased bone density, including hyperparathyroidism, renal failure, chronic gastrointestinal disorders, and long-term use of corticosteroids:

- Have you recently had a major trauma, such as a vehicle accident or a fall from a height?
- Have you ever had a medical practitioner tell you that you have osteoporosis or other disorders that could cause "weak bones"?

The PT asks the 55-year-old patient these questions and receives negative responses, which greatly reduces the suspicion of fracture as a cause of this patient's low back pain.

Finally, to rule out cauda equina syndrome associated with this patient's low back pain, the PT relies on historic and physical examination data. The PT asks the following questions:

- Have you noticed a recent onset of difficulty with retaining your urine or starting urine flow?
- Have you noticed a recent need to urinate more frequently?
- Have you noticed a recent onset of numbness in the area of your bottom where you would sit on a bicycle seat?
- Have you recently noticed your legs becoming weak while walking or climbing stairs?

A positive response to any of these questions increases the suspicion that the patient has a cauda equina syndrome. The PT follows these inquiries with a physical examination, assessing the sensory integrity of the perianal and perineal areas, as well as the L4, L5, and S1 dermatomes. The PT also assesses the motor integrity of the L4 (quadriceps and tibialis anterior), L5 (extensor hallucis longus and foot everters), and S1 (ankle plantar flexors) musculature (see Chapter 13). In our example, all of the history and physical examination findings suggesting a cauda equina lesion were negative. Table 6-2 summarizes the red flags for the low back region, and a low back medical screening questionnaire is provided in Box 6-1.

The patient's response that his pain does not ease when he rests in a comfortable position suggests a nonspinal pathology mimicking a back problem. This possibility justifies an examination for a possible serious condition in an adjacent region (see the discussion later on colon cancer). The PT found no other red flags, however, suggesting a back-related tumor or infection, spinal fracture, or cauda equina syndrome. Reviewing the function of the gastrointestinal, urogenital, and vascular systems may be especially helpful in patients with low back pain whose presentation and symptoms suggest a nonmusculoskeletal disorder.

Pelvis, Hip, and Thigh Disorders

The serious medical conditions that may mimic common musculoskeletal disorders of the pelvis, hip, and thigh include colon cancer, pathologic fractures of the femoral neck, osteonecrosis of the femoral head, Legg-Calvé-Perthes disease, and slipped capital femoral epiphysis. Colon cancer, the third most common cancer in women and men,[52] is a result of malignant neoplasms that develop in the large intestine, from the cecum to the rectum. Colon cancer is most common in individuals 50 years and older sand who have a family history of colon cancer. The initial symptoms usually are a change in bowel habits, such as blood in the stools (if the lesion is near the rectum) or black stools (if the

TABLE 6-2

Red Flags for the Low Back Region

RED FLAGS		
Condition	**Data Obtained During History**	**Data Obtained During Physical Examination**
Back-related tumor[27]	Age >50 yr	Constant pain not affected by position or activity
	Personal history of cancer	Worse at night
	Unexplained weight loss	
	Failure of conservative therapy	
Back-related infection (spinal osteomyelitis)[95]	Recent infection (e.g., urinary tract or skin infection)	Deep constant pain, increases with weight bearing
	Intravenous drug user/abuser	Fever, malaise, and swelling
	Concurrent immunosuppressive disorder	Spine rigidity; accessory mobility may be limited
Cauda equina syndrome[10]	History of spinal stenosis	Urine retention or incontinence
	History of degenerative intervertebral disk disease	Fecal incontinence
		Saddle anesthesia
		Global or progressive weakness in the lower extremities
		Sensory deficits in the feet (i.e., L4, L5, S1 areas)
		Ankle dorsiflexion, toe extension, and ankle plantar flexion weakness
Spinal fracture[10,28]	History of trauma (including minor falls or heavy lifts for osteoporotic or elderly individuals)	Exquisitely tender with palpation over fracture site
	Long-term steroid use	Increased pain with weight bearing
	Age >70 yr	Edema in local area
Abdominal aneurysm[41,59]	Back, abdominal, or groin pain	Abnormal width of aortic or iliac arterial pulses
	Presence of peripheral vascular disease or coronary artery disease and associated risk factors (age >50 yr, smoker, hypertension, diabetes mellitus)	Presence of a bruit in the central epigastric area upon auscultation
	Symptoms *not* related to movement stresses associated with somatic LBP	

LBP, low back pain.

lesion producing the bleeding is located in the more proximal portion of the colon).

Colon cancer is an especially deadly disease because malignant neoplasms can develop undetected for many years before the onset of bowel symptoms. PTs, along with other health care professionals, must stress to patients the importance of routine screening examinations for colon cancer (e.g., sigmoidoscopy and colonoscopy) for individuals with a family history of this disorder. Polyps, which are the precursor to cancerous lesions in the colon, often can be excised if they are discovered during a colonoscopy examination. In the later stages of colon cancer, a palpable mass may be felt in the abdominal cavity.

PTs often see patients with mid-back and thoracic cage pain, and the most common metastatic presentation of colon cancer includes the thoracic spine and rib cage. The following information, collected by a PT during a history or physical examination, could be red flags for colon cancer[87]:

- Age older than 50 years
- History of colon cancer in an immediate family member (first-degree relative) (see Chapter 8)
- Bowel disturbances (e.g., rectal bleeding or black stools) (see Chapter 9)
- Unexplained weight loss (see Chapter 9)
- Back or pelvic pain that is unchanged by positions or movement

Disorders of the proximal femur are another type of serious condition that the PT may encounter. As the elderly population increases, PTs will be more likely to detect and manage patients with pathologic fractures of the femoral neck. Pathologic fractures of the femoral neck occur secondary to disease and often in the absence of trauma. These fractures are most common in individuals older than 50 years (women more often than men) who have a history of metabolic bone disease, such as osteoporosis or Paget's disease. A history of a fall from a standing position is often reported, along with a feeling of a sudden, painful snap in the hip region and a giving way. Acute groin pain usually is reported, but pain also may be felt in the anteromedial thigh or in the trochanteric region. The physical examination usually reveals that the involved extremity appears shortened compared with the contralateral side and typically is held in an externally rotated position.[92]

Another serious disorder of the proximal femur is osteonecrosis (also known as *avascular necrosis*) of the femoral head. Osteonecrosis of the femoral head is a result of insufficient arterial supply to this region. This ischemic process eventually results in death of the bony tissue of the femoral head and can be associated with hip trauma, such as fractures or dislocations. It also can be associated with nontraumatic conditions, such as sickle cell disease, and with long-term corticosteroid administration,

Medical Screening Questionnaire for the Low Back Region

Question	Yes	No
1. Have you recently had a major trauma, such as a vehicle accident or a fall from a height?		
2. Have you ever had a medical practitioner tell you that you have osteoporosis?		
3. Do you have a history of cancer?		
4. Does your pain ease when you rest in a comfortable position?		
5. Have you recently had a fever?		
6. Have you recently lost weight even though you have not been attempting to eat less or exercise more?		
7. Have you recently taken antibiotics or other medicines for an infection?		
8. Have you been diagnosed as having an immunosuppressive disorder?		
9. Have you noticed a recent onset of difficulty with retaining your urine?		
10. Have you noticed a recent need to urinate more frequently?		
11. Have you noticed a recent onset of numbness in the area of your bottom where you would sit on a bicycle seat?		
12. Have you recently noticed your legs becoming weak while walking or climbing stairs?		

Adapted from Bigos S, Bowyer O, Braen G, et al: Acute lower back problems in adults. Clinical practice guideline no 14. AHCPR publication no. 95-0642, Rockville, MD, December 1994, Agency for Health Care Policy and Research, Public Health Service, US Department of Health and Human Services.

as in patients receiving corticosteroid therapy for management of rheumatoid arthritis, systemic lupus erythematosus, or asthma. Nontraumatic osteonecrosis of the femoral head may be bilateral in 60% of cases.[86]

A similar condition that occurs in children (most common in 5- to 8-year-old boys) is Legg-Calvé-Perthes disease. This condition results from an idiopathic loss of blood supply from the lateral ascending cervical artery to the femoral head. Patients with osteonecrosis and Legg-Calvé-Perthes disease often report pain in the groin, thigh, and knee that worsens with weight-bearing activities, resulting in an antalgic gait. Common clinical findings in children with Legg-Calvé-Perthes disease also include shortening of the involved extremity and limited internal rotation and abduction of the involved hip.[101] Internal rotation typically is tested in these cases with the patient prone, with both extremities simultaneously internally rotated, and with the angles of the tibial shaft relative to the table compared. Abduction is tested with the patient supine in the hook-lying position (with the knees flexed to approximately 90 degrees and both feet positioned on the table adjacent to the midline). The patient is instructed to relax his or her adductor muscles and to allow the knees to fall out to the "frog-leg" position (i.e., horizontally abducted toward the table). This test allows easy comparison of the involved and uninvolved hips; abduction is measured by using the angles of the tibial shaft relative to the table, with the femurs in approximately 45 degrees of hip flexion.[26]

A hip disorder that occurs in adolescence is slipped capital femoral epiphysis, which involves progressive displacement of the femoral head relative to the neck through the open growth plate. It is more common in boys (male-to-female ratio 2.5:1) who are typically, but not always, overweight. Patients with slipped capital femoral epiphysis usually experience groin, thigh, or knee pain that is described as diffuse and vague (i.e., difficult to pinpoint). Common findings of the physical examination are antalgic gait, involved extremity positioned in external rotation, and limitations in hip internal rotation range of motion.[18] The red flags for slipped capital femoral epiphysis and the other serious conditions of the pelvis, hip, and thigh region are listed in Table 6-3. Box 6-2 presents a self-report questionnaire that can help in screening for these conditions.

Knee, Lower Leg, Ankle, and Foot Pain

The remaining regions of the lower quarter to consider are the knee, leg, ankle, and foot regions. Two important conditions, compartment syndrome and deep vein thrombosis (DVT), are described in detail. In addition, three other potentially serious conditions of the knee, leg, ankle, and foot that a PT is likely to encounter are described: peripheral arterial occlusive disease, septic arthritis, and cellulitis.

Peripheral arterial occlusive disease, also known as *peripheral vascular disease,* is the manifestation of atherosclerosis below the bifurcation of the abdominal aorta. This disease is common because the risk factors for heart disease that are so widespread in our society (i.e., history of type 2 diabetes, smoking, sedentary lifestyle) are also the risk factors for peripheral arterial occlusive disease. Individuals who have a history of ischemic heart disease should be assumed to have peripheral arterial occlusive disease until proved otherwise. A primary clinical feature of this disease is intermittent claudication. A patient with intermittent claudication often complains of aching in the buttock and of thigh and calf pain that is precipitated by walking, intensifies with walking, and disappears with rest. In addition, the patient may complain of the distal extremities feeling cold. The physical examination findings that suggest peripheral occlusive arterial disease include decreased pedal pulses (i.e., posterior tibialis and dorsalis pedis arteries) (see Chapter 13), a unilateral cool extremity, and wounds and sores on the toes or feet.

The PT can perform two special tests that aid in confirming the presence of peripheral vascular disease: the reactive hyperemia test and the ankle-to-arm systolic pressure index (ankle-brachial index) (see Chapter 11). The reactive hyperemia test assesses the integrity of the vascular system in redistributing blood with postural changes. The PT performs this test by elevating the leg of a patient who is lying supine to 45 degrees of hip flexion (i.e., a unilateral straight leg test to 45 degrees). The lower extremity is maintained in this position for 1 to 3 minutes, or until the color of the foot, ankle, and lower leg is blanched. The examiner then lowers the limb and measures the number of seconds required for the limb to turn pink. The normal time is 1 or 2 seconds. A venous filling time of greater than 20 seconds indicates peripheral occlusive arterial disease.

The PT obtains the ankle-to-arm systolic pressure index by measuring the highest systolic blood pressure at the ankle (using the dorsalis pedis and posterior tibial arteries) with a hand-held Doppler flowmeter and dividing it by the blood pressure in the brachial artery. An ankle-to-arm systolic pressure index that is less than 0.97 indicates the presence of peripheral occlusive

TABLE 6-3

Red Flags for the Pelvis, Hip, and Thigh Region

RED FLAGS		
Condition	**Data Obtained During History**	**Data Obtained During Physical Examination**
Colon cancer[87]	Age >50 yr Bowel disturbances (e.g., rectal bleeding, black stools)	Later stages: may have hypoactive or hyperactive bowel sounds from obstruction Possible tenderness to palpation of abdomen in area of cancer
	Unexplained weight loss	May have ascites
	History of colon cancer in immediate family Pain unchanged by positions or movement	First sign may be of metastases to liver, lung, bone, or brain
Pathologic fractures of the femoral neck[92]	Older women (age >70 yr) with hip, groin, or thigh pain	Severe, constant pain—worse with movement Shortened and externally rotated lower extremity
	History of a fall from a standing position	
Osteonecrosis of the femoral head (also known as avascular necrosis)[86]	History of long-term corticosteroid use (e.g., in patients with rheumatoid arthritis, systemic lupus erythematosus, asthma)	Gradual onset of pain; may refer to groin, thigh, or medial knee that is worse with weight bearing Stiff hip joint; restrictions primarily in internal rotation and flexion
	History of osteonecrosis of the contralateral hip Trauma	
Legg-Calvé-Perthes disease[101]	5- to 8-year-old boys with groin/thigh pain	Antalgic gait Pain complaints aggravated with hip movement, especially hip abduction and internal rotation
Slipped capital femoral epiphysis[18]	Overweight adolescent	Aching in groin exacerbated with weight bearing
	History of a recent growth spurt or trauma	Involved leg held in external rotation Range of motion limitations of hip internal rotation

BOX 6-2

Medical Screening Questionnaire for the Pelvis, Hip, and Thigh Region

Question	Yes	No
1. Have you recently had a trauma, such as a fall?		
2. Have you ever had a medical practitioner tell you that you have osteoporosis?		
3. Have you ever had a medical practitioner tell you that you have a problem with the blood circulation in your hips?		
4. Are you currently taking steroids or have you received long-term steroid therapy?		
5. Does your pain ease when you rest in a comfortable position?		
6. Do you have a history of cancer?		
7. Has a member of your immediate family (i.e., parents or siblings) been diagnosed with cancer?		
8. Have you recently lost weight even though you have not been attempting to eat less or exercise more?		
9. Have you had a recent change in your bowel functioning, such as black stools or blood in your rectum?		
10. Have you had diarrhea or constipation that has lasted for more than a few days?		
11. Do you have groin, hip, or thigh aching or pain that increases with physical activity, such as walking or running?		

arterial disease.[16,67] See Chapter 11 for a detailed description of the ankle-brachial index.

A major therapy for patients with peripheral vascular disease is aerobic exercise, such as progressive walking. PTs often may help design and monitor exercise programs for patients with this disorder. When a screening examination of a lower extremity musculoskeletal disorder suggests peripheral occlusive vascular disease, however, the PT must also assume the presence of ischemic heart disease until proved otherwise. A physician evaluation (often including an exercise tolerance test) and medical management (often including medications) of the underlying cardiovascular disorder are essential so that the PT can proceed with the plan of care confident in the patient's safety.

Another serious condition of the lower extremity that may initially appear as a musculoskeletal strain is DVT. A DVT is a spontaneous obstruction of the popliteal vein of the calf and may manifest as a gradual or sudden onset of calf pain, typically intensified with standing or walking and reduced with rest and elevation. Fifty percent of patients with DVT do not experience the calf pain. The risk factors that predispose an individual to DVT are recent surgery, malignancy, trauma, prolonged immobilization of the extremities (including placement of the limb in a cast or immobilizer and a long car ride or plane trip, especially for individuals already at risk for DVT), and pregnancy. Physical examination findings that increase the suspicion of a DVT are localized calf tenderness, calf swelling and edema, and skin warmth. The diagnosis of DVT is confirmed with contrast venography or other imaging procedures. The potential that the blood clot may travel proximally toward or into the pulmonary vessels is the risk that makes a DVT a serious condition that requires referral to a physician for a medical examination and possible intervention, including anticoagulant medication.

The red flags that suggest the presence of a DVT are listed in Table 6-4. See Chapter 20 for additional information regarding DVT and pulmonary emobolism.

PTs often help in the management of patients who have experienced trauma or overuse (i.e., repetitive trauma) strains to the legs. The inflammatory phase of healing that accompanies these traumas can lead to an abnormal increase in pressure in one of the fascial compartments of the leg. This abnormal increase in pressure resulting from acute swelling inside a fascial connective tissue compartment is called a *compartment syndrome*. The vascular occlusion and nerve entrapments that are possible sequelae of a compartment syndrome make this condition a medical emergency. The PT must know the red flags that signify the presence of a compartment syndrome when examining musculoskeletal disorders of the lower extremity.

Patients with compartment syndromes have a history of a blunt trauma or crush injury or of participating in an unaccustomed physical activity involving the lower extremities, such as rapidly increasing the amount of running distance (e.g., while training for a marathon) or walking distance (e.g., while participating in a long hike). The patient often reports severe, persistent leg pain that is intensified when stretch is applied to the involved muscles. The physical examination reveals swelling, exquisite tenderness, and palpable tension (i.e., hardness) of the involved compartment. The nerve entrapment or compression found in this condition results in paresthesias and potentially in paresis or paralysis. The vascular compromise accompanying this condition results in diminished peripheral pulses (i.e., dorsalis pedis or posterior tibial) and potentially pallor. A mnemonic that clinicians use to remember the signs of a compartment syndrome are the six *P's*: *p*ain, *p*alpable tenderness, *p*aresthesias, *p*aresis, *p*allor, and *p*ulselessness.

The two remaining potentially serious conditions that may mimic lower extremity musculoskeletal disorders are related to infections. One is septic arthritis, which is an inflammation in a joint caused by a bacterial infection, and the other is cellulitis, which is an infection in the skin and underlying tissues after bacterial contamination of a wound. Patients who have septic arthritis complain of a constant aching or throbbing pain and swelling in a joint. The involved joint is usually tender and warm when palpated. Patients who develop septic arthritis often are immunosuppressed or have preexisting joint disease. This immunosuppression may be a result of corticosteroid administration, alcohol abuse, renal failure, malignancy, diabetes mellitus, intravenous drug abuse, collagen vascular disease, organ transplantation, or acquired immunodeficiency syndrome (AIDS).

Examples of preexisting joint diseases that predispose individuals to septic arthritis are rheumatoid arthritis, osteoarthritis, and psoriatic arthritis. The cause of the septic arthritis also is usually associated with a local or distant site of infection or a history of a recent joint surgery or intra-articular injection. An example of a distant infection site in a patient is a gonococcal infection. Sexually active individuals who are exposed to

---

TABLE 6-4

Red Flags for the Knee, Leg, Ankle, or Foot Region

Condition	RED FLAGS	
	Data Obtained During History	**Data Obtained During Physical Examination**
Peripheral arterial occlusive disease[16,67]	Age >60 yr	Unilaterally cool extremity (may be bilateral if aorta is site of occlusion)
	History of type 2 diabetes	Prolonged capillary refill time (>2 sec)
	History of ischemic heart disease	Decreased pulses in arteries below level of the occlusion
	Smoking history	Prolonged vascular filling time
	Sedentary lifestyle	Ankle-brachial index <0.90
	Concurrent intermittent claudication	
Deep vein thrombosis[100]	Recent surgery, malignancy, pregnancy, trauma, or leg immobilization	Calf pain, edema, tenderness, warmth
		Calf pain that is intensified with standing or walking and relieved by rest and elevation
		Possible pallor and loss of dorsalis pedis pulse
Compartment syndrome[15,88,93]	History of blunt trauma, crush injury, or unaccustomed exercise	Severe, persistent leg pain that is intensified with stretch applied to involved muscles
		Swelling, exquisite tenderness and palpable tension/hardness of involved compartment
		Paresthesia, paresis, pallor, pulselessness
Septic arthritis[100]	History of recent infection, surgery, or injection	Constant aching or throbbing pain, joint swelling, tenderness, warmth
	Coexisting immunosuppressive disorder	May have elevated body temperature
Cellulitis[100]	History of recent skin ulceration or abrasion, venous insufficiency, congestive heart failure, or cirrhosis	Pain; skin swelling; warmth; advancing, irregular margin of erythema/reddish streaks
		Fever, chills, malaise, and weakness

gonorrhea may develop gonococcal septic monarthritis or gonococcal septic polyarthritis.[102]

Infection in the tissues—cellulitis—exhibits the classic signs of pain; skin swelling; warmth; and an advancing, irregular margin of erythema or reddish streaks. On further inquiry, patients with these findings also may report other classic signs of infection: fever, chills, malaise, and weakness (see Chapter 9). Individuals with congestive heart failure, lower extremity venous insufficiency, diabetes mellitus, renal failure, liver cirrhosis, and advancing age are predisposed to developing cellulitis. The precipitating factor to developing cellulitis is typically a recent skin ulceration or abrasion.[102]

The management of septic arthritis and cellulitis includes monitored administration of antibiotic therapy, and referral of the patient to a physician should be expedited. The medical screening questionnaire for peripheral arterial occlusive disease, DVT, compartment syndrome, septic arthritis, and cellulitis is presented in Box 6-3; see Table 6-4 for red flags.

Thoracic Pain

CARDIAC AND PULMONARY DISORDERS. The thoracic spine and rib cage lie close to many organ systems that, when diseased, usually result in local or referred pain to the thoracic cage. In addition, metastatic disease and bone diseases usually manifest as pathologic fractures of the thoracic vertebrae and ribs.[46] The patient who reports "back pain" may have an underlying serious medical condition when the reported back pain is in the thoracic region. This section briefly discusses the clinical presentation and red flags of cardiac (myocardial infarction and unstable and stable angina), pulmonary (lung cancer, pneumothorax, pneumonia, pleurisy, and pulmonary embolus), gastrointestinal (peptic ulcers and cholecystitis), and urogenital (pyelonephritis) conditions.

Myocardial infarction (an acute blockage of a coronary artery resulting in death to a portion of the myocardium) has the highest mortality rate of any of the disorders discussed in this chapter

---

BOX 6-3

Medical Screening Questionnaire for the Knee, Leg, Ankle, or Foot Region

Question	Yes	No
1. Have you recently had a fever?		
2. Have you recently taken antibiotics or other medicines for an infection?		
3. Have you recently had surgery?		
4. Have you recently had an injection to one or more of your joints?		
5. Have you recently had a cut, scrape, or open wound?		
6. Have you been diagnosed as having an immunosuppressive disorder?		
7. Do you have a history of heart trouble?		
8. Do you have a history of cancer?		
9. Have you recently taken a long car ride, bus trip, or plane flight?		
10. Have you recently been bedridden for any reason?		
11. Have you recently begun a vigorous physical training program?		
12. Do you have groin, hip, thigh, or calf aching or pain that increases with physical activity, such as walking or running?		
13. Have you recently sustained a blow to your shin or any other trauma to either of your legs?		

(see also Chapter 20). A cardinal clinical feature of myocardial infarction is angina, chest symptoms that are described as discomfort, pressure, tightness, or squeezing with potential referral into the arms, neck, or jaw regions. The classic presentation of pain in the left chest and left upper extremity is not the norm for women or elderly individuals. Pain experienced in the epigastric; mid-thoracic spinal; right shoulder; or neck, jaw, and teeth regions may be the presentation for these patients. One of every three patients diagnosed with myocardial infarction did not have chest pain on initial presentation to a hospital emergency department.[20] Instead of pain as the primary manifestation, myocardial infarction may appear with the clinical features of dyspnea, nausea or vomiting, palpitations, syncope, or cardiac arrest. The risk factors for this atypical presentation of myocardial infarction are a history of diabetes, older age, female sex, nonwhite racial or ethnic group, and a history of congestive heart failure and stroke.[20]

Two related terms that PTs should understand are *stable* and *unstable angina pectoris*. Stable angina, as the name implies, is substernal chest pain or pressure with possible pain referral to the left upper extremity that occurs with predictable exertion or known precipitating events, such as exercise or exertion at an intensity level higher than usual. The chest pain that occurs with stable angina also is predictably alleviated with change in the precipitating event (e.g., rest) or with self-administration of sublingual nitroglycerin. Chest pain that occurs with stable angina is benign, especially if relief is gained with rest and administration of nitroglycerin.

Unstable angina, also as the name implies, is chest pain that occurs outside of a predictable pattern and that does not respond to nitroglycerin. Individuals experiencing unstable angina must be closely monitored (see Chapter 9). Signs suggesting myocardial infarction, such as substernal squeezing or crushing pressure, pain radiation to both arms, shortness of breath, pallor, diaphoresis, or angina lasting more than 30 minutes, should alert the PT that this is an emergency condition and that immediate transportation to an appropriate emergency department or coronary care facility is indicated. The survival rate of patients experiencing a myocardial infarction is greatly improved if therapy known to improve survival is available and used appropriately. These therapies include thrombolysis of primary angioplasty, aspirin, beta blocker therapy, and heparin.[42]

Chest pain that extends to the left shoulder and possibly down the left arm also may be pericarditis. This chest pain usually is accompanied by fever and increases with lying down, inhalation, or coughing and is alleviated with forward leaning while sitting. Pericarditis is an inflammation of the pericardium, a sac that surrounds the heart to keep it in place, to prevent overfilling with blood, and to protect the heart from chest infections. The pericardium becomes inflamed by bacterial, viral, or systemic diseases, such as kidney failure, systemic lupus, rheumatoid disease, heart failure, or increased fluid around the heart when there is leakage from an aortic aneurysm. This inflammation around the heart prevents complete expansion because the additional pressure from the inflammation results in less blood leaving the heart. To make up for the reduced stroke volume and to get enough oxygen to the tissues, the heart beats faster. If increased heart rate cannot compensate enough, the individual may start to breathe heavily, the veins in the neck may distend, and blood pressure may decrease drastically during inhalation. This condition is termed *cardiac tamponade* and is often a medical emergency. Emergency medical care is needed to remove the pressure on the heart and to restore proper cardiac output.

Pulmonary embolus (see Chapter 20) is a pulmonary condition that may produce angina-like pain. An acute massive pulmonary embolism can produce crushing chest pain that mimics myocardial infarction, especially if the blood clot, usually traveling from the calf, thigh, or pelvic veins, reaches a major pulmonary artery. The location of the chest pain usually is substernal, but the pain can be located anywhere in the thorax depending on the location of the embolus. Shoulder pain or upper abdominal pain may occur. In addition to chest pain, patients with a pulmonary embolus may develop dyspnea, wheezing, and a marked decrease in blood pressure. Factors that increase the risk of blood clots in the lower extremities or pelvis and subsequent embolus include immobilization or recent surgery; these are two patient types that PTs frequently treat. Pulmonary embolism also has a high mortality rate, so if the PT suspects this condition, he or she should immediately refer the patient to emergency care so that a definitive diagnosis can be made and appropriate anticoagulant therapy (e.g., intravenous streptokinase, heparin) can be administered.

Two other pulmonary conditions that can cause chest pain are pleurisy and pneumothorax. Pleurisy is an irritation of the pleural membranes that make up the lining between the lungs and the inner surface of the rib cage. The pain that pleurisy produces is characteristically described as sharp and stabbing and is worsened by deep inspiration and other rib cage movements, such as a cough. Passive movement testing of the rib cage and thoracic spine also may produce pleuritic pain. Pleurisy may have multiple causes, such as viral infections or tumors, and is associated with disorders such as rheumatoid arthritis. Each of these conditions requires a definitive diagnosis and intervention by a physician. Suspicion of this disorder should lead the PT to auscultate over the thorax, listening for a "pleural rub" sound. See Chapter 11 for an overview of auscultation of heart and breath sounds.

Pneumothorax—air in the thoracic cage—also produces chest pain that is intensified with deep inspiration. A pneumothorax can be a spontaneous, usually pathologic event associated with rupture of the wall of the lung lining. Such a rupture prevents the lung from maintaining negative pressure during diaphragmatic and rib cage motions. A simple pneumothorax may begin without any precipitating event, or it may follow a bout of extreme coughing or strenuous physical activity. The physical examination findings that are associated with a pneumothorax include limited ability of the affected side of the chest to expand, hyperresonance of the affected area on percussion, and markedly reduced breath sounds. A small pneumothorax may resolve within a few days without therapy. A large pneumothorax requires aspiration of the air from the lung. Factors predisposing individuals to pneumothorax are menstruation (in young women), asthma, chronic obstructive pulmonary disease, cystic fibrosis, and lung cancer.

A tension pneumothorax usually is a consequence of a trauma, such as a penetrating wound to the rib cage or a severe blow to the rib cage that may occur in contact sports or during an automobile injury (with the individual hitting the steering wheel). The signs of a tension pneumothorax include severe pleuritic-type chest wall pain, extreme shortness of breath, tracheal deviation, distended neck veins, tachycardia, hypotension, and hyperresonance to percussion of the involved (painful) side of the chest. Tension pneumothorax can be an extreme emergency requiring insertion of a chest tube with a seal or Heimlich valve.[102]

Finally, another cause of pleuritic-type chest pain is pneumonia, which is a bacterial or viral infection of the lungs. The signs of systemic infection, such as chills, fever, malaise, nausea, and vomiting, typically accompany the pleuritic pain. The fever may be absent in elderly patients, with onset or worsening of confusion being the primary manifestation (see Chapter 9). A distinguishing characteristic of pneumonia is a cough that produces sputum of varying coloration, from light green to dark brown.

GASTROINTESTINAL DISORDERS. Gastrointestinal disorders are common in the general population and may manifest as comorbidities during the examination process. The PT should routinely ask patients about bowel movement characteristics, vomiting, unexplained weight loss, or extended use of nonsteroidal antiinflammatory drugs (NSAIDs) (see Chapter 9). Common gastrointestinal disorders include gastric or peptic ulcer disease and cholecystitis. Ulcers occur when the lining of the digestive tract is exposed to digestive acids and are named according to their anatomic location. An ulcer in the duodenum is called a *duodenal ulcer* and is associated with the presence of *Helicobacter pylori* bacteria in the stomach. Duodenal ulcers manifest as dull, gnawing, or burning pain in the epigastric region, in the mid-thoracic (T6-T10) region, or in the supraclavicular region. These symptoms occur when the stomach is empty and are relieved with eating or taking antacids. Relief is temporary, however, and the symptoms return within 2 to 3 hours. If the ulcer is located in the stomach (a gastric ulcer), eating may increase, rather than relieve, the symptoms. These ulcers are more common in elderly adults secondary to increased use of NSAIDs (see Chapter 4).

In contrast to duodenal ulcers, gastric ulcers can be malignant and need the attention of a physician even if symptoms spontaneously resolve when the drugs are stopped. With esophageal ulcers, the individual experiences pain with swallowing or when lying down. Symptoms of these ulcers include black, tarry-colored stools; bright red or reddish brown clumps (coffee-ground emesis) in the vomit; relief or intensification of pain with eating; and pain in the chest, back, or supraclavicular area.

The other common gastrointestinal disorder is cholecystitis, an inflammation of the gallbladder. The initial symptom often is pain in the right upper abdominal quadrant or in the interscapular or right scapular regions,[30] which can be constant and intense. Pain usually is severe enough to cause nausea and vomiting. Murphy's sign is positive (inspiration inhibited by pain on local palpation in the right upper abdominal quadrant) in more than 50% of patients with cholecystitis.[62] Patients initially may seek pain control from a PT but should be referred to their physician or local emergency department. Inflammation of the gallbladder usually is caused by a gallstone lodged in the cystic duct, and medical help is needed to remove the gallstone.

KIDNEY DISORDERS. Disorders of the kidney such as pyelonephritis and renal stones result in pain in the posterior lateral aspect of the thoracic cage and upper lumbar area. PTs may see the terms *costovertebral angle* or *flank* in physician notes referring to this region. Both conditions manifest with chills, fever, nausea, vomiting, and renal colic. Renal colic is excruciating intermittent pain from the costovertebral angle or flank that spreads across the lower abdomen into the labia in women and into the testicles and penis in men. The pain is associated with spasms in the ureter and may extend down to the inner thighs.

Pyelonephritis is an infection in the kidney, usually caused by an infection of the ascending urinary tract. Individuals with recent or coexisting urinary tract infections are at risk for pyelonephritis. Blood-borne pathogens or conditions causing obstruction of urine flow (benign prostatic hyperplasia or kidney stones) also may cause renal infections.

Kidney stones (nephrolithiasis if in the kidney, urolithiasis if anywhere else in the urinary tract) are hard masses of salts that precipitate from the urine when it becomes supersaturated with a particular substance. Most stones are composed of calcium; less commonly, stones are composed of uric acid, cystine, or struvite (a combination of magnesium, ammonium, and phosphate). Risk factors for developing kidney stones are warm, humid atmospheric temperatures and diseases (e.g., leukemia) that involve high cell turnover. The incidence of kidney stones in men is four times greater than in women.[100] White men have three times as many stone episodes as black men. Approximately 5% to 15% of the population is expected to have kidney stones during their lifetime.[100] The best predictor for kidney stones is a past episode because approximately 50% of patients experience at least one recurrence.[76] A PT who suspects these conditions should refer the patient for medical attention. Table 6-5 summarizes the red flags for thoracic symptoms, and Box 6-4 presents a questionnaire for screening.

Shoulder and Cervical Pain

Patients with shoulder and cervical symptoms compose a large portion of an orthopedic PT's caseload.[12,29,53] Compared with the thorax, fewer serious disorders involve the shoulder and neck regions. Metastasis does not occur in the cervical region as often as in other regions of the axial skeleton.[98] PTs should be familiar with a few conditions, however, including central cord syndromes, ligamentous instability, brachial plexus neuropathies, and Pancoast's tumor.

The PT should rule out a ligamentous injury after trauma, such as a motor vehicle accident or a fall, but trauma is not the only condition that should alert the PT to the possibility of ligamentous instability. Patients with rheumatoid arthritis, Down syndrome, or ankylosing spondylitis, and women who use oral contraceptives, should be screened for ligamentous instability of the neck. The alar and transverse ligaments maintain the proper relationship of C1 on C2, whereas the ligamentum flavum, anterior and posterior longitudinal ligaments, and interspinous and intertransverse ligaments help maintain the proper alignment through the entire cervical region. Resultant instability can lead to significant neurologic and cardiovascular consequences, and PTs should routinely screen for such symptoms.

Neurologic symptoms associated with ligamentous instability can include the typical presentation of tingling, numbness, weakness, or burning pain. The PT should be concerned about possible compromise of the spinal cord if the patient has these symptoms in more than one extremity (see Chapter 20). In addition, dizziness, vertigo, or nystagmus associated with head or neck movements should alert the PT. Symptoms such as these in a patient who has been involved in a traumatic event or has a positive history of the previously mentioned disorders that can lead to instability should prompt the PT to conduct special stability tests, such as the Sharp-Purser test and the alar and transverse ligament stress tests. Other potential signs to note during the physical examination are clonus and a positive Babinski's sign.[68]

Brachial plexus neuropathies can occur secondary to repetitive overuse, postural syndromes, and trauma. Nerves affected by such neuropathies can be of three categories: sensory, motor, or mixed. The emphasis is on motor nerves, but there is no such thing as a pure motor nerve. A motor nerve carries efferent commands to the muscles but also returns with information from the muscles, joints, and associated ligamentous structures. A nerve that innervates a muscle also augments the sensation from the joint on which that muscle acts. Pain produced by a motor nerve entrapment neuropathy is not well localized, is present at rest, and has a retrograde distribution. The muscles innervated can be tender to palpate, and if the neuropathy has been present for an extended time, muscle atrophy is present, although the patient may be unaware of the weakness. The greatest challenge with entrapment neuropathies is not treatment but diagnosis. These neuropathies are more often the cumulative result of many small traumas or long-standing compression or are of mechanical origin.

With the evaluation of any new patient, the PT should conduct a thorough examination of motor and sensory function and reflexes in the area of interest (see Chapters 12 and 13). The PT should carefully observe the area, preferably with the area disrobed to allow for bilateral comparison of muscle bulk and to note possible atrophy. If the PT suspects a specific nerve, he or she should consider the muscles and sensory distribution that would be affected. The PT should palpate bilaterally along the path of the suspected nerve, looking for bone, joint, or soft tissue abnormalities. Local tenderness or a positive Tinel's sign helps identify the site of nerve entrapment. Suspicion can be confirmed by electromyography or nerve conduction studies or both.[58]

If a patient presents with weakness of shoulder abduction and cannot shrug a shoulder, the PT should suspect a nerve entrapment of the spinal accessory nerve. The patient typically has dull pain, weakness, and drooping of the shoulder. The patient has paralysis of the trapezius muscle, and winging of the scapula usually is present. The spinal accessory nerve can be injured by blunt trauma to the posterior triangle of the neck or a traction injury, or it can be a result of cervical surgery, such as for head or neck cancers.[63] The spinal accessory nerve is susceptible to trauma at the posterior triangle because of its superficial location, but the sternocleidomastoid would be spared because the injury would be distal to its innervation. A traction force that depresses the shoulder while laterally flexing the head in the opposite direction stretches the nerve and can damage the nerve.

TABLE 6-5

Red Flags for the Thoracic Spine and Rib Cage Region

	RED FLAGS	
Condition	**Data Obtained During History**	**Data Obtained During Physical Examination**
Myocardial infarction[5,19,20,22]	Presence of risk factors: previous history of coronary artery disease, hypertension, smoking, diabetes mellitus, elevated blood serum cholesterol (>240 mg/dL) Men >40 yr, women >50 yr	Chest pain Pallor, sweating, dyspnea, nausea, palpitations Symptoms lasting >30 min and not relieved with sublingual nitroglycerin
Unstable angina pectoris[42]	History of coronary artery disease	Chest pain that occurs outside of a predictable pattern Not responsive to nitroglycerin
Stable angina pectoris[42]	Common in people >65 yr More common in men History of coronary artery disease	Chest pain/pressure that occurs with predictable levels of exertion Symptoms predictably alleviated with rest or sublingual nitroglycerin
Pericarditis[102]	Often associated with autoimmune diseases (systemic lupus erythematosus, rheumatoid arthritis) History of myocardial infarction History of renal failure, open heart surgery, or radiation therapy	Sharp/stabbing chest pain that may be referred to the lateral neck or either shoulder Increased pain with left-side lying Relieved with forward leaning while sitting (supporting arms on knees or a table)
Pulmonary embolus[102]	History of, or risk factors for developing, deep vein thrombosis Immobility Trauma Cancer	Chest, shoulder, or upper abdominal pain Dyspnea Tachypnea Tachycardia
Pleurisy[102]	History of a recent or concurrent respiratory disorder (e.g., infection, pneumonia, tumor, tuberculosis)	Severe, sharp, knifelike pain with inspiration Dyspnea, decreased chest wall excursion
Pneumothorax[69]	Recent bout of coughing or strenuous exercise or trauma	Chest pain, intensified with inspiration Difficulty ventilating or expanding rib cage Hyperresonance on percussion Decreased breath sounds
Pneumonia[102]	History of bacterial, viral, fungal, or mycoplasmal infection Often follows influenza History of inhalation of toxic or caustic chemicals, smoke, dusts, or gases (smoking) History of aspiration of food, fluids, or vomitus	Pleuritic pain, may be referred to shoulder Fever, chills, headaches, malaise, nausea Productive cough
Cholecystitis[103]	Most common in middle age (particularly in women) WBC count may be elevated (12,000-15,000/mL)	Colicky pain in right upper abdominal quadrant with accompanying right scapular pain Symptoms may worsen with ingestion of fatty foods Symptoms not increased by activity or relieved by rest
Peptic ulcer[81]	Dull or gnawing pain or burning sensation in the epigastrium, mid-back, or supraclavicular regions Symptoms relieved with food History of infection (*Helicobacter pylori*) History of multiple stressors, poor coping skills, persistent anxiety and depression	Localized tenderness at right epigastrium Constipation, bleeding, vomiting, tarry-colored stools, coffee-ground emesis
Pyelonephritis[4]	More common in women Recent or coexisting urinary tract infection Kidney stone or past episode of kidney stone	Fever, chills, malaise, headache, flank pain Enlarged prostate Tenderness over costovertebral angle (Murphy's sign)

TABLE 6-5

Red Flags for the Thoracic Spine and Rib Cage Region—cont'd

RED FLAGS		
Condition	**Data Obtained During History**	**Data Obtained During Physical Examination**
Nephrolithiasis (kidney stones)[4]	Residence in hot and humid environment	Sudden, severe back or flank pain
	Past episodes of kidney stone; 50% of patients experience recurrence	Chills, fever, nausea, or vomiting
		Renal colic
		Symptoms of urinary tract infection
Spinal fracture[46]	History of fall or motor vehicle crash	Midline tenderness at level of fracture
	History of osteoporosis	Most common fracture levels are T11-L1
	Long-term steroid use	Bruising
	Age >70 yr	Lower extremity neurologic deficits
	Loss of function or mobility	Evidence of increased thoracic kyphosis

WBC, white blood cell.

BOX 6-4

Medical Screening Questionnaire for the Thoracic Spine and Rib Cage Region

Question	Yes	No
1. Do you have a history of heart problems?		
2. Have you recently taken a nitroglycerin tablet?		
3. Do you have diabetes?		
4. Do you take medication for hypertension?		
5. Have you been or are you now a smoker?		
6. Does your pain ease when you rest in a comfortable position?		
7. Have you had recent surgery?		
8. Have you recently been bedridden?		
9. Have you recently noticed that it is difficult for you to breathe, laugh, sneeze, or cough?		
10. Have you recently had a fever, infection, or other illness?		
11. Have you recently received a blow to the chest, such as during a fall or motor vehicle accident?		
12. In the past few weeks, have you noticed that when you cough, you easily cough up sputum?		
13. Are your symptoms relieved after eating?		
14. Does eating fatty foods increase your symptoms?		
15. Do you currently have a urinary tract infection, or have you had one in the past 2 months?		
16. Do you currently have a kidney stone, or have you had one in the past?		
17. Do you experience severe back or flank pain that comes on suddenly?		

The patient notices damage to the spinal accessory nerve when he or she notices a reduced ability to use his or her shoulder secondary to lack of scapular stabilization or a reduced ability to shrug the shoulder.

Weakness of shoulder abduction and flexion should raise the suspicion of a possible axillary nerve entrapment or injury. The axillary nerve arises from the posterior cord of the brachial plexus and has fibers from C5 and C6 nerve roots. After branching from the brachial plexus, the nerve travels laterally and downward, passing just below the shoulder joint and into the quadrilateral space.[63] The nerve curves around the posterior and lateral portion of the proximal humerus to innervate the deltoid and teres minor muscles, while supplying the sensation of the lateral aspect of the upper arm.[63] A typical axillary nerve injury is caused by trauma—either a direct blow to the shoulder or a dislocation that stretches the nerve where it curves around the humerus. Patients are aware of weakness with shoulder flexion and abduction, but numbness is not always present. The PT should refer such a patient to his or her physician for surgical consultation.

Scapular winging may be due to trapezius involvement or related to serratus anterior paralysis. The serratus anterior is innervated by the long thoracic nerve after it branches from the roots of C5, C6, and C7. The nerve passes down the posterolateral aspect of the chest wall, and its superficial course makes it susceptible to injury. The nerve can be damaged by excessive use of the shoulder, prolonged traction to the nerve, or trauma to the lateral chest wall. A patient with entrapment or injury of the long thoracic nerve experiences pain in the shoulder girdle, a reduction in active shoulder motions caused by a loss of scapulo-humeral rhythm, and scapular winging that becomes especially evident when doing a wall push-up.

Poorly localized shoulder pain also may be related to a rotator cuff tear or to suprascapular nerve entrapment. Suprascapular nerve entrapment often is confused with rotator cuff tear because both have wasting of the supraspinatus or infraspinatus with loss of strength in abduction and external rotation of the shoulder. The suprascapular nerve, similar to the long thoracic nerve, is a motor nerve, and pain resulting from its irritation is deep and poorly localized. The suprascapular nerve derives from the upper trunk of the brachial plexus, formed from the roots of C5 and C6. The nerve runs in the posterior triangle of the neck, sometimes passing through the body of the middle scalene, and past the anterior border of the trapezius on its way to the upper border of the scapula. After arriving at the scapula, the suprascapular nerve passes through the suprascapular notch. The notch is roofed by the transverse scapular ligament, making the U-shaped notch into a foramen. Here the nerve gives off innervation for the supraspinatus muscle, then it continues around the lateral border of the spine of the scapula. The nerve passes through the spinoglenoid notch to reach its destination in the infraspinatus muscle.[63]

Entrapment of the suprascapular nerve most often occurs at the suprascapular foramen, resulting in weakness and atrophy of the supraspinatus and the infraspinatus muscles. Entrapment also has occurred at the spinoglenoid notch, however, resulting in the isolated involvement of the infraspinatus muscle. Lajtai and coworkers[60] reported the prevalence of atrophy of the infraspinatus to be 30% among professional volleyball players. Trauma, whether in the form of repetitive microtrauma or distal trauma, causes a traction injury to the suprascapular nerve. An individual with poor scapular stability has additional motion at the suprascapular foramen against the suprascapular nerve, causing pain and inflammation through repetitive microtrauma.

A distal trauma can result from a fall onto an outstretched arm that is fully supinated, extended, and adducted. With this type of fall, the scapula remains fixed at the end of the upper extremity, while the inertia of the trunk keeps the body moving down, and the nerve is directly injured before protective crumpling or a Colles' fracture occurs. Conservative treatment of rest, NSAIDs, and physical therapy is often unsuccessful, and surgical decompression may be necessary.[63]

As stated earlier, shoulder and cervical pathologies compose a large portion of an orthopedic PT's caseload. Thoracic outlet syndrome, cervical disk disease, and intrinsic shoulder disorders (e.g., bursitis, tendinitis, or frozen shoulder) all are very common disorders. Most PTs think that they fully understand these diagnoses and can confidently guide a patient through rehabilitation, but do they understand the relationship of these diagnoses with Pancoast's tumor? All of these diagnoses are common misdiagnoses of Pancoast's tumor.

Pancoast's tumor is a malignant tumor in the upper apices of a lung; it also may be called a superior pulmonary sulcus tumor. Pancoast's tumor has the highest occurrence in men older than 50 years with a history of cigarette smoking. In more than 90% of patients, shoulder pain, rather than pulmonary symptoms, appears first.[83] Pulmonary symptoms are rare, and shoulder or disk problems are suspected because the tumor grows into the thoracic inlet, affecting the eighth cervical and first thoracic nerve roots, the subclavian artery and vein, and the sympathetic chain ganglia.

A patient with Pancoast's tumor initially has only nagging pain in the shoulder and along the vertebral border of the scapula as the tumor irritates the parietal pleura. As the tumor continues to invade the thoracic inlet, the pain becomes more burning, extending down the arm and into the ulnar nerve distribution. Over time, the intrinsic hand muscles atrophy, and the tumor occludes the subclavian vein. Occlusion causes venous distention of the ipsilateral arm. During this progressive decline, the patient seeks medical attention, and the disorder is misdiagnosed for an average of 6.8 months (ranging from 1 to 24 months).[83] As with any malignant cancer, the misdiagnosis by physicians and mistreatment by PTs and chiropractors reduce the odds of survival.

The goal is to prevent metastasis to the mediastinal lymph nodes or other peripheral sites. If a PT is treating a patient (especially one with the aforementioned profile: man older than 50 years and a smoker) for neck or shoulder diagnoses mentioned previously and does not notice any change in pain after three to four treatments, a referral back to the physician may be warranted. Table 6-6 summarizes the red flags for patients with cervical and shoulder pain, and Box 6-5 presents a medical screening questionnaire for these patients.

Craniofacial Pain

PTs have become increasingly involved in the treatment of conditions of the head, face, and temporomandibular joint. When seeing a patient for temporomandibular joint dysfunction, Bell's palsy, stroke, or conditions of the back or neck, PTs should consider the possibility of meningitis, a primary brain tumor, or a subarachnoid hemorrhage. Quick detection of all of the aforementioned conditions by an alert PT can greatly increase the chance of survival and possibly minimize morbidity.

Meningitis is a relatively rare infection that affects the meninges, causing brain swelling, bleeding, and death in 10% of cases.[17] The most serious type of meningitis is bacterial meningitis. Bacteria that are responsible for bacterial meningitis are present in the external environment and in the respiratory system. The bacteria somehow cross the blood-brain barrier after a head injury because of a depressed immune system or for some unidentifiable reason. Bacterial meningitis can cause death within hours, and a child younger than 2 years old with an unexplained fever should be seen immediately by a physician.

Viral meningitis, caused by a viral intestinal infection, mumps, or a herpes infection, is generally the least serious, clearing on its own within 1 to 2 weeks. Antiviral medications may be used in more serious cases of infection, depending on the type of viral infection. Acyclovir is effective against herpes simplex, which can cause herpes encephalitis and severe brain damage if not treated. Acyclovir, although effective against herpesvirus, does little to most other viruses and must be given before the patient lapses into a coma.

Fungal meningitis affects 10% of patients with AIDS and should be considered when seeing these patients.[17] Fungal meningitis is spread from pigeon droppings and is treated with antifungal medications after it is detected.

Meningitis is more common in individuals with compromised immune systems, such as patients with AIDS and individuals who have had a facial trauma leading to infection that spreads to the cerebrospinal fluid. Meningitis is most common in children younger than 2 years old and in individuals living in close quarters, such as college dormitories or military training camps.

If meningitis is suspected, a slump test is performed. In this test, the neck and trunk are fully flexed, causing pain that is relieved when the neck flexion ceases. Different variants are used with the trunk flexed and the leg straightened, but all forms stress the meninges.[65] If a meningeal inflammation is present, a positive test should result, as pain in the back, neck, or head is relieved when the meninges are no longer stressed. Other signs are headaches, high fever, stiff neck, nausea and vomiting, photophobia, confusion, sleepiness, and seizures. A patient with this type of presentation should be referred immediately to an emergency department or back to his or her primary care physician for proper testing. A physician must perform a lumbar puncture to obtain a sample of cerebrospinal fluid for analysis, to make the diagnosis and to determine appropriate treatment.

TABLE 6-6

Red Flags for the Cervical Spine and Shoulder Region

	RED FLAGS	
Condition	**Data Obtained During History**	**Data Obtained During Physical Examination**
Myocardial infarction[5,19,20,22]	Presence of risk factors: previous history of coronary artery disease, hypertension, smoking, diabetes, elevated blood serum cholesterol (>240 mg/dL) Men >40 yr, women >50 yr	Chest pain Pallor, sweating, dyspnea, nausea, palpitations Symptoms lasting >30 min and not relieved with sublingual nitroglycerin
Cervical ligamentous instabilities with possible cord compromise[3,24,44,85,90]	Major trauma such as a motor vehicle accident or a fall from a height History of rheumatoid arthritis or ankylosing spondylitis Oral contraceptive use	Long tract neurologic signs, especially present in more than one extremity; dizziness; nystagmus; vertigo with head/neck movements/positions; clonus; positive Babinski's sign
Cervical and shoulder girdle peripheral entrapment neuropathies	Paresthesias Pain present at rest and possibly with a retrograde distribution	Muscles innervated, can be tender to palpate Muscles and sensory distribution follow specific nerve pattern
Spinal accessory nerve[75]	History of penetrating injury, such as stab or gunshot Direct blow or stretching of the nerve during a fall or motor vehicle accident Surgical history of radical neck dissection for tumor or cervical lymph node biopsy History of a blow from a hockey stick or lacrosse stick	Asymmetry of the neck line and drooping of the shoulder Inability to shrug shoulders Lack of scapular stabilization Weakness of shoulder abduction
Axillary nerve[84]	Patients >40 yr with shoulder dislocation History of traction force or blunt trauma to shoulder History of brachial neuritis or quadrilateral space syndrome	Weakness of shoulder abduction and flexion Lack of sensation of lateral aspect of the upper arm
Long thoracic nerve[78]	Identified in players of many sports, including tennis, volleyball, archery, golf, gymnastics, bowling, weight lifting, soccer, hockey, and rifle shooting[14]	Serratus anterior weakness with scapular winging Loss of scapulohumeral rhythm
Suprascapular nerve[34,38,60]	Deep, poorly localized pain History of fracture of the scapula with involvement of the notch and blade of the scapula Traction injury mechanism Direct compression of the suprascapular nerve at the level of the scapular notch or at the spinoglenoid notch because of a ganglion cyst or a hypertrophied transverse scapular or spinoglenoid ligament	Presentation similar to rotator cuff tear because of wasting of the supraspinatus or infraspinatus muscles Loss of strength in abduction and external rotation of the shoulder
Pancoast's tumor (superior sulcus lung tumor)[54,74,83]	Men >50 yr with history of cigarette smoking	Nagging-type pain in the shoulder and along the vertebral border of the scapula Pain that has progressed from nagging to burning in nature, often extending down the arm and into the ulnar nerve distribution

Another possible intracranial disorder that requires vigilance is brain cancer. A primary brain tumor occurs infrequently, in 6 to 9 people per 100,000,[82] but the central nervous system also is a common site for metastasis. Lung cancer accounts for approximately half of all metastatic brain lesions, and breast cancer and melanomas often metastasize to the brain. PTs treating patients with a history of these primary cancers should be vigilant for symptoms suggesting central nervous system metastases. Although headache is a symptom associated with a brain tumor, neurologic deficits are a more common symptom in the early and middle stages of this disorder.[49] Change in mentation, vomiting with or without nausea, visual changes, seizures, ataxia, and speech impairment all are possible presentations, with or without headache. Symptoms of this type would warrant a detailed neurologic screening (see Chapters 12 and 13).

The third condition affecting the head, face, and temporomandibular joint region is subarachnoid hemorrhage. Hemorrhage is most often caused by a rupture of a saccular intracranial aneurysm or rupture of an arteriovenous malformation. The signs and symptoms can be very similar to the signs and symptoms of a brain tumor and of meningitis. A patient describes a headache of sudden onset that is the worst headache of his or her life, and the patient may even experience a brief loss of consciousness. Meningeal irritation symptoms and signs (nuchal rigidity, fever, photophobia, nausea, and vomiting) and brain tumor symptoms and signs (neurologic dysfunction, nausea, and vomiting) also are possible. If a PT suspects a subarachnoid hemorrhage, emergency medical care should be instituted. Early diagnosis is crucial and can prevent devastating neurologic effects. See Table 6-7 for a summary of the red flags for patients with craniofacial

BOX 6-5

BOX 6-5

Medical Screening Questionnaire for the Cervical Spine and Shoulder Regions

Question	Yes	No
1. Have you had a direct blow to your shoulder or a shoulder dislocation?		
2. Have you recently used your shoulder excessively?		
3. Have you had a traction injury to your arm?		
4. Have you had a direct blow to the lateral chest wall?		
5. Have you recently fallen onto an outstretched arm?		
6. Have you noticed difficulty lifting your arm or any other muscle weakness?		
7. Have you been experiencing pins and needles anywhere in your body?		
8. Do you experience pain that does not improve with rest?		
9. If you do have pain, where is your pain?		
10. Does your pain move into the arm?		
11. Do you currently smoke?		
12. Do you have a history of smoking?		

pain; Box 6-6 presents a medical screening questionnaire for these patients.

Elbow, Wrist, and Hand Pain

Injuries involving the elbow, wrist, and hand are common, and pain in specific locations should alert the PT to the possibility of a more serious disorder. A patient with osteoporosis or other conditions that can compromise bone density who has a fall is more likely to sustain a fracture. A patient who takes corticosteroids for chronic respiratory problems is more likely to sustain a tendon rupture or ligamentous injury secondary to the same fall. Finally, a patient who is immunosuppressed is more susceptible to a space infection in the hand. This section discusses the red flags associated with specific fractures, tendon ruptures, space infections of the hand, Raynaud's disease, and complex regional pain syndrome (reflex sympathetic dystrophy).

Fractures

A fracture at the elbow is likely to have been caused by a fall onto an outstretched arm or by direct trauma to the elbow itself. An olecranon fracture causes posterior pain, swelling, and tenderness. Elbow extension is the function most impaired, and there may be a palpable gap between the olecranon and the trochlear notch of the humerus. A fall also may cause anterolateral pain and tenderness, cause an inability to supinate and pronate the forearm, or cause the arm to be held against the side with the elbow flexed. This would be more typical of a radial head fracture, and having the elbow flexed produces the least pressure within the elbow capsule. This loose packed position of 70 degrees of ulnohumeral flexion and 10 degrees of supination also compensates for the effusion of the elbow joint that is usually present.[64] Radiographic screening often shows a positive fat pad sign, which increases the suspicion for the presence of an elbow fracture. The anterior fat pad becomes triangular in shape, and the posterior fat pad becomes visible. Either a triangular anterior fat pad or a visible posterior fat pad constitutes a positive sign. This is also known as the "sail" sign because the fat pads now resemble the sails of a ship. Immediate referral is appropriate if a fracture is suspected.

The radius also may be fractured distally during a fall onto an outstretched arm. A fracture of the distal radius, known as *Colles' fracture,* typically manifests with local pain, tenderness, swelling, and ecchymoses, and wrist extension in particular is painful.[63] The same fall onto an outstretched arm and extended wrist can cause a scaphoid fracture. The patient has similar signs and symptoms but localized to the "anatomic snuff box." The wrist also is very stiff secondary to the swelling. Radiographs, if performed with all four views plus a navicular view, have 100% diagnostic sensitivity.[102] If films are negative, the patient is put into a spica cast, and radiographs are repeated after 2 weeks. The main concern with scaphoid fractures is the possibility of avascular necrosis secondary to disruption of the blood supply.

The final type of fracture is a lunate fracture or dislocation and capitate fracture. Lunate fractures are rare and often are related to osteonecrosis. Lunate fractures can cause diffuse synovitis with generalized wrist swelling, pain, decreased motion, and decreased grip strength. The best way to identify a lunate fracture is by radiographic imaging, especially a T1-weighted MRI scan to detect loss of bone marrow. A capitate fracture is more common; patients present with similar symptoms of wrist pain, swelling, and tenderness at the mid-dorsal wrist area. Capitate fractures are the result of trauma involving maximal wrist flexion or extension, however, rather than of osteonecrosis.

Soft Tissue Injuries

Falls, traumas, and sports-related injuries cause problems not only with bones but also with local soft tissue structures. The flexor forearm muscle mass, including the pronator teres, flexor carpi radialis, palmaris longus, and flexor carpi ulnaris, can be strained or even ruptured. A grade I muscle strain is a stretching of the muscle fibers without disruption. A grade II tear is a partial tearing of the muscles with maintenance of the overlying fascia. This injury includes local tenderness, swelling, muscle spasms, a hematoma, and pain with motion and with passive elongation of the tissue. Strains of grades I and II can be treated conservatively with *RICE: r*est, *i*ce, *c*ompression, and *e*levation. Grade III tears are a complete tearing of the muscle and its investing fascia. This injury results in a total loss of motion, and surgical repair is needed. Swelling, tenderness, ecchymoses of the overlying skin, and a palpable defect in the muscle are characteristic of a grade III rupture of the flexor forearm muscle mass and warrant referral of the patient to a physician as soon as possible. The triangular fibrocartilaginous complex is an often missed source of ulnar-sided wrist pain, especially after a fall, or may be associated with concurrent Colles' fracture. Clicking with wrist motion, pain with passive ulnar deviation, or dorsal displacement of the ulna ("piano key" sign) may indicate pathology. This tissue is slow to heal and can be quite debilitating to the patient, limiting grip strength and weight bearing through the involved wrist. Referral for débridement, repair, or removal may be warranted.

Infection

The hand often is traumatized secondary to puncture wounds, abrasions, cuts, or other injuries, and a break in the skin brings the increased possibility of an infection. Hands have several spaces (e.g., mid-palmar space, web space, and thenar space) that can serve as prime areas for infection to develop and spread.

TABLE 6-7

Red Flags for the Head, Face, and Temporomandibular Joint Regions

RED FLAGS		
Condition	Data Obtained During History	Data Obtained During Physical Examination
Meningitis[6,17,23,48,71]	History of recent bacterial or viral infection (influenza)	Positive slump sign
	History of skull fracture	Headache
		Fever
		Gastrointestinal signs of vomiting and symptoms of nausea
		Photophobia
		Confusion
		Seizures
		Sleepiness
Primary brain tumor[6,36,56,104]	Age 20-64 yr	Headache
		Altered mental status
		Ataxia
		Speech deficits
		Sensory abnormalities
		Gastrointestinal signs of vomiting and symptoms of nausea
		Visual changes
		Seizures
Subarachnoid hemorrhage[43,45,61,91]	History of smoking, hypertension, and alcohol abuse	Brief loss of consciousness
	Headache of sudden onset (the worst headache of patient's life)	Brain tumor signs (neurologic dysfunction, nausea and vomiting)
		Meningeal irritation signs (nuchal rigidity, fever, photophobia, nausea and vomiting)

BOX 6-6

Medical Screening Questionnaire for the Head, Face, and Temporomandibular Joint Regions

Question	Yes	No
1. Do you have a depressed immune system?		
2. Have you recently had an intestinal infection, mumps, or herpes?		
3. Have you had recent contact with pigeons or pigeon droppings?		
4. Have you recently been living in close quarters, such as in a dormitory or military training camp?		
5. Have you recently had a head trauma?		
6. Do you currently have a high fever, or have you had a fever recently?		
7. Have you been experiencing nausea or vomiting?		
8. Have you had difficulty with light sensitivity?		
9. Have you noticed a recent inability to concentrate?		
10. Have you recently had a seizure?		
11. Do you experience abnormal sensations in the skin?		
12. Have you recently had difficulty with speaking?		
13. Have you noticed an increased clumsiness or lack of coordination?		
14. Have you recently experienced a loss of consciousness?		

Fingers also have such spaces on the volar surface, such as the pulp space of the proximal, middle, and distal phalanx. Any of these spaces can become infected after a direct puncture, formation of an abscess, or purulent tenosynovitis of tendons that pass through the space. These spaces can become infected as a result of trauma or poor nail care. A patient presents with the typical signs of local inflammation, and the swelling causes the finger pads to be tense and painful with a resultant loss of motion. Infections must be treated quickly, or the infection spreads to the adjacent web space of the hand and beyond.

If the web space becomes infected, swelling, pain, tenderness, warmth, and erythema are present in the palm and over the dorsum of the hand proximal to the involved area of the involved space. The edema can cause the metacarpal bones to become splayed, resulting in loss of the normal hand shape. The causes are similar to the causes mentioned in the previous paragraph. As mentioned, web space infection can be caused by progression of a pulp space infection.

Mid-palmar space infections appear very similar to web space infections in their presentation, with inflammation of the palm and dorsum of the hand and loss of the concavity of the palm secondary to swelling. Even the mid-palmar space can be infected by the second, third, and fourth web spaces through the lumbrical canals.[102] Direct puncture also can infect the mid-palmar space or produce tenosynovitis of the flexor tendons of the second or fourth finger.

The thenar space is the equivalent of the mid-palmar space except for the thumb. Direct puncture or tenosynovitis of the second flexor tendon or from an adjacent space, such as the mid-palmar space, can infect this area. This space is treated the same as the spaces mentioned previously—by drainage with a course of antibiotics specific to the organism causing the infection. If the patient is not seen by a physician quickly, the infection

TABLE 6-8

Red Flags for the Elbow, Wrist, and Hand Regions

Condition	RED FLAGS	
	Data Obtained During History	**Data Obtained During Physical Examination**
Fractures	Recent fall or trauma	Pain, tenderness, swelling, ecchymosis
	History of osteoporosis	
	Extended use of steroids (e.g., respiratory problems)	
	Pathologies with improper bone remodeling	
Radial head fracture[66]	Fall onto an outstretched arm that is supinated	Anterolateral pain and tenderness at the elbow
		Inability to supinate and pronate forearm
		Elbow held against the side with 70 degrees of flexion and slightly supinated
Distal radius (Colles') fracture[70]	Fall onto outstretched arm with forceful wrist extension	Wrist held in neutral resting position
		Wrist swelling
	Age >40 yr	
	Women affected more than men	Movements into wrist extension are painful
	History of osteoporosis	
Scaphoid fracture[7,72]	Fall onto outstretched arm	Wrist swelling
		Wrist held in neutral position
		Pain in the "anatomic snuff box"
Lunate fracture or dislocation[47]	Fall onto outstretched arm	Generalized wrist swelling and pain
	Diffuse synovitis	Decreased motion
		Decreased grip strength (rule out capitate fracture)
Triangular fibrocartilaginous complex tear[2]	Traumatic fall after slipping or tripping on outstretched hand with forearm pronated	Ulnar-sided wrist pain
		Tenderness and clicking with wrist movement (passive ulnar deviation)
	Commonly associated with Colles' fracture	Weakness with grip strength
		Dorsal ulnar head subluxation
Long flexor tendon rupture[31,33,47]	History of rheumatoid arthritis	*Grade I and II muscle tear:* local tenderness, swelling, muscle spasms, hematoma, pain with motion and with passive stretch
	History of corticosteroid use for chronic respiratory problems	
	History of trauma	*Grade III muscle rupture:* total loss of motion and palpable defect in the muscle, swelling, tenderness, ecchymosis of overlying skin
Space infection of the hand[99]	Recent puncture of skin	Typical signs of inflammation: swelling in palm, dorsum of hand, or finger tips
	Recent insect bite	
		Pain, tenderness, warmth, erythema
	Presence of an abscess	Signs of long-standing infection: high fever, chills, weakness, malaise
	Purulent tenosynovitis of tendons that go through a space	
Raynaud's phenomenon or Raynaud's disease[11]	Past medical history significant for rheumatoid arthritis, occlusive vascular disease, smoking, or use of beta blockers	Hands or feet that blanch, go cyanotic and then red when exposed to cold or emotional stress
		Pain and tingling in hands or feet when they turn red
Complex regional pain syndrome (reflex sympathetic dystrophy)[21,96]	Trauma including fracture, dislocation, or surgery	Severe aching, stinging, cutting, or boring pain that is not typical of injury; hypersensitivity
	Pain does not respond to typical analgesics	Area swollen (pitting edema), warm, and erythematous

could drain through a necrotic area of the skin, increasing the possibility of osteomyelitis or septic arthritis. The infection also can spread, causing high fever, chills, weakness, and malaise. Ultimately, the infection could lead to sepsis and amputation of fingers or parts of the hand.[57] As with any infection, immuno-compromised patients are at the greatest risk. Space infections also have been seen in recipients of cardiac transplants because of the need for long-term immunosuppression to prevent rejection of donor hearts.[57]

Raynaud's Disease

Another disorder that may affect patients seeing PTs is Raynaud's disease, or Raynaud's phenomenon. This disorder affects one or both hands and the feet. One or more digits may be involved, and progression of the disease involves more digits. When a person is exposed to cold or to emotional upset, the hands blanch, become cyanotic, and turn red. During the rubor stage, the patient has pain and paresthesias as the blood returns to the hands or feet. This entire phase lasts only 15 to 20 minutes, and the patient can alleviate it by running the hands under warm water. As mentioned, exposure to cold or stress usually precipitates episodes. Raynaud's phenomenon is more common in patients with rheumatoid arthritis or occlusive vascular disease; smokers; and individuals taking beta-adrenergic blocking drugs to treat migraine, angina, or hypertension.

Reflex sympathetic dystrophy (also known as *complex regional pain syndrome*) is a disorder that varies in severity but often follows trauma to the elbow, wrist, or hand. The trauma may include a fracture, sprain, dislocation, crush injury, or surgery such as a carpal tunnel procedure. There is often a lag period between the injury and the onset of the symptoms of complex regional pain syndrome. Symptoms include severe aching, stinging, cutting, or boring pain that is out of proportion to the injury, corrective surgery, or normal tissue healing.[44,94,96] The pain does not respond to typical analgesics, and regional nerve blocks usually produce only temporary relief. The hand often becomes swollen, warm, and erythematous.

Hyperhidrosis is also often present. The other hand may support the involved limb, and the patient is often resistant to let a practitioner handle the hand because of hypersensitivity. Nerve blocks are a common treatment, in conjunction with physical therapy to maintain function and assist the patient with strategies for pain management. Table 6-8 summarizes the red flags for patients with distal upper extremity pain, and Box 6-7 presents a medical screening questionnaire for these patients.

Summary

The investigation of symptoms produces information vital in determining why the patient has sought physical therapy services. As a patient describes the location, onset, and behavior of symptoms, the PT must decide whether the history makes sense based on his or her own experience and understanding of basic and clinical sciences. This information helps the PT make a diagnosis and decide whether to refer the patient to a physician. This information also helps guide the PT in choosing the body systems to screen (see Chapter 9) later during the history, helps in determining whether an upper quadrant (see Chapter 12) or lower

quadrant (see Chapter 13) screening examination is warranted, and helps identify the components of these examinations that are most relevant.

Finally, the location of symptoms should alert the PT to the possibility of certain disorders that may be responsible for the patient's symptoms. Knowledge of such disorders enables the PT to recognize the specific symptoms and warning signs for these disorders. Many of these warning signs (e.g., fever) are described in Chapter 9. The clinician also is encouraged to use the accompanying tables and figures to collect this patient information in a more effective and efficient manner.

BOX 6-7

Medical Screening Questionnaire for the Elbow, Wrist, and Hand Regions

Question	Yes	No
1. Have you recently had a trauma, such as a fall?		
2. Has a medical practitioner ever told you that you have osteoporosis?		
3. Are you currently taking steroids or have you received long-term steroid therapy?		
4. Do you have a pathology with improper bone remodeling?		
5. Have you noticed an inability to move your elbow normally?		
6. Have you noticed an inability to move your wrist normally?		
7. Do you have difficulty turning your hand upward or downward (e.g., turning a doorknob)?		
8. Have you recently had an infection?		
9. Do you have any open wounds, cuts, swelling, or redness on your hands or arms?		
10. Have you noticed weakness of your hands or frequent dropping of objects?		
11. Have you recently experienced a high fever, chills, weakness, or malaise?		
12. Do your hands or feet blanch, go blue, and then turn red when exposed to cold or emotional stress?		
13. Do you have a medical history of rheumatoid arthritis, occlusive vascular disease, or use of beta blockers?		
14. Do you currently smoke or have a history of smoking?		
15. If you have pain, does it respond to typical pain medications?		

REFERENCES

1. Acheson RM, Chan YK, Payne M. New Haven survey of joint diseases: the interrelationships between morning stiffness, nocturnal pain and swelling of the joints. J Chron Dis 1969;21:533–42.
2. Albastaki U, Sophocleous D, Gothlin J, et al. Magnetic resonance imaging of the triangular fibrocartilage complex lesions: a comprehensive clini-coradiologic approach and review of the literature. J Manip Physiol Ther 2007;30:522–6.
3. Aspinall W. Clinical testing for the craniovertebral hypermobility syndrome. J Orthop Sports Phys Ther 1990;12:47–54.
4. Bajwa ZH. Pain patterns in patients with polycystic kidney disease. Kidney Int 2004;66:1561–9.
5. Berger JP, Buclin T, Haller E, et al. Right arm involvement and pain extension can help to differentiate coronary diseases from chest pain of other origin: a prospective emergency ward study of 278 consecutive patients admitted for chest pain. J Intern Med 1990;227:165–72.
6. Berger JP, Buclin T, Haller E, et al. Does this adult patient have acute meningitis? JAMA 1999;282:175–81.
7. Bhowal B, Dias JJ, Wildin CJ. The incidence of simultaneous fractures of the scaphoid and radial head. J Hand Surg 2001;26B:25–7.
8. Bianco AJ. Low back pain and sciatica: diagnosis and indications for treatment. J Bone Joint Surg Am 1968;508:170–81.

9. Bickley LS. Bates' guide to physical examination and history taking. 10th ed. Philadelphia: Wolters Kluwer; 2009.

10. Bigos S, Bowyer O, Braen G, et al. Acute lower back problems in adults. Clinical practice guideline no 14. AHCPR publication no. 95-0642. Rockville, MD: Agency for Health Care Policy and Research, Public Health Service, US Department of Health and Human Services; December 1994.

11. Bloack J, Sequeira W. Raynaud's phenomenon. Lancet 2001;357:9237.

12. Boissonnault W. Prevalence of comorbid conditions, surgeries, and medication use in a physical outpatient population: a multicentered study. J Orthop Sports Phys Ther 1999;29:506–19.

13. Boissonnault W, DiFabio R. Pain profile of patients with low back pain referred to physical therapy. J Orthop Sports Phys Ther 1996;24:180–91.

14. Boissonnault W, Goodman C. Physical therapists as diagnosticians: drawing the line on diagnosing pathology. J Orthop Sports Phys Ther 2006;36:351–3.

15. Bourne RB, Rorabeck CH. Compartment syndromes of the lower leg. Clin Orthop 1989;240:97–104.

16. Boyko EJ, Ahroni JH, Davignon D, et al. Diagnostic utility of the history and physical examination for peripheral vascular disease among patients with diabetes mellitus. J Clin Epidemiol 1997;50:659–68.

17. Bruce M, Rosenstein N, Capparella J, et al. Risk factors for meningococcal disease in college students. JAMA 2001;286:688–93.

18. Busch MT, Morrissy RT. Slipped capital femoral epiphysis. Orthop Clin North Am 1987;18:637–47.

19. Campbell DJ. Why do men and women differ in their risk of myocardial infarction? Eur Heart J 2008;29:835–6.

20. Canto JG, Shlipak MG, Rogers WJ, et al. Prevalence, clinical characteristics, and mortality among patients with myocardial infarction presenting without chest pain. JAMA 2000;283:3223–9.

21. Ciccone DS, Bandilla EB, Wu W. Psychological dysfunction in patients with RSD. Pain 1997;71:323–33.

22. Culic V, Eterovic D, Miric D, et al. Symptom presentation of acute myocardial infarction: influence of sex, age, and risk factors. Am Heart J 2002;144:1012–7.

23. Dagi TF, Meyer FB, Poletti CA. The incidence and prevention of meningitis after basilar skull fracture. Am J Emerg Med 1983;1:295–8.

24. Delfini R, Dorizzi A, Facchinetti G, et al. Delayed post-traumatic cervical instability. Surg Neurol 1999;51:588–95.

25. Delitto A, Erhard RE, Bowling RW. A treatment-based classification approach to lower back syndrome: identifying and staging patients for conservative treatment. Phys Ther 1995;75:470–89.

26. DeRosa GP. The child. In: D'Ambrosia RD, editor. Musculoskeletal disorders: regional examination and differential diagnosis. 2nd ed. Philadelphia: Lippincott; 1986. p. 595–8.

27. Deyo RA, Diehl AK. Cancer as a cause of back pain: frequency, clinical presentation, and diagnostic strategies. J Gen Intern Med 1988;3:230–8.

28. Deyo RA, Rainville J, Kent DL. What can the history and physical examination tell us about lower back pain? JAMA 1992;268:760–5.

29. DiFabio R, Boissonnault W. Physical therapy and health-related outcomes for patients with common orthopaedic diagnoses. J Orthop Sports Phys Ther 1998;27:219–30.

30. Doran FSA. The sites to which pain is referred from the common bile duct in man and its implication for the theory of referred pain. Br J Surg 1967;54:599–606.

31. Ertel A. Flexor tendon ruptures in rheumatoid arthritis. Hand Clin 1989;5:177–90.

32. Farrell JP, Twomey LT. Acute low back pain: comparison of two conservative approaches. Med J Aust 1982;1:160–4.

33. Ferlic DC, Clayton ML. Flexor tenosynovitis in the rheumatoid hand. J Hand Surg 1978;3:364–7.

34. Ferretti A, Cerullo G, Russo G. Suprascapular neuropathy in volleyball players. J Bone Joint Surg Am 1987;69:260–3.

35. Foldes K, Balint P, Gaal M, et al. Nocturnal pain correlates with effusions in diseased hips. J Rheumatol 1992;19:1756–8.

36. Forsyth PA, Posner JB. Headaches in patients with brain tumors: a study of 111 patients. Neurology 1993;43:1678–83.

37. Fritz JM, Irrgang JJ. A comparison of a modified Oswestry Low Back Pain Disability Questionnaire and the Quebec Back Pain Disability Scale. Phys Ther 2001;81:776–88.

38. Garcia G, McQueen D. Bilateral suprascapular-nerve entrapment syndrome: case report and review of the literature. J Bone Joint Surg Am 1981;63:491–2.

39. George SZ, Fritz JM, Childs JD. Investigation of elevated fear-avoidance beliefs for patients with low back pain: a secondary analysis involving patients enrolled in physical therapy clinical trials. J Orthop Sports Phys Ther 2008;38:50–8.

40. Gorroll AH, Mulley AG. Primary care medicine. 5th ed. Philadelphia: Lippincott Williams & Wilkins; 2006.

41. Halperin JL. Evaluation of patients with peripheral vascular disease. Thromb Res 2002;106:V303–11.

42. Henderson JM. Ruling out danger: differential diagnosis of thoracic spine. Phys Sports Med 1992;20:124–31.

43. Hiroki O, Hidefumi T, Suzuki S, et al. Risk factors for aneurysmal subarachnoid hemorrhage in Aomori, Japan. Stroke 2003;34:34–100.

44. Hoffman JR, Mower WR, Wolfson AB, et al. Validity of a set of clinical criteria to rule out injury to the cervical spine in patients with blunt trauma. National Emergency X-Radiography Utilization Study Group [erratum appears in. N Engl J Med 2001;344(6):464; N Engl J Med 343:94-99, 2003.

45. Hong YH, Lee YS, Park S. Headache as a predictive factor of severe systolic hypertension in acute ischemic stroke. Can J Neurol Sci 2003;30:210–4.

46. Hsu JM, Joseph T, Ellis AM. Thoracolumbar fracture in blunt trauma patients: guidelines for diagnosis and imaging. Injury 2003;34:426–33.

47. Hunter JM, Mackin EJ, Callahan AD. Rehabilitation of the hand and upper extremity. 5th ed. St Louis: Mosby; 2002.

48. Hurwitz EL, Aker PD, Adams AH, et al. Manipulation and mobilization of the cervical spine: a systematic review of the literature. Spine 1996;21:1746–60.

49. Isaacs ER, Bookhout MR. Screening for pathologic origins of head and facial pain. In: Boissonnault WG, editor. Examination in physical therapy practice: screening for medical disease. 2nd ed. New York: Churchill Livingstone; 1995. p. 181–2.

50. Jarvik JG, Deyo RA. Diagnostic evaluation of low back pain with emphasis on imaging. Ann Intern Med 2002;137:586–97.

51. Jayson MI, Sims-Williams H, Young S, et al. Mobilization and manipulation for low back pain. Spine 1981;6:409–16.

52. Jemal A, Siegel R, Ward E, et al. Cancer statistics, 2009. CA Cancer J Clin 2009;59:225–49.

53. Jette AM, Davis KD. A comparison of hospital-based and private outpatient physical therapy practices. Phys Ther 1991;71:366–75.

54. Jett J. Superior sulcus tumors and Pancoast's syndrome. Lung Cancer 2000;42:S17–21.

55. Jonsson B, Stromquist B. Symptoms and signs in degeneration of the lumbar spine: a prospective, consecutive study of 300 operated patients. J Bone Joint Surg Br 1993;75:381–5.

56. Jukich PJ, McCarthy BJ, Surawicz TS, et al. Trends in incidence of primary brain tumors in the United States, 1985-1994. Neuro-oncology 2001;3:141–51.

57. Klein M, Chang J. Management of hand and upper-extremity infections in heart transplant recipients. Plast Reconstr Surg 2000;106:598–601.

58. Kopell H, Thompson W. Peripheral entrapment neuropathies. Malaabar, FL: Robert I Krieger Publishing; 1976.

59. Krajewski LP, Olin JW. Atherosclerosis of the aorta and lower extremities arteries. In: Young JR, Olin JW, Bartholomew JR, editors. Peripheral vascular diseases. 2nd ed. St Louis: Year Book Medical Publishers; 1996.

60. Lajtai G, Pfirrmann CWA, Aitzetmüller G, et al. The shoulders of professional beach volleyball players: high prevalence of infraspinatus muscle atrophy. Am J Sports Med 2009;37:1375–83.

61. Linn FH, Rinkel GJ, Algra A, et al. Incidence of subarachnoid hemorrhage: role of region, year, and rate of computed tomography: a meta-analysis. Stroke 1996;27:625–9.

62. Liu K, Atten M. Coping with kidney stones. Am Surg 1997;63:519–25.

63. Lorei M, Hershman E. Peripheral nerve injuries in athletes. Sports Med 1993;16:130–47.

64. Magee DJ. Orthopedic clinical assessment. 5th ed. St Louis: Saunders; 2008.

65. Maitland GD, Hengeveld E, Banks K, editors. Maitland's vertebral manipulation. 6th ed. Oxford: Butterworth/Heinemann; 2001.

66. Major N, Crawford S. Elbow effusion in trauma in adults and children: is there an occult fracture? Am J Radiol 2002;178:413–8.

67. McGee SR, Boyko EJ. Physical examination and chronic lower-extremity ischemia: a critical review. Arch Intern Med 1998;158:1357–64.

68. Meadows JTS. Orthopedic differential diagnosis in physical therapy. New York: McGraw-Hill; 1999.

69. Misthos P, Kakaris S, Sepsas E, et al. A prospective analysis of occult pneumothorax, delayed pneumothorax and delayed hemothorax after minor blunt thoracic trauma. Eur J Cardiothorac Surg 2004;25:859–64.

70. Musad T, Jordan D, Hosking D. Distal forearm fracture in an older community dwelling population: the Nottingham community osteoporosis study. Age Ageing 2001;30:255–8.

71. Pether JVS. Bacterial meningitis after influenza. Lancet 1982;8275:804.

72. Phillips TG, Reibach AM, Slomiany WP. Diagnosis and management of scaphoid fractures. Am Fam Physician 2004;70:879–84.

73. Raj PP. Prognostic and therapeutic local anesthetic block. In: Cousins MJ, Bridenbaugh PO, editors. Neural blockade in clinical anesthesia and management of pain. 2nd ed. Philadelphia: Lippincott; 1988. p. 908.

74. Robinson D, Halperin N, Agar G, et al. Shoulder girdle neoplasms mimicking frozen shoulder syndrome. J Shoulder Elbow Surg 2003;12:451–5.

75. Safran MR. Nerve injury about the shoulder in athletes, part 2: long thoracic nerve, spinal accessory nerve, burners/stingers, thoracic outlet syndrome. Am J Sports Med 2004;32:1063–76.

76. Saklayen M. Medical management of nephrolithiasis. Med Clin North Am 1997;81:785–99.

77. Schofferman L, Schoffmerman J, Zucheman J, et al. Occult infection causing persistent low back pain. Spine 1989;14:417–9.

78. Schultz JS, Leonard JA Jr. Long thoracic neuropathy from athletic activity. Arch Phys Med Rehabil 1992;73:87–90.

79. Siegmeth W, Noyelle RM. Night pain and morning stiffness in osteoarthritis: a crossover study of flurbiprofen and diclofenac sodium. J Intern Med Res 1988;16:182–8.

80. Slipman CW, Patel RK, Botwin K, et al. Epidemiology of spine tumors presenting to musculoskeletal physiatrists. Arch Phys Med Rehab 2003;84:492–5.

81. Smalley WE, Ray WA, Daugherty JR, et al. Nonsteroidal anti-inflammatory drugs and the incidence of hospitalizations for peptic ulcer disease in elderly persons. Am J Epidemiol 1995;141:539–45.

82. Snyder H, Robinson K, Shah D, et al. Signs and symptoms of patients with brain tumors presenting in the emergency department. J Emerg Med 1993;11:253–8.

83. Spengler D, Kirsh M, Kaufer H. Orthopaedic aspects and early diagnosis of superior sulcus lung tumor. J Bone Joint Surg 1973;55:1645–50.

84. Steinmann SP, Moran EA. Axillary nerve injury: diagnosis and treatment. J Am Acad Orthop Surg 2001;9:328–35.

85. Stiell IG, Clement CM, McKnight RD, et al. The Canadian C-Spine Rule versus the Nexus Low Risk Criteria in patients with trauma. N Engl J Med 2003;349:2510–8.

86. Stulberg BN, Bauer TW, Belhobek GH, et al. A diagnostic algorithm for osteonecrosis of the femoral head. Clin Orthop 1989;249:176–82.

87. Suadicani P, Hein HO, Gyntelberg F. Height, weight, and risk of colorectal cancer: an 18-year follow-up in a cohort of 5249 men. Scand J Gastroenterol 1993;28:285–8.

88. Swain R. Lower extremity compartment syndrome: when to suspect pressure buildup. Postgrad Med 1999;105(3).

89. Swartz M. Textbook of physical diagnosis: history taking and examination. 5th ed. Philadelphia: Saunders; 2006.

90. Swinkels R, Beeton K, Alltree J. Pathogenesis of upper cervical instability. Manual Therapy 1996;1:127–32.

91. Teunissen LL, Rinkel GJ, Algra A, et al. Risk factors for subarachnoid hemorrhage: a systematic review. Stroke 1996;27:544–9.

92. Tronzo RG. Femoral neck fractures. In: Steinburg ME, editor. The hip and its disorders. Philadelphia: Saunders; 1991. p. 247–79.

93. Ulmer T. The clinical diagnosis of compartment syndrome of the lower leg: are clinical findings predictive of the disorder. Orthop Trauma 2002;16:572–7.

94. Van de Vusse AC, Stomp-van den Berg SGM, de Vet HWC, et al. Interobserver reliability of diagnosis in patients with complex regional pain syndrome. Eur J Pain 2003;7:259–65.

95. Vanharanta H, Sachs BI, Spivey M, et al. A comparison of CT/discography, pain response and radiographic disc height. Spine 1988;13:321–4.

96. Veldman PH, Reynen HM, Arntz IE, et al. Signs and symptoms of reflex sympathetic dystrophy: prospective study of 829 patients. Lancet 1993;342:1012–6.

97. Waldvogel FA, Vasey H. Osteomyelitis: the past decade. N Engl J Med 1980;14:360–70.

98. Weinstein JN, McLain RF. Primary tumors of the spine. Spine 1987;12:843–51.

99. Weinzweig N, Gonzalez M. Surgical infections of the hand and upper extremity: a county hospital experience. Ann Plast Surg 2002;49:621–7.

100. Wells K. Nephrolithiasis with unusual initial symptoms. J Manip Physiol Ther 2000;23:196–205.

101. Wenger DR, Ward WT, Herring JA. Current concepts review: Legg-Calve-Perthes disease. J Bone Joint SurgAM 1991;73:778–88.

102. Wiener SL. Differential diagnosis of acute pain by body region. New York: McGraw-Hill; 1993.

103. Yusoff IF, Barkun JS, Barkun AN. Diagnosis and management of cholecystitis and cholangitis. Gastroenterol Clin North Am 2003;32:1145–68.

104. Zaki A. Patterns of presentation in brain tumors in the United States. J Surg Oncol 1993;53:110–2.

105. Zohn DA, Mennell JM. Diagnosis and physical treatment, musculoskeletal pain. Boston: Little, Brown; 1976.

Symptom Investigation, Part II: Chief Complaint by Symptom

7

William G. Boissonnault, PT, DPT, DHSc, FAAOMPT
Kristine M. Hallisy, PT, MS, OCS, CMPT, CTI

Objectives

After reading this chapter, the reader will be able to:

1. Compare and contrast conditions in terms of specific anatomic sites of involvement, patient demographics, symptom characteristics, review of systems, system review, and physical examination findings.
2. Describe current medical testing (e.g., imaging and laboratory tests) used to screen and diagnose the condition.
3. Describe common complications of each disorder to help determine the urgency of physician referral.

Chapter 6 has provided a framework for how many patients present to therapists ("I have low back pain," "My calf hurts," or "I have a headache"), followed by a description of potential causes of these local complaints. If therapists were suspicious of these, it would warrant communication with a physician. Although there will be overlap with Chapter 6, this chapter approaches the topic from a different perspective, one that is not tied to a specific location or region of symptoms but to a specific nature of the complaint. Examples for discussion include the following:

- Joint pain
- Limb (nonjoint) pain (antalgic gait)
- Dizziness

These symptoms represent some of the most common complaints addressed by physical therapists practicing in an ambulatory outpatient setting. For each of the categories, there could be a situation for which the therapist could be the primary provider, but for other causes, physician oversight and management are required. Early recognition of these potential red flags followed by a timely physician referral is critical. In the following discussion, each category includes a condition appropriate for therapist oversight, serving as a reference point for comparison with the other conditions described. For example, comparing and contrasting osteoarthritis and gout, or osteoarthritis and rheumatoid arthritis, will provide an understanding of how conditions may present to therapists—similar in some ways, but different in others.

Joint Pain

Descriptive studies have consistently demonstrated that complaints of back, neck, knee, and shoulder pain are the most common reasons for patients to seek physical therapy services.[5,25] Numerous conditions exist as potential causes, many that physical therapists can manage, but others that require

physician oversight for short- and long-term medication management or surgical intervention. Conditions covered in this section include osteoarthritis (OA), rheumatoid arthritis (RA), ankylosing spondylitis, systemic lupus erythematosus (SLE), gout, reactive arthritis (Reiter's syndrome) and septic arthritis. OA is presented as the standard for comparison because it is the most common cause of joint pain and is a condition for which physical therapists should be the primary providers of care. Therapists can also play an important role in the care of patients with the other conditions but for these, physician involvement is essential. At times, physician involvement needs to be implemented in an urgent fashion.

Anatomic Site(s) of Involvement

The number of symptomatic joints along with anatomic location (which joint[s]) provides clues about the cause of joint pain. For example, OA is the most common monoarticular joint condition, in contrast to systemic diseases with articular manifestations, such as RA, which typically present in multiple joints, often in a bilateral and symmetric presentation. Box 7-1 presents a list of joint conditions and their propensity to appear in one or multiple joints.[3,17-20,44]

It should be appreciated that these divisions of joint conditions are not absolute but represent the typical or usual pattern for these conditions. In general, when examining patients presenting with multiple joint complaints (whether symmetric or asymmetric), therapists need to consider a systemic cause of the symptoms. Timely diagnosis of these systemic conditions is paramount considering the potential for rapid irreversible joint tissue destruction. In addition, many inflammatory and systemic disorders involve other body organ systems with a potential for significant morbidity.

Similar to the number of involved joints, which joints are involved also provides clues about the underlying cause of the symptoms. Figure 7-1 provides a comparison between primary OA (most common form of OA; age-related) and RA, illustrating examples of similarities, as well as some distinct differences. For example, both OA and RA commonly involve the hips, knees, cervical spine, shoulders, hands, and feet, whereas OA rarely involves the elbow, forearm, and craniomandibular joints. Even within areas of similarities, distinct patterns emerge. For example, in the shoulder complex, RA tends to involve the sternoclavicular and glenohumeral joints, whereas OA tends to involve the acromioclavicular joint. Primary OA of the cervical spine most commonly involves the C5-6 and C6-7 motion segments, but RA involves the entire cervical spine, resulting in potentially dangerous upper cervical spine instability. In the wrist and

BOX 7-1

Joint Conditions and Associated Monoarticular or Polyarticular Presentation

Monoarticular	Polyarticular
Osteoarthritis	Rheumatoid arthritis (often symmetric)
Gout	Juvenile rheumatoid arthritis (symmetric or asymmetric)
Psoriatic arthritis	Psoriatic arthritis
Septic arthritis	Systemic lupus erythematosus (often asymmetric)
	Ankylosing spondylitis (often asymmetric)
	Reactive arthritis (often asymmetric)

hands, RA tends to involve multiple joints, including the carpal, metacarpophalangeal (MCP), and interphalangeal (IP) joints, whereas OA most commonly involves the first carpometacarpal joint and IP joints but tends to spare the MCP joints. Similarly, in the ankle-foot complex, OA usually involves the first metatarsophalangeal joint, whereas RA involves multiple joints.

Table 7-1 provides a generalized summary of sites most commonly involved with various joint conditions.[3,6,17-20,44] This will assist clinicians as they investigate the patient's complaints of joint pain and begin to develop the differential diagnosis.

Some disorders end up involving joints from multiple body regions but commonly start in a specific region. For example, although approximately one third of those with ankylosing spondylitis present with involvement of the hips, knees, and/or shoulders, classically symptoms generally start at the sacroiliac joints (SIJs), especially in males. Women with ankylosing spondylitis often present with initial involvement of the lower limb joints (knees, tarsals) and tend to have fewer spinal complaints. RA is another example; symptoms often start at the MCP and IP joints and then involve other joints.[3,4,17-20,44]

Despite the patterns that emerge when considering the number and location of joint complaints, there is overlap between OA and other conditions that require physician intervention. For example, although OA is commonly considered a monoarticular condition, someone who has a history of playing rugby or football and continues to be very active could easily have bilateral OA pain. In addition, joints such as the hip and knee are commonly involved with both OA and numerous inflammatory disorders. Therefore, what else can the clinician rely on to differentiate these conditions further?

Investigation of Joint Pain

As noted in Chapter 6, investigating patients' chief complaints includes the following: (1) location and description of symptoms; (2) onset of symptoms—insidious, traumatic, or repetitive; (3) aggravating and alleviating factors; and (4) night pain and early morning stiffness. The patient's symptomatic "story" can influence therapist's comfort level regarding the suspected cause of joint symptoms. Patterns may emerge that suggest the presence of an active inflammatory or infectious process, requiring patient referral to a physician. Table 7-2 presents a summary of most common symptomatic patterns; it should be understood that as with joint anatomic location and number of joints involved, there are exceptions to every rule.[3,4,17-20,44]

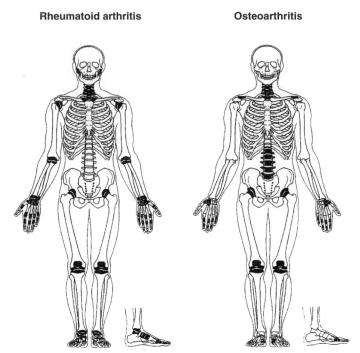

Rheumatoid arthritis   **Osteoarthritis**

FIGURE 7-1 Joints commonly involved in rheumatoid and primary osteoarthritis. (From Caldron PH: Screening for rheumatic disease. In Boissonnault WG, ed: *Examination in physical therapy practice,* 2nd ed, Churchill Livingstone, 1995, New York, p 260.)

In summary, symptom patterns unusual for OA but common for inflammatory and infectious conditions are marked by the following:

- Prolonged morning stiffness (>30 minutes), called "post–rest gel"
- Acute, severe pain; insidious onset or mild trauma
- Significant joint symptom worsening with prolonged rest, often relieved with activity
- Night pain not relieved with position change
- Joint edema, warmth, and/or redness

Finally, in terms of patient history, joint conditions associated with an inflammatory or infectious cause typically manifest with extra-articular symptoms. The systemic nature of many of these conditions results in complaints not associated with OA or other joint or soft tissue overuse or traumatic injuries. The presence of a positive review of systems finding accompanying joint pain should be a warning to clinicians that a patient referral may be indicated.

Review of Systems and Systems Review

See Chapters 9 and 10 for a detailed review of systems (ROS), including checklists of symptoms and signs associated with organ system disease and systemic illnesses. These chapters present the parameters of what makes a finding a red flag—for example, unexplained weight loss, such as a 5% to 10% loss over a 4-week to 6- to 12-month time frame, and no explanation for the loss. Starting first with a comparison between OA and RA, RA is a systemic illness marked by extra-articular manifestations, but OA is a local, nonsystemic bone and articular cartilage condition. Therefore OA manifests none of the features shown in Figure 7-2, features that can be characteristic of RA.

TABLE 7-1

Comparison of Joint Disorders and Common Anatomic Sites of Involvement[*]

Site of Involvement	OA	RA	AS	Gout	Reiter's Syndrome	SLE	Psoriatic Arthritis
Craniomandibular joint		X					
Cervical spine	X	X	X				
Shoulder	X (ACJ)	X (SCJ, GHJ)	X			X	
Elbow, forearm		X		X			X
Carpals		X		X			X
MCP		X		X	X	X	X
Hand IP	X	X		X	X	X	X
Lumbar spine	X		X		X		X
Sacroiliac joints			X		X	X	X
Hips	X	X	X		X	X	
Knee	X	X	X	X	X		X
Tarsals		X		X	X	X	X
MTP	X	X		X (first)	X (first)		X
Foot IP		X					X

[*]X indicates common site of involvement.
ACJ, acromioclavicular joint; AS, ankylosing spondylitis; GHJ, glenohumeral joint; IP, interphalangeal joint; MCP, metacarpophalangeal joint; OA, osteoarthritis; RA, rheumatoid arthritis; SCJ, sternoclavicular joint; SLE, systemic lupus erythematosus.

TABLE 7-2

Comparison of Joint Disorders and Common Symptomatic Descriptors

Parameter	OA	RA	AS	Gout	Reiter's Syndrome	SLE	Psoriatic Arthritis	Septic Arthritis
Descriptors	Dull ache	Soreness, stiffness, tightness	Stiffness, soreness	Severe excruciating pain	Soreness, stiffness	Soreness, ache, stiffness	Soreness, tenderness, stiffness	Severe excruciating pain
Symptom onset	Insidious	Insidious	Insidious	Insidious, but acute onset, often at night	Often accute	Insidious	Insidious	Insidious, but often acute
Symptomatic progression	Slow	Slow or rapid	Slow or rapid	Rapid	Slow or rapid	Slow or rapid	Slow or rapid	Rapid
Aggravating factors	WB activity	Rest and intense activity	Rest	WB activity	Rest and intense activity	Rest and intense activity	Rest and intense activity	WB activity
Alleviating factors	Rest	Short rest, mild activity	Activity, movement	Less pain with rest, but unrelenting	Short rest and mild activity	Short rest, mild activity	Short rest, mild activity	Less pain with rest, but unrelenting
Night pain	Yes		Yes, awakens typically during the second half of the night	Yes	Yes			Yes
Post–rest gel (early morning stiffness)	Short, <30 min	Severe, >30-60 min	Severe, >30-60 min		Moderate to severe	Moderate, less severe than RA	Moderate, >30 min	

AS, ankylosing spondylitis; OA, osteoarthritis; RA, rheumatoid arthritis; SLE, systemic lupus erythematosus; WB, weight-bearing.

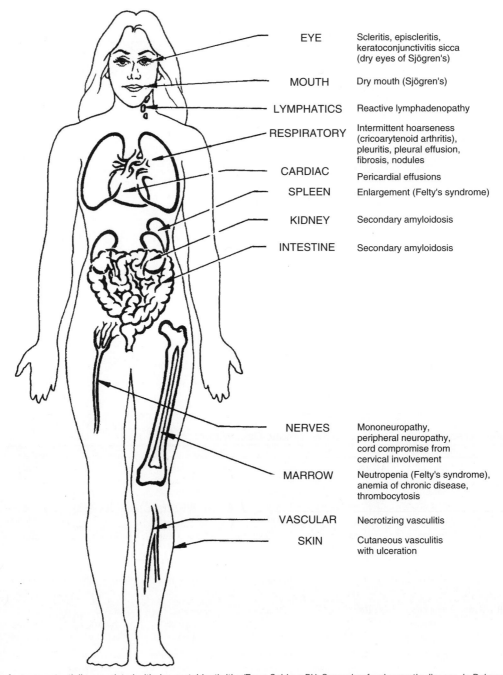

	EYE	Scleritis, episcleritis, keratoconjunctivitis sicca (dry eyes of Sjögren's)
	MOUTH	Dry mouth (Sjögren's)
	LYMPHATICS	Reactive lymphadenopathy
	RESPIRATORY	Intermittent hoarseness (cricoarytenoid arthritis), pleuritis, pleural effusion, fibrosis, nodules
	CARDIAC	Pericardial effusions
	SPLEEN	Enlargement (Felty's syndrome)
	KIDNEY	Secondary amyloidosis
	INTESTINE	Secondary amyloidosis
	NERVES	Mononeuropathy, peripheral neuropathy, cord compromise from cervical involvement
	MARROW	Neutropenia (Felty's syndrome), anemia of chronic disease, thrombocytosis
	VASCULAR	Necrotizing vasculitis
	SKIN	Cutaneous vasculitis with ulceration

FIGURE 7-2 Systemic features potentially associated with rheumatoid arthritis. (From Caldron PH: Screening for rheumatic disease. In Boissonnault WG, ed: *Examination in physical therapy practice,* 2nd ed, Churchill Livingstone, 1995, New York, p 262.)

The systemic nature of RA also accounts for constitutional complaints such as fatigue, malaise, low-grade fever, and weight loss.

Box 7-2 provides a summary of the most common ROS findings associated with various joint disorders (other than RA).[3,4,17-20,44] Note that under OA, "None" is listed, a significant distinction when compared with the other diseases.

Joint pain associated with feelings of being run down (malaise), low-grade fever, anorexia, weight loss, and fatigue should alert the therapist to the potential of a systemic illness. These complaints and the other ROS items noted may precede the joint complaints—for example, the uveitis associated with ankylosing spondylitis. This illustrates the importance of review of ROS

questioning related to the differential diagnostic process, recognizing when a physician referral is indicated.

Numerous elements of the physical examination can support concern about the cause of the joint complaints elicited during the patient history. A joint that presents with redness, warmth, and/or edema, especially in lieu of any trauma, or with minor trauma, should alert the therapist to the need for a potentially urgent physician referral. The integumentary, cardiovascular, pulmonary, and neurologic screening associated with the systems review may also reveal important findings (see Box 7-2). Figures 7-3 and 7-4 present a summary of key red flag findings associated with patients with acute and chronic joint pain.

BOX 7-2

Comparison of Joint Disorders: Common Associated Review of Systems Findings

OSTEOARTHRITIS
None

SYSTEMIC LUPUS ERYTHEMATOSUS
Skin rash (malar rash most common)
Fever, fatigue, malaise
Photosensitivity
Dyspnea, cough
Peripheral neuropathies

REITER'S SYNDROME
Urethritis
Conjunctivitis
Nausea, vomiting, diarrhea
Weight loss

ANKYLOSING SPONDYLITIS
Uveitis (20%-30% of patients)
Fatigue, weight loss, fever, malaise
Cardiac and pulmonary complications

GOUT
Fever, malaise
Tachycardia

PSORIATIC ARTHRITIS
Fever, fatigue, malaise
Psoriasis

SEPTIC ARTHRITIS
Fever, chills, malaise

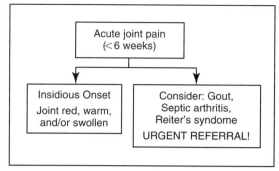

FIGURE 7-3 Classic acute joint pain red flag findings warranting an urgent physician referral.

Joint Pain: Patient Demographic and Health History Information

The details of joint pain descriptions provide the most relevant information, but patient demographics and other health risk factors can provide valuable clues about the relative risk of developing different joint conditions. Table 7-3 provides a comparison of risk factors.[3,17-20,44]

Summary

Although acute joint pain—insidious onset, accompanied by warmth, redness, and edema—provides an easy scenario leading to an urgent physician referral, many of the disorders discussed will not present so clearly and obviously. In those cases, one examination finding rarely provides enough guidance to the clinician, but a cluster of findings may. Screening criteria may be present for some disorders, but not all. For example, Rudwaleit and colleagues[40] have provide such a screening combination for ankylosing spondylitis (Box 7-3) and Arnett and associates[2] have listed classification criteria for RA (Box 7-4).

Limb Pain

Many patients also seek physical therapy services for limb non-joint-related pain. As with complaints of joint pain, certain patterns of limb symptoms suggest that physician involvement is necessary. For example, bilateral and symmetric limb complaints, or limb pain that migrates from one limb or limbs to another for no mechanical sounding reason, are unusual for conditions typically managed by physical therapists. Other conditions are more local, involving one limb (e.g., lower leg pain), but present with a pattern of worsening and potential for significant tissue compromise (bony, vascular, or neurologic). Depending on the examination findings and therapist's concerns, the patient referral to a physician may be urgent in nature. Conditions associated with limb pain covered in this section include hypothyroidism, Lyme disease, polymyalgia rheumatica, statin-related myopathies or myalgias, vascular and neurogenic claudication, tibial stress reaction injury (stress fracture), deep venous thrombosis, and

compartment syndrome. The discussion of these conditions will reveal similarities in clinical manifestations with conditions that can be effectively managed by physical therapists, complicating the differential diagnostic process. As with joint pain, a pattern will emerge of how investigating patient's health histories, review of systems, and systems review is critical to recognizing when a patient referral is necessary.

Multilimb Complaints

When patients present with bilateral limb complaints, therapists must consider a central or spinal origin—if patients complain of upper and lower limb complaints, the cervical spine must be considered—or a systemic cause. Hypothyroidism, Lyme disease, polymyalgia rheumatica, and medications such as statins can all manifest as arthralgias or myalgias. The typical distinguishing limb pain features for these conditions are listed in Box 7-5.[3,17-20,43,44]

The symptomatic pattern described in Box 7-5 is unusual for conditions that can be managed well by therapists, and should raise concern about the cause, leading to detailed review of systems screening (see Chapter 9). The presence of manifestations noted in Table 7-4, along with the accompanying nonmechanical symptom pattern, would support the decision to initiate a physician consult.[3,17-20,43,44]

As illustrated in Table 7-4, hypothyroidism affects multiple body systems and, if all the manifestations were present with the myalgias, therapists would easily recognize the need for a physician referral. Typically, however, the initial symptoms are fleeting and, in addition to the pain and stiffness, fatigue; slow, steady weight gain; constipation; dry skin; and cold intolerance tend to dominate.[43] Lyme disease is primarily found in Northeast coastal areas, upper Midwest states, and coastal Oregon and northern California. The classic erythema migrans rash is not present in all Lyme disease victims (approximately 80%); also, by the time the patient seeks therapy services for the musculoskeletal pain, the rash may have disappeared. There is also a spirochete incubation period of up to 32 days, so the outdoor (tick exposure) experience may have occurred 2 or 3 months prior to the onset of myalgia or arthralgia complaints. Polymyalgia rheumatica is marked by pain and stiffness, most commonly in the shoulder girdle regions and pelvis-thigh regions (bilateral and symmetric). The forearm, wrist, and hand regions may also be involved. As with the inflammatory joint conditions, early morning stiffness lasting 1 hour or longer is typical. The proximal involvement leads to difficulties, such as with bed mobility, transitional movements, and ambulation. Statin-induced myopathy appears to be dose-related. See Box 7-6 for a list of statins and dose thresholds associated with increased adverse events. For example, a fourfold or fivefold increase in adverse effects was noted with atorvastatin and simvastatin when daily doses were increased from 40 to 80 mg.[2,46]

The literature describing adverse muscle events associated with statins has been confusing because of the lack of consistent definitions. Four different syndromes have been documented—myopathy, myalgia, myositis, and rhabdomyolysis—with an estimated incidence of adverse events of 5% to 14%. Any of the four types can be debilitating, but rhabdomyolysis (skeletal muscle destruction) in particular carries potential serious health risks.

A timely diagnosis of these conditions is important considering the potentially serious complications that can arise if medical treatment is not initiated quickly. For example, rhabdomyolysis can be marked by azotemia, hyperkalemia, cardiac arrhythmia,

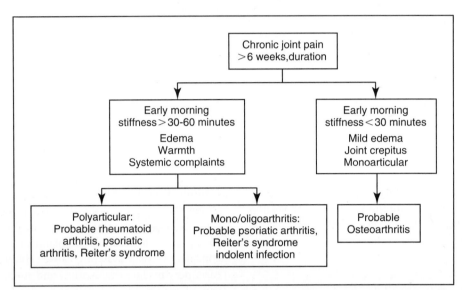

FIGURE 7-4 Classic chronic joint pain clinical manifestations comparing inflammatory arthritis with osteoarthritis conditions.

TABLE 7-3

Comparison of Patient Demographics and Health History Risk Factors

Risk Factor	Age of Symptom Onset (yr)	Sex Predilection	Family History	Health History Risk Factors
Primary osteoarthritis	Men mid-40s to early 50s; women surpass men >65	None		Joint infection, major trauma, hemarthrosis
Rheumatoid arthritis	Peak onset, 20-50	Female (2-3 times more than men)	Positive	Autoimmune thyroid disorders; history of nulliparity in women not using birth control, pregnancy and use of birth control pills lower risk
Ankylosing spondylitis	Teens through fourth decade; rare after 40	Male (2-3 times more than in women)	Positive	
Systemic lupus erythematosus	Peak onset 15-40	Female (3 times more common in African American than Caucasian women)	Positive	Infection (viral, streptococcal), sunlight or ultraviolet light exposure, medications (e.g., hydralazine, anticonvulsants, penicillins)
Gout	30; peak incidence in fifth decade	Male; incidence increases in women typically >15 yr postmenopause	Positive	Renal disorders associated with increased levels of uric acid, leukemia, lymphoma, psoriasis, chemotherapy, hypothyroidism, heavy alcohol consumption, taking diuretics and salicylates
Psoriatic arthritis	Psoriasis—peak onset in second and third decades, with arthritis following up to 20 yr later	None	Positive	Psoriasis
Reiter's syndrome	Peak onset, third decade	More common in males		Venereal or dysenteric infection
Septic arthritis				Systemic corticosteroid use, diabetes, infection elsewhere, direct penetrating joint trauma

renal failure, and disseminated intravascular coagulation. In addition to the organ failure, the local edema can cause neurovascular compromise similar to compartment syndrome, necessitating a fasciotomy to avoid tissue necrosis. Polymyalgia rheumatica has a strong association with giant cell arteritis, with up to 20% of patients developing this vasculitis condition. The resultant vascular stenosis can result in permanent visual loss if the cranial arteries are involved, and the inflammation can lead to aortic dissection.[2,46] Blood vessels typically involved include the medium and large vessels originating from the aortic arch. The inflammation is likely to be segmental, skipping portions of the vessel. See Box 7-7 for a summary of clinical manifestations associated with giant cell arteritis, with an emphasis on the two most common locations involved—the cranial-temporal and aortic arch vessels.[3,17-20,44]

Dizziness

General Considerations

Dizziness (impairment in spatial perception and stability) and vertigo (spinning sensation) rank among the most common complaints in medicine, affecting approximately 20% to 30% of persons in the general population.[21,22,27] An estimated 7.5 million patients with dizziness are examined each year in ambulatory care settings, and dizziness is one of the most common complaints in the emergency department.[28] The top three settings in which those with dizziness present are primary care clinics (medical offices, physical therapy, and/or chiropractic clinics), emergency departments, and specialized dizziness clinics (otolaryngology, neurologic and vestibular clinics).[11] Although common in adults, especially in those older than 60 years (almost 20%), dizziness in children is rare.[27] Age is a significant contributor to dizziness; with every 5-year increase in age, there is a 10% increase in the probability of dizziness.[11] Table 7-5 outlines dizziness across the life span, key diagnoses to watch for, and recommendations for the primary care provider.

The nonspecific subjective complaint of dizziness has a multitude of pathophysiologic causes (e.g., vestibular, cardiovascular, craniovertebral junction disorders, neurologic, psychiatric) and deserves follow-up questioning by the primary care physical therapist. Serious pathologic neck conditions should be considered when evaluating for sources of dizziness (Box 7-8).[13]

A precise description of the nature of dizziness is the most crucial factor in identifying a specific diagnosis.[11] A timeline of symptoms (acute versus gradual onset), duration (seconds versus minutes versus hours versus days), dizziness related to positional changes, and any associated complaints (e.g., hearing loss, tinnitus, aural pressure, central nervous system (CNS) or cerebellar signs) are essential to ascertain. Accurate and timely diagnosis and management are essential in life-threatening cases of dizziness (e.g., intracranial bleeds, cardiac arrhythmias, brain tumor) and can significantly improve long-term quality of life.[11,27]

Questions regarding dysequilibrium and function (walking, hearing, vision) are pertinent. If head and neck movements generate cardinal signs of dizziness (e.g., bilateral or quadrilateral paraesthesia, perioral [lip] numbness, nystagmus, drop attacks), either cord compression caused by atlantoaxial instability (AAI) or vertebrobasilar artery insufficiency should be considered.[34,37] If trauma to the head and neck has induced dizziness, a full examination for traumatic brain injury (see later, "Traumatic Brain

---

BOX 7-3

Classification Criteria for Ankylosing Spondylitis

Individual parameters
- Morning stiffness >30 min in duration
- Improvement in back pain with exercise, but not with rest
- Night pain during second half of night only
- Alternating buttock pain
  If at least two of four criteria present:
- Sensitivity = 36.6% (95% confidence interval [CI], 27.9-46.4)
- Specificity = 83.9% (95% CI, 76.0-89.6)
- Positive likelihood ratio = 2.3 (95% CI, 1.4-3.7)
- Post-test probability = 10.8%
  If at least three of four criteria present:
- Sensitivity, 33.6% (95% CI, 25.1-43.3)
- Specificity, 97.3% (95% CI, 92.4-99.1)
- Positive likelihood ratio = 12.4 (95% CI, 4.0-39.7)
- Post-test probability = 39.4%

BOX 7-4

Classification Criteria for Rheumatoid Arthritis*

Criterion	Description
Morning stiffness[†]	In and around the joints, lasting at least 1 hr before maximal improvement
Arthritis of three or more joint areas[†]	Simultaneously has soft tissue swelling or fluid observed by clinician; 14 possible areas include right or left PIP, MCP, wrist, elbow, knee, ankle, and MTP joints
Arthritis of hand joints[†]	Minimum of one area swollen in wrist, MCP, or PIP joints
Symmetric arthritis[†]	Simultaneous involvement of same joint areas as defined in criterion 2 (bilateral involvement of PIP, MCP, or MTP joints acceptable without absolute symmetry)
Rheumatoid nodules	Subcutaneous nodules, over bony prominences or extensor surfaces or in juxta-articular regions, observed by clinician
Serum rheumatoid factor	Abnormal amounts of serum rheumatoid factor determined by any method for which result has been positive in <5% of normal control subjects
Radiographic changes	Posteroanterior hand and wrist radiographs, including erosions, unequivocal bony decalcification localized in or most marked adjacent to involved joints (OA changes alone do not qualify)

*Duration of disease <1 yr. If at least four of seven criteria are present for disease of <1 yr, sensitivity is 85%, specificity is 90%.
†These four criteria must be present for at least 6 weeks.
MCP, metacarpophalangeal; *MTP,* metatarsophalangeal; *OA,* osteoarthritis; *PIP,* proximal interphalangeal.

Injury") and a trauma algorithm for examination of the neck (Box 7-9) should be undertaken by the primary care provider.

The patient's past medical history, medications, and lifestyle factors (e.g., smoking, alcohol, exercise, sleep hygiene) should all be considered as possible sources or contributors to dizziness. Many medications (e.g., antibiotics, antineoplastics, diuretics) and environmental toxins (e.g., toluene or methylbenzene, mercury, tin, lead, carbon monoxide) are ototoxic—that is, they have a deleterious effect on the vestibular or cochlear division of cranial nerve (CN) VIII. Other medications (e.g., antihistamines, anticholinergics, antidepressants, opioids) have sedative influences on the vestibular system and/or the CNS.[14] Neurologic red flags (e.g., numbness, tingling, weakness, slurred speech, loss of consciousness [LOC], rigidity, visual field loss, memory loss, cranial nerve dysfunction, progressive hearing loss, tremors, poor coordination, upper motor neuron signs) all warrant further investigation.[34] All medical examinations and tests to date, as well as living situation, work, and functional status, should be ascertained.

The Dizziness Handicap Inventory (DHI) can be a helpful outcome tool to ascertain baseline; monitor symptoms; and differentiate physical (P), functional (F), and emotional (E) factors associated with dizziness (Figure 7-6).[23] Possible scores for the DHI range from 0 to 100, with higher scores indicating a worse handicap. Subscores for each domain (P, F, and E) can also be calculated. Whitney and colleagues have proposed that DHI scores correlate well to levels of functional balance impairment.[53]

Categories of Dizziness

Dizziness can be classified into four broad categories (Figure 7-7) but, like many generalized classification systems, this has its shortcomings. First, it must be understood that these categories best

---

BOX 7-5
Clinical Features of Pathologic Origins of Limb Pain

Symptom Descriptors
- Typically aching, cramping, weakness, stiffness

Symptom Location
- Often multiple limbs involved
- Symptoms may migrate from one area to another

Symptom Onset
- Insidious onset

Symptom 24-Hour Report
- Nonmechanical pattern—aggravating or alleviating factors. Although symptoms may increase with general activity, they are not consistently associated with specific movements, postures, or positions.
- Prolonged early morning stiffness—possibly >30 min

TABLE 7-4
Pathologic Origins of Limb Symptoms: Patient Demographics, Risk Factors, and Review of Systems

Parameter	Primary Hypothyroidism	Lyme Disease	Polymyalgia Rheumatica	Statin-Related Myopathy*
Age	Typically, from 30-60 yr	Any	Rare <50 yr	Advanced age
Sex	Female-to-male ratio, 4:1	Either	Female-to-male ratio, 2-3:1; much more common in whites, non-Hispanics	Women > men
Pain characteristics			Bilateral pain and stiffness, stiffness severe in early morning	
Medical history risk factors	Hashimoto's thyroiditis, thyroid ablation (radioiodine, surgical), radiation therapy for head or neck cancer, medications (e.g., lithium, methimazole, amiodarone)	Exposure to tick (*Ixodes* sp.)		High dose (see Box 7-6), concurrent use of immunosuppressant drugs, frail health, hypothyroidism, chronic renal impairment, alcohol abuse, ingestion of grapefruit juice (typically, >0.95 L/day)
Review of systems—constitutional complaints	Fatigue, unexplained weight gain, weakness, subjective paresthesia	Early stages—fatigue, malaise, fever, chills, lethargy	Fatigue, weight loss, malaise, low-grade fever	Weakness; if associated with rhabdomyolysis, dark tea-colored urine, nausea, fever
Review of body systems	Cold intolerance, dyspnea, constipation, menstrual irregularities, hair loss, brittle nails	Peripheral neuritis complaints and radiculopathies		
Systems review	Bradycardia, pallor, cold skin, obesity, proximal muscle weakness, slow lethargic movements, hyporeflexic, slowed deep tendon reflex (DTR) relaxation phase, hair loss, nonpitting edema (eyes, hands, feet), change in mentation	Early stages—erythema migrans (but rash tends to fade by wk 3 or 4); later stages—cranial neuropathies, encephalitis (headache, neck stiffness with flexion)	Diffuse edema, possible pitting edema in dorsum of hands or feet	If associated with rhabdomyolysis, muscle edema possibly associated with neurovascular compromise—numbness, weakness, pallor, lack of pulses

*Statins include atorvastatin (Lipitor), fluvastatin (Lescol), lovastatin (Mevacor), pravastatin (Pravachol), and simvastatin (Zocor).

represent the patient's chief complaint, not the patient's differential diagnosis. Similarly, these categories are not mutually exclusive. A subject can have a presyncopal cause of dizziness (vascular compromise to the cerebellum) and experience vertigo (sensation of spinning), dysequilibrium (imbalance), and psychophysiologic (panic/anxiety) symptoms all at the same time. Furthermore, these groupings are not specific to a particular body system.

VERTIGO. Vertigo, the illusion of rotatory movement, is caused by asymmetric involvement of the vestibular system.[27] The vestibular system consists of peripheral components (CN

BOX 7-6

Dose-Related Thresholds for Stain-Induced Myopathy

Atorvastatin (Lipitor), 80 mg
Simvastatin (Zocor), 80 mg
Pravastatin (Pravachol), 160 mg
Rosuvastatin (Crestor), 80 mg

BOX 7-7

Common Clinical Manifestations of Giant Cell Arteritis

CRANIAL OR TEMPORAL ARTERITIS
- Headache, unilateral—temporal area, throbbing, piercing, sudden onset, intense
- Jaw claudication
- Visual disturbances—flashing lights, diplopia, and/or field deficits may precede blindness
- Acute hearing loss and vertigo

AORTIC ARCH SYNDROME
- Upper extremity claudication
- Reynaud's phenomenon

POSSIBLE ACCOMPANYING SYSTEMIC COMPLAINTS
- Fever, fatigue, malaise, weight loss

VIII, semicircular canal, and otolith [utricle and saccule]) and central components (vestibular nuclear complex, vestibulocerebellum, brain stem, spinal cord, and vestibular cortex). Oscillopsia, an illusion of linear motion (e.g., up and down, side to side, or forward and backward bobbing of the visual field), is most commonly associated with vestibular dysfunction (vestibular labyrinth, CN VIII, cerebellum, vestibular nuclei, or their neurologic projections) but can also be caused by extraocular muscle paresis (CN III, IV, and VI).[21] Autonomic symptoms, such as diaphoresis, pallor, nausea, and vomiting, are commonly associated with vertigo (peripheral greater than central) and are typically less prominent with other types of dizziness.[27]

Peripheral Vestibular Disorders. Peripheral vestibular problems are common (40% of dizziness problems) and implicate damage to CN VIII and its end-organs.[27] Despite the fact that persons with peripheral vestibular lesions tend to have more pronounced nausea and vomiting, more prominent movement illusions (sensation of horizontal environment spin or clear self-rotation), and auditory symptoms (hearing loss, tinnitus, fullness or pain in the ear), most of these conditions are benign and readily treatable.[12,27] Physical therapy is advocated to help patients accommodate to unilateral or bilateral peripheral vestibular loss.[14,21]

Benign paroxysmal (sudden-onset) positional vertigo (BPPV) is the most common peripheral vertigo. The condition occurs when debris (otoconia) from the utricle accidently circulates within the endolymphatic system (semicircular canals), causing positional irritation of the cupula and stimulating vertigo and nystagmus.[12] The condition comes in two forms—canalilithiasis (loose debris) and cupololithiasis (attached debris); the latter is more difficult to manage. The Epley maneuver has been proven to be 85% to 95% effective in treating patients with BPPV.[12,21]

TABLE 7-5

Dizziness Across the Life Span: Diagnoses and Recommendations

Age (yr)	Key Differential Diagnoses that Can Cause Complaint of Dizziness	Recommended Action by Primary Care Provider
Infants and toddlers, 0-3	Benign paroxysmal positional vertigo (BPPV) of childhood; vestibular migraine; vestibular neuronitis (labyrinthitis); brain stem or cerebellar tumor; traumatic brain injury (see "Traumatic Brain Injury")	BPPV and vestibular migraine account for 50% of cases; symptoms can include headache, fever, nausea, and/or vomiting.[24] Given the prevalence of brain tumor in children, MRI may be warranted. Children 0-4 yr of age are at high risk for TBI.[29]
Children and adolescents, 3-18[3]	Vertiginous migraine (39%); BPPV (15%); vestibular neuronitis (ear infection) (14%); anxiety (13%); orthostatic hypotension (9%); concussion (3%); seizure (3%); syncope (2%); nonspecific dizziness (2%)	More judicious use of laboratory tests, electroencephalography, electronystagmography, and MRI is suggested for diagnosing children with dizziness or vertigo.*
Adults, 19-65	Vestibular neuronitis (labyrinthitis); BPPV (typically traumatic onset); presyncopal conditions	Vestibular neuronitis (inner ear infection) with acute onset of dizziness, with or without associated hearing loss, necessitates same-day referral to ENT specialist (audiography). Attempt to differentiate between central and peripheral vestibular.
Older adults, >65	BPPV (insidious onset because of aging), presyncopal conditions	Must rule out presyncopal conditions (orthostatic hypotension, vascular disease, arrhythmia) in this age group because many can be life-threatening or result in high morbidity.

*Ravid and colleagues[38] have developed a questionnaire and a computer-assisted algorithm (Figure 7-5) to aid in diagnosing children with dizziness or vertigo. The sensitivity of the questionnaire in reaching the correct diagnosis was calculated to be 92%. The sensitivity of the computer algorithm was 84%.

ENT, ear, nose, and throat; *MRI,* magnetic resonance imaging; *TBI,* traumatic brain injury.

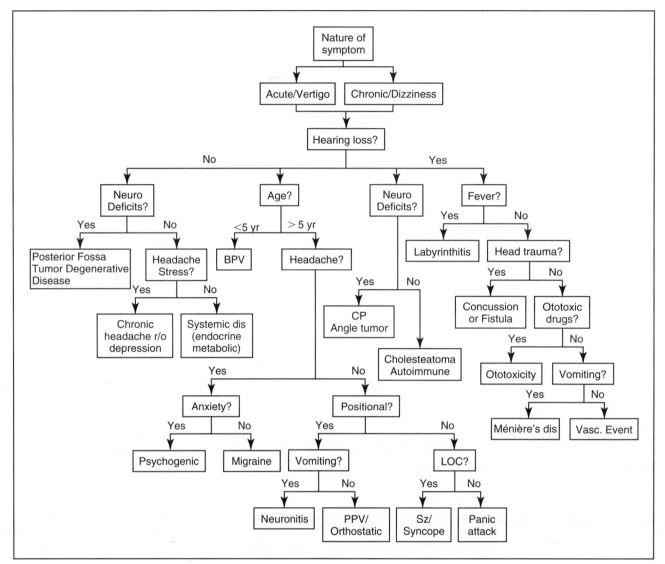

FIGURE 7-5 Diagnostic algorithm for dizziness in children and adolescents (3-18 years of age). *BPV*, Benign paroxysmal vertigo; *CP*, cerebellopontine; *Dis*, disease; *LOC*, loss of consciousness; *PPV*, paroxysmal positional vertigo; *r/o*, rule out; *Sz*, seizure; *Vasc*, vascular.

BOX 7-8

Manifestations of Serious Pathologic Neck Conditions

Cervical Myelopathy	Neoplastic Conditions	Upper Cervical Ligamentous Instability	Vertebral Artery Insufficiency	Inflammatory or Systemic Disease
Sensory disturbances of the hands	Age >50 yr	Occipital headache and numbness	Drop attacks	Temperature >37° C
Muscle wasting of hand intrinsic muscles	Previous history of cancer	Severe limitation during neck active range of motion in all directions	Dizziness or lightheadedness related to neck movement	Blood pressure >160/95 mm Hg
Unsteady gait	Unexplained weight loss	Signs of cervical myelopathy	Dysphasia	Resting pulse >100 beats/min
Hoffman's reflex	Constant pain, no relief with bed rest		Dysarthria	Resting respiration >25 breaths/min
Hyperreflexia	Night pain		Diplopia	Fatigue
Bowel and bladder disturbances			Positive cranial nerve signs	
Multisegmental weakness and/or sensory changes				

Modified from Childs JD, Fritz JM, Piva SR, Whitman JM: Proposal of a classification system for patients with neck pain, *J Orthop Sport Phys Ther* 34:686-700, 2004.

BOX 7-9

Sequencing the Examination of the Patient With Post-Traumatic Neck Injury

History of cardinal signs → physician
- Bilateral or quadrilateral limb paresthesia
- Perioral (lip) numbness
- Nystagmus
- Drop attacks

Fracture tests → physician
- Canadian cervical spine rules (see Chapter 14, "Diagnostic Imaging")
- Gross loss of active or passive range of motion
- Observation of mastoid or facial ecchymosis
- Light cranial compression painful
- Abnormal end feel on ligamentous testing
- Painful weakness on resisted isometric contraction
- Tuning fork (pain with vibration)

Neurologic tests positive → physician
- Cranial nerve signs
- Long tract signs—evaluate neurologic systems, including sensation (light touch, pain, temperature), mechanoreception (conscious proprioception, vibration, stereoagnosis), motor (strength, spasticity, coordination), deep tendon reflexes, clonus, and nociceptive reflex tests (Babinski, Oppenheimer, Hoffman)

Ligament tests positive → physician
- Tectorial membrane (Pettman's distraction test)
- Alar rotation and side-bending tests
- Transverse ligament stress test
- Sharp-Purser test

Vertebral artery test positive → physician

Modified from Meadows JTS: *Orthopedic differential diagnosis in physical therapy: a case study approach*, New York, 1999, McGraw-Hill.

Otitis media (middle ear infection) can cause acute onset of vertigo. Patients with otitis media are at risk for permanent hearing loss if left untreated. Early use of antibiotics and treatment of the underlying otitis should negate complications.[12]

Labyrinthitis (inflammation the canals of the inner ear) can be the result of unmanaged otitis media or an upper respiratory infection (URI), or can have an unknown cause (viral or bacterial agent). It may also follow allergy, cholesteatoma (abnormal skin growth in the middle ear behind the eardrum), or ingestion of ototoxic drugs. Severe vertigo, hearing loss, nausea, and fever are hallmarks. Bacterial labyrinthitis is one of the few causes of peripheral vertigo that requires early and aggressive management (transfer to the emergency department, possible hospitalization for intravenous antibiotics) to prevent progression to meningitis or the need for surgical débridement of the internal auditory canal.[12]

Vestibular neuritis usually results as a complication of a viral URI. The virus affects the vestibular nuclei and causes sudden and severe vertigo, nausea, and vomiting that is debilitating. Auditory symptoms are usually absent. The peak age is 40 to 50 years. Aggressive treatment with prednisone in the first 10 days after onset may shorten the course of illness. Ramsay Hunt syndrome is a variant of vestibular neuritis (varicella zoster) that affects CN VII (facial paralysis) and CN VIII (tinnitus, hearing loss, vestibular defect). In addition to prednisone, a course of acyclovir is recommended for these patients.[12]

Cholesteatoma is a benign skin growth in the middle ear behind the eardrum, usually caused by repeat infection. Over time, the cholesteatoma can increase in size and destroy the delicate bones of the middle ear (malleus, incus, stapes), causing hearing loss and transient severe vertigo (few seconds). Surgical resection is indicated for symptomatic patients.[12]

Trauma to the head and neck is a significant source of dizziness and dysequilibrium, causing from 40% to 60% of cases. There are numerous causes, including blunt trauma to the head causing concussion of the membranous labyrinth and an explosive blast (pressure sound waves) or barotrauma (atmospheric pressure change seen in pilots and deep-sea divers). The latter is rare but can rupture the membrane between the middle ear and perilymphatic space. Perilymph fistulas from barotraumas cause sudden severe vertigo and dizziness and typically require 1 to 2 weeks of bed rest and avoidance of the Valsalva maneuver. A few cases will require surgery.[12]

Endolymphatic hydrops presents with a classic triad of tinnitus, fluctuant sensorineural hearing loss, and severe vertigo (minutes to an hour). Ménière's disease is the most common variant. The condition usually starts unilaterally, becomes more frequent over time, and progresses to bilateral symptoms in 50% of cases. Strict salt restriction and diuretics are cornerstones of treatment, used for 90% of cases. One in 10 patients requires surgical intervention (e.g., endolymphatic sac decompression or shunting, vestibular nerve resection, labyrinthectomy). Chemical ablation of the vestibular apparatus can be performed but carries a greater risk of hearing loss.[12]

Vestibular schwannoma or acoustic neuroma is a benign tumor of the vestibular nerve and accounts for 5% to 10% of all intracranial tumors.[27] Vertigo is the most common presenting symptom, and progressive unilateral hearing loss, tinnitus, and ataxia are common.[12,27] Gadolinium-enhanced magnetic resonance imaging (MRI) should be ordered when intracranial tumors are suspected, because MRI detects intracanalicular abnormalities with 100% sensitivity (gold standard).[12] Because the tumor can expand intracranially (become a CNS problem), radiotherapy or surgical removal is advocated.[12]

Central Vestibular Disorders. Central causes are responsible for almost 25% of the dizziness experienced by patients.[27] Central vertigo is generally associated with severe imbalance (inability to stand or walk), additional neurologic signs, less prominent movement illusion and nausea, and central nystagmus (involuntary rhythmic oscillations of the eyes).[27]

Cerebrovascular disorders that affect the blood supply to the inner ear, brain stem, and cerebellum (vertebrobasilar system) can cause vertigo. Primary care providers should watch for the five Ds—*d*izziness, *d*iplopia, *d*ysarthria, *d*ysphagia, and *d*ystaxia.[27,34,37] The five Ds cluster, along with ipsilateral cranial nerve deficits and contralateral sensorimotor deficits, is typically seen in persons with posterior circulation compromise (Box 7-10) and warrants medical referral (marker for impending stroke).[30] Symptoms may range from asymptomatic to comatose (locked-in syndrome), depending on the severity of the vascular ischemia.

Although complaints of dizziness, vertigo, and balance deficits can impair quality of life, the overall prognosis for posterior

Dizziness Handicap Inventory

Name: _____ DOB: _____ Date: _____

Instructions: The purpose of this scale is to identify difficulties that you may be experiencing because of your dizziness or unsteadiness. Please answer "yes", "no", or "sometimes" to each question.
Answer each question as it applies to your dizziness or unsteadiness only.

Item	Question		Y	N	S
1	Does looking up increase your problem?	P			
2	Because of your problem, do you feel frustrated?	E			
3	Because of your problem, do you restrict your travel for business or recreation?	F			
4	Does walking down the aisle of a supermarket increase your problem?	P			
5	Because of your problem, do you have difficulty getting into or out of bed?	F			
6	Does your problem significantly restrict your participation in social activities such as going out to dinner, to movies, dancing, or to parties?	F			
7	Because of your problem, do you have difficulty reading?	F			
8	Does performing more ambitious activities like sports, dancing, or household chores such as sweeping or putting dishes away increase your problem?	P			
9	Because of your problem, are you afraid to leave your home without having someone accompany you?	E			
10	Because of your problem, have you been embarrassed in front of others?	E			
11	Do quick movements of your head increase your problem?	P			
12	Because of your problem, do you avoid heights?	F			
13	Does turning over in bed increase your problem?	P			
14	Because of your problem, is it difficult for you to do strenuous housework or yard work?	F			
15	Because of your problem, are you afraid people may think you are intoxicated?	E			
16	Because of your problem, is it difficult for you to walk by yourself?	F			
17	Does walking down a sidewalk increase your problem?	P			
18	Because of your problem, is it difficult for you to concentrate?	E			
19	Because of your problem, is it difficult for you to walk around your house in the dark?	F			
20	Because of your problem, are you afraid to stay at home alone?	E			
21	Because of your problem, do you feel handicapped?	E			
22	Has your problem placed stress on your relationship with members of your family or friends?	E			
23	Because of your problem, are you depressed?	E			
24	Does your problem interfere with your job or household responsibilities?	F			
25	Does bending over increase your problem?	P			
			X 4	X 0	X 2
		=			
		TOTAL			

P _____ E _____ F _____

100-70 = Severe perception of having a handicap,
69-40 = Moderate perception of handicap, 39-0 = Low perception of handicap

FIGURE 7-6 Dizziness Handicap Inventory. Adapted from Jacobson GP, Newman CW: The development of the dizziness handicap inventory. *Arch Otolaryngol Head Surg* 1990; 116:414-7.

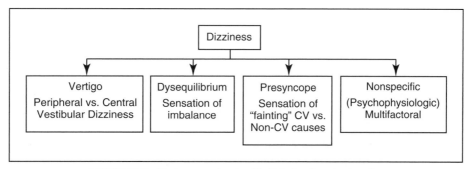

FIGURE 7-7 Dizziness can be classified into four broad categories.

Syndromes of Posterior Circulation Stroke

Location	Name of Syndrome	Ipsilateral	Contralateral
Cerebrum	Anton's (top of the basilar artery)	Bilateral loss of vision with denial of blindness, somnolence, confusion	
Midbrain	Weber's	CN III palsy (oculomotor nerve)	Hemiplegia
Pons	Millard-Gubler	CN VII palsy (facial nerve)	Hemiparesis
Medulla	Wallenberg's	Nystagmus, vertigo, Horner's syndrome, facial sensory loss	Pain and temperature loss

From Lewandoski C, Santhakumar S: Posterior circulation stroke. Foundation of Education and Research in Neurological Emergencies. http://www.uic.edu/com/ferne/pdf/posterior0501.pdf. Accessed March 11, 2010.
CN, cranial nerve.

circulation stroke is good (4% to 10% mortality) with the exception of locked-in syndrome (basilar artery occlusion), which has a more than 90% mortality.[7,30] It is noteworthy that 60% of persons with basilar artery thrombosis have prodromal symptoms (stuttering or progressive onset of symptoms 2 weeks before emergency department presentation). The prodromal symptom, in order of frequency, includes vertigo and nausea (30%), headache or neck ache (20%), hemiparesis (10%), dysarthria (10%), diplopia (10%), and hemianopia (6%).[15,30]

Migraine (periodic unilateral headaches, with or without photophobia, phonophobia, and aura) is estimated to occur in 18% to 29% of women, 6% to 20% of men, and 4% of children. Migraine and vertigo are two clinical features that tend to occur together.[27] Typically, adult migraine is temporal and unilateral. The clinical features of migraine in the pediatric population include frontal or periorbital headache usually lasting 2 hours, with associated vertigo, nausea, vomiting, and visual disturbances. According to the International Classification of Disease guide for headaches, benign paroxysmal vertigo of childhood is a disorder characterized by "multiple, brief, sporadic episodes of dysequilibrium, anxiety, nystagmus or vomiting in the context of a normal neurologic exam and an unremarkable electroencephalogram."[51] The exact mechanism of dizziness or vertigo from migraine is unknown, making management difficult.[12] Pharmacologic treatments include symptomatic medications (nonopioid analgesics, antinausea) and preventive therapy (amitriptyline, beta blockers, calcium channel blockers, acetazolamide).[12] Amelioration of triggers (diet, stress, alcohol) can be helpful in prevention.

Multiple sclerosis (MS) is a disease of the CNS fatty myelin sheaths (demyelination and scarring) leading to a broad spectrum of signs and symptoms depending on the site of the lesion.[36]

Vertigo is the initial symptom in 5% of patients with MS and occurs at some time during the disease in 50% of patients. It can be central in nature, but BPPV can also be a complication of MS treatment. MS affects young adults, women more frequently than men.[27]

Central positional vertigo/nystagmus (CPV/N) can be caused by various CNS lesions located in the region of the fourth ventricle, dorsal vermis, or vestibular nuclei. There are three forms of CPV/N—positional downbeat nystagmus, positional nystagmus without concurrent vertigo, and positional vertigo with nystagmus. The most common causes include cerebrovascular disorders, spinocerebellar atrophy, MS, Arnold-Chiari type I malformations, tumors of the brain stem and cerebellum, and some drugs.[27]

Spontaneous and positional vertigo, tinnitus, hearing loss, dysarthria, dysphonia, ataxia, shortness of the neck, lower neck hair line, limited range of motion in the neck, lower cranial nerve signs, and sometimes hydrocephalus are typically seen in craniovertebral junction (CVJ) anomalies.[27] Vertebrobasilar artery (VBA) compromise is the main threat with these disorders. CVJ disorders with AAI can be congenital, disease-produced, or traumatic. Congenital fusion of the atlas and foramen magnum, platybasia (flat base of skull), achondroplasia (underdevelopment) of the dens, achondroplasia dwarfism, trisomy 21 (Down syndrome), and Arnold-Chiari malformations are common congenital causes of AAI.[27] The latter can also be induced by trauma. Certain conditions (e.g., RA, ankylosing spondylitis, Ehlers-Danlos syndrome, Marfan's syndrome, Grisel's syndrome) and trauma can also pose a threat to the VBA via AAI instability.

Neoplastic tumors (primary and metastatic) can cause central or peripheral vertigo. Vestibular schwannoma was discussed earlier (peripheral vertigo). Cerebellar tumors include astrocytomas, ependymomas, hemangioblastomas, medulloblastomas, and metastases. Medulloblastomas are most common in children, and metastases are most common in adults.[27] The typical presentation includes progression of neurologic symptoms (e.g., ataxia, oculomotor disorders, occipital headache, positional vertigo, nystagmus) over weeks or months.[27] Lung, colon, and renal cancers account for 80% of metastatic brain tumors in men.[32] Breast, lung, and colon cancers and melanomas account for 80% of metastatic brain tumors in women.[32]

Paraneoplastic cerebellar degeneration syndromes are nervous system disorders caused by cancer but not metastatic disease, vascular or metabolic deficits, infections, or nutritive deficiency. They are a rare complication of cancer, most frequently associated with ovarian, breast, and lung cancer, as well as Hodgkin's lymphoma.[27]

Differentiating Between Central and Peripheral Vestibular Vertigo.
Differentiating central versus peripheral vertigo is an integral part of the differential diagnosis of dizziness (Table 7-6).[27] Although signs and symptoms are usually distinct, patients should be referred to an otolaryngologist or ear, nose, and throat (ENT) doctor for special testing (e.g., audiography, caloric testing, electronystagmography) and precise medical diagnosis. Nystagmus, which is named by the direction of the fast phase, can also be helpful in identifying the source of vertigo (Table 7-7).[27] There are numerous types and variations of nystagmus, but the key variants include the following:

- Gaze-evoked nystagmus—elicited by changes in gaze position (movement of eyes)
- Head-shaking nystagmus—elicited by vigorous rotation of the head in the horizontal plane (indicates a unilateral vestibular hypofunction)
- Positional nystagmus—elicited by changes in head position (relationship of the inner ear to gravity); implicates peripheral vestibular issue
- Spontaneous nystagmus—occurs in seated patients, eyes in primary position, and without movement of the head; implicates central vestibular issue if optic fixation does not stop nystagmus

DYSEQUILIBRIUM. Dysequilibrium refers to dizziness, imbalance, or unsteadiness without vertigo. It often signals a dysfunction in the vestibular, somatosensory, and visual systems and/or frontal lobes, cerebellum, and/or basal ganglia.[27] Degenerative changes in the brain, alterations in central processing (integration), biomechanical constraints of aging (decreased range of motion, muscle weakness and stiffness), and changes from disease processes (neuropathy, spasticity, motor incoordination) can help explain dysequilibrium and loss of postural control.

There are three primary afferent systems contributing to the postural control system: the somatosensory (70%), vestibular (20%), and visual pathways (10%).[21] Somatosensory system input includes data from the three primary ascending systems, with conscious proprioception (kinesthesia) and subconscious proprioception recognized the most.

Peripheral inputs are integrated by the CNS to create efferent (motor) outputs such as reactive postural responses (ankle, hip, and stepping strategies) and proactive (anticipatory) postural adjustments. Abnormalities of the balance triad are commonly measured by physical therapists via platform posturography (computerized dynamic posturography [CDP]). Posturography testing has two components, the sensory organization test (SOT), which tests the subject's ability to use the individual components of the balance triad, and the limits of stability (LOS) test.

PRESYNCOPE. Presyncope (near-faint) refers to the lightheaded sensation that occurs just before fainting or losing consciousness; the absence of an illusion of motion distinguishes it from vertigo.[27] Presyncopal signs and symptoms, including generalized weakness, giddiness, headache, blurred vision, diaphoresis, paresthesia, pallor, nausea, and vomiting are usually present for seconds or minutes before LOC.[27] The mechanism is almost always a reduction in blood flow to the entire brain, and symptoms may be spontaneous or positional (orthostatic hypotension) or have specific triggers (head injury, hypoglycemia).[27]

Cardiovascular causes of presyncopal dizziness include structural heart disease, coronary heart disease, and arrhythmia. Cardiovascular causes warrant sound medical history and physical examination, including general screening for peripheral vascular disease; blood pressure testing with the patient in supine, sitting,

---

TABLE 7-6

Differential Diagnosis of Central and Peripheral Vertigo

Signs and Symptoms	Central	Peripheral
Nausea	None or mild	Severe
Movement illusion	Less prominent	More prominent
Worse with head movement	No	Yes
Neurologic signs	Common	Rare
Imbalance	Severe	Mild to moderate
Hearing loss	Rare	Common
Oscillopsia	Severe	Mild
Caloric test (per ENT)	Hyperexcitability	Canal paresis
Recovery	Months or longer	Days to weeks

ENT, ear, nose, and throat specialist.
From Karatas M: Central vertigo and dizziness: epidemiology, differential diagnosis, and common causes, *Neurologist* 14:355-364, 2008.

TABLE 7-7

Differentiation Between Spontaneous Nystagmus of Central and Peripheral Origin*

Parameter	Central Origin	Peripheral Origin
Appearance	Pure vertical or torsional PAN, multidirectional, disconjugate or dissociated; may change direction with changes in gaze	Torsional—horizontal unidirectional in all gazes, conjugated
Suppression with OF	No or minimal	Yes
Alexander law	No	Yes
Direction, fixed	No	Yes
Localization	Medulla	Labyrinth
	Pontine tegmentum	Vestibular nerve (CN VIII)
	Cerebellum	

*An exception is the patient with a multiple semicircular canal (SCC), who may have a composite nystagmus.
OF, optic fixation; *PAN*, periodic alternating nystagmus.
From Karatas M: Central vertigo and dizziness: epidemiology, differential diagnosis, and common causes, *Neurologist* 14:355-364, 2008.

and standing positions (orthostatic hypotension screening); and auscultation for carotid bruits.[18,27] The examination, including cardiac auscultation, electrocardiography, Holter monitoring, tilt-table test, and blood glucose and hematocrit analyses are the most important parts of the evaluation for suspected presyncope.[27]

Non cardiovascular causes of presyncopal dizziness include orthostatic hypotension, postural orthostatic tachycardia syndrome, hypovolemia, hypoglycemia (metabolic), and hyperventilation syndrome.[27] Neurocardiogenic (vasovagal) presyncope is an unexplained cause associated with painful or emotionally stressful situations, such as anxiety or fear with prolonged standing or specific trigger situations (psychiatric).[27] Iatrogenic (caused by medication) dizziness is seen most often in individuals receiving sympathetic blocking agents and vasodilator drugs for hypertension, older patients receiving tranquilizers, and patients with anemia.[27,35]

The American Autonomic Society and the American Academy of Neurology define orthostatic hypotension as a systolic blood pressure decrease of at least 20 mm Hg or a diastolic blood pressure decrease of at least 10 mm Hg within 3 minutes of standing. This is most commonly the result of peripheral vascular vasoconstriction or reduction of intravascular volume.

NONSPECIFIC (PSYCHOPHYSIOLOGIC) DIZZINESS. Psychophyslogic dizziness refers to a combination of symptoms reported as floating, rocking, or swimming sensations; giddiness; internal spinning; or a feeling of being removed from one's body. Symptoms may worsen with stress, fatigue, and some daily activities. It may also develop after labyrinthine disorders.[27] This category of dizziness is multifactorial, typically has an emotional component (anxiety) when tested with the DHI (see Figure 7-6), and is often accompanied by a complaint of motion sensitivity (e.g., car sickness, difficulty in crowds). Rarely is a true nystagmus found. There tends to be an overreliance on the vision component or the balance triad, frequently causing the patient to be fooled and overreact to visual stimuli.[14]

Psychogenic diagnoses of dizziness include pain disorder with agoraphobia, generalized anxiety and personality disorders, and depression. Patients with these diagnoses have dizziness at social events and inappropriately excessive anxiety or fear, and no spontaneous nystagmus can be detected. It is noteworthy that primary vestibular disorders also induce secondary psychiatric symptoms.[27]

Another category of psychiatric dizziness is phobic postural vertigo. Patients with phobic postural vertigo have a combination of nonrotational dizziness and subjective disturbance in upright posture and gait, despite normal results of clinical balance tests. Increased unsteadiness when looking at moving scenes (motion sensitivity), accompanied by anxiety and panic, leads to deconditioning, generalization, and fear-avoidance behaviors. Subjective postural imbalance without falls is typical and commonly coincides with psychosocial stress. Behavioral therapy and regular physical activity can be effective, but failure to treat can lead to hypofunctioning (deconditioning) of the vestibular system, chronicity, and considerable societal impairment (work, school, family).[14,27]

Cervicogenic Dizziness. Cervicogenic dizziness (CD) is a unique form of nonspecific (somatosensory) dizziness that must be differentiated from AAI and vestibular dysfunction; it is a diagnosis of exclusion. It was first described as a nonspecific sensation of altered orientation in space and dysequilibrium originating from abnormal afferent activity from the neck.[54] The mismatch among cervical afferent inputs and the vestibular and visual systems leads to dysequilibrium. CD is characterized by dizziness and disequilibrium associated with neck pain in patients with cervical pathology.[54] Conditions that have been linked to CD include whiplash-associated disorders (WADs), AAI, and degenerative changes of the cervical spine.[34,37]

A variety of clinical tests can be used to rule out vestibular dysfunction and to rule in CD. A modified vertebral artery test is advocated so as not to stimulate the posterior semicircular canals (BPPV) while testing for potential VBA insufficiency.[31,54] Hautant's test is used to differentiate a somatosensory (cerebellar) source of dizziness from a vascular problem.[31] The head-fixed, body-turned maneuver[21] is the clinical equivalent to the smooth pursuit neck torsion test, which is considered the definitive test for CD.[47] A study of the smooth pursuit neck torsion test in subjects with persistent whiplash, both with and without dizziness, compared with healthy control subjects has suggested that the test is not influenced by a patient's level of anxiety but by disturbed cervical afferentation.[48]

A history of WADs, particularly posterior impact whiplash,[50] is frequently seen with CD, suggesting that damage to the myofascioligamentous system of the craniovertebral region (occiput, atlas, axis) may be contributory. Some (e.g., the North American Institute of Orthopedic Manual Therapy) have advocated that trigeminal facilitation (CN V) from craniovertebral dysfunction is an explanation for CD. Symptoms of trigeminal facilitation include, but are not restricted to, the following[34,37]:

- Pain felt in the sensory distribution of CN V—head (frontal, occipital, parietal), jaw, face, eye (similar to conjunctivitis), orbit (retro-ocular), middle ear, and teeth
- Dizziness (disequilibrium) associated with neck motion
- Tinnitus (because CN V innervates the tensor tympani)
- Paresthesia of the tongue, face, or head (must be clearly distinguished among facial, oral, and perioral paresthesia)
- Tongue sensitivity changes (e.g., acidic, metallic tastes)
- Feelings of anxiety associated with neck or head symptoms (stress attacks)
- Medically unsubstantiated subjective complaints of visual problems (e.g., fuzzy vision, black spots)

See Box 7-9 for an overview of patients with dizziness and post-traumatic neck injury.

Traumatic Brain Injury

Brain injury can occur via a variety of mechanisms—CNS infections, noninfectious disorders (e.g., epilepsy, hypoxia, ischemia, genetic or metabolic disorders), tumors, vascular abnormalities, and trauma (e.g., sports activities, motor vehicle accident, bicycle or pedestrian accident, falls, assault).[26] Common signs and symptoms of traumatic brain injury (TBI), including dizziness, are listed in Box 7-11.[31]

EXAMINATION. The most prevalent (75%) form of TBI (mild) is often missed at the time of the initial injury. Signs and symptoms of mild TBI can include fatigue, headaches, visual disturbances, sensitivity to light or sound, memory loss, poor attention and concentration, getting lost or confused, slowness in thinking,

Common Signs and Symptoms of Concussion (Traumatic Brain Injury)

Acute	Late (Delayed)
Lightheadedness	Persistent low-grade headache
Delayed motor and/or verbal responses	Easy fatigability
Memory or cognitive dysfunction	Sleep irregularities
Disorientation	Inability to perform daily activities
Amnesia	Depression/anxiety
Headache	Lethargy
Balance problems/incoordination	Memory dysfunction
Vertigo, dizziness	Lightheadedness
Concentration difficulties	Personality changes
Loss of consciousness	Low frustration tolerance/irritability
Blurred vision	Intolerance to bright lights, loud sounds
Vacant stare (befuddled facial expression)	
Photophobia	
Tinnitus	
Nausea	
Vomiting	
Increased emotionality	
Slurred or incoherent speech	

From Magee DJ: *Orthopedic physical assessment*, ed 5, Philadelphia, 2008, Saunders-Elsevier, p 79.

sleep disturbances, dizziness and loss of balance, irritability and emotional disturbances, feelings of depression, and seizures. Patients may also complain of nausea or loss of smell. Of those with mild TBI, 15% have symptoms that last 1 year or longer.[45]

A patient who receives a blow or incurs an acceleration-deceleration injury of the head should be thoroughly evaluated. Vital signs (pulse, respiration rate, blood pressure) should be taken to determine baseline and monitor physiologic status changes over time. Deviations from the normal heart rate (60 to 80 beats/min for adults) include slow weak pulse (decreased stroke volume or increased peripheral resistance), short rapid pulse (heart failure or shock), slow bounding pulse (increased intracranial pressure), and accelerated pulse (more than 150 beats/min indicates pressure on the base of the brain). Bradyapnea, or slow respiration (fewer than 12 breaths/min), may indicate intracranial pressure.[1]

History and mental status testing are used to assess for confusion and amnesia, the hallmarks of a concussion. Although disorientation may be present, the cardinal features of confusion include the following: (1) disturbance of vigilance, with heightened distractibility; (2) inability to maintain a coherent stream of thought; and (3) inability to carry out a sequence of goal-directed movements.[1] Mental status testing includes questions regarding orientation (person, place, time, circumstances surrounding the mechanism of injury), tasks of concentration and memory, observation of behavior (irrational, inappropriate, or belligerent behavior), questions regarding other symptoms (headache, tinnitus, nausea, diplopia, dizziness), and quantification of LOC.[1,31]

In regard to observational findings, the health care provider should specifically look for leakage of cerebrospinal fluid (CSF). A basilar skull fracture may result in blood or CSF leaking from the ear, whereas a cribriform (facial) fracture may result in blood and CSF leaking from the nose. Discoloration about the eyes (raccoon's eyes) or behind the ears (Battle's sign) may indicate skull fracture, hematoma, or laceration. Overall skin color and level of moisture (sweat) should be monitored for signs of shock (e.g., pale cool skin is a sign of systemic shock). Irritability, aggressive behavior, or uncontrolled crying for no apparent reason may signal cerebral dysfunction.[1] Observation also includes assessing the integrity of certain cranial nerves (see Chapter 10 for details of cranial nerve screening), pupil size, and accommodation to light; gaze abnormalities may be noted. Such findings would lead to continued neurologic assessment for strength and upper motor neuron tests (e.g., deep tendon reflexes, Babinski and Hoffman reflexes, clonus).

Coordination and balance is the final area of testing for the patient with head injury. Although generally considered cerebellar testing, tests of coordination and balance also assess other portions of the brain, including afferent pathways, CNS integration, and efferent outputs. A basic cluster of tests for the head injured and/or dizzy patient includes gait, Romberg, sharpened Romberg (tandem stance), alternating finger-to-nose, heel-to-shin gait, and stork stand (single-leg balance), all with eyes open and closed for comparison.

Dizziness leading to a history of falls and head trauma should suggest an intracranial bleed. There are four potential intracranial bleeds that could cause the aforementioned symptoms: (1) epidural (above the dura mater); (2) subdural (below the dura, within the arachnoid layer); (3) subarachnoid (bleeding into the CSF); and (4) cerebral hemorrhage (intraparenchymal bleeding), which can occur after head trauma.[52]

Epidural bleeds (talk and die syndrome) are fortunately rare (less than 1%) but have a 15% to 20% mortality, even with appropriate care. Symptoms tend to develop rapidly and are most commonly caused by laceration of the middle meningeal artery.[52] Symptoms of subdural hematoma mirror those of epidural bleeding but have a much more subtle progression. It often takes a more experienced or alert clinician to trace the presenting symptoms back to the initial head injury.[52] Depending on the time between the initial insult and development of symptoms, subdural hematoma can be classified as acute (within 24 hours), subacute (2 to 6 days), or chronic (after 2 weeks). Mortality rates are time-dependent, with the first 24 hours having the highest mortality—acute (50% to 80%), subacute (25%), and chronic (20%). Subdural hematomas ultimately need to be surgically evacuated.[52]

Subarachnoid hemorrhage results in bloody CSF and intense meningeal irritation. Patients will have a sudden, localized, and severe headache that spreads into a more diffuse, dull, throbbing headache. Neurologic symptoms include dizziness, nausea, severe neck pain, unequal pupils, confusion, seizures, and unresponsiveness. Urgent medical care is needed to decompress the brain.[52]

Finally, after head or neck trauma, patients should be closely monitored for signs and symptoms of vertebrobasilar artery insufficiency (VBI) or altered posterior brain circulation. From a traumatic perspective, VBI can be caused by several mechanisms:

- Early contact sports (age)—the dens is skeletally immature until the age of 11 or 12 years (supplies the rationale for noncontact [touch] football and/or the issue of weight restrictions in youth football leagues)

- Atlantoaxial ligamentous instability—traumatic damage to the tectorial membrane, alar ligament, and/or transverse ligament, or a rim lesion from flexion-extension whiplash
- Craniovertebral fracture—basilar (occipital) skull fracture, or atlas or axis (odontoid process) fracture of the transverse processes of vertebrae C1-6 (location of transverse foramen)
- Vertebral artery dissection (VAD), which can result spontaneously or with musculoskeletal torsional trauma to the cervical spine

A latent period of up to 3 days between the onset of pain and the development of CNS manifestations can occur. Severe occipital headaches and posterior nuchal pain are often the initial chief presenting complaints. In addition to vertigo and dysequilibrium, other manifestations include ipsilateral facial dysesthesia, dysarthria or hoarseness, diplopia, dysphagia, hiccups, nausea and vomiting, unilateral hearing loss, contralateral loss of pain and temperature sensations in trunk and limbs, and ipsilateral loss of taste.

Summary

Numerous published examples exist describing patients seeking physical therapy services with common complaints (e.g., joint pain or dizziness) and the therapist's examination findings detecting potentially serious health issues. The ability to compare and contrast health risk factors and clinical manifestations of conditions that physical therapists can manage versus those that require physician involvement is critical to the early detection of disease processes. Concern about many of these conditions would warrant an urgent patient referral. The aforementioned information combined with material in Chapter 6 provides readers with a list of conditions to "think" about as a patient describes his or her symptoms. The therapist's interpretation of the examination findings will determine whether the "thinking" turns into "worrying" about the underlying cause of symptoms.

REFERENCES

1. Anderson MK, Hall SJ, Martin M. Foundations of athletic training—prevention, assessment and management. 3rd ed. Philadelphia: Lippincott, Williams & Wilkins; 2005.
2. Arnett FC, Edworthy SM, Bloch DA, et al. The American Rheumatism Association 1987 revised criteria for the classification of rheumatoid arthritis. Arthritis Rheum 1988;31:315–24.
3. Backes JM, Howard PA, Ruisinger JF, Moriarty PM. Does simavastatin cause more myotoxicity compared to other statins? Ann Pharm 2009;43:2012–20.
4. Bickley LS. Bates' guide to physical examination and history taking. 10th ed. Philadelphia: Lippincott Williams & Wilkins; 2009.
5. Boissonnault W. Prevalence of comorbid conditions, surgeries, and medication use in a physical therapy outpatient population: A multi-centered study. J Orthop Sport Phys Ther 1999;29:506–25.
6. Caldron PH. Screening for rheumatic disease. In: Boissonnault WG, editor. Examination in physical therapy practice. 2nd ed. New York: Churchill Livingstone; 1995. p. 257–75.
7. Caplan LR, Chung C-S, Wityk RJ, Glass TA, et al. New England Medical Center posterior circulation stroke registry: I. Methods, data base, distribution of brain lesions, stroke mechanisms, and outcomes. J Clin Neurol 2005;1:14–30.
8. Centers for Disease Control and Prevention (CDC). Facts about concussion and brain injury—where to get help, http://www.cdc.gov/ncipc/tbi/; [accessed December 6, 2009]. Chestnut R, Kelly JP, Kozeny D, et al. are the authors.
9. Centers for Disease Control and Prevention (CDC). Sports-related recurrent brain injuries—United States. MMWR Morbid Mortal Wkly Rep 1997;46:224–77.
10. Centers for Disease Control and Prevention (CDC). Traumatic brain injury in the United States: emergency department visits, hospitalizations, and deaths. Atlanta: Centers for Disease Control and Prevention, National Center for Injury Prevention and Control; 2006.
11. Chan Y. Differential diagnosis of dizziness. Curr Opin Otolaryngol Head Neck Surg 2009;17:200–3.
12. Chawla N, Olshaker JS. Diagnosis and management of dizziness and vertigo. Med Clin North Am 2006;90:291–304.
13. Childs JD, Fritz JM, Piva SR, Whitman JM. Proposal of a classification system for patients with neck pain. J Orthop Sport Phys Ther 2004;34:686–700.
14. Dewane JA, Shea T, Grove C, Hallisy KM. Clinical decision making in vestibular and balance rehabilitation. Madison, WI: University of Wisconsin–Health Continuing Education Symposium; 2007.
15. Frebert A, Bruckmann H, Drummen R. Clinical features of proven basilar artery occlusion. Stroke 1990;21:1135–42.
16. Goleburn CR, Golden CJ. Traumatic brain injury outcome in older adults: a critical review of the literature. J Clin Geropsychol 2001;7:161.
17. Goldman RL, Bennett JC, Goldman L, editors. Cecil textbook of medicine. 21st ed. Philadelphia: Sauders; 2000.
18. Goodman CC, Fuller KS. Pathology: implications for the physical therapist. 3rd ed. St. Louis: Sauders; 2009. p. 1265–83.
19. Goodman CC, Snyder TE. Differential diagnosis for physical therapists: screening for referral. 4th ed. St. Louis: Saunders; 2007.
20. Goroll AH, Mulley AG, editors. Primary care medicine. 5th ed. Philadelphia: Lippincott Williams & Wilkins; 2006. p. 1043–51.
21. Herdman SJ. Vestibular rehabilitation. 3rd ed. Philadelphia: FA Davis; 2007.
22. Huijbregts P, Vidal P. Dizziness in orthopaedic physical therapy: classification and pathophysiology. J Manipulative Physiol Ther 2004;12:199–214.
23. Jacobson GP, Newman CW. The development of the dizziness handicap inventory. Arch Otolaryngol Head Surg 1990;116:424–7.
24. Jahn K. [Vertigo in children. Clinical presentation, course and treatment.]. Nervenarzt 2009;80:900–8.
25. Jette AM, Davis KD. A comparison of hospital-based and private outpatient physical therapy practices. Phys Ther 1991;71:366–75.
26. Johnson AR, DeMatt E, Salorio CF. Predictors of outcome following acquired brain injury in children. Dev Disabil Res Rev 2009;15(2):124–32.
27. Karatas M. Central vertigo and dizziness: epidemiology, differential diagnosis, and common causes. Neurologist 2008;14:355–64.
28. Kerber KA, Brown DL, Lisabeth LE, et al. Stroke among persons with dizziness, vertigo, and imbalance in the emergency department: a population-based study. Stroke 2006;37:2484–7.
29. Langlois JA, Rutland-Brown W, Thomas KE. Traumatic brain injury in the United States: emergency department visits, hospitalizations, and deaths. Atlanta: Centers for Disease Control and Prevention, National Center for Injury Prevention and Control; 2004.
30. Lewandoski C, Santhakumar S. Posterior circulation stroke. Foundation of Education and Research in Neurological Emergencies, http://www.uic.edu/com/ferne/pdf/posterior0501.pdf; [accessed March 11, 2010].
31. Magee DJ. Orthopedic physical assessment. 5th ed. Philadelphia: Saunders Elsevier; 2008.
32. Metastatic tumors to the brain and spine, American Brain Tumor Association, 1993 (website), http://neurosurgery.mgh.harvard.edu/abta/mets.htm#about_1; [accessed February 6, 2010].
33. McClune T, Burton AK, Waddell G. Whiplash associated disorder: a review of the literature to guide patient information and advice. Emerg Med J 2002;19:499–506.
34. Meadows JTS. Orthopedic differential diagnosis in physical therapy: a case study approach. New York: McGraw-Hill; 1999.
35. Merck Manual of Geriatrics. Ch. 86 Hypotension. Available at: http://www.merck.com/mkgr/mmg/sec11/ch86/ch86b.jsp; [accessed December 8, 2009].
36. Multiple sclerosis (website). http://en.wikipedia.org/wiki/Multiple_sclerosis; [accessed February 6, 2010].
37. Pettman E: Stress tests of the craniovertebral joints, J Manipulative Physiol 19:185-194, 194
38. Ravid S, Bienkowski R, Eviator L. A simplified diagnostic approach to dizziness in children. Pediatr Neurol 2003;29:317–20.
39. Reid SA, Rivett DA. Manual therapy treatment of cervicogenic dizziness: a systematic review. Man Ther 2005;10:4–13.
40. Rudwaleit M, Metter A, Listing J, et al. Inflammatory back pain in ankylosing spondylitis: A reassessment of the clinical history for application as classification and diagnostic criteria. Arthritis Rheum 2006;54:569–78.
41. Schenk R, Coons LB, Bennett SE, Huijbregts PA. Cervicogenic dizziness: a case report illustrating orthopaedic manual and vestibular physical therapy comanagement. J Man Maninipulative Ther 2006;14:E56–68.

42. Shumway-Cook A, Wollacott M. Motor control: theory and practical applications. Baltimore: Williams & Wilkins; 1995.

43. Slovik DM. In: Goroll AH, Mulley AG, editors. Primary care medicine. 5th ed. Philadelphia: Lippincott Williams & Wilkins; 2006. p. 745–50.

44. Swartz MH. Textbook of physical diagnosis history and examination. 5th ed. Philadelphia: Saunders Elsevier; 2006.

45. Traumatic Brain Injury.com. http://www.traumaticbraininjury.com/; [accessed December 15, 2009].

46. Thompson PD, Clarkson P, Karas RH. Statin-associated myopathy. JAMA 2003;289:1681–90.

47. Tjell C, Rosenhall U. Smooth pursuit neck torsion test: a specific test for cervical dizziness. Am J Otol 1998;19:76–81.

48. Treleaven J, Jull G, LowChoy N. Smooth pursuit neck torsion test in whiplash-associated disorders: relationship to self-reports of neck pain and disability, dizziness and anxiety. J Rehabil Med 2005;37:219–23.

49. Vegso IJ, Torg JS. Field evaluation and management of intracranial injuries. In: Torg JS, editor. Athletic injuries to the head, neck and face. St. Louis: Mosby-Year Book; 1991.

50. Walton DM, et al. Risk factors for persistent problems following whiplash injury: results of a systematic review and meta-analysis. J Orthop Sports Phys Ther 2009;39:334–50.

51. Weisleder P, Fife TD. Dizziness and headache: a common association in children and adolescents. J Child Neurol 2001;16:727–30.

52. Whitehead S. Types of brain hemorrage (website), http://theemtspot.com/2009/07/13/types-of-brain-hemorrhage; [accessed February 6, 2010].

53. Whitney SL, Marchetti GF, Morris LO. Usefulness of the dizziness handicap inventory in the screening for benign paroxysmal positional vertigo. Otol Neurol 2004;25:139–43.

54. Wrisley DM, Sparto PJ, Whitney SL, Furman JM. Cervicogenic dizziness: a review of diagnosis. J Orthop Sports Phys Ther 2000;30:755–66.

Patient Health History Including Identifying Health Risk Factors

William G. Boissonnault, PT, DPT, DHSc, FAAOMPT

Objectives

After reading this chapter, the reader will be able to:

1. Identify categories of patient health history information to be collected during the initial visit.
2. Explain the relevance of patient health history information to physical therapists' clinical decision making in the areas of examination, evaluation, diagnosis, prognosis, and provision of effective and safe interventions.
3. Explain how patient health history information combined with patient symptoms and signs and systems review can effectively screen patients for depression, domestic violence, and chemical dependency.
4. Collect patient health history information effectively and efficiently during an initial patient visit using patient-administered questionnaires.

As part of a comprehensive examination, physical therapists (PTs) routinely collect patient health history information in inpatient and outpatient settings.[2] Although this information may or may not be directly related to why physical therapy has been initiated, it is often crucial to establishing a safe and effective patient plan of care. Many diseases manifest in very similar fashions to impairment-driven conditions, or conditions amenable to physical therapy intervention (see Chapters 6 and 7). Skeletal spinal cancers typically manifest initially as backache; the average length of time between when this ache begins and when the diagnosis of cancer is made is 9 months.[34] The finding that is most predictive of the presence of an underlying tumor causing back pain is a previous history of cancer.[12] In another scenario, a patient with a recent history of an infection presents with complaints of chills, fatigue, and a low-grade fever. The chills, fatigue, and low-grade fever could be related to a "benign" virus that is self-limited and not a serious concern, but with the history of a recent infection, this patient should be seen by a physician to ensure that the "recent infection" has not returned or spread to another body region.

In a patient presenting with mid-thoracic pain who has a comorbidity associated with loss of bone density (e.g., chronic renal failure), the PT may choose to assess joint play of the thoracic spine by a method other than applying posterior-to-anterior pressure over the thoracic spinous processes with the patient in a prone (lying) position. This type of technique with the patient prone could cause "bowing" of the ribs, with the potential for fracture. The joint play information must be collected, but choosing a technique that places less mechanical load on the bony thorax would be in the patient's best interest.

Another patient is taking beta blockers for hypertension, and the PT needs to monitor the patient's general well-being during a conditioning activity. Something other than the patient's heart rate should be assessed because of the physiologic effect beta blockers have on the cardiovascular system. Finally, the presence of specific comorbid conditions (e.g., diabetes) can have an effect on the patient's prognosis—with the potential for prolonged or suboptimal recovery.

Patient Health History Data

The following categories of health history information are important to the PT in clinical decision making:

- Patient demographics (age, sex, race, marital status, and level of education)
- Social history (cultural and religious customs and beliefs, occupation and work status, living environment, and family and social support)
- Current and past personal medical history (illnesses, allergies, surgeries, injuries, and medication use)
- Social habits (exercise—yes/no, frequency, intensity) including substance use (tobacco use, alcohol intake, and caffeine intake)
- Family medical history

Patient Demographics

Patient demographics and identifying data are important to the medical screening component of the examination. Certain diseases are associated more often with specific age ranges and specific genders. Women account for 99% of breast cancer cases, and women 60 years old or older are the highest risk group.[22] Prostate cancer accounts for more than one third of all male cancers, and men aged 60 years or older are the highest risk group.[22] In general, adults older than 50 years of age are at highest risk for developing cancer.[22] Other disorders also are more common in one gender but occur at younger ages. Thyroid disease, rheumatoid arthritis, and depression all are more common in women; the age of initial onset is approximately 20 to 40 years.

Race also may predispose groups to higher incidences of certain disorders. Prostate cancer and sickle cell disease are found more often in African Americans, whereas skin cancer is more common in whites. These examples show that not all patients carry the same risk for diseases, so the degree of medical screening and concern about potential health risk issues should vary in part based on the patient's age, race, and other demographics.

Patient Social History

The patient's occupation, leisure activities, customs, and beliefs all expose the patient to various health risks. In addition, this information may reveal potential obstacles to a successful rehabilitation outcome. An occupation that includes repetitive activity or prolonged static body postures or positions or a leisure activity that places similar demands on the body carries the risk of development of repetitive, overuse conditions, such as stress fractures or tendinitis. If work demands cannot be altered, or the patient is unwilling to modify the leisure activity, recovery from the condition may be hampered. A change in occupation or in the intensity of leisure activities may account for the onset or worsening of symptoms. A new occupation may carry higher levels of emotional stress that may account for current health issues being faced.

Customs, beliefs, and value systems can vary considerably among individuals and can dictate how a person responds to the PT's requests or instructions. Chapter 3 presents several examples to raise one's awareness of how such issues may be the key to rehabilitation outcome. Finally, investigating the patient's living environment and family and social support network may identify challenges to the delivery of care. The living environment may present obstacles to patient mobility, and many patients depend on others for needs at various points during illness or surgery recovery. Issues such as these may prompt the PT to initiate a consultation or referral for various social services.

Personal Medical History

A review of a patient's medical history includes investigating illnesses, surgeries, injuries, and medication use. Health history questions should include distant past events but with emphasis on current or recent episodes during the initial visit. Follow-up questions to positive health history findings are key to determining the clinical relevance of this information. If a patient acknowledges a heart problem, the PT should ask, "What type of heart problem, and is it something for which you are currently being treated?" The condition may be a heart arrhythmia, mitral valve prolapse, or ischemic heart disease, all of which are associated with different precautions or clinical guidelines. A patient may state he or she has angina, but the PT should not assume this means chest pain. The author had a patient who, when asked where her angina was, pointed to her throat and jaw—she never experienced left-sided chest pain (see Chapter 6 and 20 for pain patterns associated with heart disease).

A description of the usual symptoms associated with the heart condition gives the PT baseline information that can be used for comparison with new and possibly related complaints. A worsening of ischemic heart disease may result in new or different symptoms, and instead of the usual left-sided chest pain, the patient may now complain of epigastric pain, or symptoms now occur at rest compared with previously being associated with physical exertion. The patient may associate this new pain with indigestion, not the heart problem, but an astute PT is vigilant for all possible symptoms (see Chapters 6, 9, 11, and 20) associated with ischemic heart disease, including upper abdominal pain.

Routine follow-up questions related to illnesses should include the following:

- Can you describe the condition to me (e.g., what type of heart problem is it)?
- Are you currently receiving care for the illness or condition, or is it something from the past that has fully resolved?

- How is the condition currently being managed (e.g., diet, exercise, medication), and by whom?
- If the condition is current, what symptoms or warning signs do you typically have? Are you limited or restricted by the condition?
- Have the symptoms recently changed (e.g., intensity, frequency) in any way?

A patient report of recent surgery or major trauma should alert the PT to the potential risk of infection or venous thrombosis. Knowing the possible symptoms (see Chapters 6, 7, 9, and 20) associated with these conditions is paramount to early suspicion and report of concerns to the physician. Investigating surgeries from long ago can focus on whether the patient is limited or restricted in any way because of the surgery or the reason for the surgery.

Finally, current medical treatment (e.g., medications) for a condition may be as relevant as the condition itself. Patients seeking services from PTs take a variety of medications,[5,6] some of which may require the PT to alter or modify his or her usual examination or intervention schemes. PTs should monitor items other than heart rate during physical activity for patients taking beta blockers because these drugs dampen heart rate response to exertion. Many of these drugs also carry significant risk for adverse drug events; PTs can screen for these risks by using the review of systems checklists described in Chapters 4 and 9.[7] Understanding the physiologic events associated with medications and their common side effects can help the PT identify the symptoms and signs to watch for. An important principle to guide this screening process is that approximately 80% of adverse drug events are an extension of the therapeutic effects of the drug (see Chapter 4). The primary adverse drug event associated with antihypertensive medications is hypotension. Appendix 8-1 presents a summary of drugs and potential adverse events for each of the body systems, and Chapter 4 describes additional strategies for screening drug side effects.

Important follow-up questions about the use of medications include the following:
- What is the reason you are taking the medication?
- Do you feel the medication is helping you?
- What is the dose and schedule for taking the medication? Are you following the dosage schedule?
- Who prescribed the medication?
- Have you noticed any side effects from taking the medication?

Starting with asking why a medication is being taken can provide important illness information that may not be acknowledged earlier in the history. The most common example the author has encountered is a patient denying a history of any illness but who is taking a diuretic or beta blocker. When asked why the medication is being taken, the response is "for my blood pressure." In these situations, from the patients' perspective, they do not have a blood pressure problem—as long as they take the medication!

For patients taking over-the-counter (OTC) medications (medications *not* prescribed by a physician), important additional questions are as follows:
- Is your physician aware that you are taking this medication?
- Have you recently needed to take more of the medication than usual?

Boissonnault and Meek[7] described an example of how OTC drug use can raise suspicion of serious drug complications. Of 1817 surveyed patients taking nonsteroidal anti-inflammatory drugs (NSAIDs), 28% also were taking OTC antacids, and another 10% were taking histamine (H_2) antagonists (e.g., cimetidine [Tagamet], ranitidine [Zantac]). These drugs are taken for symptoms such as indigestion and heartburn, which could be related to NSAID-induced gastrointestinal ulcers. If a patient reports needing to increase a drug dosage (that is not curative of gastrointestinal ulcer) to get the same degree of relief as in the past, this may be a signal that a serious gastrointestinal condition is worsening.

Finally, PTs should identify patients who need counseling from their physician or pharmacist about proper use of medications. Encouraging patients to keep their primary care physician informed of any medication, remedy, or supplement they are using and to buy medication at the same pharmacy or pharmacy chain promotes appropriate medication usage.

Social Habits

The investigation of social habits includes questions about caffeine and alcohol intake and tobacco use. This baseline patient information not only identifies risk factors for disease but also may have an effect on the patient prognosis and alert the PT to symptom etiology. *Caffeine intoxication* can occur with ingestion of 100 mg of caffeine per day and may be marked by several manifestations. Diagnostic criteria for caffeine intoxication as described by the *Diagnostic and Statistical Manual of Mental Disorders*[3] (can be used by PTs as a screening tool) include the following:

- Recent consumption of caffeine, usually more than 250 mg (the equivalent of two to three cups of coffee or more)
- Five or more of the following developing during or shortly after caffeine consumption:
  Restlessness
  Nervousness
  Excitement
  Insomnia
  Flushed face
  Diuresis
  Gastrointestinal disturbance
  Muscle twitching
  Rambling flow of thought or speech
  Tachycardia or cardiac arrhythmia
  Periods of inexhaustibility
  Psychomotor agitation and
- The aforementioned effects cause clinically significant distress or impairment in social, occupational, rehabilitation, school, or other settings.
- The aforementioned manifestations are *not* due to a general medical condition.

PTs also should be aware of caffeine withdrawal manifestations, including headache, lethargy, fatigue, muscle pain and stiffness, and dysphoric mood changes. Research has suggested that these symptoms can occur in people who drink 2.5 cups (or the equivalent of 235 mg of caffeine) of coffee per day.[33] Studies have shown that a patient's postoperative headaches could be related to caffeine withdrawal.[15]

Approximately 3 in 10 U.S. adults consume alcohol at levels that carry increased risk for physical, mental health, and social problems.[26] Quantity of *alcohol intake* alone, although important to document, is not the key issue in determining whether someone is alcohol dependent. Figure 8-1 illustrates a continuum of alcohol use and definitions. Patients in the at-risk use, abuse, and dependence categories are candidates for intervention. The consequences associated with use are what distinguish these categories from low-risk use. For dependency, the magnitude of the consequences and the neurobiologic changes separate this category from the others.

PTs can use the following guidelines, published by the National Institute on Alcohol Abuse and Alcoholism (NIAAA),[27] to identify at-risk drinking:

- Men: >14 drinks/week or >4 drinks/occasion
- Women: >7 drinks/week or >3 drinks/occasion
- Elderly (>65 years old) men and women: >7 drinks/week or >1 drink/occasion
- One drink = 12 oz of beer, 5 to 6 oz of wine or 1 to 1.5 oz of liquor

The at-risk drinking criteria from the NIAAA correspond to the World Health Organization's category of *hazardous use*.[32] Potential health risks associated with the described levels of alcohol intake include the following[19,30]:

- Hypertension
- Hepatitis
- Cirrhosis
- Gastritis
- Sleep disorders
- Major depression
- Hemorrhagic stroke
- Pancreatitis
- Impotence/loss of libido
- Cardiomyopathy

Beyond the at-risk drinking guidelines, *alcohol abuse* is defined by the American Psychiatric Association in the *Diagnostic and Statistical Manual of Mental Disorders*[3] as a maladaptive pattern of alcohol use leading to clinically significant impairment or distress manifested within a 12-month period by one or more of the following:

- Failure to fulfill role obligations at work, school, or home (or rehabilitation)
- Recurrent use in hazardous situations
- Legal problems related to alcohol
- Continued use despite alcohol-related social or interpersonal problems

In general, alcohol abuse is marked by repetitive consequences associated with use. If PTs note a potential issue associated with alcohol use—the admitted level of use or the presence of conditions that could be alcohol-related—additional screening tools can be used. Appendix 8-2 contains three questions related to alcohol intake: how many heavy drinking days in the past year, how many days per week one drinks, and on those days, how many drinks one has. If one meets or exceeds the aforementioned at-risk drinking levels or has exceeded the heavy drinking threshold (five or more drinks for men, four or more drinks for women), a consultation for intervention should be considered.[26]

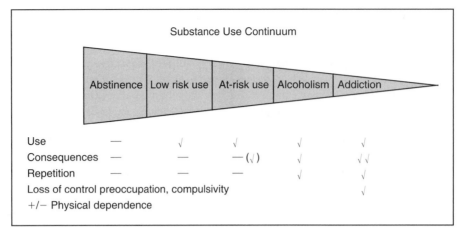

FIGURE 8-1 Categories of alcohol use. Adapted from Brown RL. Module 3: Screening and Assessment. In Pfeifer J (ed): Project Mainstream Syllabus. Providence, RI, Association for Medical Education and Research in Substance Abuse, 2005. Accessed at http://www.projectmainstream.net/projectmainstream.asp?cid=23 on March 2, 2010.

Other screening tools exist. The CAGE instrument is one example to help determine the need for a consultation and consists of the following four questions:

- Have you ever felt you should **C**ut down on your drinking?
- Have people **A**nnoyed you by criticizing your drinking?
- Have you ever felt bad or **G**uilty about your drinking?
- Have you ever had a drink first thing in the morning to steady your nerves or get rid of a hangover (**E**ye-opener)?

The sensitivity of the CAGE questions for identifying lifetime alcohol problems in patients ranges from 60% to 95%, and the specificity ranges from 40% to 95% when the cutoff is set at two or more positive responses.[11,16,25]

In addition to the aforementioned tools, PTs may note a pattern of patients being repetitively late or missing appointments, inappropriate behaviors directed toward staff members or inappropriate interactions with staff members, outbursts of anger or mood swings, and undue defensiveness when asked about alcohol (or drug) use.[4] A key item to consider when investigating this aspect of the patient health history is to avoid using one's own level of use (or nonuse) as a reference point to "judge" a patient's level of intake. If the PT drinks no alcohol, he or she may think that drinking one or two drinks per day most days is at-risk drinking, when evidence suggests that one or two alcoholic drinks per day may reduce the risk of adverse cardiovascular events in certain populations. A PT who drinks four to five drinks 5 days per week might think that drinking any less than that is not a problem, when long-term consumption of more than seven drinks per week (for women) is considered at-risk drinking. Initiating a consultation when at-risk drinking or alcohol abuse is suspected is crucial because brief intervention strategies have been shown to be effective in individuals who have not yet progressed to the stage of alcohol dependence.[28]

Tobacco use is associated with increased risk for numerous disorders, including cardiovascular and pulmonary conditions and kidney and bladder cancers. Tobacco use also can impede patients' recovery from injury or surgery, because delayed bone and soft tissue healing has been reported in tobacco users.[10,24] PTs see many patients after injury or surgery and use many factors to establish the initial prognosis for recovery. Tobacco use in these patients does not preclude a recovery from the trauma, but

a patient might not progress at the expected speed; this tendency might prompt the PT to modify goals when developing the plan of care.

Family History

Collecting family history at the initial visit, especially of first-degree relatives (parents and siblings), is important to identify potential patient health risks. Identifying patients with significant family histories, such as individuals whose parents were diagnosed in their 40s with heart disease, could prompt PTs to help patients establish relationships with family practice physicians. Although positive family history by itself would rarely warrant referring a patient to a physician, asking detailed follow-up questions when the PT has significant concerns about the patient's current health status is relevant. At this point, the decision to contact a physician about the health concerns essentially has been made, so gathering pertinent information supporting the referral is important. If a patient reveals a family history of heart disease, the following questions become relevant:

- Who in your family has the heart disease?
- What type of heart disease do (did) they have?
- At what age was he or she diagnosed?
- What is his or her current health status? If the person has died, was it from the heart problem, and at what age?

The age of diagnosis is an important factor in the risk for the patient. The risk of someone developing heart disease increases with a younger age of onset for the parents (e.g., diagnosed at age 40 versus age 75). Knowing the health status of the family member also reveals information about the patient's support system or may reveal demands that the patient faces in providing care for family members.

Methods Used to Collect Patient Health History Information

A challenge to all clinicians is collecting the necessary information effectively and efficiently. Patient health history data can be gathered from many sources and through a variety of methods. In inpatient settings, patient medical records should contain current health histories; in outpatient settings, access to computerized health records, including physician reports, can produce the information. The PT must consider, however, whether the information found in these sources is accurate and up-to-date.

In outpatient settings, having patients complete health history questionnaires before starting the interview can save time. The form can be completed by the patient before the actual start time of the scheduled appointment, and the PT can scan the questionnaire before beginning the interview. This practice allows for identification of health issues that may or may not be related to the primary reason for the physical therapy visit. Knowledge of such issues before investigating the chief complaint (see Chapters 6 and 7) allows the clinician to adjust the interview format to ensure that time is available to address the potential health issues adequately.

Patient self-reports have long been advocated for use in ambulatory medical settings[9,18,20,31]; self-reports show reliability and validity in most cases and may save time by improving the efficiency of data collection.[1,17,21,23,29] Care must be taken when developing the questionnaire, however, because open-ended and medication-related questions can lead to suboptimal accuracy of patient answers. Boissonnault and Badke[8] reported that of 98 health history questionnaire items (illnesses, surgeries, medication use, and demographics) completed by outpatients with orthopedic conditions, 11 showed poor-to-fair accuracy (per kappa statistics). Of these 11 questionnaire items, 5 were open-ended questions (list "other illnesses") and 5 were inquiries about specific medications (e.g., Tylenol, "yes or no"). To avoid such open-ended questionnaire items, the clinician would need to add an all-inclusive list of items, such as illnesses, producing a form that is unrealistically long. General U.S. disease incidence/prevalence data and survey research describing the medical history profile of adult outpatients (primarily with orthopedic conditions) seeking physical therapy services[5,6] can serve as a basis for items to include on a health history questionnaire. Discussing the content of the form with staff members and with physician and pharmacist colleagues is highly recommended, followed by piloting the survey-getting feedback from patients.

As described earlier, the questionnaire presented in Appendix 8-2 allows for the collection of information beyond the patient health history because it includes screening elements for issues such as depression and domestic violence. At the top of the second column of Appendix 8-2 are four questions that fall within the category of *review of systems* for depression and domestic violence. All patients should be asked questions about these particular issues because PT screening tools should address conditions and situations that PTs are likely to see most frequently and that have significance for patients' general well-being, morbidity, and mortality. In the author's clinic, many of the female patients are in their childbearing years, warranting the question, "Are you currently pregnant?" as a part of the form. The two questions for depression ("depressed mood or apathy") have been shown to be a useful instrument in screening for depression.[35] These questions have been found to have a sensitivity of 96% and a specificity of 57% for the diagnosis of depression; a negative response to both questions makes the presence of depression very unlikely, but a yes answer to one or both of the items would warrant further screening (see Chapter 20). Major

clinical depression has a lifetime prevalence of 10% to 25% for women and 5% to 12% for men; in addition, 15% of patients with major clinical depression may commit suicide.[3] Screening for this condition warrants priority on any questionnaire. Screening questions for this issue include the following:

- Are you currently under the care of a psychiatrist/psychologist?
- Have you ever been diagnosed with depression?
- The two-question case-finding instrument: Have you experienced depressed mood or apathy?
- Is there a family history of mental illness?
- Have you recently noted fatigue, sleep difficulties, or weight change—all potentially associated with major depression (see Chapter 20)?

The remaining two-part question ("Do you ever feel unsafe at home," and "Has anyone at home hit you or tried to injure you in any way?") screens for domestic violence. This is an extremely common health issue (>90% of cases involve women being abused by men), as indicated by the following statistics:

- One in four women seeking care in an emergency department is a victim of domestic violence.
- One in six pregnant women is abused during the pregnancy.
- One in four women seen in primary care settings has been abused at some point in her life.

The two-part screening question for domestic violence has a sensitivity of 71% and a specificity of 85% in detecting domestic violence.[13,14] In most cases, a victim is not likely to volunteer a "yes" reply to this question to someone (the PT) during the initial meeting, but at least the subject has been broached, and a window of opportunity is available to the victim. Even with a "no" response, the PT can affirm the patient's response; state that if the patient is ever in a threatening situation, there are resources available; and then briefly describe the resources. If the patient answers "yes" to either of these questions, the PT should follow up by investigating the following:

- The nature of the abuse
- The dates and times of the abusive events
- The circumstances of the events
- Any previous assaults and resultant injuries
- Detailed documentation of any bruises, lacerations, or other signs

All health care facilities should have a specific procedure in place for situations such as this. The American Physical Therapy Association website (www.apta.org) is a good resource for more information on this topic.

The appendices in this chapter present examples of patient self-report questionnaires designed to collect patient health history information. Appendix 8-2 presents a questionnaire used by the author for more than 15 years in adult outpatient orthopedic clinics. Experience has shown that patients take 6 to 8 minutes to complete the form. This form not only enables the PT to collect health history information but also allows the PT to begin the review of systems (see Chapter 9). The list of symptoms at the end of the questionnaire provides a general screen of all body systems and systemic illnesses—the key identifying symptoms that are new, unusual, or atypical for the patient. Appendix 8-3 presents a similar adult questionnaire in Spanish. Appendix 8-4 presents a form designed for pediatric patients; parents or other caregivers complete this questionnaire.

Finally, the *Guide to Physical Therapist Practice*[2] contains comprehensive templates for data collection in inpatient and outpatient settings. At our facility, many of the patient social history questions and others found in the *Guide to Physical Therapist Practice* are documented in other required facility paperwork, so we do not use the templates.

Review of the Health History during the Patient Interview

As noted previously, ideally the PT can review the patient's health history before beginning the interview, but the interview itself should begin with a discussion of what has precipitated the physical therapy examination (see Section Two Prologue). Discussing the patient's chief presenting complaint and primary goals gives the PT important guidance for the remainder of the examination. After this discussion, the pertinent elements of the patient's health history can be discussed.

Summary

Integrating patient demographic and health history information with the additional data collected during the history gives the PT tools that guide all aspects of clinical decision making during the initial visit. Developing an effective and efficient method for collecting patient health history information should be a priority of all practitioners. Being able to access patients' medical records or physicians' notes produces valuable information, but these sources may not contain all of the available reports, and the patient's health status may have changed since the patient last saw the physician. PTs working in any setting should collect patient health history information themselves at the initial visit. One result of this detailed information gathering is that the PT often is able to add new, important information to the patient's permanent medical record.

REFERENCES

1. Abrahamson JH. The Cornell medical index—as an epidemiological tool. Am J Public Health 1966;56:287–98.
2. American Physical Therapy Association. Guide to physical therapist practice. 2nd ed. Phys Ther 2001;81:9–744.
3. American Psychiatric Association. Diagnostic and statistical manual of mental disorders. 4th ed, text revision. Washington, DC: American Psychiatric Association; 2000.
4. Bilkey WJ, Koopmeiners MB. Screening for psychological disorders. In: Boissonnault W, editor. Examination in physical therapy practice: screening for medical disease. New York: Churchill Livingstone; 1995. p. 277–302.
5. Boissonnault W, Koopmeiners MB. Medical history profile: orthopaedic physical therapy outpatients. J Orthop Sports Phys Ther 1994;20:210.
6. Boissonnault W. Prevalence of comorbid conditions, surgeries, and medication use in a physical therapy outpatient population: a multicentered study. J Orthop Sports Phys Ther 1999;29:506–25.
7. Boissonnault WG, Meek PD. Risk factors for anti-inflammatory drug-or aspirin-induced gastrointestinal complications in individuals receiving outpatient physical therapy services. J Orthop Sports Phys Ther 2002;32:510–17.
8. Boissonnault W, Badke MB. Collecting patient health history information: the accuracy of a self-administered questionnaire in an orthopedic outpatient population. Phys Ther 2005;85:531–43.
9. Brodman K, Erdmann AJ. The Cornell medical index, an adjustment to medical interview. JAMA 1949;140:530–4.
10. Brown CS, Orune TJ, Richardson HD. The rate of pseudoarthrosis (surgical nonunion) in patients who are smokers and patients who are nonsmokers: a comparison study. Spine 1988;11:942–3.
11. Buschbaum DG, Welsh J, Buchanan RG, et al. Screening for alcohol abuse using CAGE scores and likelihood ratios. Ann Intern Med 1991;115:774–7.
12. Chou R, Qaseem A, Snow V, et al. Diagnosis and treatment of low back pain: a joint clinical practice guideline from the American College of Physicians and the American Pain Society. Ann Intern Med 2007;147:478–91.
13. Eisenstat SA, Bancroft L. Domestic violence. N Engl J Med 1999;341:886–92.
14. Feldhaus KM, Kozial-McLain J, Amsbury HL, et al. Accuracy of 3 brief screening questions for detecting partner violence in the emergency room. JAMA 1997;277:1357–61.
15. Fennelly M, Galletly DC, Purdie GI. Is caffeine withdrawal the mechanism of postoperative headache? Anesth Analg 1991;72:449–53.
16. Fleming MF, Barry KL. The effectiveness of alcoholism screening in an ambulatory care setting. J Stud Alcohol 1991;52:33–6.
17. Gilkison CR, Fenton MV, Lester JW. Getting the story straight: evaluating the test-retest reliability of a university health history questionnaire. J Am Coll Health 1992;40:247–52.
18. Hall GH. Experiences with outpatient medical questionnaires. BMJ 1972;1:42–5.
19. Hanna EZ. Approach to the patient with alcohol abuse. In: Goroll AH, Mulley AG, editors. Primary care medicine. 4th ed. Baltimore: Lippincott Williams & Wilkins; 2000. p. 1169–77.
20. Hershberg PI. Medical diagnosis: the role of a brief, open-ended medical history questionnaire. J Med Educ 1969;44:293–7.
21. Inui TS, Jared RA, Carter WB, et al. Effects of a self-administered health history questionnaire on new-patient visits in a general medical clinic. Med Care 1979;17:1221–8.
22. Jemal A, Siegel R, Ward E, et al. Cancer statistics, 2008. CA Cancer J Clin 2008;58:71–96.
23. Katz JN, Chang LC, Sangha O, et al. Can comorbidity be measured by questionnaire rather than medical interview? Med Care 1996;34:73–83.
24. Lind J, Kramhoft M, Bodtker S. The influence of smoking on complications after primary amputations of the lower extremity. Clin Orthop 1991;267:211–17.
25. Liskow B, Campbell J, Nickel EJ, et al. Validity of the CAGE questionnaire in screening for alcohol dependence in a walk-in (triage) clinic. J Stud Alcohol 1995;56:277–81.
26. National Institute on Alcohol Abuse and Alcoholism. Unpublished data from the 2001-2002 National Epidemiology Survey on Alcohol and Related Conditions (NESARC), a nationwide survey of 43,093 U.S. adults aged 18 or older, 2004.
27. National Institute on Alcohol Abuse and Alcoholism. Helping patients who drink too much—a clinician's guide. Washington, DC: US Department of Health & Human Services, Government Printing Office; 2005.
28. O'Connor PG, Schottenfeld RS. Patients with alcohol problems. N Engl J Med 1998;338:592–602.
29. Pecoraro RE, Inui TS, Chen MS, et al. Validity and reliability of a self-administered health history questionnaire. Public Health Records 1979;94:231–8.
30. Rehm J, Room R, Graham K, et al. The relationship of average volume of alcohol consumption and patterns of drinking to burden of disease: an overview. Addiction 2003;98:1209–28.
31. Rockart JF, McLean ER, Hershberg PI, et al. An automated medical history system. Arch Intern Med 1973;132:348–58.
32. Saunders JB, Aasland OG, Babor TF, et al. Development of the alcohol use disorders identification test (AUDIT): WHO collaborative project on early detection of persons with harmful alcohol consumption—II. Addiction 1993;88:791–804.
33. Silverman K, Evans SM, Strain EC, et al. Withdrawal syndrome after the double-blind cessation of caffeine consumption. N Engl J Med 1992;327:1109–14.
34. Slipman CW, Patel PK, Botwin K, et al. Epidemiology of spine tumors presenting to musculoskeletal physiatrists. Arch Phys Med Rehabil 2003;84:492–5.
35. Whooley MA, Avins AL, Miranda J, et al. Case-finding instruments for depression: two questions are as good as many. J Gen Intern Med 1997;12:439–45.

Appendix **8-1** **Review of Systems: Drug Side Effects/Subjective Complaints***

1. Gastrointestinal (dyspepsia, heartburn, nausea, vomiting, abdominal pain, constipation, diarrhea, bleeding)
   Salicylates
   Nonsteroidal anti-inflammatory drugs (NSAIDs)
   Opioids
   Corticosteroids
   Beta blockers
   Calcium channel blockers
   Skeletal muscle relaxants
   Diuretics
   Angiotensin-converting enzyme (ACE) inhibitors
   Digoxin
   Nitrates
   Cholesterol-lowering agents
   Antiarrhythmic agents
   Antidepressants (tricyclic antidepressants [TCAs], monoamine oxidase [MAO] inhibitors, lithium)
   Neuroleptics
   Antiepileptic agents
   Oral contraceptive agents (OCAs)
   Estrogens and progestins
   Theophylline
2. Pulmonary (bronchospasm, shortness of breath, respiratory depression)
   Salicylates
   NSAIDs
   Opioids
   Beta blockers
   ACE inhibitors
3. Central nervous system (dizziness, drowsiness, insomnia, headaches, hallucinations, confusion, anxiety, depression, muscle weakness)
   NSAIDs
   Skeletal muscle relaxants
   Opioids
   Corticosteroids
   Beta blockers
   Calcium channel blockers
   Nitrates
   ACE inhibitors
   Digoxin
   Antianxiety agents
   Antidepressants (TCAs and MAO inhibitors)
   Neuroleptics
   Antiepileptic agents
   OCAs
   Estrogens and progestins
4. Dermatologic (skin rash, itching, flushing of face)
   NSAIDs
   Corticosteroids
   Beta blockers
   Opioids
   Calcium channel blockers
   ACE inhibitors

Nitrates
Cholesterol-lowering agents
Antiarrhythmic agents
MAO inhibitors and lithium
OCAs
Estrogens and progestins
Antiepileptic agents
5. Musculoskeletal (weakness, fatigue, cramps, arthritis, decreased exercise tolerance, osteoporosis)
   Corticosteroids
   Beta blockers
   Calcium channel blockers
   ACE inhibitors
   Diuretics
   Digoxin
   Antianxiety agents
   Antiepileptic agents
   Antidepressants
   Neuroleptic agents
6. Cardiac (bradycardia, ventricular irritability, atrioventricular block, premature ventricular contractions, ventricular tachycardia)
   Opioids
   Diuretics
   Beta blockers
   Calcium channel blockers
   Digoxin
   Antiarrhythmic agents
   TCAs
   Neuroleptics
   Oral antiasthmatic agents
7. Vascular (claudication, hypotension, peripheral edema, cold extremities)
   NSAIDs
   Corticosteroids
   Diuretics
   Beta blockers
   Calcium channel blockers
   ACE inhibitors
   Nitrates
   Antidepressants (TCAs and MAO inhibitors)
   Neuroleptics
   OCAs
   Estrogens and progestins
8. Genitourinary (sexual dysfunction, urinary retention, urinary incontinence)
   Opioids
   Diuretics
   Beta blockers
   Antiarrhythmic agents
   Antidepressants (TCAs and MAO inhibitors)
   Neuroleptics
   OCAs
   Estrogens and progestins

9. Head, eyes, ears, nose, and throat (tinnitus, loss of taste, head-ache, lightheadedness, dizziness)
   Salicylates
   NSAIDs
   Opioids
   Skeletal muscle relaxants
   Beta blockers
   Nitrates
   Calcium channel blockers
   ACE inhibitors

Digoxin
Antiarrhythmic agents
Antianxiety agents
Antidepressants (TCAs and MAO inhibitors)
Antiepileptic agents

---

*In order of most common occurrence.

From Boissonnault W: *Examination in physical therapy practice: screening for medical disease,* ed 2, New York, 1995, Churchill Livingstone.

Appendix **8-2**

To ensure you receive a complete and thorough evaluation, please provide us with the important background information on the following form. If you do not understand a question, leave it blank and your therapist will assist you. Thank you!

NAME: _____

LEISURE ACTIVITIES: _____

OCCUPATION: _____

ALLERGIES: List any medication(s) you are allergic to:

_____

Are you latex sensitive?   YES   NO

List any other allergies we should know about:

_____

Please check (√) any of the following whose care you are under

___ Medical doctor   ___ Psychiatrist/   Other _____
     (MD)   Psychologist

___ Osteopath   ___ Physical therapist

___ Dentist   ___ Chiropractor

Date of last physical examination: _____

If you have seen any of the above during the past 3 months, please describe for what reason (e.g., illness, medical condition, physical): _____

_____

_____

Have you EVER been diagnosed as having any of the following conditions?

YES   NO   Cancer. If *Yes,* what kind: _____
YES   NO   Heart problems. If *Yes,* what kind: _____
YES   NO   High blood pressure
YES   NO   Circulation problems
YES   NO   Asthma
YES   NO   Stomach ulcers
YES   NO   Chemical dependency
           (e.g., alcoholism)
YES   NO   Thyroid problems
YES   NO   Diabetes
YES   NO   Multiple sclerosis
YES   NO   Rheumatoid arthritis
YES   NO   Other arthritic conditions
YES   NO   Depression
YES   NO   Hepatitis
YES   NO   Tuberculosis
YES   NO   Stroke
YES   NO   Kidney disease. If *Yes,* what kind: _____
YES   NO   Blood clots
YES   NO   Osteoporosis
YES   NO   Other: _____

During the past month have you been feeling down, depressed, or hopeless? YES NO

During the past month have you been bothered by having little interest or pleasure in doing things? YES NO

Do you ever feel unsafe at home or has anyone hit you or tried to injure you in any way? YES NO

Have you ever been threatened, hurt, or made to feel afraid or humiliated by your partner or someone close to you? YES NO

Please list any surgeries or other conditions for which you have been hospitalized, including the approximate date and reason for the surgery or hospitalization:

SURGERIES/HOSPITALIZATIONS
(INCLUDE DATE AND REASON)

1. _____ _____
2. _____ _____
3. _____ _____
4. _____ _____
5. _____ _____
6. _____ _____

Please describe any significant injuries for which you have been treated (including fractures, dislocations, or sprains) and the approximate date of injury:

DATE	INJURY	DATE	INJURY
_____	_____	_____	_____
_____	_____	_____	_____

Has anyone in your immediate family (parents, brothers, sisters) ever been treated for any of the following?

YES   NO   Diabetes
YES   NO   Heart disease
YES   NO   High blood pressure
YES   NO   Stroke
YES   NO   Inflammatory arthritis (rheumatoid, ankylosing)
YES   NO   Cancer
YES   NO   Alcoholism (chemical dependency)
YES   NO   Depression
YES   NO   Kidney disease

Which of the following medications have you taken in the last week?

	Physician Prescribed	Not Prescribed by Physician
Aspirin	YES/NO	YES/NO
Tylenol	YES/NO	YES/NO
Anti-inflammatories (Advil, Motrin, Ibuprofen)	YES/NO	YES/NO
Stomach ulcer medications	YES/NO	YES/NO
Vitamins/mineral supplements	YES/NO	YES/NO
Herbal remedies	YES/NO	YES/NO

Others NOT prescribed by a physician: _____

Please list any other physician-prescribed medication you are currently taking (including pills, injections, or skin patches):

1. _____ 2. _____ 3. _____
4. _____ 5. _____ 6. _____

How much caffeinated coffee or other caffeine-containing beverages do you drink per day? _____

Tobacco use: How many packs do you smoke per day_____, for how many years_____? If quit, when?_____

How many days per week do you drink alcohol? _____

If 1 drink equals 1 beer or glass of wine, how much do you drink at an average sitting? _____

How many times in the past year have you had: for men, 5 or more drinks in a day_____; for women, 4 or more drinks in a day_____

Please circle any of the following that are NEW, UNUSUAL, or ATYPICAL for you.

YES	NO	Weight loss/gain
YES	NO	Nausea/vomiting
YES	NO	Dizziness/lightheadedness
YES	NO	Fatigue
YES	NO	Weakness
YES	NO	Fever/chills/sweats
YES	NO	Numbness or tingling
YES	NO	Tremors
YES	NO	Seizures
YES	NO	Double vision
YES	NO	Loss of vision

YES	NO	Eye redness
YES	NO	Skin rash
YES	NO	Problems sleeping
YES	NO	Sexual difficulties
YES	NO	Night sweats
YES	NO	Hearing problems
YES	NO	Recently fallen down
YES	NO	Joint/muscle swelling
YES	NO	Easy bruising
YES	NO	Excessive bleeding
YES	NO	Difficulty breathing
YES	NO	Regular cough
YES	NO	Arm/leg swelling
YES	NO	Heart racing in your chest
YES	NO	Difficulty swallowing
YES	NO	Heartburn/indigestion
YES	NO	Constipation/diarrhea
YES	NO	Blood in stools
YES	NO	Postmenopause
YES	NO	Problems urinating (e.g., difficulty starting, painful)
YES	NO	Urinary incontinence
YES	NO	Blood in the urine
YES	NO	Pregnant or think you might be pregnant
YES	NO	Stress at home or work
YES	NO	Problems with balance

_____   _____
Therapist signature   Date   Patient signature   Date

Apéndice **8-3**

Para asegurarnos de que usted recibe una evaluación completa, sea tan amable de proveernos con la información más importante de su historial médico. Si usted no entiende alguna de las siguientes preguntas, déjelas sin contestar, y su terapista físico le ayudará. Gracias por su cooperación.

NOMBRE: _____

PASATIEMPOS: _____

TRABAJO: _____

> **ALERGIAS**: Indique aquellos medicamentos a los que usted es alérgico: _____
>
> ¿Es usted sensible o alérgico al látex?   SÍ   NO
> Mencione aquellas alergias que usted entiende debemos conocer: _____

¿Ha declarado usted el "Directiva Avanzada Médica" de no resucitar?
SÍ: _____ NO: _____

Favor de marcar (√) a aquellos de los siguientes especialistas que manejan el cuidado de su salud:

___ Doctor en Medicina   ___ Siquiatra/Sicólogo
      (MD)   ___ Terapista Físico
___ Osteópata   ___ Quiropráctico
___ Dentista   Otro _____

Si usted ha visitado alguno de los especialistas arriba mencionados en los últimos 3 meses, por favor indique cuál fue la razón de la visita (e.j., enfermedad, condición médica, examen físico):

_____

_____

¿Ha sido usted diagnosticado ALGUNA VEZ con cualquiera de las siguientes condiciones?

SÍ   NO   Cáncer. Si es *Sí*, indique cuál tipo: _____
SÍ   NO   Problemas cardíacos. Si es Sí, indique cuál típo: ___
SÍ   NO   Alta presión sanguínea
SÍ   NO   Problemas circulatorios
SÍ   NO   Asma
SÍ   NO   Emfisema/Bronquitis
SÍ   NO   Dependencia química
                  (e.j., alcoholismo)
SÍ   NO   Problemas de la tiroide
SÍ   NO   Diabetes
SÍ   NO   Esclerosis múltiple
SÍ   NO   Artritis reumatoide
SÍ   NO   Otras condiciones artríticas
SÍ   NO   Depresión
SÍ   NO   Hepatitis
SÍ   NO   Tuberculosis
SÍ   NO   Infarto cerebral
SÍ   NO   Enfermedad renal (riñón). Si es *Si*, indique
                  cual tipo: _____
SÍ   NO   Anemia
SÍ   NO   Epilepsia
SÍ   NO   Otro: _____

¿Se ha sentido triste, deprimido(a), o desesperado(a) en el pasado mes? SÍ NO

En el pasado mes, ¿se ha preocupado porque siente que tiene poco interés o placer haciendo actividades que normalmente goce? SÍ NO

¿Se has sentido alguna vez inseguro(a) en su propia casa, o alguna vez alguien le ha golpeado o tratado de lastimar de alguna manera? SÍ NO

Solo Mujeres: ¿Está embarazada o piensa que podría estarlo? SÍ NO

Favor indicar cualquier tipo de cirujía u otro tipo de condición por la cual usted haya sido hospitalizado(a), incluyendo la fecha aproximada y la razón para la cirujía/hospitalización:

FECHA Y RAZÓN PARA CIRUJÍA/HOSPITALIZACIÓN

1._____ _____
2. _____ _____
3._____ _____
4. _____ _____

Por favor, indique si usted ha recibido alguna lesión grave por la cual haya sido tratado (incluya fracturas, dislocaciones, desgarre/estiramiento de ligamentos/tendones) y la fecha aproximada de la lesión:

FECHA	LESIÓN	FECHA	LESIÓN
_____	_____	_____	_____
_____	_____	_____	_____

¿Ha sido un miembro de su familia inmediata (padres, hermanos[as]) tratado alguna vez por alguna de las siguientes condiciones?

SÍ   NO   Diabetes
SÍ   NO   Tuberculosis
SÍ   NO   Enfermedad cardíaca
SÍ   NO   Alta presión sanguínea
SÍ   NO   Infarto cerebral
SÍ   NO   Enfermedad renal (riñón)
SÍ   NO   Alcoholismo (dependencia química)
SÍ   NO   Cáncer
SÍ   NO   Artritis
SÍ   NO   Anemia
SÍ   NO   Dolor de cabeza
SÍ   NO   Epilepsia
SÍ   NO   Enfermedad mental

¿Cúal de los siguientes medicamentos SIN PRESCRIPCIÓN usted ha tomado en la última semana?

SÍ   NO   Aspirina
SÍ   NO   Tylenol
SÍ   NO   Advil, Motrin, Ibuprofen
SÍ   NO   Descongestionantes
SÍ   NO   Antihistamínicos

SÍ   NO   Laxantes
SÍ   NO   Antiácido
SÍ   NO   Suplementos vitamínicos/minerales
SÍ   NO   Otros: _____
Favor de indicar los medicamentos bajo PRESCRIPCIÓN que usted está actualmente tomando (INCLUYA pastillas, inyecciones, cremas medicadas, y/o parchos de piel):

1._____   2._____   3._____

4._____   5._____   6._____

¿Cuánto café cafeinado o bebidas carbonatadas con cafeína usted consume por día?_____

¿Cuántos paquetes/cajetillas de cigarrillos usted fuma al día?_____

¿Cuántos días a la semana usted toma bebidas alcohólicas?_____

Si una bebida es equivalente a una cerveza o copa de vino, ¿cuánto usted toma al día?_____

¿Ha notado recientemente:
SÍ   NO   Aumento/pérdida de peso?
SÍ   NO   Nauseas/vómitos?
SÍ   NO   Fatiga?
SÍ   NO   Debilidad?
SÍ   NO   Fiebre/sudores/escalofrios?
SÍ   NO   Adormecimiento u hormiguilleo?

_____   _____

Firma del Terapista   Fecha   Firma del Paciente   Fecha

Appendix **8-4** Gibson-Pike-Warrick Special Education Cooperative– General Health Form

To ensure your child receives a complete and thorough evaluation, please provide us with the important background information on the following form. If you do not understand a question, your therapist will assist you. Thank you.

Child's name _____

Birth date _____

School _____

Teacher _____

Parent/guardian _____

Home phone _____

Address _____

Work phone _____

Has the child seen any of the following in the past 3 months? If *Yes,* who?

YES   NO   Medical doctor _____

YES   NO   Psychiatrist/Psychologist _____

YES   NO   Orthopedist _____

YES   NO   Eye doctor _____

YES   NO   Osteopath _____

YES   NO   Physical therapist _____

YES   NO   Dentist _____

YES   NO   Chiropractor _____

Please describe the reason the child visited the above provider (illness, medical, surgery):

_____

_____

_____

_____

_____

_____

For what problem is the child being evaluated by the therapist?

_____

_____

_____

Has the child EVER been diagnosed as having any of the following?

YES   NO   Cancer

YES   NO   Heart problems

YES   NO   High blood pressure

YES   NO   Asthma/breathing problems

YES   NO   Thyroid problems

YES   NO   Diabetes

YES   NO   Arthritis

YES   NO   Depression

YES   NO   Hepatitis

YES   NO   Tuberculosis

YES   NO   Stroke

YES   NO   Kidney disease

YES   NO   Anemia

YES   NO   Epilepsy

YES   NO   Seizures

YES   NO   Cerebral palsy

YES   NO   Muscular dystrophy

YES   NO   Spina bifida/myelomeningocele

YES   NO   Attention-deficit disorder/attention-deficit hyperactivity disorder (ADD/ADHD)

YES   NO   Other

Please list any surgeries or other conditions for which the child has been in the hospital:

_____

_____

_____

_____

_____

_____

Has anyone in the child's immediate family (parents, brothers, sisters) ever been treated for any of the following?

YES   NO   Diabetes

YES   NO   Tuberculosis

YES   NO   Heart disease

YES   NO   High blood pressure

YES   NO   Stroke

YES   NO   Kidney disease

YES   NO   Cancer

YES   NO   Arthritis

YES   NO   Anemia

YES   NO   Headaches

YES   NO   Epilepsy

YES   NO   Mental illness

YES   NO   Alcoholism or chemical dependency

Please list all of the prescription medications and the dosage that the child is currently taking:

_____

_____

_____

_____

_____

_____

List any over-the-counter medications the child frequently takes:

_____

_____

Has the child recently experienced any of the following?

YES   NO   Weight loss or gain

YES   NO   Nausea/vomiting

YES   NO   Fatigue

YES   NO   Unusual weakness

YES   NO   Fever/chills/sweats

How many caffeine-containing beverages does the child drink daily?

_____

Does the child have allergies?

_____
_____

Does the child have special equipment? What?

_____
_____
_____

What functional problems is the child having at home?

_____
_____
_____
_____
_____
_____

Person completing form: _____

Date _____

Form reviewed by therapist with parent/guardian? Yes No

Date _____

_____

(Therapist)

Date _____

Review of Systems

William G. Boissonnault, PT, DPT DHSc, FAAOMPT

Objectives

After reading this chapter, the reader will be able to:

1. Create screening checklists for general health and for each of the body organ systems.
2. Describe strategies for determining whether a "yes" answer to any checklist item is a red flag (warrants physician contact) or a yellow flag (warrants monitoring only).
3. Discuss the types of patients and for which of the patient visits (initial or follow-up) each of the checklists is appropriate.
4. Describe strategies to integrate the review of systems checklists efficiently into a patient examination scheme.

The review of systems (ROS) is an important category of data collected during the patient interview. These data, in conjunction with a patient's medical history and symptoms and signs, are vital to the role of the physical therapist (PT) in medical screening and differential diagnosis, as described in the *Guide to Physical Therapist Practice.*[3] Investigating a patient's health history along with the ROS provides therapists with a well-rounded, more complete picture of the patient's health statuses. The ROS investigation includes using checklists of symptoms associated with each of the body systems. The purpose of the ROS is to identify symptoms unusual for impairment-related conditions, such as sprains and strains, which may have been overlooked during the investigation of the patient's chief presenting complaints.[8,39] The underlying assumption is that these symptoms are not why a PT's services have been sought—in essence, they are secondary complaints.

The systematic review of each body system may reveal symptoms related to the reason the patient initiated physical therapy. For example, back and leg symptoms, and accompanying urinary dysfunction, may be related to cauda equina syndrome. Equally important, the checklists may identify symptoms that are unrelated to the patient's chief presenting complaint; that is, they are adjunct symptoms that may be associated with one or more existing comorbid conditions, occult disease, or adverse drug reactions. Detecting such symptoms, which were not previously reported to the patient's physician or that represent a worsening of preexisting manifestations of a comorbid condition or medication use, would prompt contact with the appropriate health care provider. These checklists are *not* intended to rule out specific systemic or visceral diseases; this is the role of the physician. They are based on the physiology of each body system so that, if the system is malfunctioning in some way, the patient may report the symptoms identified in these checklists, assuming that the therapist has asked the appropriate questions.

To promote efficiency, including the initial ROS screening on a health history questionnaire can save considerable time and provide guidance as to which body systems need to be screened in detail. Box 9-1 contains the initial ROS screening from Chapter 8, Appendix 8-2.

"Yes" responses to any of the screening questions, and the location and description of patients' symptoms and medical history, will determine the need to carry out a more complete ROS and systems review screening. A significant challenge for the PT is deciding whether a positive response ("yes" response) truly constitutes a red flag (requiring communication with another care provider) or a yellow flag (something to note in the PT's documentation that should be monitored, but not something that warrants immediate communication with a physician). This is especially challenging with general findings such as fatigue; everyone gets tired, so what would make fatigue a red flag? Concern should be raised about these findings; for any "yes" answer, determine the following:

1. Does the complaint represent something new, different, or unusual for the patient?
2. Is there an explanation for it that would minimize concern?
3. Has the patient mentioned this to a physician?
4. If a physician is aware of it, has it become worse?

This chapter discusses additional guidelines that clinicians can use to make this important decision, including follow-up questions for the various checklist items.

The addition of the ROS checklists to the PT's examination scheme may cause some therapists to ask, "Where do I find time to add even more questions to the patient interview?" A literature review on low back pain associated with cancer has revealed that unexplained weight loss is a statistically relevant examination finding associated with an increased risk of cancer.[25] Similarly, complaints of fever, chills, or sweats with low back pain increases the risk of the presence of back pain–related infection.[25] As described in Chapter 6, there is considerable commonality of pain complaints between disease and impairment-driven conditions. Without ROS questioning and patient health history investigation, clinicians are at risk of overreporting or underreporting patient health concerns.

This chapter will present an ROS screening for all body systems. Checklist items found in Box 9-1 will be included in the more comprehensive screening list.

General Health and Constitutional Screening

The first seven items found in Box 9-1 (left column), along with malaise and mentation changes, are complaints that can result from the following: (1) many diseases in different body systems;

BOX 9-1
Initial Review of Systems Screening

Please circle any of the following that are *new*, *unusual*, or *atypical* for you.

YES NO Weight loss, gain
YES NO Nausea, vomiting
YES NO Dizziness, lightheadedness
YES NO Fatigue
YES NO Weakness
YES NO Fever, chills, sweats
YES NO Numbness or tingling
YES NO Tremors
YES NO Seizures
YES NO Double vision
YES NO Loss of vision
YES NO Eye redness
YES NO Skin rash
YES NO Problems sleeping
YES NO Sexual difficulties
YES NO Night sweats
YES NO Hearing problems
YES NO Recently fallen down

YES NO Joint, muscle swelling
YES NO Easy bruising
YES NO Excessive bleeding
YES NO Difficulty breathing
YES NO Regular cough
YES NO Arm, leg swelling
YES NO Heart racing in your chest
YES NO Difficulty swallowing
YES NO Heartburn, indigestion
YES NO Constipation, diarrhea
YES NO Blood in stools
YES NO Postmenopause
YES NO Problems urinating (e.g., difficulty starting, painful)
YES NO Urinary incontinence
YES NO Blood in the urine
YES NO Pregnant or think you might be pregnant
YES NO Stress at home or work
YES NO Problems with balance

BOX 9-2
General Health Component of Review of Systems

1. Fatigue
2. Malaise
3. Fever, chills, sweats—significant if 99.5° F or higher for more than 2 weeks
4. Weight loss, gain—5%-10% of body weight increase, decrease, unexplained
5. Nausea, vomiting
6. Dizziness, lightheadedness
7. Paresthesia, numbness
8. Weakness
9. Change in mentation, cognitive abilities

BOX 9-3
Conditions Presenting as Chronic Fatigue

PSYCHOLOGICAL
- Depression
- Anxiety
- Somatization disorder

ENDOCRINE OR METABOLIC
- Hypothyroidism
- Diabetes mellitus
- Pituitary insufficiency
- Addison's disease
- Chronic renal failure
- Hyperparathyroidism

INFECTIOUS
- Endocarditis
- Tuberculosis
- Mononucleosis
- Hepatitis
- HIV infection

NEOPLASMS
- Occult malignancy
- Cardiopulmonary
- Congestive heart failure
- Chronic obstructive pulmonary disease

CONNECTIVE TISSUE DISEASE
- Rheumatic disorders

SLEEP DISTURBANCES
- Sleep apnea
- Esophageal reflux
- Allergic rhinitis

Adapted from Bickley LS: *Bates' guide to physical examination and history taking*, 10th ed, Philadelphia, 2009, JB Lippincott.

(2) multisystem disorders; (3) systemic illnesses; and (4) adverse drug reactions. Some of these symptoms (e.g., fatigue and malaise) are extremely vague but may be the initial manifestation of a very serious illness. These checklist items provides PTs with a valuable first level of medical screening (general health screening; Box 9-2) and should be included in the initial patient visit.

Fatigue

Patients presenting with fatigue is extremely common in primary care practice, annually accounting for approximately 20% of U.S. primary care office visits.[21,29] Fatigue can be associated with many serious illnesses, including some psychological disorders, infections, cancers (typically advanced disease), and endocrine disorders (Box 9-3). In addition, fatigue may be associated with medication use, including antihypertensives, cardiovascular and psychotropic agents, and antihistamines, all commonly prescribed medications.[29] The challenge to the PT is differentiating fatigue associated with daily life from a potentially serious disorder. After the patient reports fatigue, the PT should ask the following questions:

- "What do you mean by fatigue? Describe your fatigue to me. Is it interfering with your daily activities?"
- "When did the fatigue begin?"
- "Was the onset slow and gradual or fast?"

This will provide clues about the potential acuteness of the underlying disorder, possibly making the referral more urgent in nature.

- "Do you know why you are so tired?"
- "In addition to the fatigue, have you noticed any other unusual symptoms (e.g., nausea, fever, weight loss, symmetric joint pain, and early morning stiffness)?"

The presence of these accompanying complaints suggests possible malignancy, infection, or rheumatic disorder.

Fatigue becomes a red flag when the tiredness interferes with a patient's ability to carry out daily activities at home, work, or school, or in a social setting or during rehabilitation, and when it has lasted for 2 to 4 weeks or longer.[4,29] For example, a patient may say that up until 3 weeks ago, she typically worked 8 to 9 hours every day, went home, helped take care of dinner, and then was active until she went to bed at 11 PM. Now she struggles to make it through her workday, and she went home early twice this week because of her fatigue. When she comes home from work now, she barely makes it through dinner, and has been going to bed by 9 PM. This report represents a change in the patient's ability to carry out her daily activities. When communicating concerns about fatigue to the physician's office, the PT must describe the specifics of the condition. Simply reporting that the patient is tired will not alarm anyone, but describing the functional limitations associated with the fatigue will.

Malaise

Malaise is a sense of uneasiness or general discomfort, an out of sorts feeling. Patients may describe this uneasiness as an intuition that "something isn't right" or that they are "coming down with something." Malaise is often noted with systemic conditions that typically generate fever (e.g., infectious disorders).[21,22] A patient may describe malaise by saying, "I felt like I was coming down with the flu for weeks, but haven't gotten sick." Another patient with an existing history of heart problems or cancer might start experiencing new symptoms or a return of previous symptoms. This patient may say, "I am worried that the cancer has come back." On review of Chapter 8, Appendix 8-2 and Box 9-1, malaise is not included in the checklist. Most patients will not recognize the term, so this symptom is generally identified by the therapist, based on patient comments.

Fever, Chills, and Sweats

Fever, chills, and sweats are symptoms and signs most often associated with systemic illnesses such as infections, cancers, and connective tissue disorders such as rheumatoid arthritis.[7,30] Fever associated with a pathologic condition is a result of the release of pyrogens into the bloodstream by toxic bacteria or from degenerating body tissues. These events will cause the set point of the hypothalamic thermostat to rise. When the blood temperature is lower than the hypothalamic set point, the body reacts by increasing core body temperature via the normal responses, including cutaneous vasoconstriction (Figure 9-1). This superficial vasoconstriction produces a drop in skin temperature that can lead to shaking chills or rigor. If the body temperature reaches 39.5° C (103° F), however, the patient typically no longer feels chilled or hot.[24] If the patient answers "yes" to fever on the questionnaire, follow-up questions are in order. As with any other "yes" answer on these checklists, the therapist should determine whether the patient knows why he or she has the fever (e.g., "I have the flu or a sinus infection"). If the patient complains of persistent chills or sweats but does not know whether he or she has a fever, the therapist should take the patient's temperature.

When assessing fever, the PT should understand that normal body temperature is not defined by a single value, 37° C (98.6° F) at a single point in time. Body temperature (mean rectal temperature) typically follows a circadian rhythm, ranging from approximately 36.1° C (97° F) in the morning to 37.4° C (99.3° F) in the late afternoon.[22] Therefore fevers tend to be highest in the evenings. In addition, activities and physiologic events such as exercise and menstruation can also alter body temperature. This, along with the fact that symptoms and signs associated with fever can vary tremendously, ranging from some patients being asymptomatic and others overtly ill, creates challenges for clinicians.

Fever of unknown origin has been defined as a body temperature higher than 37.5° to 38.3° C (99.5° to 101° F).[13,22] To qualify as a red flag, the fever should have been present for a long time, as with the symptom of fatigue. If the fever has been present for 2 to 3 weeks or longer and a physician has not seen the patient during that time frame, the patient should be referred to a physician. The 3-week window accounts for the common self-limited

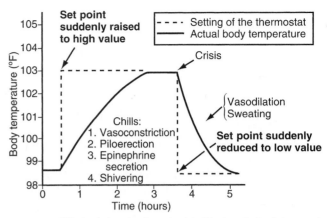

FIGURE 9-1 Effects of changing the set point of the hypothalamic temperature controller. (From Guyton AC, Hall JE: *Textbook of medical physiology,* 10th ed, Philadelphia, 2000, WB Saunders, p 831.)

viruses that can be accompanied by a fever but of shorter duration. If the patient does not know whether he or she has a fever, the therapist can ask the patient whether he or she feels the same today as he or she has felt for the past 2 weeks or more. If the answer is yes and the patient has a temperature of 37.5° to 38.3° C or higher via the clinical reading, the therapist should assume that the patient has had this fever for 3 or more weeks, unless proven otherwise. The referral takes on a more urgent nature if the therapist gets a reading of 39° C (102° F) or higher. Such a fever may require hospitalization.[13]

Normal body temperature also varies among age groups. Studies have shown that the amount of fluctuation in the circadian body temperature was lower in an older population, as was the baseline body temperature.[42] Therefore screening guidelines may vary, depending on the population in question. One study[11] of an older population found that an oral temperature of 37.2° C (98.9° F) carried a sensitivity of 83% and a specificity of 89% for the detection of infection. Thus, the authors recommended that a persistent oral temperature higher than 37.2° C, or an increase of 1.3° C above the patient's baseline body temperature in an older person, be considered as cause for concern. Therapists can use this guideline to help determine whether to contact a physician about a patient's health.

Finally, therapists should remember that a perceived absence of fever does not preclude the possibility that the patient has an infection. The older adult population is especially vulnerable to this. Reduced thermoregulatory responses in older people may be responsible for the differences in fever response to infection between older and younger populations.[30] This finding is in part responsible for the increased morbidity and mortality associated with infectious processes. For example, pneumonia is the most common cause of infectious death in the geriatric population because of the frequent absence of the expected fever, productive cough, and pleuritic pain.[1,17] The PT must watch for other warning signs (see later, "Change in Mentation") that may be present, suggesting to the PT that the patient may have a serious condition. Other symptoms commonly accompanying conditions that may generate a fever include malaise, fatigue, myalgias, chills, sweats, tachycardia, confusion, and delerium.[22] In addition, in infants and children, high fevers (104° to 106° F) can be associated with convulsions.

Unexplained Weight Change

Unexplained weight loss or gain is also a red flag potentially associated with multiple disorders. Involuntary weight loss is more common that weight gain but, much like fatigue, is a sensitive but nonspecific finding. The potential causes of weight loss can be summarized by physiologic categories (Table 9-1). Not all these disorders occur with equal frequency.

Thompson and Morris[40] have investigated unexplained weight loss in an older population (63 years and older; 67% female), identifying those who had lost 7.5% or more of their baseline body weight over a 6-month period. The patients then were followed for up to 24 months or until the definitive cause of the weight loss had been determined. The disorders most frequently associated with the weight loss were depression (18%), cancer (16%), and gastrointestinal (GI) disease other than cancer (11%).

Marton and colleagues[28] have investigated involuntary weight loss in a patient population (mean age, 59 ± 17.5 years; 99% male) at a Veterans Medical Center, identifying those who had lost at least 5% of their usual body weight during the previous 6 months. The causes most often noted included cancer (19%), GI disorders (14%), and psychiatric and cardiovascular disorders (9%). The definition of a significant weight loss varies. Goroll and Mulley[21] used a loss of more than 5%, and Swartz[39] suggested a loss of 5% or 10% of body weight over 6 to 12 months, respectively, as a warning sign of underlying disease. This author's personal communications with physicians have led to my suggesting the use of a loss of 5% to 10% of body weight as a guideline. The exception to this general rule is women who are pregnant; a loss of more than 5% of body weight during the first trimester should be reported.[8] See Chapter 17 for additional information related to women who are pregnant.

If a patient reports weight loss during the examination, appropriate follow-up questions include the following:

- "How much weight have you lost?"
- "Over what period of time have you lost weight?"
- "Have you noted any other new or unusual symptoms during this time?"
- "Do you know why you have lost weight?"

The third question is the most important in determining the importance of the weight loss. If the patient has purposely changed the diet or increased physical activity during the time of the weight loss, the therapist's concern can drop considerably—now there is a reason, an explanation for the weight loss. If the patient reports a loss of 5% to 10% of body weight with no purposeful change in diet or activity level, the weight loss becomes a red flag and should be reported to the patient's physician. The patient may say that he or she is eating less because, "I'm just not as hungry as I used to be," or "I have been sick to my stomach." If this is the only explanation that the patient offers, the therapist must be concerned, especially if the patient has risk factors for serious disease (see Chapter 8).

Although weight gain is not as commonly noted as a red flag compared with weight loss, excessive weight gain also can be a manifestation of serious disease. Rapid weight gain often is associated with fluid retention (e.g., edema, ascites) that can be a manifestation of conditions such as congestive heart failure, liver or renal disease, and preeclampsia.[12,39] In these conditions, the

TABLE 9-1

Physiologic Categories Associated with Weight Loss

Category	Symptoms	Diseases
Decreased caloric intake	Anorexia or satiety Loss of sense of taste Dry, sore mouth Difficulty with chewing, swallowing Nausea, vomiting	Depression, dementia, anxiety disorders Poor dentition Upper gastrointestinal tract disease Malignancies Infections Alcoholism Chronic congestive heart failure Medications—NSAIDs, amphetamines, antitumor drugs, digitalis excess
Maldigestion, malabsorption	Diarrhea Fatty malodorous stools Food particles in stools	Gallbladder, pancreatic disorders Infection (giardiasis) Small bowel disease, Crohn's disease
Excessive demand, requirements	Fever Change in appetite	Infection Hyperthyroidism Malignancies Manic disorders
Increased loss, excretion	Diarrhea Increased urination Excessive vomiting	Uncontrolled diabetes Burns Occult gastrointestinal bleeding

Adapted from Goroll AH, Mulley AG: Evaluation of weight loss. In Goroll AH, Mulley AG, eds: *Primary care medicine*, 5th ed, Philadelphia, 2006, Lippincott Williams & Wilkins, p 54; and from Swartz MH: *Textbook of physical diagnosis*, 5th ed, Philadelphia, 2006, Saunders, p 95.

therapist may detect the initial warning sign of a relatively rapid onset of edema and then check the patient's weight. This assumes that the therapist knows the patient's usual weight and can compare it with the new weight (see Chapter 11), assuming that the patient's weight is determined at the initial visit.

The extremities are the areas most often affected by dependency-related edema, but the face and neck regions can also be involved in patients with preeclampsia.[12,34] Other conditions that can manifest as unexplained weight gain are depression, hypothyroidism, and Cushing's syndrome. The same general guideline used to qualify weight loss as a red flag (i.e., 5% to 10% unexplained loss of body weight) can be used for weight gain. An exception to this rule for weight gain would be a gain of 5 lb or more over a 1-week period during pregnancy. This is a warning sign and is potentially associated with preeclampsia[12] (see Chapter 17).

Nausea and Vomiting

Like being tired (fatigue) or occasionally catching a virus, nausea is experienced by many people. The challenge once again becomes deciding whether this complaint is a red flag. The PT may intuitively link nausea with the GI checklist rather than the general health checklist, but nausea can be a manifestation of primary disease of other organ systems, systemic illnesses (metastatic disease), or an adverse drug reaction (Box 9-4). In most cases of patients vomiting over time, the physician already has been contacted, but low-level or mild nausea may go unreported

Common Causes of Nausea and Vomiting*

AS ACUTE PREDOMINANT OR INITIAL SYMPTOM:
- Ketoacidosis
- Inferior myocardial infarction
- Hepatitis
- Drug withdrawal
- Early pregnancy
- Medication use—opiates, digitalis, cancer chemotherapeutic agents

RECURRENT OR CHRONIC:
- Psychogenic disorders (bulimia)
- Metabolic disorders (adrenal insufficiency, uremia)
- Bile reflux after gastric surgery
- Pregnancy

IN ASSOCIATION WITH NEUROLOGIC SYMPTOMS:
- Increased intracranial pressure
- Vestibular disturbances
- Migraine headaches
- Midline cerebellar hemorrhage

*Other than primary gastrointestinal disorders.
Adapted from Swartz MH: *Textbook of physical diagnosis*, 5th ed, Philadelphia, 2006, Saunders, pp 484-485.

for several months. The PT must ask follow-up questions when a patient reports nausea:

- "Describe your nausea to me (constant or intermittent, how frequent?)."
- "How long have you been experiencing the nausea?"
- "In addition to the nausea, have you experienced any other new or unusual symptoms during this time?"
- "Do you know why you are nauseated?"
- "Is your physician aware of the nausea? (If the answer is yes, "Has it gotten any worse since your last physician contact?")
- "Is the nausea associated with vomiting or any other symptoms?"
- "Do you have vomiting without nausea?"
- "How are you treating the nausea?"

Vomitus greenish-yellow in color represents biliary colic, whereas intestinal obstruction can cause bilious vomit followed by feculent-smelling fluid. Coffee-ground vomitus represents blood (hematemesis).[8,39]

The initial warning sign may be related to medication use. A patient may report taking over-the-counter treatments for nausea and indigestion; patients coming in for physical therapy commonly use antacids and histamine (H_2) antagonists (e.g., cimetidine, ranitidine).[10] If the patient reports such use, the therapist must ask why the patient is taking these medications, for how long, and whether the patient's physician knows about this drug use. The PT also should ask, "Do you need more of the medication to feel comfortable compared with a few weeks or months ago?" An affirmative answer may reveal a serious condition that is worsening.

Paresthesia, Numbness, or Weakness

In addition to primary neurologic disorders, several other conditions can be manifested as paresthesia, numbness, and weakness, including certain renal and endocrine diseases, as well as adverse

drug reactions. As described in Chapters 4 and 6, the therapist should ask all patients questions about changes in sensation and strength during the first visit because of the possible urgency of a progressive neurologic loss. For example, Jarvik and Deyo[25] have stated that an important goal of the diagnostic process in patients with low back pain who are being seen in primary care settings is to determine whether the patient has a neurologic impairment that requires surgical evaluation. The primary red flags for this patient population include progressive sensory or strength deficits (based on patient report and detection of a deficit during the physical examination; see Chapters 12 and 13) and any symptoms of saddle anesthesia, urinary retention, increased urinary frequency, and overflow incontinence.[9]

In addition to the progressive neurologic symptoms, which represent a spinal nerve root or peripheral nerve entrapment lesion, the PT should screen for descriptions unusual for the orthopedic outpatient population. These include the following:

- Glove and stocking distribution of altered sensation
- Bilateral extremity deficits (sensory, motor)
- Combination of upper extremity and lower extremity deficit patterns (sensory, motor)

Chronic renal failure, multiple sclerosis, hypothyroidism, and adverse drug events are examples of disorders that could present with these findings. Any subjective complaints of numbness or tingling require further investigation as the clinician moves into the neurologic screening of the physical examination.

Many patients may report weakness but, much like the symptom of fatigue, this finding often is not a red flag. These scenarios often include general symptoms of weakness ("I feel run down"), or reports such as "My back goes out and feels weak" or "My knee goes out on me." Further questioning reveals local sharp pain that precipitates these symptoms, a scenario that lessens the concern regarding the possible presence of a primary neurologic deficit. If the patient reports an inability to carry out usual activities (e.g., difficulty navigating stairs, leg giving out in the absence of pain, tripping over one's feet) because of weakness, a detailed neurologic screening of the upper and/or lower quarters would be warranted (see Chapters 12 and 13. If the patient has no other neurologic symptoms such as sensation changes; balance problems; visual symptoms; or taste, smell, or hearing deficits, and if the results of the neurologic screening are negative, the symptom of weakness becomes a yellow flag—something to monitor—and not a red flag.

Dizziness and Lightheadedness

Patients can interpret the feeling of dizziness in many ways, such as leading to difficulty differentiating between feeling lightheaded or faint, or the room spinning around. In addition, some patients suffer from a combination of these complaints. It is important for therapist to try to distinguish among these potentially serious symptoms. Dizziness can be associated with disorders of most body systems and with multisystem disease or adverse drug reactions. For certain types of disorders, physical therapy should be the primary treatment, but some causes of dizziness require a physician's management (Box 9-5). The following questions can be asked to elicit a precise description of what the patient means by dizzy:

- Do you feel lightheaded or faint?
- Is there a spinning sensation in your head?

Potential Causes of Dizziness

NEUROLOGIC DISORDERS
- Multiple sclerosis
- Benign positional vertigo
- Ménière's disease
- Acoustic neuromas
- Ototoxic drugs
- Aminoglycoside antibiotics (streptomycin, gentamicin)
- Antineoplastics (cisplatin, vincristine)
- Diuretics (furosemide, bumetanide, mannitol)
- Environmental toxins (mercury, tin, lead, carbon dioxide)
- Basilar insufficiency

CARDIAC AND VASCULAR DISORDERS
- Critical aortic stenosis
- Carotid sinus hypersensitivity
- Volume depletion
- Severe anemia
- Diminished vascular reflexes (older adults)

OTHER CAUSES
- Diabetes mellitus
- Cervical spondylosis
- Anxiety
- Psychosis
- Hypoxia

Adapted from Allison L, Fuller K: Balance and vestibular disorders. In Umphred DA, ed: *Neurological rehabilitation*, 5th ed, St Louis, 2007, Mosby, pp 732-774; and from Pruitt AA: Evaluation of dizziness. In Goroll AH, Mulley AG, eds: *Primary care medicine*, 5th ed, Philadelphia, 2006, Lippincott, Williams & Wilkins, p 1087.

- Is the room spinning around you?
- Is it associated with specific postures or movements?
- Is it associated with nausea, vomiting, diaphoresis, hearing loss, tinnitus, visual disturbance, or hemiparesis?
- Have you fallen because of the dizziness?

Vestibular disease often manifests with sensations of the head spinning or the room spinning around the patient. Symptoms may also be described as headache, weaving, seasickness, rocking, sensation of things moving, or a feeling that the ground is rising and falling. Nausea and vomiting can be associated with severe vestibular disorders and migraine headaches. The associated hearing loss and tinnitus could be manifestations of Ménière's disease and labyrinthitis. Finally, symptoms of visual disturbance or hemiparesis along with the dizziness could be signs of vertebral basilar insufficiency.[2,31,39] See Chapter 7 for details related to differentiating common causes of dizziness.

Lightheadedness or a feeling of faintness often is associated with cardiac and vascular insufficiency or with conditions such as arrhythmias, orthostatic hypotension, vertebral artery insufficiency, and impaired ventricular function. Such symptoms typically worsen on standing and improve with lying down. In addition, anxiety and emotional distress can be associated with this complaint. Assessing patients' vital signs along with auscultation for heart and lung sounds (see Chapter 11), and incorporating special tests related to dizziness, such as the Dix-Hallpike, Hautant, and Romberg tests, can provide the therapist with information leading to the appropriate diagnosis.

Change in Mentation

The onset of confusion or disorientation, or a worsening of these symptoms, can be a manifestation of multiple disorders, including delirium, dementia, head injury, adverse drug reactions, and infection. If these problems are discovered during the history-taking process, the PT should point out the observation to the patient, caregiver, and/or family member and ask whether he or she noted the difficulties. The observations may include the following[8]:

- Level of consciousness—alertness or state of awareness
- Attention—ability to focus on a task or activity
- Memory—short-term versus long-term
- Orientation—personal identity, place, and time
- Thought processes—logical and coherent thoughts leading to selected goal
- Judgment—ability to evaluate alternatives and follow appropriate values while choosing a course of action

If the patient or family member reports that these issues have been present since the head injury or stroke, and they have not worsened since the last visit to the physician, the observation becomes a yellow flag. If the difficulties represent a new onset or worsening, follow-up questions are in order:

- When did you first note the changes?
- Do you know the cause (e.g., a fall, blow to the head, a new medication)?
- Did the problem come on quickly, or slowly and gradually?
- Have you noted the onset of any other problems or difficulties associated with the mentation difficulties?

The onset of confusion can be a particularly challenging and important finding in older patients.[1] For example, pneumonia is the most common cause of death from infection in older adults because of its atypical clinical presentation. The expected productive cough, pleuritic pain, and fever often do not appear in this group, and confusion and mental deterioration are the primary manifestations.[17,26] Because altered mentation and confusion are such general terms, the onus is on the PT to be as specific as possible when collecting these data and communicating these concerns to a physician. The more detail that the PT can provide about the situation, the more likely the physician will take these concerns seriously.

General Health Checklist Summary

Because the general health checklist covers symptoms associated with a number of body systems, disease states, and adverse drug reactions, the PT can use this tool for an initial screen of the entire body. These items, along with the more system-specific items, will provide therapists with a more comprehensive picture of a patient's general health status. A significant number of "yes" responses will direct the therapist to complete a more detailed systems review and special tests. The following sections are organized by body system (e.g., cardiovascular) or region (e.g. eyes, ears, nose and throat).

Checklist For Cardiac and Peripheral Vascular Systems

Some items listed in Box 9-1 (including dyspnea, cough, and palpitations) overlap with the checklist for of the cardioperipheral vascular and pulmonary systems (see Box 9-6). Dyspnea is the

---

BOX 9-6

Cardio/peripheral Vascular and Pulmonary System Checklists

- Dyspnea
- Cough (duration, positional, productive, sputum?)
- Palpitations
- Syncope
- Sweats
- Edema
- Cold distal extremities
- Skin discoloration
- Open wounds/ulcers
- Clubbing of the nails
- Wheezing, stridor

TABLE 9-2

Possible Causes of Positional Dyspnea

Type	Possible Causes
Orthopnea	Congestive heart failure
	Mitral valve disease
	Severe asthma (rarely)
	Emphysema (rarely)
	Chronic bronchitis (rarely)
	Neurologic diseases (rarely)
Trepopnea	Congestive heart failure
Platypnea	Status postpneumonectomy
	Neurologic diseases
	Cirrhosis (intrapulmonary shunts)
	Hypovolemia

---

subjective sensation of difficult or uncomfortable breathing and is most often associated with chronic heart and lung disease. This entity must be distinguished from tachypnea, or rapid breathing. Dyspnea can be related to activity, exertion, or body position. Examples include orthopnea, difficulty breathing when recumbent (lying flat), and platypnea, difficulty breathing when sitting upright and ease of breathing when recumbent. Finally, trepopnea is ease of breathing that is improved by assuming a side-lying position. Typically, difficulty with breathing would be associated with activity or exertion, so if a therapist asks about dyspnea only in this context, patients may not volunteer that they get short of breath when they lie down. Important follow-up questions for the patient with dyspnea include the following[39]:

- When did the shortness of breath (SOB) begin?
- Did the SOB begin suddenly or slowly over time?
- Do you wake up suddenly at night with severe SOB (paroxysmal nocturnal dyspnea)?
- Do you know why the SOB started?
- Is the SOB constant?
- Does SOB occur with exertion only? At rest? Or when in certain positions, such as lying flat (orthopnea) or when sitting up (platypnea)?

See Table 9-2 for causes of shortness of breath.

Palpitations are described as uncomfortable sensations in the chest and are associated with a variety of arrhythmias. Patients may use terms such as *fluttering*, *jumping*, *pounding*, *irregularity*, *stopping*, or *skipping beats* to describe this sensation. The PT should ask follow-up questions about frequency; duration; and associated symptoms such as chest pain, syncope, lightheadedness, and dyspnea when investigating this report.[18]

Syncope is a sudden loss of consciousness accompanied by an inability to maintain postural tone, followed by spontaneous recovery, which patients often describe as fainting.[37] These blackouts usually are caused by a reduction in blood flow to the brain, but other potential causes of syncope have metabolic and psychogenic origins.[8] The incidence of syncope increases with age, marked by a sharp increase in patients older than 70 years.[37] Most patients or their caregivers will be sufficiently alarmed to report any episodes of fainting or blackouts to the physician, but the incident may simply be described as a fall. During the history portion of the examination, one patient may report that he has fallen four times in the past 6 months and it is unclear whether the physician knows of the number of recent falls. The therapist must consider the many possible reasons for the repeated falls, including the presence of syncope, especially in patients with risk factors for reduced cerebral blood flow.

Investigation of pain was discussed in Chapter 6, and the topic of sweats was covered earlier (see "General Health Checklist"). The onset of pain with sweats is relevant when the PT screens the cardiovascular system. Diaphoresis is a common finding associated with an acute myocardial infarction. If the patient has chest pain or tightness extending into the left upper extremity along with the onset of diaphoresis, the patient and PT probably will grasp the seriousness of these symptoms. However, in addition to this classic presentation, the location of pain associated with ischemic heart disease can vary considerably (see Chapters 6 and 20) and can include the jaw, neck, tooth, right shoulder, epigastric, and midthoracic regions. Women and older adults are the two groups most likely to present with pain patterns such as these. A patient with pain in these locations, accompanied by reports of sweats, should raise the PT's suspicion, especially in a patient who has risk factors for cardiac disease.

Like dyspnea, the presentation of a cough should trigger concern about the pulmonary system, but this finding is associated with disorders of the cardiovascular system as well. Cough, especially at night (nocturnal cough), can be associated with heart failure[18] and is also a side effect of some calcium channel-blocking agents.[15] A cough can be considered chronic if the duration is 3 weeks or longer.[21] The most common causes of cough are cigarette smoking (as a result of the direct bronchial irritation), allergies, and postnasal drip. The finding also may be associated with very serious disorders such as asthma, pneumonia, cancer, and heart failure. How does the PT determine the seriousness of a cough? Follow-up questions are the key, including the following:

- What is the duration?
- What is the cause (from the patient's perspective)?
- Is it constant and persistent or intermittent?
- Is the cough related to position or posture?
- Is it a productive cough (including color and odor of sputum)?
- Is there pain accompanying the cough?
- Are there associated symptoms (dyspnea and items from the general health checklist)?

A productive cough that has lasted 3 weeks or longer and is associated with any other relevant symptoms should raise the PT's concern. Sputum should be odorless and clear to whitish gray in color. Sputum that is yellow, red or bloody (hemoptysis), pink, rust, green, or a combination of these colors suggests the presence of pathology. A cough associated with heart failure typically will be noted with a recumbent position.[18,39] A PT concerned with a cough should auscultate the chest (see Chapter 11).

Peripheral edema may be observed at any point during the history-taking process. This finding can be associated with many serious disorders, including venous insufficiency, congestive heart failure, deep venous thrombosis (DVT), and pulmonary hypertension. The PT must note whether the edema is unilateral or bilateral. Unilateral edema may be associated with DVT, whereas a bilateral presentation is associated more often with the other disorders listed earlier. Important follow-up questions to ask include the following:

- What was the onset of the edema (slow versus fast)?
- Is it related to dependent limb position?
- Is it related to time of day—morning versus end of the day?
- Are there any other associated symptoms or signs (e.g., pain, cyanosis, jaundice, redness of the limb[s], clubbing of the nails)?

After the PT has gathered the aforementioned information, he or she should palpate the limb(s) during this patient visit. Does the patient have pitting edema (Figure 9-2), local tenderness, altered skin temperature (cold or warmth), or a palpable cord along a vein? Is there any discoloration of the limb? The PT should take circumferential measurements of the limb. Unilateral edema is marked by a difference of 1 cm or more just above the ankle or 2 cm or more at the midcalf region.[8] Correspondingly, patients should be asked about skin temperature: whether the limb(s) feel cold, warm, or hot. Related to the peripheral vascular system, the most likely complaint would be the limbs feeling cool or cold, related to arterial insufficiency, whereas localized warmth or feeling hot could be associated with DVT. (See later, "Integumentary System," for more details about skin assessment.)

Pulmonary System Checklist

Box 9-6 is the checklist of screening items for the pulmonary system. See the earlier discussion of dyspnea and cough ("Checklist for Cardiac and Peripheral Vascular Systems") and see Chapter 10 for a discussion of clubbing of the nails (digital clubbing). Stridor and wheezing are abnormal respiratory sounds audible to the ear. Wheezing is a high-pitched noise caused by a partial obstruction of the airway; stridor is a high-pitched sound that is also associated with obstruction of the larynx or trachea. The wheezing may be resolved by the opening of the airway or a further narrowing of the airway. The PT should watch for additional signs of general and pulmonary distress and perform auscultation to identify the reason for the decrease in the wheezing.

Follow-up questions relevant to this finding include the following[39]:

- Have you noticed this noise?
- Do you know why the sound exists?
- How long has it been present?
- How often does it occur?
- What are the precipitating factors (e.g., odors, food, animals, exertion, emotions)?
- Are there any associated symptoms?

Hematologic System Checklist

Blood disorders include erythrocyte, leukocyte, and platelet conditions and bleeding disorders. Considering the physiologic role that red and white blood cells play, along with platelets, it

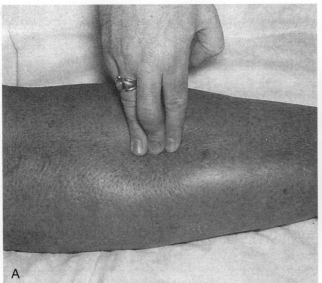
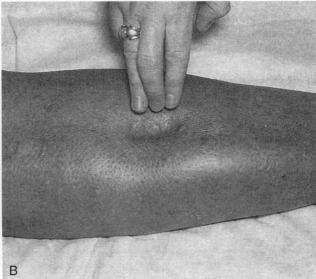

FIGURE 9-2 A, Palpating for pitting edema. The examiner is pressing into the lower leg. **B,** Indentation that remains after the pressure is removed from the limb, demonstrating the pitting edema. (From Swartz MH: *Textbook of physical diagnosis,* 4th ed, Philadelphia, 2002, Saunders, p 381.)

is not surprising that disease-related symptoms and signs are numerous and varied. Box 9-7 provides a list of manifestations, indicating potentially serious underlying disease.[8,19] Abnormal bleeding, in addition to cuts and scrapes that demonstrate prolonged bleeding, may be noted as menorrhagia (excessive menstruation), hematemesis (vomiting blood), melena (see later, "Gastrointestinal System Checklist"), gingival bleeding, and hemarthrosis.

Chapter 15 includes details of clinical laboratory values for the complete blood count and platelet assessment. Normal values and ranges are presented, with rehabilitation guidelines and potential symptoms and signs associated with low and high values. The symptoms and signs listed earlier may alert the therapist to communicate with the patient's physician, leading to laboratory tests being performed or, where allowed, directing the therapist to send the patient for laboratory testing.

Gastrointestinal System Checklist

Upper Gastrointestinal System

Box 9-8 presents the GI system checklist. Two items obviously missing from this checklist are nausea and vomiting, but note that they are part of the general health checklist given earlier. Swallowing difficulties (dysphagia) typically are a result of a loss of coordinated local muscle activity or a mechanical obstructive disorder. Myasthenia gravis, multiple sclerosis, amyotrophic lateral sclerosis, and Parkinson's disease are disorders that could result in local muscle incoordination. Tumors, thyroid goiter,

osteophytes of the cervical spine, and aortic aneurysm could be causes of the mechanical obstruction.[39] Table 9-3 provides a comparison of manifestations of motor versus obstructive causes of dysphagia. Follow-up questions about the swallowing difficulties should determine the presence or absence of each manifestation. Other questions include where the patient senses the difficulty (e.g., back of the throat, behind the sternum); whether it is associated with swallowing solids, liquids, or both; and whether pain accompanies the difficulty (odynophagia).

Indigestion and heartburn are common symptoms that fall under the category of dyspepsia, which can have an organic cause (e.g., peptic ulcer, gastroesophageal reflux disease) or a functional source (no ascertainable cause). Use of nonsteroidal anti-inflammatory drugs (NSAIDs) also has been associated with these upper GI tract symptoms.[38,39] The patient usually feels these symptoms retrosternally or in the epigastric region. Important follow-up questions for these symptoms include the following:

- How long have you had these symptoms?
- Do you know what is causing them?
- Are they constant or intermittent?
- How are you treating the symptoms?
- Are there any associated symptoms (e.g., fatigue, weakness, shortness of breath)?

These questions may reveal important information, such as the fact that the symptoms have become more persistent or more intense and that the need for self-treatment has increased. Many over-the-counter medications, such as antacids (e.g., Milk of Magnesia, Alu-Tab, Tums, Maalox) and histamine (H_2) antagonists (e.g., Tagamet, Zantac, Pepcid AC), are designed to relieve heartburn and indigestion.[15] Even though these drugs may provide symptomatic relief, they do not cure the underlying organic cause. Therefore, if the patient reports the need to take increasing amounts of the drug to obtain relief, the PT should communicate with the patient's physician.

Food intolerance associated with the provocation of symptoms can be a warning sign of underlying pathology. A patient who realizes that symptoms appear only after ingesting certain

---

BOX 9-7
Potential Manifestations of Hematologic Disorders

- Exertional dyspnea
- Palpitations
- Anginal pain patterns
- Fatigue
- Pallor
- Digital clubbing
- Lightheadedness
- Syncope
- Drowsiness
- Confusion
- Easy bruising and bleeding
- Fever, chills, sweats
- Malaise

BOX 9-8
Gastrointestinal System Checklist

- Swallowing difficulties
- Indigestion, heartburn
- Food intolerance
- Bowel dysfunction
  - Color of stool
  - Shape, caliber of stool
  - Constipation
  - Diarrhea
  - Difficulty initiating
  - Incontinence

TABLE 9-3
Comparison of Symptoms—Motor Versus Mechanical Cause of Dysphagia

Manifestation	CAUSE OF DYSPHAGIA	
	Motor	**Mechanical**
Onset	Gradual onset	Faster onset
Progression	Slow	Faster
Swallowing solid food versus liquids	Equal difficulty	More difficulty swallowing solids
Swallowing cold substances	Worsening of swallowing difficulties	Swallowing difficulties not affected by temperature
Bolus passage	Facilitated by repeated swallowing, Valsalva maneuver, throwing back the head and shoulders	Can be accompanied by regurgitation

foods probably will report this to a physician but, if the symptoms appear only as pain in the back (not in the anterior chest wall or abdominal area), the patient might not associate the symptoms with the food. A classic example is pain referred from gallbladder disorders, often noted in the midthoracic or right scapular region.[14,41] The patient may relate the onset of these symptoms to his or her posture or excessive time spent at the computer rather than to the ingestion of fatty foods, which stimulates gallbladder activity. Another example in which the ingestion of a certain food may precipitate symptoms is the tendency of cheese, chocolate, citrus fruits, nuts, and red wine to trigger migraine headaches in some people. In addition, gastric ulcer symptoms may be worsened by meals or provoked by food, whereas ingestion of food may relieve symptoms of other conditions. For example, duodenal ulcer symptoms may be relieved by food.[21]

One element of bowel function relates to upper GI system screening—the color of the stool, which is an indicator of potentially serious health issues. Melena, or the passage of black, tarry stools (sticky and shiny), represents GI bleeding (most likely from upper GI structures, such as the esophagus, stomach, and duodenum), with a blood loss of 150 to 200 mL or more being necessary to produce a consistent or regular occurence.[35] If the patient reports melena, the PT should ask these important follow-up questions:

- How long have you been having black, tarry stools?
- Have you felt lightheaded?
- Have you had any nausea, vomiting, diarrhea, fatigue, lightheadedness, abdominal or back pain, or sweats associated with these stools?

With such reports, the PT should check the patient's heart rate and blood pressure (see Chapter 11). These questions produce important information for the physician about the urgency of the situation.[39] In addition to an upper GI bleed, black but nonsticky stools can be associated with the ingestion of iron and bismuth salts (e.g., Pepto-Bismol), black licorice, and some commercial chocolate cookies.[8]

In addition to melena, light gray or pale stools (*acholic*, without bile) can be associated with obstructive jaundice.[8] If this is reported, the PT should ask the following:

- How long have you noticed the light, pale-colored stools?
- Have you noticed an atypical color (e.g., dark) of your urine? (See the genitourinary system checklist in Box 9-9.)
- Have you noticed any associated symptoms, such as fatigue, fever, chills, unexplained weight change, or nausea?

Lower Gastrointestinal System

The screening of the lower GI tract is based on questions about bowel function, including color of stools, shape and caliber of stools, constipation, diarrhea, difficulty initiating a bowel movement, and incontinence. The PT may initiate this line of questioning with a general question, such as "Have you recently noted any problems or difficulties with bowel function?" Regardless of the patient response, however, the PT must complete the entire checklist in Box 9-8. Many patients initially answer the general question by reporting "no problems," but later answer "yes" when the PT asks specific questions from the list. Many of these patients assume that if no pain is associated with defecation, there are no problems.

BOX 9-9

Genitourinary System Checklist

URINARY SYSTEM
- Color
- Flow—frequency, urgency, output, retention, dysuria
- Reduced caliber or force of urine stream
- Difficulty initiating urine stream
- Incontinence

REPRODUCTIVE SYSTEM
Male
- Urethral discharge
- Sexual dysfunction
- Pain during intercourse, ejaculation

Female
- Vaginal discharge
- Pain with intercourse
- Menstruation—frequency of periods, length of cycle, dysmenorrhea, blood flow
- Number of pregnancies and deliveries
- Menopause—perimenopausal, postmenopausal vaginal bleeding or spotting

---

HEMATOCHEZIA. Hematochezia, or the passage of bright blood-red stools, usually originates in the left side of the colon or the anorectal area.[33] With this symptom, the PT should ask the following questions:

- How long have you noticed bright red blood in your stools?
- Is the red blood mixed within the stools (red streaks) or not?
- Are there any associated symptoms, such as difficulty in initiating bowel movements or a feeling of lightheadedness or fatigue?

As noted earlier with melena, the PT should check the patient's heart rate and blood pressure (see Chapter 11). In addition, as with black stools, reddish stools may be nonbloody stools, caused by ingestion of beets.[8] The PT can broach the subject of atypical stool color by asking, "Have you noticed any unusual color of your stools recently, such as black, tarry; bloody red; or light pale-colored stools?"

A change in shape or caliber of stools is also a potentially significant finding. Stools that are pencil thin in diameter or flat and ribbon-like are suggestive of a space-occupying mass, including an anal or distal colon carcinoma. As with the bleeding, there may be no pain associated with these types of lesions, so again no pain may be interpreted as no problems being present.

CONSTIPATION AND DIARRHEA. Constipation and diarrhea are conditions that most everyone experiences for relatively brief periods at various times in their lives but, for some patients, these symptoms can represent a serious underlying pathology. Table 9-4 lists potential causes of constipation and diarrhea. When a patient reports constipation, the PT should ask what the patient means by being constipated. A report of "hard stools that are difficult or painful to push out" warrants follow-up questions by the PT, including the following:

- How long have you been constipated?
- When was the last time you had a bowel movement?
- Do you ever have periods of constipation alternating with periods of diarrhea (a pattern noted in some patients with colon cancer or diverticulitis)?

TABLE 9-4
Potential Causes of Constipation and Diarrhea

Mechanism	Cause
CONSTIPATION	
Impaired motility	Inadequate dietary fiber
	Inactivity
	Diverticulitis
	Hypothyroidism
	Hypercalcemia
	Scleroderma
Neurologic dysfunction	Multiple sclerosis
	Spinal cord injury
Psychosocial dysfunction	Depression
	Situational stress
	Anxiety
DIARRHEA	Infectious agents
	Laxative abuse
	Colon cancer
	Irritable bowel syndrome
	Crohn's disease
	Ulcerative colitis
	Diabetic enteropathy

- Do you have any associated symptoms, such as malaise, a sensation of abdominal fullness or bloating, fever, agitation, or altered mental status?

The associated symptoms described in the last question represent potential manifestations of fecal impaction and should prompt immediate communication with the patient's physician.[1] Impaction in older adults may also be manifested by confusion or change in mentation. If the patient reports that the constipation is caused by a current medication that he or she has been taking, such as an opiate, the PT must ask whether the constipation has gotten worse since the last physician visit. If the patient is having bowel movements and the constipation is not getting worse, the PT should document the information provided by the patient and, in the following 1 or 2 weeks, ask whether the constipation has changed. The PT may learn a few weeks after the initial visit that the condition has worsened and now warrants physician contact.

Diarrhea is described as excessively frequent passage of watery and unformed stools.[8] Episodes that are brief and self-limited do not require reporting, but diarrhea that becomes severe raises concern about the underlying cause and may carry the risk of dehydration. With a patient report of diarrhea, the PT should ask these follow-up questions[39]:
- How many episodes do you have each day?
- How long have you had diarrhea?
- Do you ever have periods of diarrhea alternating with periods of constipation?
- Is the diarrhea worse at certain times of the day?
- Do family members or companions have similar symptoms?
- Do you have any associated symptoms, such as fever, chills, nausea, vomiting, confusion, or abdominal pain or distention?

Manifestations of dehydration include the following[19]:
- Thirst and dry mouth
- Postural hypotension
- Rapid breathing
- Rapid pulse (higher than 100 beats/min)

- Confusion, irritability, lethargy
- Headache

The last two items on the checklist are related to difficulty initiating a bowel movement and incontinence. Difficulty initiating a bowel movement may be part of the patient's description of the constipation. It also may be associated with a condition called tenesmus, in which the patient has an intense urge to defecate but with little or no result. This painful and ineffective straining can be associated with inflammation or cancer of the anorectal region.[39] Fecal incontinence may bring the patient to physical therapy, depending on the nature of the therapist's practice but, in most settings, reports of this nature should raise considerable concern. The therapist should approach this symptom like all others. If the patient does not provide a good explanation for the finding, if the physician is unaware of the symptoms, or if the condition has worsened since the last communication with the physician, then this finding becomes a red flag.

Genitourinary System Checklist

The checklist illustrated in Box 9-9 represents two physiologic functions, urination and reproduction. As with the screening of bowel function, the PT may want to start with a general question, "Do you have any trouble with urination?" Regardless of the patient's response, the PT must ask the patient to complete a detailed checklist. Color of urine (reddish or dark-brown, tea-colored) can be an important indicator of pathology. Dark urine can be associated with hepatic or biliary obstructive disease and with acute exertional rhabdomyolysis. A case report by Baxter and Moore[6] has described a patient presenting to physical therapy with shoulder pain and weakness and a report of dark urine. Laboratory tests led to the diagnosis of acute exertional rhabdomyolysis.

Hematuria, or blood in the urine, can be a manifestation of almost every disease of the genitourinary (GU) tract.[16] Reddish-colored urine also may be present for reasons other than the presence of blood, including ingestion of vegetable dyes, heavy ingestion of beets, and use of medications such as phenazopyridine (Pyridium).

Important follow-up questions to better identify the symptoms include the following:
- How long have you noticed the red urine?
- Do you have a history of bleeding problems (see Chapter 8)?
- What medications are you currently taking (see Chapter 8)?
- Do you currently have or have you recently recovered from an upper respiratory infection or sore throat?

Red urine noted 1 to 2 weeks after an upper respiratory tract infection may be associated with acute glomerulonephritis.[39]
- Have you noticed whether the urine starts red and then clears, starts clear and then turns red, or is red throughout?
- Do you have any associated symptoms, such as items on the general health checklist, including fever, weight loss, fatigue, or flank or abdominal pain?

Urinary frequency, urgency, output, and dysuria also are important indicators of GU system disorders, with urinary frequency being the symptom most often reported.[39] Increased frequency may be most noticeable with nocturia (urination at night) because most patients recognize when a pattern of not waking to urinate changes to waking two to three times a night to urinate. In general, for those younger than 50 years to wake once per night, and for those older than 50 years to wake once or twice per night, is within normal limits. Urinary urgency, the intense and immediate sensation of the need to urinate, can be associated with infection or irritation. Dysuria, pain on urination, can occur with inflammation, infection, and sudden distention of a structure.[8,39] Polyuria, increased amounts of urine, can be associated with diabetic conditions. The PT should ask these follow-up questions after reports of a change in urinary flow:

- Have these changes occurred quickly or over a long period of time?
- Have you been drinking more fluids (with an excessive thirst) than usual lately?
- What medications are you taking (diuretics)?
- Have you noticed that, despite the urge to urinate, you cannot start urination?
- After urine flow has stopped, do you experience the sensation of still needing to urinate?
- Do you have any associated symptoms, such as headaches or visual problems (possibly diabetes-related), or items on the general health checklist, such as fever, nausea, and weight loss?

Symptoms of a reduced force or caliber of urine flow and difficulty in starting the urine stream are common symptoms associated with obstructive disorders, including benign prostatic hyperplasia (BPH). For patients already diagnosed with BPH, the physician will be aware of the urinary difficulties, but the PT should forward any reports that the urinary flow problems may be worsening. The term *benign* can be misleading, because BPH can result in complications of hydroureter and renal failure.[5] True urinary retention is associated with serious conditions such as cauda equina syndrome. A recent onset of urinary dysfunction (problems of retention, frequency, or overflow incontinence) and saddle anesthesia is a red flag in patients with low back pain.[9]

The final urinary disorder to consider is incontinence, a very common disorder in the adult population for which many patients receive physical therapy services. When incontinence is not the reason for the physical therapy intervention, the same screening principles apply to this symptom. For example, important follow-up questions to ask patients who report incontinence include the circumstances, causes, timing, frequency, and volume of urine loss; presence of any additional warning signs; and intactness of perineal and bladder sensation.[20] See Chapter 17 for a related discussion of incontinence in the obstetric population.

Reproductive function is the other important GU aspect to screen. Areas of overlap among men and women are discharge and sexual dysfunction. Discharge from the penis or vagina suggests the possibility of infection. The PT should follow such reports by asking the following questions:

- What is the frequency?
- Is it a continuous flow, spotting, or sporadic episodes?
- What is the color of the discharge?
- Is the discharge accompanied by an odor?
- Are there associated symptoms, such as pruritus (itching), local pain or inflammation, fever, nausea, or dyspareunia?

Early treatment of urinary tract infections and sexually transmitted infections is important, because untreated infections may increase the risk of developing an ectopic pregnancy and may lead to infertility.[21,27,32]

Some patients presenting with mechanical low back, sacroiliac, and hip joint conditions report dyspareunia, pain during or after sexual intercourse. One way to help differentiate pain of mechanical dysfunction from pain of internal pelvic disease or disorders is to investigate the pain pattern (see Chapter 6). Pain of mechanical origin (nonacute) is typically associated with specific intercourse positions, whereas pain associated with pelvic organ disease likely will occur regardless of position. If pain is present regardless of position, another follow-up question to ask is "Is the pain provoked with initial insertion or with deep vaginal penetration?" If the complaint is the former, the pelvic floor may be the source of pain, warranting referral to a physical therapist for an examination. Regardless, if the patient reports that a physician has examined her and ruled out disease, then the PT should refer the patient to a PT who specializes in women's health (see Chapter 17).

In addition to pain during intercourse, sexual dysfunction may include erectile dysfunction (inability to achieve or maintain an erection), which can be associated with neurologic conditions resulting from spinal cord injury, herniated disk, postsurgical complications (radical prostate, bladder, or colon procedures), diabetes mellitus, medication side effects, or psychogenic disorders.[21]

The PT should ask these important follow-up questions:

- How long has the condition been present?
- How constant or intermittent is the problem?
- Have you noticed any other difficulties with bowel and bladder function or any neurologic complaints, such as numbness, tingling, or weakness?

Questions about menstruation have the same goal as the investigation of cough and bowel and bladder function, identifying a change from the usual pattern. The items to assess include frequency and length of periods, dysmenorrhea, and blood flow. Abnormal vaginal bleeding is described as bleeding at an inappropriate time or in excessive amounts. The general time frame for inappropriate bleeding is less than 21 days and more than 36 days since the last period.

As a general rule, blood flow lasting more than 7 days should be considered excessive. The menstrual cycle tends to shorten as menopause approaches. Menopause can be associated with hot flashes, flushing, sweats, and sleep disturbances. Postmenopausal bleeding—that is, vaginal bleeding noted 6 to 8 months or longer after the cessation of periods—warrants a consultation with the physician.[8,39]

Dysmenorrhea (pain with menstruation) is common, but a screening that reveals pain that is atypical in location, in the cycle in which it occurs, in intensity, in quality, and in duration should raise suspicion about the underlying cause. Another challenge in the screening of menstruation is that some women do not generally experience a regular pattern. In such a case, a primary care physician should regularly monitor the woman's health. The PT should ask the following questions about menstruation:

- When was your last period?
- Was it a normal period for you (timing of the period compared with her normal cycle, pain pattern, blood flow)?
- Have you experienced any vaginal bleeding between periods?

Cessation of periods (amenorrhea) has been associated with female long distance runners, anorexia, and diseases of the endocrine system.[8,21] The patient may also be pregnant so, if the amenorrhea is not explained by existing health history factors, inquiring whether she might be pregnant would be appropriate. If the patient cannot present a convincing reason "it's not possible," then asking about the presence of symptoms associated with early pregnancy should follow. See Box 9-10 for common manifestations during early pregnancy.[8]

The PT also should investigate the woman's obstetric history. Depending on the nature of the PT's practice, the PT should at minimum learn the number of pregnancies and any residual complications or limitations associated with the pregnancies and deliveries. In a women's health practice, the questioning is much more extensive (see Chapter 17).

Other Systems

Nervous System

The PT routinely screens the nervous system during the investigation of symptoms (see Chapter 6), which takes place before the specific ROS questioning. Using the entire body diagram and noting the locations of any symptoms (including pain, numbness, pins and needles, and weakness) are key elements of the examination process. In addition, investigating the onset of symptoms may reveal a history of falling, which may be related to a neurologic condition; when the PT is investigating levels of function, information about difficulty with stairs or bed mobility may be elicited. In addition, a number of items found in Box 9-1 can potentially be associated with the neurologic system:

- Numbness, tingling
- Weakness
- Tremors
- Seizures
- Vision changes
- Sexual difficulties
- Hearing problems
- Difficulty swallowing
- Urinary incontinence
- Vomiting without nausea
- Dizziness
- Recent falls
- Balance problems

In addition, the PT performs a routine nervous system screening during the patient observation that begins with the interview process (see Chapter 10) and continues with the upper or lower quadrant examination (see Chapters 12 and 13).

Endocrine System

Considering the physiology of the endocrine system, one can understand that malfunction in this system could lead to symptoms involving a number of body systems. For example, people who have hypothyroidism may experience any or all of the following[21]:

- Joint or muscle pain
- Paresthesias
- Dry, scaly skin or brittle hair and nails
- Cold intolerance
- Reduced sweating
- Weight gain
- Constipation
- Fatigue
- Dyspnea
- Periorbital edema
- Bradycardia
- Hoarseness of voice
- Slow reflex relaxation

Many of the items on this list would be noted during parts of the data collection process other than the ROS. The paresthesia and joint and muscle pain would be noted on the body diagram during symptom investigation (see Chapter 6). An atypical symptom pattern (e.g., insidious onset, symptoms that come and go for no apparent mechanical reason, no consistent time of day when symptoms are better or worse) may raise the suspicion that the endocrine system is involved. See Box 9-11 for a summary checklist for the endocrine system.

Integumentary System

Much of the integumentary system screening takes place through observation during the physical examination. As with general screening of the nervous system, screening of the integumentary system begins when the patient interview begins (see Chapter 10), and it continues throughout the physical examination as more skin becomes visible in the postural assessment and regional examinations. Chapter 10 contains an extensive discussion of skin cancer and descriptions of various skin lesions. The PT can note wounds, abrasions, and bruises on the body diagram used during the symptom investigation and then can examine these findings in more detail during the physical examination.

In addition to what is observed regarding skin, hair, and nails, see Box 9-12 for a list of integumentary system screening items. The guiding principle, as with other body systems, is to ask the

---

BOX 9-10

Early Pregnancy Manifestations

- Increased urinary frequency
- Breast tenderness
- Fatigue
- Weight loss (associated with nausea and vomiting)
- Heartburn
- Constipation
- Leukorrhea (white, yellowish vaginal discharge)

BOX 9-11

Endocrine System Checklist

- General health (fatigue, unexplained weight change, weakness)
- Psychological, cognitive (personality changes, memory loss, confusion, irritability)
- Gastrointestinal (nausea, vomiting, anorexia, dysphagia, diarrhea, constipation)
- Urogenital (impotence, intermittent urine stream, dribbling, straining to void, impotence)
- Musculoskeletal (muscle weakness and cramps, arthralgias, myalgias, stiffness, bone pain)
- Sensory (paresthesia, numbness)
- Dermatologic (foot ulcerations; edema; dry, coarse skin; impaired wound healing)
- Miscellaneous (temperature intolerance, visual changes, orthostatic hypotension, increased bruising, increased thirst)

BOX 9-12

Screening the Integumentary System

- Changes in skin—color, sores, moles, rashes, lumps
- Changes in nails—discoloration, thickening, ridges, splitting or separation from nail bed
- Changes in hair—hair loss, increase in hair, change in thickness or distribution
- Pruritis (itching)
- Change in sweating or dryness of skin

---

patient whether she or he has noticed or experienced any unexplained or unusual changes in the skin, hair, or nails.[8,39]

Pruritis can be associated with a number of conditions and disorders, including pregnancy, lymphomas, leukemia, drug reactions, uremia, biliary cirrhosis, and renal failure.

Psychological System

The range of mental disorders is so extensive that providing screening protocols for this entire category of illness is beyond the scope of this text. The *Diagnostic and Statistical Manual of Mental Disorders*, 4th edition, is an excellent resource for the clinician in screening this system.[4]

The general health checklist and other manifestations noted in Box 9-1 will act as a general screen for many of these disorders. Fatigue; unexplained weight change; a change in mentation; or an onset of confusion, difficulty concentrating, and sleep disturbance are symptoms associated with many psychological disorders. Three specific mental disorders—major clinical depression, chemical dependency, and abuse—are discussed in this text because of their incidence and their potential for serious complications, such as morbidity and mortality. (See Chapters 8 and 20 for a detailed discussion of screening for these disorders.)

Musculoskeletal System

The checklist for the musculoskeletal system consists primarily of items extensively discussed in Chapters 6 and 7. Items such as onset of symptoms; how and when symptoms change with the time of day, posture, and activity; night pain (positional or not?); post–rest gel[36]; ease or lack of ease of decreasing the symptom intensity; and correlation of symptoms with the findings of the physical examination are key elements for screening this system. Determining whether a symptom story from the patient makes sense according to our understanding of basic and clinical sciences, along with existing risk factors for cancer, infection, fractures, and inflammatory disorders, is the basis for deciding whether to communicate with the physician. In addition are the pain complaints accompanied by ROS complaints suggestive of a systemic illness (e.g., weight loss, fever, chills, fatigue, malaise). The detailed screening of musculoskeletal disorders, including cancer, infection, inflammatory disorders, and fractures (e.g., traumatic, stress, pathologic[23]) is described in Chapters 6, 7, 14, 16, and 20.

Other Considerations

Adverse Drug Reactions

Adverse drug reactions are screened with the same tools (checklists) described for the screening of potential occult disease. Ultimately, physicians will determine whether the symptoms or signs PTs bring to their attention are related to disease, medications, or both. The challenge to PTs is to decide which checklists are relevant for each group of medications, remembering that the general health checklist screens many medications to some degree. Chapters 4 and 8 include a detailed description of potential adverse drug reactions associated with commonly used drugs, as well as medication screening.

Checklist Use

BASED ON SYMPTOM LOCATION OR PATTERN. Not all checklists must be used with every patient in their entirety. The location and pattern of symptoms can help guide these choices, because part of the rationale for use of the checklist is that individual organs making up each particular body system are potential symptom generators (see Chapter 6). Because of this, the PT will use more checklists when examining a patient with symptoms located in the trunk (including pelvis) than with patients who have symptoms located only from midhumerus to fingers and midfemur to toes, because more non-neuromusculoskeletal structures are located in the trunk than at the periphery of the body (Box 9-13).

Certain body systems may not present with a predictable pain location (local or referred) but present with an atypical pattern of symptoms that move from one body region to another. The symptoms may be inconsistent in their intensity, increasing and decreasing regardless of time of day, posture, and physical activity (see Chapters 6 and 7). In addition to the location of symptoms, the checklist provided in Box 9-1 provides an initial screening of all body systems. Patients' "yes" responses to any of those items will guide therapists toward consideration of specific body systems to be screened in detail.

BASED ON PATIENT MEDICAL HISTORY. The patient's report of current illnesses also will guide the PT in selecting the body systems to screen. For example, if the patient reports heart problems, one of the follow-up questions to ask is, "What symptoms do you have with your heart problem?" If the patient replies, "Chest pain and shortness of breath," the PT should ask whether the patient has ever experienced any of the other items on the cardiovascular checklist to make sure that the patient has not omitted any important information. This provides a baseline from which therapists may recognize worsening of an existing disease. The same approach applies if the patient reports a GI or GU disorder.

AT FOLLOW-UP VISITS? It is not necessary to repeat the entire ROS at every single visit but, at times, asking questions again at a follow-up visit is appropriate. If the patient reports worsening of symptoms or onset of new symptoms for no apparent mechanical-sounding reason, suspicion must be raised about the origin of these complaints. A helpful question to ask the patient could be, "In addition to this new pain, has anything else changed, or is anything else new or different for you?" The therapist can use the general health checklist as a starting point for follow-up. In addition, the location of new complaints should suggest body systems to think about, based on understanding visceral local and pain referral patterns (see Chapter 6). Another question that would be appropriate would be whether the patient has a history of difficulty starting the urine stream and increased frequency because of benign prostatic hyperplasia. If therapy continues longer than 4 to 6 weeks, revisiting urinary problems is warranted, noting

---

BOX 9-13

Selection of Body Systems to Screen Based on Symptom Location

ALL PATIENTS, FIRST VISIT
- General health checklist

CERVICAL AND LEFT, RIGHT SHOULDER PAIN (INCLUDING SHOULDER GIRDLE REGION)
- Cardiovascular
- Pulmonary
- Gastrointestinal (potential referral to scapular and shoulder strap regions)

THORACIC SPINE PAIN
- Cardiovascular
- Pulmonary
- Gastrointestinal
- Genitourinary (thoracolumbar junction)

LUMBAR-PELVIC PAIN
- Gastrointestinal
- Urogenital
- Peripheral vascular

MIDHUMERUS, FEMUR TO DIGITS PAIN
- Peripheral vascular

INCONSISTENT SYMPTOM PATTERN
- Psychological
- Endocrine
- Neurologic
- Rheumatic disorders
- Adverse drug reaction

---

any worsening of the difficulties. If acknowledged, then having the patient call his or her physician to report the changes would be appropriate.

Summary

Considering the amount of data that PTs collect during symptom investigation, review of the patient's medical history, and ROS, the medical screening examination is extensive. The ROS is a very important component of the examination because it enables the PT to recognize clinical manifestations, other than the patient's chief presenting complaints, that require referral to another health care provider. At the same time, the PT should avoid raising a false alarm about a patient's health status whenever possible. Asking specific follow-up questions about the patient's symptoms, learning whether the patient's physician is aware of the symptoms and if whether the symptoms have worsened, and finally, judging the patient's ability to give an accurate history (does this complaint represent something new, different, or unusual?) all contribute to the ability to distinguish between a red flag and a red herring. Erring on the side of patient safety, however, should always be the priority.

REFERENCES

1. Ahronheim JC. Special problems in the geriatric patient. In: Goldman L, Bennett JC, editors. Cecil textbook of medicine. 21st ed. Philadelphia: WB Saunders; 2000. p. 22–5.

2. Allison L, Fuller K. Balance and vestibular disorders. In: Umphred DA, editor. Neurological rehabilitation. 5th ed. St. Louis: Mosby; 2007. p. 723–74.

3. American Physical Therapy Association. Guide to physical therapist practice. 2nd ed. Alexandria, VA: American Physical Therapy Association; 2001.

4. American Psychiatric Association. Diagnostic and statistical manual of mental disorders. 4th ed. Washington, DC: American Psychiatric Association; 2000, p.317-328.

5. Barry MJ, Goodson JD. Approach to benign prostatic hyperplasia. In: Goroll AH, Mulley AG, editors. Primary care medicine. 5th ed. Philadelphia: Lippincott, Williams & Wilkins; 2006. p. 909–13.

6. Baxter RE, Moore JH. Diagnosis and treatment of acute exertional rhabdomyolysis. J Orthop Sports Phys Ther 2003;33:104–8.

7. Berland B, Gleckman RA. Fever of unknown origin in the elderly. Postgrad Med 1992;92:197–210.

8. Bickley LS. Bates' guide to physical examination and history taking. 10th ed. Philadelphia: JB Lippincott; 2009.

9. Bigos S, Bowyer O, Braen G, et al. Acute low back problems in adults. Clinical practice guideline (AHCPR Publication No. 95-0643). Rockville, MD: U.S. Department of Health and Human Services, Public Health Service, Agency for Health Care Policy and Research; 1994.

10. Boissonnault WG, Meek PD. Risk factors for anti-inflammatory drug or aspirin-induced gastrointestinal complications in individuals receiving outpatient physical therapy services. J Orthop Sports Phys Ther 2002;32:510–7.

11. Castle SC, Yeh M, Toledo S, et al. Lowering the temperature criterion improves detection of infections in nursing home residents. Aging Immunol Infect Dis 1993;4:67–76.

12. Chesley LC. Hypertensive disorders in pregnancy. New York: Appleton-Century-Crofts; 1978.

13. Dale DC. The febrile patient. In: Goldman L, Bennett JC, editors. Cecil textbook of medicine. 21st ed. Philadelphia: Saunders; 2000. p. 1564–5.

14. Doran FSA. The sites to which pain is referred from the common bile duct in man and its implication for the theory of referred pain. Br J Surg 1967;54:599–606.

15. Drug facts and comparisons 2009. St. Louis: Facts and Comparisons, pocket version; 2009. p. 815.

16. Fang LS. Evaluation of the patient with hematuria. In: Goroll AH, Mulley AG, editors. Primary care medicine. 5th ed. Philadelphia: Lippincott Williams & Wilkins; 2006. p. 861–4.

17. Gladman JRF, Barer D, Venkatesan P, et al. The outcome of pneumonia in the elderly: a hospital survey. Clin Rehabil 1991;5:201–4.

18. Goldman L. Cardiovascular diseases. In: Goldman L, Bennett JC, editors. Cecil textbook of medicine. 21st ed. Philadelphia: Saunders; 2000, p. 160–2, 212–3.

19. Goodman CC, Snyder TE. Differential diagnosis for physical therapists. 4th ed. St. Louis: Saunders Elsevier; 2007. p. 96, 261–71.

20. Goodson JD. Approach to incontinence and other forms of lower urinary tract dysfunction. In: Goroll AH, Mulley AG, editors. Primary care medicine. 5th ed. Philadelphia: Lippincott Williams & Wilkins; 2006. p. 889–96.

21. Goroll AH, Mulley AG. Primary care medicine: office evaluation and management of the adult patient. 5th ed. Philadelphia: Lippincott Williams & Wilkins; 2006. Chapters 41, 68, 101, 104, 132.

22. Goroll AH, Mulley AG. Primary care medicine: office evaluation and management of the adult patient. 5th ed. Philadelphia: Lippincott Williams & Wilkins; 2006. Chapter 11.

23. Gunta K. Alterations in skeletal function: trauma and infection. In: Mattson-Porth C, editor. Pathophysiology: concepts of altered health states. 4th ed. Philadelphia: JB Lippincott; 1994. p. 1203–9.

24. Guyton AC, Hall JE. Textbook of medical physiology. 10th ed. Philadelphia: Saunders; 2000, 830–32.

25. Jarvik JG, Deyo RA. Diagnostic evaluation of low back pain with emphasis on imaging. Ann Intern Med 2002;137:586–97.

26. Johanson WG. Overview of pneumonia. In: Goldman L, Bennett JC, editors. Cecil textbook of medicine. 21st ed. Philadelphia: Saunders; 2000. p. 436–8.

27. Kumar V, Cotran RS, Robbins SL, et al. Robbins basic pathology. 7th ed. Philadelphia: Saunders; 2003. p. 701–2.

28. Marton KI, Sox HC, Krupp JR. Involuntary weight loss: diagnostic and prognostic significance. Ann Intern Med 1981;95:568–74.

29. Morrison RE, Keating HJ. Fatigue in primary care. Prim Prev Care Obstet Gynecol 2001;28:225–40.

30. Norman DC. Fever in the elderly. Clin Infect Dis 2000;31:148–51.

31. Pruitt AA. Evaluation of dizziness. In: Goroll AH, Mulley AG, editors. Primary care medicine. ed 5. Philadelphia: Lippincott Williams & Wilkins; 2006. p. 1087.

32. Rebar RW, Erickson GF. Menstrual cycle and fertility. In: Goldman L, Bennett JC, editors. Cecil textbook of medicine. 21st ed. Philadelphia: Saunders; 2000. p. 1338–9.

33. Richter JM. Evaluation of gastrointestinal bleeding. In: Goroll AH, Mulley AG, editors. Primary care medicine. 5th ed. Philadelphia: Lippincott Williams & Wilkins; 2006. p. 466.

34. Roberts JM. Pregnancy-related hypertension. In: Creasy RK, Resnick R, editors. Maternal-fetal medicine. 4th ed. Philadelphia: Saunders; 1999. p. 837.

35. Rockey DC. Occult gastrointestinal bleeding. N Engl J Med 1999;341:38–46.

36. Smith-Pigg J, Bancroft DA. Alterations in skeletal function: rheumatic disorders. In: Mattson-Porth C, editor. Pathophysiology: concepts in altered health status. 4th ed. Philadelphia: JB Lippincott; 1994. p. 1246–9.

37. Soteriades ES, Evans JC, Larson MG, et al. Incidence and prognosis of syncope. N Engl J Med 2002;347:878–85.

38. Straus WL, Ofman JJ, Maclean C, et al. Do NSAIDs cause dyspepsia? A meta-analysis evaluating alternative dyspepsia definitions. Am J Gastroenterol 2002;97:1951–8.

39. Swartz MH. Textbook of physical diagnosis. 5th ed. Philadelphia: Saunders; 2006.

40. Thompson MP, Morris LK. Unexplained weight loss in the ambulatory elderly. J Am Geriatr Soc 1991;39:497–500.

41. Tucker LE. Back pain due to visceral disease. Hosp Med 1985;25–145.

42. Weitzman ED, Moline ML, Czeisler CA, et al. Chronobiology of aging: temperature, sleep-wake rhythms, and entrainment. Neurobiol Aging 1982;3:299–309.

Patient Interview: The Physical Examination Begins   10

William G. Boissonnault, PT, DPT, DHSc, FAAOMPT

Objectives

After reading this chapter, the reader will be able to:

1. Describe findings from patient observation that suggest the presence of underlying disease.
2. Provide follow-up questions to ask after concerning observations are noted.
3. Provide follow-up physical examination screening tools to implement after concerning observations are noted.

The goals of the initial patient visit include establishing rapport with the patient (and caregiver), collecting sufficient examination data, establishing a diagnosis, initiating an intervention program, establishing a prognosis, and formulating a plan of action with the patient. Having to do all this in a 30- to 45-minute visit can be overwhelming to any clinician. One characteristic that master clinicians tend to exhibit[14] that can enhance efficiency is the ability to multitask during the visit. An example of multitasking is starting the physical examination (patient observation) when first meeting the patient and continuing to do so throughout the history-taking process.

Patient data collected by observation, although general in nature, can affect the remainder of the history taking and the physical examination. During the interview of a patient with low back pain, the physical therapist (PT) may observe asymmetric pupil size. This observation warrants follow-up questioning regarding the patient's vision and a cranial nerve screening, items that are not routinely incorporated into the examination of patients with low back pain. This chapter discusses potential observational findings relevant to making the decision of whether to initiate a referral to, or consultation with, another health care practitioner. Observational findings include an integumentary systems screen, atypical surface anatomy, and a general nervous system screen. The description includes the examination data to be collected and the evaluation of these data relating to clinical decision making.

General Observation: Integumentary System

The skin performs many roles in maintenance of homeostasis. Functions of this important organ system include moderating body temperature; safeguarding deeper tissues from daily exposure to microorganisms, radiation, and trauma; and synthesizing vitamin D. The epidermis, the most superficial layer, is very thin and lacks blood vessels, whereas the dermis has a rich blood supply and contains various glands and hair follicles (Figure 10-1). Skin conditions noted by the PT may represent changes associated

with aging, exposure to the environment, local skin disease or trauma, or a manifestation of organ disease and systemic illness. The elements of the integumentary system most relevant to observation during the interview include exposed skin, hair, and nails. Observation continues during the remainder of the physical examination, including the postural and regional examination.

Skin Color and Condition

Skin color varies considerably from individual to individual and is generally determined by the presence of melanocytes, carotene, oxygenated hemoglobin, and local blood flow. Melanocytes, found in the deep basal layer of the epidermis, contain brown granules called *melanin*. In addition to contributing to skin color, melanin also provides protection during episodes of sun exposure. Carotene found in subcutaneous fat tissue contributes to the yellowish color of the skin. This substance is especially concentrated in the palms of the hands and soles of the feet. Last, the normal reddish color of skin is attributed to the presence of oxygenated blood being transported through the arteries and capillaries. Certain skin colors may represent serious disease, including pale (pallor), blue (cyanosis), yellow (jaundice or icterus), gray, and brown (hyperpigmentation). Table 10-1 summarizes these abnormal states, including the underlying physiologic features and associated causes of the color.

CYANOSIS. Increased levels of deoxyhemoglobin in cutaneous tissues results in bluish discoloration called *cyanosis*. Oxyhemoglobin "loses" oxygen as blood courses through the capillary beds converting to deoxyhemoglobin, (which has a darker and bluer pigment). There are two forms of cyanosis: central and peripheral. *Central cyanosis* results from inadequate pulmonary gaseous exchange causing significantly low arterial oxygen levels and is most noticeable in the oral mucosa, lips, tongue, and frenulum but can also be detected in hands and nails. Causes of central cyanosis include advanced pulmonary disorders, acute airway obstructions, congenital heart diseases, intracardiac shunts, and hemoglobinopathies. *Peripheral cyanosis* results from a decrease or slowing of cutaneous blood flow, which allows for tissues to extract increased levels of oxygen from the circulating blood. The cyanosis is noted primarily in the toes, fingers, nails and nail beds, or nose but may appear on outer surfaces of lips. Venous obstruction and congestive heart failure are potential causes of peripheral cyanosis. Peripheral cyanosis tends to dissipate when local warming occurs, whereas central cyanosis does not dissipate.[4,33] An associated change might be digital clubbing (Figure 10-2).[37]

JAUNDICE. Jaundice or icterus, associated with excessive levels of bilirubin, is manifested by a yellow discoloration of sclera (often more easily noted here), skin, and mucous membranes.

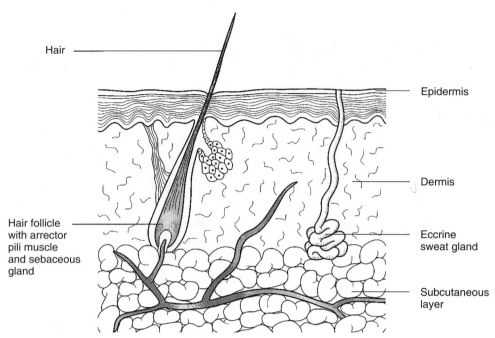

Hair

Epidermis

Dermis

Hair follicle
with arrector
pili muscle
and sebaceous
gland

Eccrine
sweat gland

Subcutaneous
layer

FIGURE 10-1 Normal human skin, including hair and associated vascular supply. (From Shapiro C, Skopit S: Screening for skin disorders. In Boissonnault W, ed: *Examination in physical therapy practice: screening for medical disease,* 2nd ed, New York, 1995, Churchill Livingstone.)

TABLE 10-1

Abnormal Color Changes of the Skin

Color Change	Physiologic Change	Common Causes
White, pale (pallor)	Absence of pigment or pigment change; blood abnormality; temporary interruption or diversion of blood flow; internal disease	Albinism (albinos); lack of sunlight; anemia; lead poisoning; vasospasm; syncope; stress; internal bleeding; chronic gastrointestinal disease; cancer; parasitic disease; tuberculosis
Blue (cyanosis)	Decreased oxygen in blood (deoxyhemoglobin)	Methemoglobinemia (oxidation of hemoglobin); high blood iron level; cold exposure; vasomotor instability; cerebrospinal disease
Yellow	Jaundice, excess bilirubin in blood (2-2.5 mg/100 mL), excess bile pigment; high levels of carotene in blood (carotenemia); high levels of metals in body	Liver disease; gallstone blockage of bile duct; hepatitis (conjunctiva also yellow); ingestion of food high in carotene and vitamin A
Gray	Disturbances of adrenocortical hormones	Increased iron, bronze/gray; increased silver, blue/gray
Brown (hyperpigmentation)	Disturbances of adrenocortical hormones	Adrenal or pituitary glands, Addison's disease

From Shapiro C, Skopit S: Screening for skin disorders. In Boissonnault W, ed: *Examination in physical therapy practice: screening for medical disease,* 2nd ed, New York, 1995, Churchill Livingstone.

Hemolytic anemia (excessive bilirubin production), extrahepatic obstruction (gallstones, tumor, or stricture that impedes bile flow), and hepatic diseases (e.g., hepatitis) are examples of conditions linked to the onset of jaundice. Severely jaundiced individuals may have a greenish hue to the skin resulting from the oxidation of bilirubin to biliverdin.[24,27] As the blood levels of unconjugated bilirubin increase, urine may turn dark yellow or a tea color, and if the biliary obstruction is severe, stools may become light-colored or gray (absence of bile).[4,24,33]

PALLOR. Pallor, or paleness associated with decreased levels of oxyhemoglobin and local blood flow, can occur throughout the body or involve a local anatomic area depending on the underlying cause. Arterial insufficiency, anemias, compartment syndrome, and Raynaud's disease can result in pallor. Associated

symptoms depend on the etiology: (1) arterial insufficiency—intermittent claudication, cool skin temperature, and trophic changes in skin (including hair loss, skin cracking, fissuring); (2) anemias—exertional dyspnea, fatigue, weakness, and pica (often includes a craving for ice); (3) compartment syndrome—local pain with activity, paresis, paresthesia, pulselessness, and palpatory pain and tissue hardness; and (4) Raynaud's disease—the digits turn pale in response to cold, then a bluish purple, followed by a reactive erythema.[4,12]

In addition to general skin color changes, local alterations can indicate a condition that should be reported to a physician. Local redness accompanied by local heat, edema, and tenderness that develops within a few days may be a manifestation of an underlying infection or inflammation, such as cellulitis, a

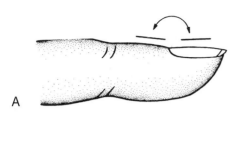

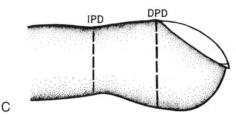

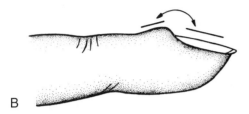

FIGURE 10-2 Clubbing of nails. **A,** Normal nail configuration. **B,** Mild digital clubbing with increased hyponychial angle. **C,** Severe digital clubbing. *DPD,* distal phalangeal diameter; *IPD,* interphalangeal diameter. (From Wilkins RL, Sheldon RL, Krider SJ: *Clinical assessment in respiratory care,* 4th ed, St. Louis, 2000, Mosby.)

bacterial infection. This infection may be accompanied by red streaks extending proximally, which are associated with secondary lymphangitis.[29] Other local skin changes could also be a result of chronic arterial insufficiency. Ischemic ulcers, thin and shiny skin, hair loss, paleness of an elevated extremity, and intense rubor when the limb assumes a dependent position all are possible manifestations of this condition. Last, although cuts and bruises are common, their presence on the head, face, and neck may be an indication of physical abuse. In addition, similar findings on the forearms may be indicative of defensive injuries sustained while trying protect oneself.[8,20] Chapter 8 contains additional information regarding screening for domestic abuse. Easy bruising may also indicate an underlying bleeding disorder.

Skin Cancer

Although many skin lesions are benign, skin cancer was projected to be the most common malignancy in the United States during 2009. The American Cancer Society projected more than 1 million new cases of basal and squamous cell carcinomas in 2009, more than five times the estimates for breast and prostate cancers. In addition, more than 55,000 new cases of melanoma were projected over the same period,[13] with the incidence increasing at a rate of 4% annually, faster than all other malignancies.[23] The PT's role does not include differentiating a melanoma from squamous cell cancer, but it does include recognizing atypical skin lesion characteristics that require a physician

BOX 10-1
Risk Factors for Melanoma (HARMM)

Risk Factor	Relative Increased Risk
History of previous melanoma	3.3 (95% CI 2.9-3.8)
Age >50 years	1.2 (95% CI 1.1-1.3)
Regular dermatologist absent	1.4 (95% CI 1.3-1.5)
Mole changing	2.0 (95% CI 1.9-2.2)
Male gender	1.4 (95% CI 1.3-1.5)

CI, confidence interval.

BOX 10-2
ABCD Screening for Melanoma

A—Asymmetry
B—Borders (irregularity, blurred)
C—Color (multiple variants, black)
D—Diameter (>6 mm)

Data from Koh HK: Cutaneous melanoma, *N Engl J Med* 325:171–182, 1991.

consultation. This consultation may lead to a lesion undergoing biopsy and being diagnosed earlier in the course of the disease. PTs are rarely included in discussions of secondary prevention and skin cancer,[15] but considering how much skin PTs tend to "see" during a patient visit and the high incidence of skin cancer, PTs could be valuable members of the health care team screening for such lesions. A patient case has been published demonstrating PT recognition of unusual skin lesion characteristics leading to an earlier diagnosis of skin cancer.[38]

Of the skin cancers, melanoma is the most aggressive type in terms of metastasis, and metastasis to the spine seems to be increasing.[31] Early detection is crucial for a positive prognosis; the long-term survival rate is 92% for a localized lesion but only 5% for metastatic melanoma.[19] Early detection can be accomplished by identifying relative risk for the disease and unusual lesion characteristics. Goldberg and colleagues[11] described a melanoma risk model called the *HARMM model* (Box 10-1). Individuals with four or five of the risk factors mentioned in the HARMM model were 4.4 times more likely to have a diagnosis of melanoma (95% confidence interval 3.8-5.1).[11] In addition, a history of melanoma in a first-degree relative carries an 8- to 12-fold increased risk.[23]

The presence of moles also carries increased risk for melanoma development; Fears and associates[10] reported a relative risk estimate of 4.6 in men with 17 or more moles and 5.2 in women with 12 or more moles. The "*ABCD* rule" is related to warning signs of moles and melanoma (Box 10-2).[16] Studies have noted this tool to have sensitivities approaching 100%, with specificity less well noted, but each criterion is not weighted equally. For example, a lesion 3 mm in diameter, but black and having indistinct or blurred borders, needs to be examined by a physician. Authors state that the sensitivity values using this screening tool may be increased if all four criteria are not required to be present, citing that early melanomas are often less than 6 mm in diameter.[36] More recently, authors have promoted adding an "*E*" to the acronym, standing for evolving or changing.[1,23] A unique distribution pattern has been reported in people with dark skin, with the plantar surface of the feet being a common location for melanomas to appear.[34]

Table 10-2 summarizes characteristics typical of a benign versus a malignant (melanoma and nonmelanoma) skin lesion. Friability and ulceration imply weakened or damaged tissue and may be represented by an area that is scabbed over or by a lesion that is bleeding. The PT may note a spot of blood showing through the patient's clothing. These are findings more commonly associated with basal and squamous cell carcinomas. Basal cell carcinomas (which constitute approximately 80% of skin cancers) also frequently have a depressed center surrounded by a raised, firm border, and squamous cell cancers often manifest with scaling, crusty nodules or plaques. The most common site for basal and squamous cell lesions include the head and face, ears, neck, and hands, but reports describe squamous cell lesions also occurring on lower extremities of African American women.[4] There also seems to be an association between nonmelanomas and postoperative organ transplant recipients. The increased risk ranges from 65 to 250 times for squamous cell carcinomas and 10 times for basal cell carcinomas. The common time frame for appearance of cancer varies depending on patient age; for patients older than 60 years, the risk occurs up to 3 years postoperatively, whereas for patients in their 40s the risk occurs up to 8 years postoperatively.[9]

See the Evolve website for examples of benign and malignant skin lesions. If any atypical characteristics are observed by the PT, follow-up questions should be asked:

- Have you noticed this skin lesion?
- Has it recently changed in terms of size, color, shape, or surface appearance?
- Has a physician looked at the lesion? If so, what did the physician say about it?

If the patient states that a physician has not looked at the lesion, or the patient is unsure whether the lesion has changed since the physician has checked it, the PT should refer the patient to his or her primary care physician. If the patient states the lesion has been there as long as he or she can remember, and no change in the lesion has occurred, a referral is unnecessary as long as the PT has confidence in the patient being an accurate historian. If the skin lesion is on a body part that is not readily visible to the patient, the PT should assume that a physician should examine the lesion.

Two common benign vascular skin lesions that PTs may observe include spider and cherry angiomas. Both lesions tend to be small, with a cherry angioma measuring up to 3 mm in diameter and a spider angioma measuring up to 2 cm. These lesions are marked by a bright or fiery red color. A cherry angioma is round with smooth borders, whereas a spider angioma has a central body surrounded by radiating red "legs." Pressure applied to the central body of a spider angioma causes blanching of the "legs." Spider angiomas can occur in women who are pregnant and may be a manifestation of liver disease or vitamin B deficiency. Although cherry angiomas may increase in size and number as the patient ages, they are not typically associated with a pathologic condition.[4,33]

Skin Rash

When a rash is noted, important follow-up questions should be asked (Box 10-3). The general rule should be followed: A referral is warranted if the lesion is new, the lesion is unexplained, the patient's physician is unaware of the lesion, or the lesion is worsening. Numerous causes of rashes exist—some benign and others requiring a more urgent referral. A more urgent referral is in order if the rash seems to be spreading quickly; is accompanied by systemic complaints such as fever, fatigue, or malaise (see Chapter 9); or is accompanied by complaints such as joint pain.

Nails

As with skin color, changes in the nails may indicate the presence of occult disease. The changes may occur in the nail itself or in the surrounding tissues. Figure 10-3 illustrates normal nail anatomy,[26] and Figure 10-4 compares normal and abnormal nail appearances.[28] The PT may also observe "clubbing" of the digits, an abnormality associated with cystic fibrosis, chronic hypoxia, and lung cancer[4] (see Figure 10-2). *Clubbing* is manifested by three abnormal appearances: the distal phalanx appears rounded and bulbous, the nail plate is convex-shaped, and the proximal nail fold and plate angle (Lovibond's angle) increases to 180 degrees or more.[4,33]

Hair

Hair is normally found over the entire body except for the soles of the feet, palms of the hands, and portions of the genitalia. A vascular network located in the dermal layer of the

---

TABLE 10-2

Skin Characteristics: Benign versus Cancerous Lesions

Characteristics	Benign	Malignant
Size	<6 mm	>6 mm
Color	Uniform	Varied/black
Borders	Distinct/smooth	Irregular/indistinct
Shape	Symmetric	Asymmetric
Consistency	Soft to firm	Firm to hard
Friability	None	Often
Ulceration	Seldom	Often
Mobility	Mobile	Mobile/nonmobile
Rate of change (color, shape, size, surface)	Slow	Slow or rapid

---

BOX 10-3

Follow-up Questions Related to Observation of Rash

- Do you know what has caused the rash?
- Was the rash initially flat, raised, or blistered?
- Has the rash changed, spread, or developed in other body sites?
- What seems to alleviate or aggravate the rash?
- Does the rash feel numb or painful; does it itch or burn?
- Have you traveled recently? If so, where?
- Have you been in contact with anyone who had a similar rash?
- Have you noted fever, fatigue, joint pain, or any other new symptoms along with the rash?

From Swartz MH: *Textbook of physical diagnosis: history and examination*, 5th ed, Philadelphia, 2006, Saunders, p 371.

skin provides the necessary nourishment to hair follicles (see Figure 10-1). If the local circulation is compromised, as in arterial insufficiency, hair loss occurs along with the other manifestations previously mentioned. If the disorder has progressed so that these skin changes have occurred, the patient is likely to state that the extremity is cold. Hair loss (alopecia) of the scalp,

although most often associated with male-pattern and female-pattern baldness, can result from various diseases or be a side effect of medication use[21,30] (Box 10-4). In general, hair loss that occurs quickly or that does not begin in the frontoparietal scalp should cause concern.[30] Brittle hair leading to hair breakage can also indicate illness, such as hypothyroidism.[22] The broken hair may be noted later in the examination after the patient sits up after lying on a sheet or pillow case.

Observation: Surface Anatomy and Body Contour

During the interview, the face, neck, anterior shoulder girdle, hand, and maybe lower legs are typically visible. In addition to observing the elements associated with skin, the PT should also be vigilant for abnormal body contours that may be manifestations of masses or abnormal fluid accumulation (edema). Masses may not be manifested by a lump or bump on the body surface but instead by the absence of a notch or body concavity. Enlarged tissues located within a fossa or notch may simply "fill in" the notch. Examples include the sternal notch completely or partially filled in by an enlarged thyroid gland or the supraclavicular fossa filled in by an enlarged supraclavicular lymph node. Cervical masses may also be manifested by a tracheal deviation. When the patient is observed from the front, the trachea should be vertically oriented. If a mass is present, the trachea may appear to be "pushed" to one side. The observation of any abnormality should

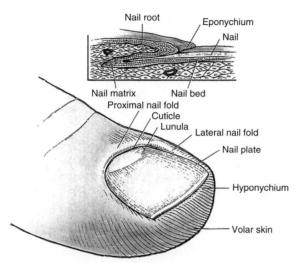

FIGURE 10-3 Nail anatomy. (From Sams WM Jr: Structure and function of the skin. In Sams WM, Lynch PJ, eds: *Principles and practice of dermatology,* 2nd ed, New York, 1996, Churchill Livingstone.)

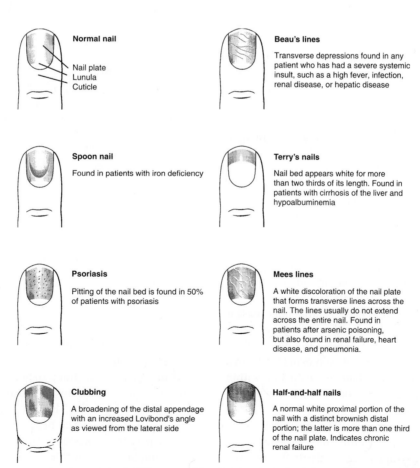

FIGURE 10-4 Normal nail appearance and common systemic diseases manifested in changes in the nail. (From Shapiro C, Skopit S: Screening for skin disorders. In Boissonnault W, ed: *Examination in physical therapy practice: screening for medical disease,* 2nd ed, New York, 1995, Churchill Livingstone.)

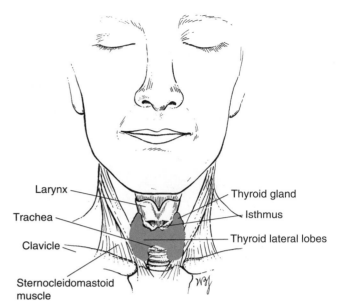

FIGURE 10-5 The thyroid gland located in the sternal notch. (From Swartz MH: *Textbook of physical diagnosis,* 5th ed, Philadelphia, 2006, Saunders, p 196.)

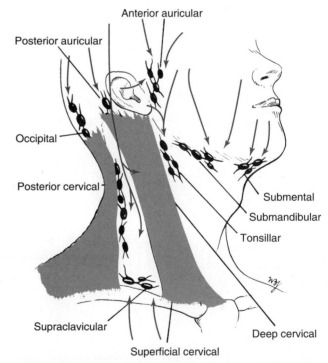

FIGURE 10-6 Lymph nodes of the neck and their drainage. (From Swartz MH: *Textbook of physical diagnosis,* 5th ed, Philadelphia, 2006, Saunders, p 197.)

direct the PT to palpate the area when the physical examination begins and then ask follow-up questions:

- Are you aware of this lump?
- Is the lump painful (if so, could be an inflammatory process or infection)?
- Has the lump changed within the past few months (size, shape, consistency)?
- Is your physician aware of the lump? If so, what did he or she say about it?

As with skin lesions, if the physician is unaware of the finding or if the mass has changed since the last physician visit, the PT should initiate a referral.

Neck Masses (Palpation)

The structures most likely to manifest as a neck mass include the thyroid, parotid, and submandibular glands and the local lymph nodes (Figures 10-5 and 10-6). Glandular surfaces tend to be lobulated and irregular compared with the smaller lymph nodes, which tend to be round or ovoid in shape and smooth. Glands normally tend to be nontender and soft to firm to touch, and hard nodules should not be present within the structure. Table 10-3 summarizes characteristics of normal versus abnormal lymph nodes. Abnormal lymph nodes may be exquisitely tender in the presence of acute inflammation but may also be nontender if the mass is slow to moderate growing. This nontender lymph node would be firm to hard. A nontender mass is often the initial manifestation of head and neck cancers.[6] Pain generated from an inflamed lymph node often is a dull, diffuse, nonlocalized ache instead of the pinpoint pain expected from a structure that is a few centimeters in diameter. Palpation within the area of the ache reveals a local lump that is exquisitely painful and firm to hard in consistency.

During a patient examination, questions may arise as to whether the palpable mass is a band within a muscle belly or is an adjacent superficial involved lymph node. To clarify the involved structure, the PT can elicit a light contraction of the local muscle while palpating the lump. If the lump does not change from a palpation perspective, the mass is probably superficial to the muscle belly. If the lump changes or disappears under the fingers palpating the area, the lump may be within the muscle belly or deep to the muscle. In this scenario, palpating posterior to the muscle belly (if possible) is warranted to discern whether the mass is within the muscle belly. Palpable bands within a muscle belly may be associated with a trigger point as described by Travell and Simons.[35] If this is the PT's conclusion, the patient's response to treatment is key in terms of deciding whether a physician needs to be contacted.

TABLE 10-3
Characteristics of Normal and Abnormal Lymph Nodes

Characteristics	Normal	Abnormal
Size	<1.5 cm	Can be >1.5 cm
Consistency	Soft, squishy	Firm to hard
Mobility	Mobile	Mobile to nonmobile
Pain/tenderness	Nontender	Tender or nontender

Anterior Shoulder Girdle Masses (Palpation)

If the patient is not wearing a shirt or has a tank top or sports bra on, the PT may be able to observe the supraclavicular, infraclavicular, and anterior glenohumeral joint regions. Figure 10-7 illustrates palpation of the infraclavicular fossa, in which lymph nodes are located.[5] Enlarged local lymph nodes or a breast mass may "fill in" this fossa. Breast tissue extends up toward the anterior glenohumeral joint region (upper and outer quadrant of the breast), and in some women the tissue can extend into the axilla (Figure 10-8). The upper and outer breast quadrant is often the site of neoplasms.[7] As described earlier, a PT who palpates a lump in this region should attempt to determine whether the mass is within the local musculature (e.g., pectoralis major muscle) or within tissue superficial to the muscle (e.g., breast tissue). If the mass is superficial to the muscle, the PT would probably not note a change in the lump while eliciting a gentle contraction of the local musculature. If the PT has any concerns about the nature of the noted mass, follow-up questions should be asked:

- Have you noticed this lump?
- Has a physician examined this area?

If the patient is unaware of the lump, a referral is warranted, and if the answer to the second question is no, or the patient states the lump may have changed since the physician examined it, the following questions are warranted:

- Has the lump changed (shape, size, consistency, number of)?
- Is the lump tender?
- Have you noticed any changes of the skin overlying the breast (color, puckering, scaliness, dimpling, peau d'orange)?
- Have you noticed any nipple discharge or retraction?

Approximately 1% of breast cancers occur in men, so the same principles apply to finding a mass in this region in a male patient.[13]

Observation: General Nervous System Screen

A general nervous system screen can also begin as soon as the PT sees and starts interacting with the patient, including observation of the following:

- Gross movement patterns
- Gait
- Balance
- Tremors
- Asymmetric facial features
- Pupils
- Ptosis
- Strabismus
- Facial contour
- Hearing

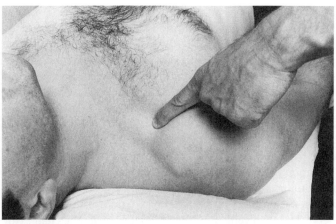

FIGURE 10-7 Palpation of infraclavicular fossa. (From Boissonnault W: *Examination in physical therapy practice: screening for medical disease,* 2nd ed, New York, 1995, Churchill Livingstone.)

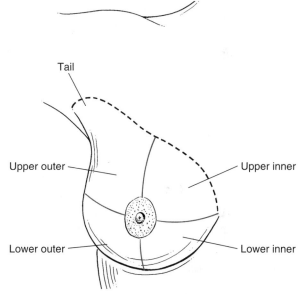

FIGURE 10-8 Four breast quadrants. (From Swartz MH: *Textbook of physical diagnosis,* 5th ed, Philadelphia, 2006, Saunders, p 466.)

If the PT meets the patient in the waiting area, watching the patient rise from the chair and walk back to the treatment area provides information about gross muscle strength, coordination, and balance. When the patient interview begins, the PT can be vigilant for tremors, areas of muscle atrophy, and asymmetric facial features.

Facial Inspection

Careful inspection of the face, including the pupils, eyelids, gaze, and movement of the eyes, during the interview can reveal important findings associated with nervous system function. Figure 10-9 shows normal external landmarks of the eye. Although a small percentage of the population has a normal anatomic variant of up to 1 mm in diameter, pupils are normally equal in size and round, with smooth margins.[25,33] An abnormal pupil may be enlarged (mydriasis) or constricted (miosis). Mydriasis may be associated with medication use (sympathomimetics and dilating drops; see Chapter 4) or conditions such as acute glaucoma.

Miosis may be associated with parasympathomimetic medications (see Chapter 4) or conditions such as Horner's syndrome and inflammation of the iris. Table 10-4 summarizes common pupillary abnormalities. Although not associated with a nervous system disorder, a specific pattern of eye redness should alert the PT to ask follow-up questions (see subsequent list). An intense circle of redness (vasodilated vessels) around the iris, called *ciliary flush,* is associated with inflammation of the iris or cornea or acute glaucoma.[3] Observation of ciliary flush warrants an immediate consultation with the patient's physician.

Drooping of the upper eyelid (ptosis) may also be a manifestation of a normal anatomic variant or of a pathologic condition, including myasthenia gravis, lesion of the oculomotor nerve, and involvement of the cervical sympathetic chain. Normally, the upper eyelid covers the upper margin of the iris and the sclera above, whereas a thin strip of the sclera is usually visible between the lower lid and the bottom margin of the iris. The space between the upper and lower eyelids is called the *palpebral fissure.* Because of connective tissue changes in the skin associated with aging, elderly patients may have bilateral drooping of the upper eyelids (senile ptosis).[17] Unilateral ptosis is a classic component of Horner's syndrome. To maintain the visual field, the patient may compensate by contracting the frontalis (resulting in wrinkling the forehead) to raise the upper eyelid.[25] Bilateral ptosis in a nonelderly patient and unilateral ptosis in any patient should concern the PT.

The final component of the static assessment of the eyes is gaze. Normally, both of the patient's eyes should meet the PT's during the interview process. Misalignment of the two eyes—one eye is focused on the PT, but the other is not—is called *strabismus.* Observation of any of the earlier described abnormalities would warrant follow-up questions:

- Have you noticed the abnormality (ptosis, pupil asymmetry, strabismus)? If so, how long has the abnormality been present, and what brought it on?
- Have there been any recent changes in your vision, including acuity or sharpness of vision, flashes, photophobia, loss of visual field, diplopia or double vision, colored halos around lights, difficulty seeing in dim light, or altered colored vision? (See Box 10-5 for a summary of visual abnormalities and potential disease states.)
- Is there any pain in or around your eye?
- Is your physician aware of the condition?

Additional follow-up questions regarding nervous system status should also be asked:

- Have you noticed any recent changes in your ability to smell, taste, swallow, talk, or hear?
- Have you noticed any recent changes in your balance, memory, ability to concentrate, or attention span?

If the patient states that he or she is unaware of the abnormality of the eyes or gives equivocal answers to the that aforementioned questions, the PT should include some tests in the physical

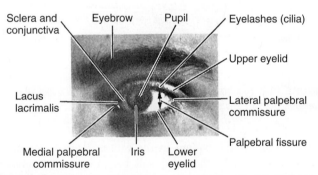

FIGURE 10-9 External features of the eye. (From Magee DJ: *Orthopedic physical assessment,* 5th ed, Philadelphia, 2008, Saunders, p 109.)

BOX 10-5
Common Visual Symptoms and Possible Disease States

Symptom	Disease States
Loss of vision	Optic neuritis, detached retina, retinal hemorrhage, central retinal vascular occlusion, central nervous system disease
Spots	Impending retinal detachment, fertility drugs
Flashes	Migraine headaches, retinal detachment, posterior vitreous detachment
Loss of visual field, presence of shadows	Retinal detachment, retinal hemorrhage
Glare, photophobia	Iritis, meningitis
Distorted vision	Retinal detachment, macular edema
Impaired vision in dim light	Myopia, vitamin A deficiency, retinal degeneration
Colored halos around lights	Acute narrow-angle glaucoma, opacities in lens or cornea
Colored vision changes	Cataracts, medication such as digitalis (increases yellow vision)
Double vision (diplopia)	Extraocular muscle paresis or paralysis

Adapted from Swartz MH: *Textbook of physical diagnosis: history and examination,* 5th ed, Philadelphia, 2006, Saunders.

TABLE 10-4
Pupillary Abnormalities

	Adie's Tonic Pupil	Argyll Robertson Pupil	Horner's Syndrome
Etiology	Unknown	Diabetes, tertiary syphilis	Lesions of brain stem, cervical root, carotid artery dissection, apex of the lung, orbit
Laterality	Often unilateral	Bilateral	Unilateral
Reaction to light	Minimally reactive	Nonreactive	Reactive
Accommodation	Sluggishly reactive	Reactive	Reactive
Pupillary size	Mydriatic	Miotic	Miotic
Other signs	Absent or diminished tendon reflexes	Absent knee-jerk reflexes	Slight ptosis and anhidrosis

Adapted from Swartz MH: *Textbook of physical diagnosis: history and physical examination,* 5th ed, Philadelphia, 2006, Saunders.

examination to gather more information about the status of the relevant cranial nerves. The pupillary reaction test can be used to test elements of the second and third cranial nerves (Figure 10-10). The pupils of both eyes should constrict briskly and to the same degree in response to the light stimulus. In addition, ocular movements can be used to assess function of the third, fourth, and sixth cranial nerves and associated muscles (Figure 10-11). The PT holds a finger approximately 10 to 15 inches from the patient's nose[18,33] and slowly traces a large "H" in front of the patient's face (Figure 10-12). The patient is asked to follow the finger with his or her eyes, and the eyes should track together. The PT asks the patient to follow the finger as it moves toward the tip of the patient's nose; the eyes should converge together. If the eyes do not track together, or, in the presence of strabismus, the degree of misalignment

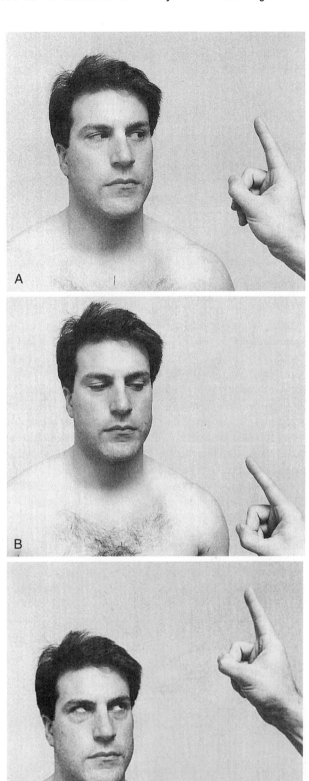

FIGURE 10-12 Assessment of ocular movements. **A,** The PT's finger moving laterally to the patient's left. **B,** The PT's finger moving down and away from the patient's nose. **C,** The PT's finger moving up and away from the patient's nose. All three movements are repeated to the patient's right side. (From Boissonnault W: *Examination in physical therapy practice: screening for medical disease,* 2nd ed, New York, 1995, Churchill Livingstone.)

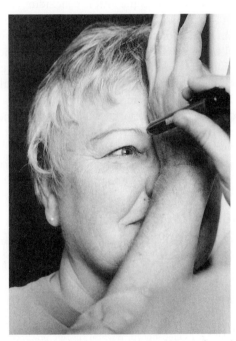

FIGURE 10-10 Pupillary light reaction test should be performed in a dimly lit room with the patient told to look at a distant object. The PT's hand divides the patient's visual field and shines the light into one eye, watching that pupil for the response (direct response). The PT then shines the light in the *same* eye, watching the *opposite* pupil for the response (consensual response). This process is repeated while shining the light in the other eye.

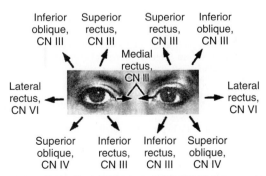

FIGURE 10-11 Six cardinal fields of gaze with associated eye muscles and cranial nerves responsible for the movements. (From Magee DJ: *Orthopedic physical assessment,* 4th ed, Philadelphia, 2002, Saunders.)

varies depending on which direction the eyes are moving (paralytic strabismus), especially when accompanied by diplopia, the patient's physician should be contacted. Abnormalities of which the patient or physician is unaware or abnormalities that have worsened since that last physician visit warrant communication with the patient's physician.

Hearing

During the interview, a hearing deficit may be suspected by the PT or reported by a concerned patient. Impaired hearing has many potential causes, including neurologic conditions. There are three types of hearing loss: conductive (involvement of the middle ear, outer ear, or both), sensorineural (involvement of the inner ear), or a combination of both. Ultimately, the patient's physician determines the type of hearing loss when the PT refers the patient with a suspected occult hearing impairment. If the patient reports the suspected hearing loss is of new onset or has recently worsened, tests should be included in the physical examination. The recommended auditory acuity test is the *whispered voice test,* not the bone conduction–tuning fork tests (Weber and Rinne tests).[2] The PT whispers familiar letters, numbers, or words (e.g., 5, B, 13, hot dog) and asks the patient to repeat the words that were whispered. To test one ear at a time and to ensure the patient cannot lip read, the PT should stand approximately 2 feet (arm's length) behind and off to one side of the patient while whispering. To ensure unilateral assessment, the patient should place the tip of the finger in the external auditory canal of the ear not being tested and move (rub) that finger in the canal (Figure 10-13). If a unilateral or bilateral deficit is noted or if the findings are equivocal, follow-up testing is warranted by a specialist.[2,32]

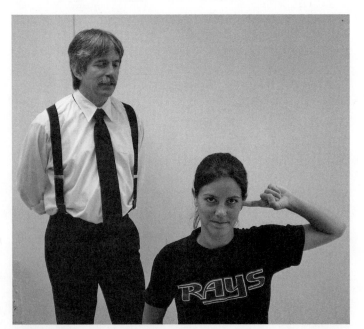

FIGURE 10-13 "Whispered voice" screening test for hearing impairment. The PT stands at arm's length behind the patient off to one side. The patient places the index finger into the ear not being tested and moves/rubs the finger tip inside the ear. The PT then whispers three to four words asking the patient to repeat the words.

Summary

Although one of the goals of this chapter is to foster efficient clinical practice, it might seem that the recommended observations, follow-up questions, and physical examination techniques could disrupt the natural flow of the initial visit. Depending on the makeup of the PT's patient population, the abnormal observations noted in this chapter may often have nothing to do with the health issues that have precipitated the physical therapy visit. In that case, following the normal examination scheme and organization is important for the sake of efficiency, but at some point during the visit (often toward the end), the observation warranting concern needs to be addressed. For example, a patient comes to physical therapy for upper body pain, and a suspicious-looking skin lesion is noted on the lower leg. The PT can complete the usual examination for the upper body pain and associated functional limitation, but as the visit is concluding the PT could state, "Before we finish for the day, I would like to talk to you about a spot I noticed on the outside of your right leg." This statement could be followed up by the questions and the physical examination techniques described throughout this chapter. The observations described are not just germane to the initial patient visit. The PT should make an effort to remain vigilant during any subsequent visits for the surface anatomy, skin, and nervous system findings that were described. Clinical manifestations can be easily overlooked during a hectic initial visit, especially when they are not directly related to the reason for the physical therapy visit, and new manifestations can develop after the initial visit.

REFERENCES

1. Abbasi NR, Shaw HM, Rigel DS, et al. Early diagnosis of cutaneous melanoma: revisiting the ABCD criteria. JAMA 2004;292:2771–6.
2. Bagai A, Thavendiranathan, P, Detsky AS. Does this patient have hearing impairment? JAMA 2006;295:416–28.
3. Berson FG. Basic ophthalmology for medical students and primary care residents. San Francisco: American Academy of Ophthalmology; 1993.
4. Bickley LS. Bates' guide to physical examination and history taking. 10th ed. Philadelphia: Lippincott Williams & Wilkins; 2009, p. 164–8.
5. Boissonnault W. Examination in physical therapy practice: screening for medical disease. 2nd ed. New York: Churchill Livingstone; 1995.
6. Concus AP, Singer MI. Head and neck cancer. In: Goldman L, Bennett JC, editors. Cecil textbook of medicine. 21st ed. Philadelphia: Saunders; 2000. p. 2257–61.
7. Damjanov I. Pathology for the health-related professions. 2nd ed. Philadelphia: Saunders; 2000.
8. Eisenstat SA, Bancroft L. Domestic violence. N Engl J Med 1999;341:886–92.
9. Euvrard S, Kanitakis J, Claudy A. Skin cancers after organ transplantation. N Engl J Med 2003;348:1681–91.
10. Fears TR, Guerry DT, Pfeiffer RM, et al. Identifying individuals at high risk of melanoma: a practical predictor of absolute risk. J Clin Oncol 2006;24:3590–6.
11. Goldberg MS, Doucette JT, Lim HW, et al. Risk factors for presumptive melanoma in skin cancer screening: American Academy of Dermatology National Melanoma/Skin Screening Program experience 2001-2005. J Am Acad Dermatol 2007;57:60–6.
12. Gorroll AH, Mulley AG. Primary care medicine. 5th ed. Philadelphia: Lippincott Williams & Wilkins; 2006, p. 1062–1065.
13. Jemal A, Siegel R, Ward E, et al. Cancer statistics, 2009. CA Cancer J Clin 2009; 59:225–49.
14. Jensen GM, Shepard KF, Gwyer J, et al. Attribute dimensions that distinguish master and novice physical therapy clinicians in orthopedic settings. Phys Ther 1992;72:711–22.
15. Koh HK, Geller AC, Miller DR, et al. Prevention and early detection strategies for melanoma and skin cancer. Arch Dermatol 1996;132:436–43.
16. Koh HK. Cutaneous melanoma. N Engl J Med 1991;325:171–82.
17. Lewis CB, Bottomley JM. Geriatric physical therapy: a clinical approach. Norwalk, CT: Appleton & Lange; 1994.

18. Magee DJ. Orthopedic physical assessment. 5th ed. Philadelphia: Saunders; 2008.

19. Miller BA, Ries LAG, Hnakey BF, et al, editors. Cancer statistics review: 1973-1990. National Institutes of Health publication no. 93-2789, Bethesda, MD: National Cancer Institute; 1993.

20. Muelleman RL, Lenaghan PA, Pakieser RA. Battered women: injury locations and types. Ann Emerg Med 1996;28:486–92.

21. Parker F. Skin diseases of general importance. In: Goldman L, Bennett JC, editors. Cecil textbook of medicine. 21st ed. Philadelphia: Saunders; 2000. p. 2293–4.

22. Porth CM, Jurwitz LS. Alterations of endocrine controls of growth and metabolism. In: Porth CM, editor. Pathophysiology: concepts of altered health states. 4th ed. Philadelphia: Lippincott; 1994. p. 915–7.

23. Rager EL, Bridgeford EP, Ollila DW. Cutaneous melanoma: update on prevention, screening, diagnosis, and treatment. Am Fam Physician 2005;72:269–76.

24. Richter JM. Evaluation of jaundice. In: Goroll AH, Mulley AG, editors. Primary care medicine. 5th ed. Philadelphia: Lippincott Williams & Wilkins; 2006. p. 461–6.

25. Ross RT. How to examine the nervous system. 3rd ed. Stamford, CT: Appleton & Lange; 1999.

26. Sams Jr WM. Structure and function of the skin. In: Sams WM, Lynch PJ, editors. Principles and practice of dermatology. 2nd ed. New York: Churchill Livingstone; 1996.

27. Scharschmidt BF. Bilirubin metabolism, hyperbilirubinemia, and the approach to the jaundiced patient. In: Goldman L, Bennett JC, editors. Cecil textbook of medicine. 21st ed. Philadelphia: Saunders; 2000. p. 770–5.

28. Shapiro C, Skopit S. Screening for skin disorders. In: Boissonnault W, editor. Examination in physical therapy practice: screening for medical disease. 2nd ed. New York: Churchill Livingstone; 1995.

29. Shellow WVR, Craft N. Approach to bacterial skin infections. In: Goroll AH, Mulley AG, editors. Primary care medicine. 5th ed. Philadelphia: Lippincott Williams & Wilkins; 2006. p. 1206–10.

30. Shellow WVR, Rotunda AM. Approach to the patient with hair loss. In: Goroll AH, Mulley AG, editors. Primary care medicine. 5th ed. Philadelphia: Lippincott Williams & Wilkins; 2006. p. 1177–81.

31. Spiegel DA, Simpson JH, Richardson WJ, et al. Metastatic melanoma to the spine: demographics, risk factors, and prognosis in 114 patients. Spine 1995;20:2141–6.

32. Swan IRC, Browning GG. The whispered voice as a screening test for hearing impairment. J Roy Coll Gen Pract 1985;35:197.

33. Swartz MH. Textbook of physical diagnosis. 5th ed. Philadelphia: Saunders; 2006.

34. Toombs E. A global perspective on dark-skinned people. Skin Cancer Found J 2006;24:65–7.

35. Travell J, Simons DG. Myofascial pain and dysfunction. vol. 2. Baltimore: Williams & Wilkins; 1992.

36. Whited JD, Grichnik JM. The rational clinical examination: does this patient have a mole or a melanoma? JAMA 1998;279:696–701.

37. Wilkins RL, Sheldon RL, Krider SJ. Clinical assessment in respiratory care. 4th ed. St. Louis: Mosby; 2000.

38. Wills M. Skin cancer screening. Phys Ther 2002;82:1232–7.

Review of Cardiovascular and Pulmonary Systems and Vital Signs

11

Steven H. Tepper, PT, PhD
D. Michael McKeough, PT, EdD

Objectives

After reading this chapter, the reader will be able to:

1. Provide a rationale for the need to measure, monitor, and record vital signs at rest, during activity, and during recovery from activity.
2. Provide a rationale for the need to measure, monitor, and record body mass index.
3. Define blood pressure, heart rate, ventilatory rate, and heart and breath sounds, and describe accurate, reliable, and valid clinical tests for each of these measurements.
4. Describe the expected normal and potential abnormal changes in blood pressure, heart rate, ventilatory rate, and heart and breath sounds at rest and in response to acute activity—or long-term training.
5. Describe how abnormal measures of vital signs and body composition are potential risk factors for the development of pathologic conditions, impairment, functional limitation, and disability.
6. Describe how measures of vital signs and body composition can be used to establish treatment goals, assist with the development of a treatment plan, and assess response to intervention (verify treatment effectiveness).

Physiologic measures of the cardiovascular and respiratory systems and body composition are important because they may accurately reflect the patient's general health and wellness. Simply, health can be defined as "[a] state of being associated with freedom from disease and illness that also includes a positive component (wellness) that is associated with a quality of life and positive well-being," and wellness can be defined as "[a] multidimensional state of being describing the existence of positive health in an individual as exemplified by quality of life and a sense of well-being."[2a] Blood pressure (BP), heart rate (HR), and ventilatory rate are basic physiologic measures of the cardiovascular and pulmonary systems. Heart and lung sounds also help delineate normal function or potential disease. The locations of these and other physiologic measures are shown in Figure 11-1. Body mass index (BMI) is a measure of body composition and has been shown to be related to the risk of developing many of the diseases commonly seen in the physical therapy clinic.

Normal values and ranges have been established for these physiologic measures at rest and during activity in various age groups. Significant deviations from these norms may indicate an abnormal condition and are valuable in assessing the patient's risk of developing a disease or disorder. The ability to provide quality health care depends in part on the practitioner's ability to assess and interpret accurately measures of these important physiologic parameters (vital signs) at rest and during activity and recovery. Despite the demonstrated value of these measures in assessing a patient's general health and risk of developing disease and the recommendation by the *Guide to Physical Therapy Practice*,[2] more recent evidence indicates that they have not yet become a routine part of assessment by the physical therapist (PT).[17,49]

For most patients, a baseline measurement of vital signs and body composition should be established so that changes in these values related to exercise, diet, medications, or other factors can be determined. If abnormal values are found at rest, the cause of these abnormal values should be determined before initiating any activity that involves significant physical or psychological stress. Individuals with abnormal resting values are often less able to tolerate physical activity or other stress-producing events. Depending on the extent of these abnormalities, significant life-threatening sequelae may occur.

Measurements of these physiologic parameters can be used to determine the need to refer the patient to a physician, establish intervention goals, assist in developing an intervention plan, and assess the individual's response to intervention (establish treatment effectiveness). Patients being seen for complications associated with diabetes mellitus (DM) (elevated blood glucose levels) are often found to have hypertension (elevated BP), hypercholesterolemia (elevated total cholesterol), impaired cardiovascular and muscular endurance, and obesity (elevated BMI). These risk factors and complications for DM are related to the disease process and lifestyle and usually lead to a more sedentary lifestyle. An intervention plan should be developed that may include drug therapy to help control blood glucose level, hypertension, and cholesterol; an exercise program to help control blood glucose level, hypertension, cholesterol, lack of endurance, and obesity; and dietary modifications to help control blood glucose level, hypertension, cholesterol, and obesity. At 4 weeks into the intervention (e.g., a walking program), the short-term goals should include better control of blood glucose level, reduced total cholesterol, reduced resting and submaximal HR and BP, and a reduction in BMI.[11] By discharge, the patient should have accepted responsibility for controlling his or her comorbidities. Controlling comorbidities involves a permanent change in lifestyle, including medications (which over time may be reduced or eliminated), regular exercise, and eating a healthyful diet.[13] The intervention plan is deemed effective if, by discharge, the measures of physiologic parameters are closer to or within normal limits.[4]

Body Mass Index

It has been estimated that 66.3% of the U.S. population is overweight or obese, a condition that leads to increased risks for cardiopulmonary, musculoskeletal, neurologic, and integumentary

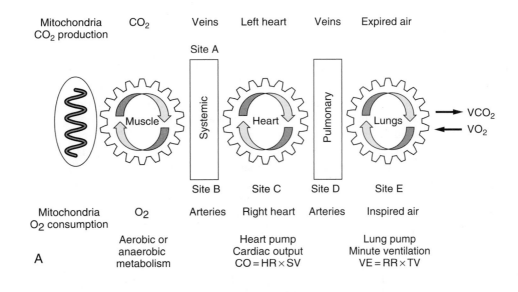

Measurements at Sites

- **Site A**
  - Jugular venous distention
  - Venous pulse
  - Central line
    - Central venous pressure
    - PvO_2

- **Site B**
  - Pulse palpation for:
    - Heart rate
    - Heart rhythm
    - Patency of blood vessel
  - Blood pressure
  - Pulse oxygen or O_2 saturation
  - Arterial line
    - BP
    - PaO_2
    - Cardiac output or index

- **Site C**
  - ECG
  - Heart rate
  - Heart rhythm
  - Heart sounds

- **Site D**
  - Swan-Ganz catheter
    - Pulmonary artery BP
    - Pulmonary capillary wedge pressure

- **Site E**
  - Breath frequency
  - Tidal volume
  - Lung sounds

FIGURE 11-1 Anatomic sites for physiologic measurements. **A,** Oxygen transport system. **B,** Measurements obtained at sites *A* through *E. BP,* blood pressure; *CO₂,* carbon dioxide; *CO,* cardiac output; *ECG,* electrocardiogram *PaO₂,* partial arterial oxygen pressure, *PvO₂,* partial oxygen pressure in mixed venous blood; *RR,* respiratory rate; *SV,* stroke volume; *TV,* tidal volume; *VCO₂,* carbon dioxide output; *VE,* ventricular ejection; *VO₂,* oxygen consumption. (Adapted from Wasserman K, Hansen JE, Sue DY, et al: *Principles of exercise testing and interpretation,* Philadelphia, 1987, Lea & Febiger.)

disorders (Box 11-1).[37] Disorders in any of these functional systems may lead to functional limitations and disability that motivate these patients to seek the assistance of health care professionals, including PTs.[45] Comprehensive health care for these patients cannot be achieved without addressing the issue of overweight as an underlying cause of their functional limitations. The National Institutes of Health National Heart, Lung, and Blood Institute has developed clinical guidelines for adults who are overweight or obese. A free downloadable copy of "Clinical Guidelines for the Identification, Evaluation, and Treatment of Overweight and Obesity in Adults" is available at http://www.nhlbi.nih.gov/guidelines/obesity/ob_home.htm.

How to Measure Body Mass Index

BMI (body weight in kilograms divided by the square of the height in meters; Box 11-2) is the recommended measurement for assessing a patient's level of overweight or obesity and risk

---

BOX 11-1

Comorbid Risks Associated with Being Overweight or Obese

- Hypertension
- Dyslipidemia (abnormalities of blood lipids)*
- Type 2 diabetes*
- Coronary heart disease*
- Stroke
- Gallbladder disease
- Osteoarthritis
- Sleep apnea and respiratory problems
- Endometrial, breast, prostate, and colon cancer

*Primary risk factor.
From National Institutes of Health: *Clinical guidelines on the identification, evaluation, and treatment of overweight and obesity in adults,* NIH publication no. 98-4083 (website), http://www.nhlbi.nih.gov/guidelines/obesity/ob_home.htm. Accessed August 13, 2009.

for disease. Although the validity of the BMI varies, and it is not useful in individuals who have enlarged muscle mass, this simple clinical measure is endorsed for use by health care professionals. BMI has been correlated with percent body fat and the risk of disease. By coupling the BMI with waist measurement, an even more valid measure of the risk of disease in adults (≥20 years old) can be achieved (Table 11-1). Waist measurement should be taken at the iliac crest parallel to the floor. Individuals who carry a greater percentage of their weight in the abdominal region (women with waist measurement >35 inches and men with waist measurement >40 inches) have a higher risk of developing disease.[16,43]

When to Measure Body Mass Index

As part of a shift from a disease-oriented approach to health care to a wellness approach, and because of its value in predicting the risk of developing debilitating disorders, BMI should be assessed as part of the initial examination of all patients older than 2 years old, regardless of the reason for the visit. For individuals 2 to 20 years old, Figure 11-2 is used for evaluation. Children with BMI greater than 85% are deemed overweight, and children with BMI greater than 95% are deemed obese. For adults 20 years old and older, the classification provided in Table 11-1 is used.

After BMI is established, it can serve as part of the health profile monitored at follow-up visits. Increased physical activity is one approach that has been shown to be effective in reducing BMI.[1] Behavior modification, dietary modification, and pharmacologic and surgical approaches have also been shown to be effective.[12] Reduction in BMI has been associated with a reduction in the development of disease.[12]

Role of the Physical Therapist

By focusing exclusively on the impairments causing a patient's chief complaint, PTs risk overlooking the role of excess body weight in the patient's condition. Excess body weight can cause various musculoskeletal disorders, such as low back, hip, knee, and ankle impairments, and may lead to various pathologic conditions, such as hypertension; stroke; DM; breast, endometrial, prostate, or colon cancer; and coronary heart disease. Joint degeneration may be the direct cause of a patient's hip replacement; however, obesity may have been the original cause of the joint degeneration. Failure to address the excess body weight may shorten the life expectancy of the prosthesis or cause additional joint degeneration, leading to the need for additional hip or knee joint replacements.

The current epidemic of obesity in the United States requires that the role of BMI be considered in all cases.[12] It is the professional duty of the PT to inform patients that if they want to reduce their overweight or obesity and risk of disease, the PT can recommend an activity program and help them seek nutritional counseling.[14, 46, 53] A study of overweight and obese individuals who were at high risk of developing DM reported that mild changes in diet and physical activity (walking 30 minutes a day at >3 mph for 5 days of the week) reduced the occurrence of type 2 DM by 58% compared with a control group.[31]

Heart disease is the leading cause of death in the United States today. Because the risk of heart failure increases with an increasing BMI, strategies to promote optimal body weight may reduce the incidence of heart failure.[28] During a 14-year follow-up of the 5881 participants in the Framingham Heart Study, initiated in 1948 under the direction of the National Heart Institute, 496 subjects (258 women and 238 men) developed heart failure. After adjusting for established risk factors, there was an increase in the risk of heart failure of 7% for women and 5% for men for each increment of 1 in BMI. Obese subjects had double the risk of heart failure of subjects with normal BMI. A study of male physicians found that for every increase in BMI, there was an 11% increase in the likelihood of congestive heart failure (CHF).[29]

BOX 11-2

Calculation of Body Mass Index (BMI)[43]

- BMI gives comparative weight for height information that is "significantly correlated with total body fat"
  - Nonmetric formula = weight (lb)/height (inches)^2 × 704.5
  - Metric formula = weight (kg)/height (m)^2
- Subject is female—weight 183 lb, height 5 feet 4 inches, waist 32 inches
- BMI = [183/64^2] × 704.5 = 31.5
- Using table, subject is at high risk for disease

TABLE 11-1

Classification by Body Mass Index (BMI), Waist Circumference, and Associated Disease Risks[*]

	BMI (kg/m^2)	Obesity Class	DISEASE RISK[*] RELATIVE TO NORMAL WEIGHT AND WAIST CIRCUMFERENCE	
			Men ≤102 cm (≤40 inches); women ≤88 cm (≤35 inches)	Men >102 cm (>40 inches); women >88 cm (>35 inches)
Underweight	<18.5		—	—
Normal[†]	18.5-24.9		—	—
Overweight	25-29.9		Increased	High
Obesity	30-34.9	I	High	Very high
	35-39.9	II	Very high	Very high
Extreme obesity	≥40	III	Extremely high	Extremely high

[*]Disease risk for type 2 diabetes, hypertension, and cardiovascular disease.
[†]Increased waist circumference can also be a marker for increased risk even in individuals of normal weight.
From National Institutes of Health: *Clinical guidelines on the identification, evaluation, and treatment of overweight and obesity in adults,* NIH publication no. 98-4083 (website), http://www.nhlbi.nih.gov/guidelines/obesity/ob_home.htm. Accessed August 13, 2009.

Blood Pressure

BP is the force driving the blood through the vascular tree (see Figure 11-1). This pressure is usually measured in the systemic arteries. BP is usually divided into systolic BP (SBP) and diastolic BP (DBP). SBP is the peak lateral force primarily caused by the contraction of the heart ejecting blood, or stroke volume (milliliters of blood ejected from the left ventricle), into the systemic vascular tree. DBP is the minimal lateral force found in the arteries and is primarily related to resistance (total peripheral resistance) to blood flowing through systemic arterioles into the capillaries. Capillaries are the functional unit of the vascular tree that enables the exchange of materials, whereas pressure maintains blood flow.

BP is usually expressed as SBP/DBP in millimeters of mercury (mm Hg). Mean arterial BP (MABP) is related to cardiac output (HR × stroke volume, which is the amount of blood being ejected from the heart per beat; see Figure 11-1) × total peripheral resistance. Figure 11-3 shows factors affecting MABP. MABP can be estimated by DBP + ⅓ SBP − DBP (or pulse pressure), which shifts the pressure closer to DBP because more time is spent in diastole (Figure 11-4). A minimal MABP of approximately 70 mm Hg is needed to ensure adequate flow of blood to tissues and organs. Pressures lower than this level may lead to complications related to inadequate blood flow. Inadequate blood flow to the brain may result in lightheadedness or reduced mentation, and inadequate blood flow to other organs may result in ischemic disorders and shock. BP is controlled by multiple mechanisms (e.g., baroreceptors, chemoreceptors, hormones that control fluid balance) under a negative feedback control system. In adults, excessive

BP, or hypertension, is defined as a resting SBP of more than 140 mm Hg or a resting DBP of more than 90 mm Hg. Hypertension leads to damage to tissues (blood vessels) and organs (e.g., renal failure, stroke, myocardial infarction, blindness).

How to Measure Blood Pressure

BP can be *directly* measured through a catheter placed into an artery. This technique is used in more severely ill patients in the acute care setting. Most of the time BP is *indirectly* measured with a sphygmomanometer (BP cuff) and a stethoscope. The reason BP can be indirectly assessed is that the turbulent flow of fluid moving under pressure through a vessel produces an audible sound (bruit). Listening with a stethoscope (auscultation) over a normal artery, usually no sound is heard because of laminar (smooth) flow. When cuff pressure exceeds SBP (Figure 11-5), all blood flow ceases in the artery distal to the occlusion, and no sound is heard. As cuff pressure gradually decreases, there comes a point where SBP exceeds cuff pressure, and blood flow is restored. When the pressure in the artery exceeds the pressure in the cuff, blood squirts through the artery, creating a bruit. The bruit continues until smooth laminar flow is returned.

The technique for measuring brachial artery BP is as follows:

- Explain the procedure if the patient is unaware of this measurement.
- Obtain a resting BP after a 5-minute rest period.
- Place the cuff on the patient's arm 2 to 4 cm above the antecubital area.
- Palpate the brachial artery (medial to the biceps tendon).
- Place the diaphragm of the stethoscope over the brachial artery.

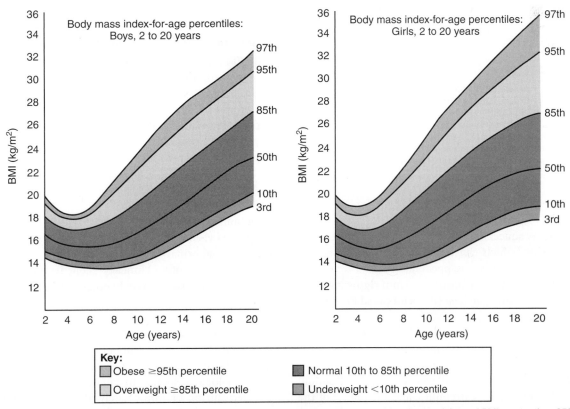

FIGURE 11-2 Body mass index (BMI) for girls and boys 2 to 20 years old. BMI greater than 85% is considered overweight, and BMI greater than 95% is considered obese.

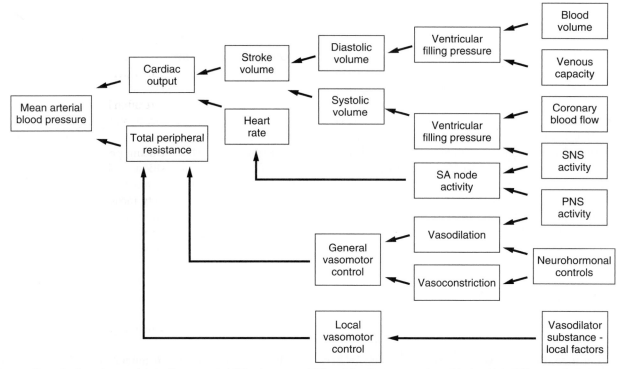

FIGURE 11-3 Cascade of events associated with mean arterial blood pressure. *PNS,* peripheral nervous system; *SA,* sinoatrial; *SNS,* sympathetic nervous system.

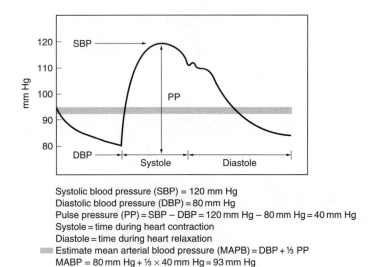

Systolic blood pressure (SBP) = 120 mm Hg
Diastolic blood pressure (DBP) = 80 mm Hg
Pulse pressure (PP) = SBP – DBP = 120 mm Hg – 80 mm Hg = 40 mm Hg
Systole = time during heart contraction
Diastole = time during heart relaxation
Estimate mean arterial blood pressure (MAPB) = DBP + ⅓ PP
MABP = 80 mm Hg + ⅓ × 40 mm Hg = 93 mm Hg

FIGURE 11-4 Example of estimation of mean arterial blood pressure.

- Inflate the cuff by squeezing the pressure bulb to greater than the patient's SBP (which can be assessed by palpating the radial artery until the pulse disappears).
- Reduce the cuff pressure at a rate of 2 to 3 mm Hg/heartbeat.[30]
- Listen for the first sound you hear (the bruit called *Korotkoff 1,* considered SBP).
- Listen for the sound to continue (*Korotkoff 2 to 4*).
- Listen for the last sound (DBP, or *Korotkoff 5*).
- Express BP in even numbers (e.g., 136/92 mm Hg).
- If this is the first time assessing BP in a patient, the BP should be assessed in both upper extremities, and the higher of the two pressures should be used in subsequent pressure measurements (denoted by *R* or *L*).

Common Errors in Measuring Blood Pressure

Table 11-2 lists common errors in BP determination. The most common errors include use of an inappropriate cuff size, inability to hear the bruits (e.g, listening through clothing, stethoscope is placed in the ears incorrectly, stethoscope is not correctly set for diaphragm), and an uncalibrated aneroid sphygmomanometer.[3,8,9,41]

When Blood Pressure Should Be Assessed

RESTING. Resting BP should be assessed during the systems review portion of the examination. Because a large percentage of the population has hypertension that usually occurs without symptoms (the "silent killer"), resting BP should be assessed with all new patients. BP should also be assessed if a patient has any of the symptoms of hypertension or hypotension. Signs of hypertension include the following[18]:
- Headache (usually occipital and present in the morning)
- Vertigo (dizziness)
- Flushed face
- Spontaneous epistaxis (nosebleed)
- Blurred vision
- Nocturnal urinary frequency

Hypertension is often clinically silent in the early and middle stages of the disease. Signs of hypotension include the following[18]:
- Lightheadedness
- Syncope
- Mental or visual blurring
- Sense of weakness or "rubbery" legs

ACTIVITY. BP can also be used as an objective assessment of physiologic response to changes in activity.[15] BP may be assessed during or immediately after the activity. With every metabolic equivalent increase in activity, SBP should increase by 8.5 ± 1.5 mm Hg. DBP should remain the same or decrease with

Blood pressure

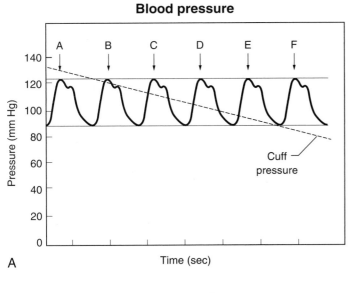

A

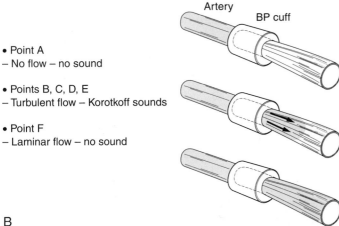

B

FIGURE 11-5 Assessment of blood pressure. **A,** Relationship of systolic blood pressure to cuff pressure. **B,** Indirect assessment of blood pressure auscultating over a normal artery. *BP cuff,* blood pressure cuff.

- Point A
  – No flow – no sound

- Points B, C, D, E
  – Turbulent flow – Korotkoff sounds

- Point F
  – Laminar flow – no sound

activity.[47] Changes in BP can also serve as an objective outcome measure of the effectiveness of interventions such as aerobic exercise training. Prolonged aerobic training has been associated with a reduction in BP at rest and during submaximal exertion. Guidelines indicate that activity of moderate intensity (40% to 60% oxygen consumption reserve or walking briskly) performed more than 30 minutes on most, if not all, days of the week leads to a significant reduction in BP.[42]

MEDICAL CONSULTATION OR EMERGENCY SITUATION. BP can also be used to distinguish between a medical emergency (calling a code or dialing 911) and a suggested medical consultation. With a high BP (e.g., 180/98 mm Hg), the PT can ask the patient whether he or she could contact the patient's physician to set up an appointment or ensure that the patient contacts his or her physician. If the patient agrees, the PT should contact the physician. If the patient does not want the PT to contact the physician, the PT can educate the patient about the potential consequences of high BP and document the educational intervention. A medical emergency would include (1) no BP or an extremely low BP in which a lack of normal mentation or unconsciousness exists and (2) an elevated BP greater than 200/110 mm Hg at rest.

RELIABILITY AND VALIDITY OF BLOOD PRESSURE MEASUREMENT. The validity of BP measurements is determined by comparing values obtained with direct (gold standard) and indirect techniques. Measurements of resting BP vary from 3 to 24.6 mm Hg.[3,8,9,15,30] Resting BP taken by a trained person is usually within 3 to 5 mm Hg for SBP and 5 mm Hg for DBP. Measurements of BP during exercise or activity are often less valid and reliable. When comparing direct and indirect methods on a cycle ergometer, SBP levels of −2.3 to 12.9 mm Hg and DBP levels of −4.3 to 18.2 mm Hg were found.[20,52] During peak anaerobic activity, direct and indirect measures of SBP were found to be highly correlated ($r = 0.87$; direct, 197 ± 11 mm Hg; indirect, 191 ± 9 mm Hg). During peak anaerobic activity, measures of DBP were found to be invalid.[21,48] After exercise, BP decreases precipitously (in healthy individuals) and may not reflect actual BP during the activity. (Griffin and colleagues[19] provide a good review of this topic.)

RESTING BLOOD PRESSURE VALUES (NORMAL AND ABNORMAL). Normal resting SBP and DBP ranges are determined by age. Table 11-3 lists normal and elevated pressure ranges for children, young adults, and adults. Table 11-4 lists the ranges of resting BP for optimal; normal; high normal; and hypertension stages 1, 2, and 3 in adults.

VALUES THAT MAY CONTRAINDICATE ACTIVITY OR REQUIRE TERMINATION OF ACTIVITY. BP values that contradict initiating activity vary by practice setting. Guidelines from the American College of Sports Medicine (ACSM)[1] suggest exercise testing is contraindicated for individuals whose resting SBP is greater than 200 mm Hg or less than 80 mm Hg and DBP is greater than 100 mm Hg. In some practice settings, such as the coronary care unit, where PTs work with patients immediately after myocardial infarction, these critical BP values would be significantly less than those suggested by the ACSM, whereas after a stroke, BP recommendations might be significantly higher (to increase cerebral perfusion pressure). Termination of exercise is warranted with an increase in SBP to greater than 250 mm Hg or DBP greater than 110 mm Hg. Because SBP during activity increases above resting values, a decrease in SBP by more than 10 to 20 mm Hg with maintenance or increase of activity or increasing the load of activity is another reason to terminate activity. Depending on the type of patient and practice setting, ACSM guidelines may need to be modified.

OTHER EXAMPLES OF BLOOD PRESSURE MEASUREMENT. The ankle-brachial index (ABI) is a useful means of assessing the likelihood of peripheral arterial vascular disease. Peripheral arterial vascular disease is caused primarily by atherosclerosis (deposition of fibrous fatty plaque in the lining layer [intima] of the artery). Arteries of the lower extremities that are commonly affected include the iliac, femoral, and popliteal. With the patient in the supine position, the SBP is measured in all four extremities. In the upper extremities the SBP is measured at the level of the heart (brachial pressure). In the lower extremities, the SBP is measured in either the posterior tibial artery or the dorsalis pedis artery. The ABI is calculated by dividing each ankle pressure by the highest brachial pressure (Figure 11-6). ABI measurements less than 0.96 are considered abnormal, with lower values representing worsening of the disease (Box 11-3).

If ABI is less than 0.8, or the mean of three readings is less than 0.9, the predictive validity of the patient having significantly altered vessel lumen (e.g., peripheral vascular disease) is 95% as

TABLE 11-2
Common Problems in Measuring Blood Pressure

Problem	Result	Recommendation
EQUIPMENT		
Stethoscope		
Earpieces plugged	Poor sound transmission	Clean earpieces
Earpieces poorly fitting	Distorted sounds	Angle earpieces forward
Bell or diaphragm cracked	Distorted sounds	Replace equipment
Tubing too long	Distorted sounds	Length from earpieces to bell should be 30-38 cm (12-15 inches)
Aneroid Manometer		
Needle not at 0 at rest	Inaccurate reading	Recalibrate
BLADDER CUFF		
Too narrow for arm	Blood pressure too high	Use cuff length 80% of circumference
Too wide for arm	Unable to fit on arm	Use regular but longer cuff
Inflation System		
Faulty valves	Inaccurate reading	Replace equipment
	Difficulty inflating and deflating bladder	
Leaky tubing or bulb	Inaccurate reading	Replace equipment
Observer		
Digit preference	Inaccurate reading	Be aware of tendency; record blood pressure to nearest 2 mm Hg
Cutoff bias	Inaccurate reading	Record to nearest 2 mm Hg
Direction bias	Inaccurate reading	Record to nearest 2 mm Hg
Fatigue or poor memory	Inaccurate reading	Write down reading immediately
Subject		
Arm below heart level	Reading too high	Place patient with midpoint of upper arm at heart level
Arm above heart level	Reading too low	Place patient with midpoint of upper arm at heart level
Back unsupported	Reading too high	Avoid isometric exercise during measurement
Legs dangling	Reading too high	Avoid isometric exercise during measurement
Dysrhythmia	Blood pressure level variable	Take multiple measurements and average
Large or muscular arm	Reading too high	Use appropriate cuff size
Calcified arteries	Reading too high	Note presence of positive Osler's sign in record
TECHNIQUE		
Cuff		
Wrapped too loosely	Reading too high	Rewrap more snugly
Applied over clothing	Inaccurate reading	Remove arm from sleeve
Manometer		
Below eye level	Reading too low	Place manometer at eye level
Above eye level	Reading too high	Place manometer at eye level
Stethoscope Head		
Not in contact with skin	Extraneous noise	Place head correctly
Applied too firmly	Diastolic reading too low	Place head correctly
Not over artery	Sounds not well heard	Place head over palpated artery
Touching tubing or cuff	Extraneous noise	Place below edge of cuff
Palpatory pressure omitted	Danger of missing auscultatory gap	Routinely check systolic pressure by palpation first
	Underestimation of systolic pressure	
Inflation level too high	Patient discomfort	Inflate to 30 mm Hg above palpatory blood pressure
Inflation level too low	Underestimation of systolic pressure	Inflate to 30 mm Hg above palpatory blood pressure
Inflation rate too slow	Patient discomfort	Inflate at even rate
	Diastolic pressure too high	

TABLE 11-2

Common Problems in Measuring Blood Pressure—cont'd

Problem	Result	Recommendation
Stethoscope Head—cont'd		
Deflation rate too fast	Systolic pressure too low	Deflate at 2 mm Hg/sec or 2 mm Hg/beat
	Diastolic pressure too high	
Deflation rate too slow	Forearm congestion	Deflate at 2 mm Hg/sec or 2 mm Hg/beat
	Diastolic pressure too high	Completely deflate cuff at end of measurement

Note: In patients in whom Korotkoff sounds are faint and difficult to hear, the following technique may help: Have the subject raise the arm over the head and make a fist several times. Inflate the cuff to 50 mm Hg above expected systolic level while the arm is still overhead but the hand is relaxed. Have the patient lower the arm rapidly and measure the blood pressure in the usual manner. Draining the venous blood in this fashion often amplifies the Korotkoff sounds and makes weak sounds, particularly diastolic sounds, more audible.

Modified from Perloff D, Grim C, Flack J, et al: Human blood pressure determination by sphygmomanometry, *Circulation* 88(5 pt 1):2460-2470, 1993.

TABLE 11-3

Normal Ranges for Blood Pressure by Patient Age

	Age (yr)	SYSTOLIC (mm Hg)		DIASTOLIC (Mm Hg)	
		Maximum	Minimum	Maximum	Minimum
Children	3-6	116	80	76	50
	6-9	122	84	78	55
Young adults	10-13	126	90	82	55
	14-19	142	90	86	60
Adults	20-60	150	90	90	60
	>60	160	90	95	60

From Blumenthal S: Report on the Task Force on Blood Pressure Control in Children, *Pediatrics* 59(suppl):797, 1977; and The 1988 Report of the Joint National Committee on Detection, Evaluation, and Treatment of High Blood Pressure, *Arch Intern Med* 148:1023-1038, 1988.

TABLE 11-4

Classification of Blood Pressure for Adults 18 Years or Older[*][†]

Category	Systolic (mm Hg)		Diastolic (mm Hg)
Optimal[‡]	<120	*and*	>80
Normal	120-129	*and*	80-84
High normal	130-139	*or*	85-89
HYPERTENSION			
Stage 1	140-159	*or*	90-99
Stage 2	160-179	*or*	100-109
Stage 3	≥180	*or*	≥110

[*]Not taking antihypertensive drugs and not acutely ill. When systolic and diastolic blood pressure (BP) fall into different categories, the high category should be selected to classify the individual's BP status. In addition to classifying stages of hypertension based on average BP levels, clinicians should specify the presence or absence of target organ disease and additional risk factors. This specificity is important for risk classification and treatment.

[†]Based on the average of two or more BP readings taken at each of two or more visits after an initial screening.

[‡]Optimal BP regarding cardiovascular risk is <120/80 mm Hg. Unusually low readings should be evaluated for clinical significance, however.

Modified from The seventh report of the Joint National Committee on Prevention, Detection, Evaluation, and Treatment of High Blood Pressure, *JAMA* 289:2560-2572, 2003.

determined by angiography.[22,51] Conversely, if ABI is greater than 1.1, or the mean of three measurements is greater than 1, peripheral vascular disease can be ruled out 99% of the time.[22,51] SBP in the lower extremity is usually measured with a pocket Doppler; however, it may also be measured in the dorsalis pedis using a stethoscope.[23,38] The determination of an abnormal ABI should be followed by a systematic search to locate the vessel lesion (abnormality in tissue structure). The BP cuff is moved progressively up the lower extremity for subsequent segmental SBP measurements (Figure 11-7). Measurements taken below and above the knee help locate the lesion site, which is revealed by a significant change (>20 to 30 mm Hg) in SBP from one location to another.

Finally, measurements of segmental BP can be used to examine local blood flow. Adequate blood flow is a critical variable in wound healing. Healing of an arterial ulcer requires SBP more than 60 mm Hg for a patient without DM and greater than 80 mm Hg for a patient with DM.

Common Conditions Related to Blood Pressure and the Physical Therapist's Role

Orthostatic Hypotension

Often in clinical situations, patients report a symptom of lightheadedness on rising from supine to sitting or standing. This rapid change in body position causes blood to pool in the abdomen and lower extremities because of gravity. The resulting

Abnormal ABI

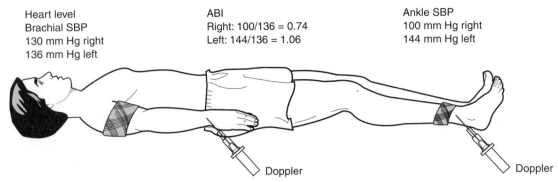

Heart level
Brachial SBP
130 mm Hg right
136 mm Hg left

ABI
Right: 100/136 = 0.74
Left: 144/136 = 1.06

Ankle SBP
100 mm Hg right
144 mm Hg left

Doppler   Doppler

FIGURE 11-6 Calculation of ankle-brachial index *(ABI)*. *SBP,* systolic blood pressure.

BOX 11-3

Ankle-Brachial Index Interpretation

>0.96	Normal
<0.95	Abnormal; stress testing is appropriate
<0.8	Probably claudication
<0.5	Multilevel disease of long segment occlusion
<0.3	Ischemic rest pain; possible tissue necrosis

From *Integrated ultrasound reference guide,* Plano, TX, 1996, Society of Diagnostic Medical Sonographers Education Foundation.

---

reduction in venous return leads to a reduced stroke volume and cardiac output and a lowering of the BP. This decrease in BP leads to a lack of activation of the baroreceptors. Reduced baroreceptor firing causes activation of the cardiorespiratory area of the medulla, which leads to an increased sympathetic discharge. This discharge may help increase BP by increasing total peripheral resistance, venous return and cardiac output, and HR. Sometimes the sympathetic compensation is not enough, and BP still decreases.

Reduction in BP by 10 to 20 mm Hg in either SBP or DBP or an increase in HR by 10 to 20 beats/min reveals orthostatic signs. Symptoms of orthostasis include lightheadedness, "rubbery legs," and feelings of syncope. HR and BP should be monitored in patients experiencing these symptoms when going from supine to sitting or standing. When a patient reports orthostatic symptoms, or orthostatic signs are revealed, the PT should have the patient sit or lie down. Performing "ankle pumps" while supine may help equilibrate pressures and facilitate successful standing on the next attempt. If orthostatic signs or symptoms persist, notifying other medical personnel is warranted, and standing activities should be discontinued.

Hypertension and Prehypertension

Hypertension can produce serious consequences, including the following:
- Stroke
- Myocardial infarction
- CHF
- Peripheral vascular disease
- Renal failure
- Blindness

In adults, hypertension at rest is defined as either SBP greater than 140 mm Hg or DBP greater than 90 mm Hg. Increasing grades of hypertension are shown in Table 11-4. If the pressures are high enough (e.g., >200/100 mm Hg), a single measure of BP is enough to diagnose hypertension. If the pressures are elevated only slightly (e.g., 146/92 mm Hg), three consecutive measures are needed to diagnose this borderline hypertension. After a diagnosis of hypertension, it is sometimes difficult to convince patients to comply with drug therapy. Hypertension usually occurs without symptoms, and medications often produce side effects. Although hypertension is usually clinically silent, some associated symptoms may include morning headache, dizziness, and blurred vision. The benefits of routine physical activity (a walking program) should be discussed with patients and their physicians. Although treatment, including dietary modifications, routine aerobic activities, weight loss, and medications, has been shown to reduce hypertension, this regimen has not yet become the standard of care.

New guidelines established by the National Institutes of Health have defined *prehypertension*.[10,24] This new diagnostic category establishes a population with a strong potential of becoming hypertensive. This category helps begin medical management with dietary alterations and increased activity level. People whose BP is more than 120/80 mm Hg fall into the prehypertensive range and should be counseled to increase their physical activity, reduce their weight (if increased), and reduce their salt intake.

Congestive Heart Failure: Jugular Venous Pressure, Palpation, and Engorgement

Right-sided CHF leads to elevated right atrial and systemic venous pressure (see Figure 11-1). If severe, the elevated pressure results in engorgement and distention of the jugular veins. Estimating jugular venous pressure has been shown to be an insensitive and nonspecific test for disease. When right atrial pressure increases to more than 15 mm Hg, the jugular vein distends, a reliable measure of heart failure if the person is known to have impaired heart function.[7] Other signs and symptoms associated with this increase in systemic venous pressure include increased fluid retention as evidenced by weight gain, dependent and pitting edema, and increased fatigue with activity.

Segmental BP

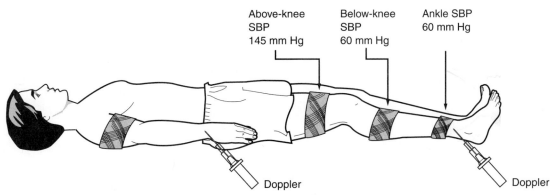

Above-knee
SBP
145 mm Hg

Below-knee
SBP
60 mm Hg

Ankle SBP
60 mm Hg

Doppler

Doppler

FIGURE 11-7 Segmental blood pressure *(BP)* assessment. *SBP,* systolic blood pressure.

Pulse Palpation for Heart Rate, Rhythm, and Patency of Blood Vessels

The heart pumps blood to the lungs for the exchange of gases and to the body for distribution of oxygen, nutrients, and other vital components in blood. The amount of blood pumped by the heart per minute is referred to as *cardiac output* and is calculated by multiplying HR by stroke volume (see Figure 11-1). The rate and rhythm of blood pumped during myocardial contraction can be sensed by lightly placing the fingertips over the skin covering peripheral arteries (see Figure 11-1). As the myocardium contracts, a volume of blood is ejected from the left ventricle. The forward-rushing blood produces a pressure wave that extends from the aorta through the arterial system. This traveling pressure wave can be felt by the fingertips as a change in tension in the peripheral vessel. The rate and rhythm of the pressure wave are determined by the rate and rhythm of myocardial contractions.

The strength of the peripheral pulse is determined by the difference between SBP and DBP (pulse pressure) and the elasticity of the blood vessels. Pulse pressure can vary from stroke volume (amount of blood ejected per beat) and the resistance to blood flow. With increased filling time, blood volume, or strength of contraction, the stroke volume increases and the pulse becomes stronger. With increased vascular resistance, reduced stroke volume, or hypovolemia (reduced blood volume), there is a reduction in pulse strength.

Because of the electrophysiologic properties of the pacemaker cells of the heart (sinoatrial node and atrioventricular node), the rate and rhythm of myocardial contraction at rest are usually stable. HR increases or decreases in response to changes in energy demands, but rhythm usually remains regular because of the sinoatrial node. Box 11-4 lists factors affecting pulse and HR. Dysrhythmias (alterations in rate or rhythm) produce variations in the time of the myocardial contraction (interpulse interval). Unequal time in filling the heart increases the variation in stroke volume and pulse pressure. A delay in filling leads to a stronger pulse because of increased stroke volume and pulse pressure, and a shortened time of filling leads to a reduced stroke volume and pulse pressure and a weaker or missed pulse. Factors leading to dysrhythmias are presented in Box 11-5.

BOX 11-4
Factors Affecting Pulse Rate

- Age—increased in infants and decreased in adults >65 years
- Gender—male < female
- Environmental, core temperature, hydration
- Physical activity
- Emotional status
- Medications (beta-receptor blocker, calcium channel blocker, or beta-receptor stimulators), chemicals (caffeine), hormones (thyroid hormones)
- Pain
- Pathology—anemia, congestive heart failure, autonomic dysfunction (e.g., diabetes, spinal cord injury, fever)
- Physical condition

From Pierson F, Fairchild S: *Principles and techniques of patient care,* 3rd ed, Philadelphia, 2002, Saunders.

BOX 11-5
Causes of Dysrhythmias or Ectopic Pacemakers

- Ischemia/hypoxia of the myocardium
- Sympathetic discharge—anxiety, exercise
- Acidosis
- Alterations in electrolytes (primary ↓ K^+ <3.2 mEq/dL)
- Excessive stretch of the myocardium (e.g., congestive heart failure)
- Pharmacologic agents
  - Sympathomimetics—caffeine
  - Antiarrhythmic drugs
  - Digitalis

How to Measure the Pulse

The pulse can be measured wherever the artery is large enough and close enough to the body surface to be felt with the fingertips. Common sites for pulse palpation include the radial, brachial, carotid, femoral, temporal, popliteal, and posterior tibial arteries. The examiner lightly palpates in the appropriate area for a change in tension. It is recommended that the examiner palpate with the second, third, or fourth digit of the dominant hand. The thumb is a less desirable digit for palpation because it has a particularly strong pulse of its own that sometimes interferes with accurately assessing the patient's pulse.[26,30,44]

Pulse Assessment Scales

PULSE 0-4 SCALE*

0	Absent pulse
1	Markedly reduced pulse
2	Slightly reduced pulse
3	Normal pulse
4	Bounding pulse

PULSE 0-3 SCALE†

0	Absent
1	Weak, thready
2	Normal
3	Full, bounding

*Greenberger NJ, Hinthorn DR: *History taking and physical examination,* St Louis, 1993, Mosby.

†Jarvis C: *Examination and health assessment,* Philadelphia, 1992, Saunders.

Terms commonly used to describe pulse strength include *bounding* or *full* when the pulse is strong and *thready* or *weak* when the pulse volume is reduced. Pulse strength can also be quantified with a pulse scale. Two pulse scales are shown in Box 11-6. To date, no validity or reliability studies have been performed with these scales. The rhythm of the pulse is often classified into one of the following three categories:
1. *Regular*—similar rate (equal interpulse intervals) and volume (e.g., normal sinus rhythm or sinus tachycardia)
2. *Regularly irregular*—the periodic nature of the irregularity comes at a specific time (interpulse intervals are unequal, but the pattern is periodic and stable), such as bigeminy (one normal, one abnormal heart contraction) or trigeminy (two normal and one abnormal heart contraction)
3. *Irregularly irregular*—no specific pattern, and rate and volume vary widely (interpulse intervals are unequal, and the pattern is unstable), such as atrial fibrillation or multiple premature ventricular contractions not in a row or sequence

Common Errors in Palpating the Pulse

When palpating for HR and rhythm, the most common problem is examiner error. The inability to locate a pulse can be caused by anatomic variation, but more often the examiner's fingers are placed in the wrong area or are pressing too strongly. Box 11-7 lists common causes of false-positive or false-negative results when assessing pulse rate and rhythm. When a patient has a dysrhythmia, such as atrial fibrillation or a premature beat, a pulse deficit may be found. The pulse deficit is the difference between the number of heart contractions and the HR as determined by pulse palpation. The mechanism is shown in Figures 11-8 and 11-9. If the heart contracts before the left ventricle has filled completely because of changes in filling time, the volume of blood ejected (and the pulse pressure) is reduced. The weakened pulse pressure may be below threshold by the time the pressure wave has traveled down the vascular system to the point where the examiner is palpating, causing the examiner to miss feeling the beat. When a person has an irregularly irregular pulse, HR should be determined by electrocardiogram (ECG) or auscultation (listening to the heart [apical pulse] with a stethoscope).[50]

Potential Errors in Pulse Assessment

FALSE-POSITIVE ERRORS
- Anorexia
- Examiner error (e.g., examiner's digital pulse)

FALSE-NEGATIVE ERRORS
- Obesity
- Edema
- Scar tissue
- Thickened skin
- Examiner error (e.g., palpation in wrong area)

When Heart Rate Should Be Assessed

RESTING HEART RATE. HR should be assessed during the systems review in all patients at an initial visit. HR is an objective, indirect measure of the status or condition of the cardiovascular system. Baseline measurements should be taken only after a 2- to 5-minute rest period (sitting or reclining). The rest period ensures baseline metabolic conditions. Table 11-5 lists normal resting values of HR by age. A 15- to 30-second monitoring period should be used to determine resting HR.[30]

HEART RATE DURING ACTIVITY. During activity, HR is an objective, indirect measure of work intensity. HR responds to changes in workload in a linear fashion. Exercise HR should be assessed with a 10-second monitoring period because of the rapid decline in HR with cessation of the activity.[44] During training, HR should be assessed to ensure training intensity is within the guidelines set forth by the American Heart Association (target HR) or ACSM for specific conditions. One effect of prolonged aerobic training (weeks to months) is a reduction in HR under resting and submaximal working conditions. HR can serve as an outcome measure indicating the effectiveness of long-term aerobic training.

Target HR as a measure of exercise intensity must be used in reference to some expected maximal value. In the healthy, normal population, maximal HR can be estimated by subtracting the subject's age from 220. Newer calculations are also available and may improve the prediction of maximal HR.[25] This estimate should not be used in patients with underlying pathologic conditions or patients taking medications that affect HR (e.g., beta blockers, calcium channel blockers).

EMERGENCY SITUATIONS. HR should be assessed in an emergency situation. The HR may differentiate "calling a code" in a hospital situation or dialing 911 in an outpatient setting from merely initiating a medical consultation (a dysrhythmia is found without significant symptoms). When signs or symptoms of circulatory decompensation arise in a patient (Box 11-8), palpation of the pulse is useful but is neither sensitive nor specific. Auscultation of the heart may often aid in determining HR in patients with a weak or irregular pulse. Clinical vascular testing with a Doppler device can be useful for assessing patency of the arteries. This procedure may also be coupled with a sphygmomanometer for determining SBP.

VALIDITY OF MEASUREMENT. The gold standard for determining HR is an ECG. HR should be assessed as an objective measure of resting metabolic activity. At rest, palpation measurement of

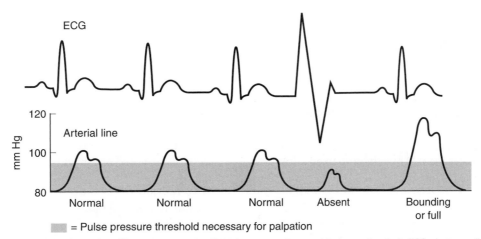

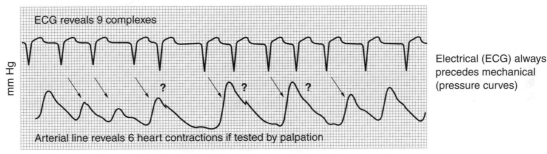

FIGURE 11-8 Palpating pulse with premature contractions (e.g., premature ventricular contraction). *ECG,* electrocardiogram.

FIGURE 11-9 Pulse "inaccuracy" deficit. *ECG,* electrocardiogram.

HR performed by trained personnel can vary by 3 to 5 beats/min compared with the gold standard. During activity, palpation measurement of HR performed by trained personnel can vary by 3 to 10 beats/min compared with the gold standard. The validity of exercise HR requires the measurement to be taken quickly and immediately after the cessation of activity because HR decreases precipitously after exercise in a healthy person.[30,39]

Common Conditions Related to Heart Rate and Rhythm and the Physical Therapist's Role

Dysrhythmias

The PT may be the first health care practitioner to assess the patient's HR and rhythm at rest and during activity. Dysrhythmias can be an alteration in HR or rhythm. Many dysrhythmias are common and of little concern under certain circumstances. Sinus tachycardia (HR >100 beats/min) is usual in a person performing physical activity or in an infant at rest. Sinus tachycardia at rest can be abnormal in a healthy person without any other contributing factors. Sinus bradycardia (HR <60 beats/min) is normal in a well-trained aerobic athlete or in a patient taking beta-receptor–blocking medication. Consequently, sinus bradycardia of 45 beats/min in an individual who is 65 years old and not in good shape or taking medications that affect HR can be an ominous sign.

A sudden change in HR (>20 to 40 beats/min), either an increase or a decrease, at rest or during activity may be a signal of an ectopic pacemaker or conduction abnormality. A patient's resting HR that is 76 beats/min and suddenly increases to 166 beats/min without any physiologic or psychological stress is abnormal. Likewise, a sudden decline in HR with maintained or increasing activity is also abnormal. Changes in rhythm can also be either a normal response to changes in workload or a life-threatening malfunction in cardiac regulation.

In general, if a patient has a normal sinus rhythm and the heart rhythm suddenly becomes irregular, the patient should be asked whether he or she has a history of cardiac dysrhythmia and be monitored for signs and symptoms of cardiac decompensation. If the patient is not showing signs or symptoms of cardiac decompensation, referral to a physician is warranted. Usually more than six abnormal beats in 1 minute, such as with premature ventricular contractions (the most common type of ectopic beat), requires medical attention. Depending on the severity of the symptoms caused by the dysrhythmia, if the patient shows signs of severe cardiac compromise (see Box 11-8), this may be a medical emergency. If there is no pulse, calling a code or dialing 911 and starting cardiopulmonary resuscitation (CPR) are necessary. If a patient is known to have a dysrhythmia, accurate HR measurement is determined by ECG or auscultation.[15,33]

Ventilatory Rate and Rhythm

The ventilatory musculature pumps air into and out of the lungs for the exchange of gases (oxygen and carbon dioxide). The amount of air moved by the lungs per minute is referred to as *minute ventilation* and is calculated by multiplying ventilatory rate by tidal volume (see Figure 11-1). The rate and rhythm of air moved during ventilation can be sensed by observing the chest rise and fall in correlation to time. Normal rate for an adult is 12 to 20 breaths/min. Normal tidal volume in an adult is approximately 500 mL, with expiration being twice as long as inspiration. Tidal volume can be greater or less depending on body size. Observing the rate, volume, and rhythm is necessary during the systems review in the pulmonary screen. Terms to describe ventilatory rate and rhythm or breathing patterns include the following[15]:

- *Apnea*—no breathing
- *Tachypnea*—rate greater than 20 breaths/min in an adult
- *Bradypnea*—rate less than 12 breaths/min in an adult
- *Hyperpnea*—normal rate but increased volume
- *Hypopnea*—normal rate but decreased volume
- *Hyperventilation*—increased rate and volume
- *Hypoventilation*—decreased rate and volume
- *Cheyne-Stokes*—hyperventilation followed by hypoventilation, then apnea, with the cycle repeating
- *Orthopnea*—difficulty breathing while horizontal, with easing of breathing with more vertical positioning
- *Dyspnea*—labored or difficult breathing

How to Measure Ventilation

Ventilation is observed by watching the chest rise and fall in relation to time. Usually this is assessed in a 30-second to 1-minute time interval. Because ventilation is under involuntary and voluntary control, awareness by the patient of the PT's observation may cause ventilation to be modified from the usual resting pattern. A trick that is often used is to appear as though taking a pulse measurement but actually to observe the rise and fall of the chest.[30,36] Shallow breathing also makes this assessment more difficult. Ventilatory rate and rhythm should be assessed on the first patient visit during the systems review portion of the examination. If the patient reveals any abnormality in ventilatory rate or rhythm, further examination (auscultation and examination of symptoms) is required.[6]

VALIDITY OF MEASUREMENT. A study performed on nurses assessing ventilatory rate revealed a 20% error by the nurses one third of the time.[32] Another study on interobserver reliability in physicians, nurses, and respiratory therapists revealed an excellent kappa value when observing children who were being extubated.[27]

Resting Values (Normal and Abnormal)

Normal resting values for breathing rate change with age. See Table 11-6 for normal values by age.

Activity Values

With activity, ventilatory rate and volume increase to supply the needed oxygen to the active tissues and remove synthesized carbon dioxide. The more strenuous the activity, the greater

---

TABLE 11-5
Resting Pulse Rate

	NORMS	
	Average (beats/min)	Limits
Fetal	120-160	—
Newborn	120	70-190
1 yr	120	80-160
2 yr	110	80-130
4 yr	100	80-120
6 yr	100	75-115
8-10 yr	90	70-110
12 YR		
Girls	90	70-110
Boys	85	65-105
14 YR		
Girls	85	65-105
Boys	80	60-100
16 YR		
Girls	80	60-100
Boys	75	55-95
18 YR+		
Women	75	55-95
Men	70	50-90
Well-conditioned athlete	50-60	50-100
Adult	—	60-100
Aging	—	60-100

Adapted from Jarvis C: *Physical examination and assessment,* Philadelphia, 1992, Saunders, p 202.

BOX 11-8
Classic Cardiac Symptoms and Signs of Decompensation

Symptoms	Signs
Angina	Dysrhythmias
Palpitations	Syncope
Dyspnea or shortness of breath	Dyspnea or shortness of breath (using scale)
Fatigue	Dependent edema
	Hemoptysis (coughing blood)
	Cyanosis

Adapted from Swartz MH: *Textbook of physical diagnosis: history and examination,* 4th ed, Philadelphia, 2002, Saunders, pp 345-390.

TABLE 11-6
Normal Resting Respiratory Rates

Age	Breaths/min
Neonate	30-40
1 yr	20-40
2 yr	25-32
4 yr	23-30
6 yr	21-26
8-10 yr	20-26
12-14 yr	18-22
16 yr	16-20
18 yr	12-20
Adult	10-20

Adapted from Jarvis C: *Physical examination and assessment,* Philadelphia, 1992, Saunders, p 203.

the oxygen demand. When a person is performing an activity that is above his or her anaerobic/ventilatory threshold, lactic acid begins accumulating in muscles and produces metabolic acidosis. The normal ventilatory response is to increase ventilatory depth and rate (hyperventilation leading to a respiratory alkalosis in an attempt to balance the lowered pH). The inability to converse during exercise is an indirect measure that the performer has reached anaerobic/ventilatory threshold. Anaerobic threshold decreases with deconditioning such that severely deconditioned patients may reach anaerobic threshold and become unable to hold a conversation during slow ambulation down the hallway.

Values that May Contraindicate Activity or Require Termination of Activity

ACSM[1] recommends not performing an endurance test if the patient's resting respiratory rate is more than 45 breaths/min. If the patient reports dyspnea with activity, the Ranchos Los Amigos Physical Therapy Department recommends the following tool to quantify the level of involvement. The patient is asked to inhale normally and then count to 15 aloud over a 7.5- to 8-second time period:

Level 0: on a single breath
Level 1: requires two breaths
Level 2: requires three breaths
Level 3: requires four breaths
Level 4: unable to count

If the dyspnea is severe enough or a new onset, this may be a reason to decrease or stop activity level. For patients with chest discomfort, see the questions outlined in Box 11-9.

Another dyspnea scale that has been validated in patients with chronic obstructive pulmonary disease is the Borg Dyspnea Scale[35]:

0	Nothing at all
0.5	Very, very slight (just noticeable)
1	Very slight
2	Slight (light)
3	Moderate
4	Somewhat severe
5	Severe
6	
7	Very severe
8	
9	
10	Very, very severe (almost maximal)
*	Maximal

Measures of Oxygen Delivery

Oxygen saturation (Sao_2), or pulse oxygen, is a useful measurement to assess the adequacy of ventilation. Pulse oxygen reveals the saturation of oxygen on hemoglobin contained in arterial blood erythrocytes (red blood cells). This measurement tells one piece of the oxygen delivery equation: the percentage of oxygen on hemoglobin. To get the full picture of oxygen delivery, the patient's hematocrit and hemoglobin levels must also be known. A patient may have normal oxygen saturation, but if he or she is anemic, the delivery of oxygen to tissue can be impaired. Normal values for oxygen saturation are 90% to 100% in systemic arterial blood. If a patient has *no known lung pathology* and an oxygen saturation of less than 90%, the PT needs to do the following:

- Stop performing any physical activity
- Check that the device is on properly
- Retake the measurement with the patient being still
- Notify medical personnel, if the measurement is valid
- Continue to monitor the patient

BOX 11-9

Guidelines for Patients with Onset of Chest Pain or Discomfort

- Stop any activity and place patient in comfortable position (sitting or lying)
- Monitor vital signs
- Ask whether patient has been diagnosed with heart disease
- If *yes*, then
  - Ask whether this symptom is usual or different
  - Ask whether patient has medication (e.g., nitroglycerin)
  - Allow administration of three tablets in a 10-minute period, and if symptoms do not resolve, get patient to emergency department or seek medical attention
- If *no*, then
  - Ask patient to describe discomfort
  - Ask what precipitated discomfort
  - Ask whether discomfort is getting worse or better
  - If signs and symptoms improve and do not appear to be musculoskeletal (movement or revealed by palpation) in origin, have patient see his or her physician
  - If signs and symptoms are worsening, get patient to the emergency department
- Assess for common changes in vital signs with chest discomfort from coronary artery disease
  - Pulse may change from normal sinus rhythm to dysrhythmia (ischemia of heart cells leads to overexcitability and ectopic pacemakers), causing pulse to change in rhythm
  - Pulse rate may increase (anxiety and pain) or decrease (damage to pacemaker cells)
  - Blood pressure may increase (anxiety and pain) or decrease (damage to myocardium)
  - Ventilatory rate usually increases (anxiety and pain) with tidal volume declining (anxiety and pain)

- Auscultate heart for changes in rate, rhythm, or sound (S_3)
- Ask whether patient has been diagnosed with lung disease
- If *yes*, then
  - Ask whether this symptom is usual or different
  - Ask whether patient has medication (inhaler)
  - Allow use of inhaler and see whether symptoms resolve. If symptoms do not resolve and are worsening, get patient to emergency department or seek medical attention
- If *no*, then
  - Ask patient to describe the discomfort
  - Ask what precipitated the discomfort
  - Ask whether discomfort is getting worse or better
  - If signs and symptoms are improving and do not appear to be musculoskeletal (movement or revealed by palpation) in origin, have patient see his or her physician
  - If signs and symptoms are worsening, get patient to emergency department
- Assess for common changes in vital signs with chest discomfort from lung disease
  - Ventilatory rate usually increases when tidal volume increases
  - Pulse rate usually increases
  - Blood pressure may increase (anxiety and pain) or decrease (lack of normal blood flow through lungs or retention of CO_2, which is a potent vasodilator)
  - Auscultate lung for changes in ventilatory sounds (crackles, wheezes, lack of normal ventilation)

If the patient has known lung disease, a resting value of less than 90% is often found. PTs should stop activity if SaO_2 decreases by 5% below resting value or is less than 88% in patients with right-sided heart failure (cor pulmonale). Patients with lung disease should not have a resting SaO_2 of less than 80%. Patients whose lung disease causes SaO_2 to be less than 88% usually receive supplemental oxygen. Depending on state laws, it is often advisable when performing activity to increase the patient's flow of oxygen to maintain oxygen saturation if needed. Maximal flow rate with a nasal cannula cannot exceed 6 L/min O_2. The PT must remember to lower the oxygen flow level back to the normal flow when activity has ended.

Auscultation of the Heart and Lungs

Differentiating the various heart and lung sounds that accompany disorders or pathologic conditions requires skill beyond reading this text. When compared with a gold standard, even physicians who are trained in this skill are often no better than chance at detecting true abnormalities in heart and lung sounds.[34,40] PTs should familiarize themselves with normal heart and lung sounds. The ability to differentiate abnormal from normal sounds is an important first step in using auscultation to detect pathologic conditions. Differentiating the type of pathologic feature is beyond the scope of physical therapy practice. Some PTs are skilled in auscultation, particularly PTs who have received specialized training or practice in settings that use these techniques.

Using a Stethoscope

The head of a stethoscope usually contains a bell and a diaphragm (Figure 11-10). The smaller diameter bell is more effective in discriminating low-frequency heart sounds (S_3), whereas the larger diameter diaphragm is more effective in discriminating high-frequency heart sounds (S_1 and S_2), BP, and lung sounds. The bell and diaphragm can be switched by rotating the head of the stethoscope. The price of the stethoscope is determined, in part, by the quality of the head and the sound transmission. Less expensive stethoscopes tend to have poorer quality sound resolution, and more expensive stethoscopes tend to have higher quality sound resolution. A shorter, thicker tube connecting the head of the stethoscope to comfortable, well-fitting earpieces aids in sound quality along with reduced environmental noises.

When a stethoscope is used for auscultation of either heart or lung sounds, proper anatomic placement is essential. Firmness of pressure of the stethoscope head onto the body is crucial. The pressure should be sufficient to ensure that the entire head of the scope (either diaphragm or bell) is in direct contact with the underlying skin. Excessive or inadequate pressure leads to extraneous noise and potential inaccuracy of measurement.

When to Measure Heart and Lung Sounds

Measurement of heart and lung sounds should occur in all patients with a history of chronic cardiac or pulmonary conditions or signs or symptoms of cardiopulmonary distress. Differentiation of normal sounds from abnormal should be a goal.

Normal Heart Sounds

The normal heart sound of "lub dub," or S_1 and S_2, is attributed to the vibrations caused by the closure of the heart valves. With the increased pressure caused by contraction of the heart muscle (systole), the right and left atrioventricular valves (commonly called the tricuspid [T_1] and mitral [M_1] valves) slam shut. This closing of the atrioventricular valves causes the S_1 heart sound, or the characteristic "lub." This is followed by the opening of the semilunar valves, which are the aortic and pulmonic valves. No heart sound occurs with the opening of normal valves. At the end of systole or the ejection phase of the contraction, the closing of the aortic and pulmonic valves causes the S_2 heart sound, or the characteristic "dub."

These sounds can be heard with varying intensity over different areas on the chest (Figure 11-11). Probably the best site

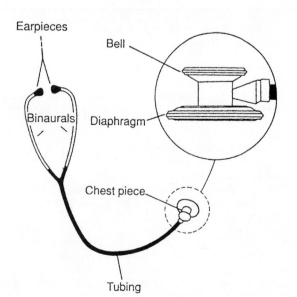

FIGURE 11-10 Components of a stethoscope. (From Boissonnault WG: *Examination in physical therapy practice: screening for medical disease,* 2nd ed, Philadelphia, 1995, Churchill Livingstone, p 76.)

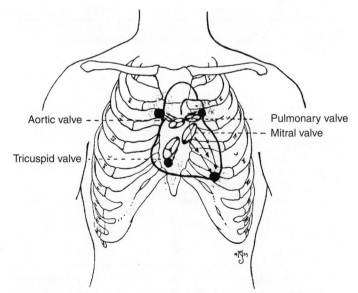

FIGURE 11-11 Anatomic location of heart valves and areas where sounds are best heard. (From Boissonnault WG: *Examination in physical therapy practice: screening for medical disease,* 2nd ed, Philadelphia, 1995, Churchill Livingstone, p 76; and Delp M, Manning R: *Major physical diagnosis,* 8th ed, Philadelphia, 1979, Saunders.)

for hearing S_1 and S_2 is the apex of the heart. With deep inhalation, the S_2 sound can be differentiated into two components, aortic (A_2) and pulmonic (P_2). Deep inhalation creates an interval between A_2 and P_2 because of basic cardiac physiologic characteristics. During deep inhalation, thoracic pressure is decreased. During the decreased thoracic pressure, venous return to the heart is increased. The increased venous return produces an increased filling of the right side of the heart. The increased venous return produces an increased stroke volume and delays the closure of the pulmonic valve, separating the A_2 and P_2 sounds. Depictions and recordings of these sounds may be found at http://blaufuss.org.

Abnormal Heart Sounds

Reliable detection of abnormal heart sounds requires considerable practice. Even with considerable experience, reliability and validity of measurement by physicians are limited.[34,40] Murmurs, S_3 or gallop, and pericardial friction are three frequently occurring abnormal heart sounds that PTs should be able to detect.

Murmurs are caused by abnormal vibrations through stenotic valves (narrowed opening), incompetent valves (leaky valves), high flow, or abnormal communication between blood vessels (e.g., patent ductus arteriosus) or heart chambers (ventricular septal defects). Murmurs can be divided into systolic, which produce a "lub-swish-dub" sound; diastolic, which produce a "lub-dub-swish" sound; and continuous, which produce a "lub-swish-dub-swish" sound. A stenotic aortic valve can produce a systolic murmur, whereas an incompetent aortic valve can produce a diastolic murmur. Detection of a murmur is based on a complete understanding of normal anatomy and physiologic characteristics of the heart and its valves. Depending on type and severity of murmur, certain types of physical activity might be contraindicated. If a patient is unaware of an existing murmur and the PT detects an abnormal heart sound, a medical consultation is in order. Signs and symptoms of moderate to severe murmurs may include cardiopulmonary compromise at rest or with increasing physical activity (see Box 11-8).

S_3, or gallop, is caused by an excessive amount of high-pressure blood from the atrium hitting a distended ventricular wall during diastole. The S_3 sound is found with either right-sided or left-sided CHF. This sound is normal in children and young adults until their 20s, but abnormal in adults older than 40 years. The mnemonic "Ken-tuk-ee" is often used to mimic the sound of S_3, which is often compared with a horse galloping. In patients with CHF, this sound may occur at rest or with increasing activity. S_3 can be accompanied by the symptoms of shortness of breath or dyspnea found with left-sided heart failure. Excessive physical activity is contraindicated when the S_3 sound is present.

The pericardial friction rub sound is caused by friction between the outer wall of the heart (epicardium or the visceral layer of the serous pericardium) and the pericardium (parietal layer of the serous pericardium) that occurs with pericarditis. Excessive physical activity is contraindicated with this sign because inflammation would be potentially worsened by increased HR and BP, causing more rubbing of the two surfaces. Examples of normal and abnormal heart sounds may be found at http://depts.washington.edu/physdx/heart/demo.html.

Normal Lung Sounds

Normal breath sounds occur because of the turbulence of air flow. This turbulence is related to the volume of air moving and the diameter of the lung passageways. The diameter of the lung passageways determines the resistance to the flow, which leads to the turbulence. Depending on the patient's position and anatomic location of assessment, auscultation of normal breath sounds varies. The three major normal breath sounds are as follows[44]:

1. *Vesicular sounds* are heard over the lung parenchyma, primarily alveoli or smaller air passageways. These sounds, heard primarily on inhalation, are described as "soft," with exhalation occurring without a break (continuous) and lasting only about a third of the inspiratory time. In a normal healthy person, vesicular sounds are heard with auscultation over the peripheral lung fields on the anterior, posterior, and lateral chest walls.

2. *Bronchial sounds* are heard over the trachea and major bronchi. These sounds are much louder than the vesicular breath sounds because of the large volume of air moving. They have a higher pitch and last for an equal time during inhalation and exhalation. There is a notable pause between inhalation and exhalation (discontinuous). In a normal healthy person, bronchial breath sounds are heard with auscultation over the trachea.

3. *Bronchovesicular sounds* are heard over the junction of the major bronchi as air moves into the smaller segmental bronchi. These sounds are similar to bronchial sounds but occur without any pause between inhalation and exhalation. In a normal healthy person, bronchovesicular breath sounds are heard with auscultation over the posterior chest wall (lateral to the thoracic spine) at the level of the scapula.

With various pathologic conditions, normal breath sounds may be heard in anatomic areas where they should not occur. Listening over the peripheral lung fields in a normal healthy person should reveal vesicular sounds. In the presence of a pathologic condition that causes consolidation within the lung (e.g., pneumonia, significant atelectasis), vesicular sounds are replaced by bronchial sounds in the peripheral lung fields. This is because with consolidation of the lung parenchyma, movement of air in the large airways is transmitted through the nonventilated consolidated areas.

Abnormal "Adventitious" Lung Sounds

The use of auscultation to detect abnormal breath sounds reliably requires considerable practice. PTs, despite practice and experience, have shown limited reliability and validity in using auscultation to detect abnormal breath sounds.[5,6] Abnormal or adventitious (extra) sounds are caused by pathologic alterations in the respiratory process. Because the reliable detection of abnormal breath sounds is difficult, PTs should begin by differentiating abnormal sounds from normal sounds. Three abnormal sounds are of particular importance: crackles, wheezes, and pleural friction rubs.

Crackles are a discontinuous "popping" sound most often heard during inhalation. During inhalation, crackles are caused by the reinflation of closed alveoli. Crackles may also occur

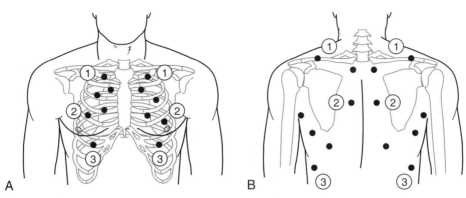

FIGURE 11-12 One method of auscultating the chest. **A,** Anterior chest wall. **B,** Posterior chest wall. (From Buckingham EB: *A primer of clinical diagnosis,* 2nd ed, New York, 1979, Harper & Row.)

TABLE 11-7

Guidelines for the Documentation and Interpretation of Auscultated Sounds

Type of Sound	Nomenclature	Interpretation
Breath sound	Normal	Normal, air-filled lung
	Decreased	Hyperinflation in chronic obstructive pulmonary disease
		Hypoinflation in acute lung disease (e.g., atelectasis, pneumothorax, pleural effusion)
	Absent	Pleural effusion Pneumothorax Severe hyperinflation Obesity
	Bronchial	Consolidation Atelectasis with adjacent patent airway
	Crackles	Secretions, if biphasic Deflation, if monophasic
	Wheezes	Diffuse airway obstruction if polyphonic; localized stenosis if monophonic
Extrapulmonary adventitious sounds	Pleural rub	Pleural inflammation or reaction
	Pericardial rub	Pericardial inflammation

Adapted from Irwin S, Tecklin JS: *Cardiopulmonary physical therapy,* 2nd ed, St Louis, 1990, Mosby, p 289.

during exhalation as air moves over the secretions present in pneumonia and CHF. Crackles are present in pathologic conditions that cause restriction or obstruction of the lung and during deep breathing in patients with atelectasis. Differentiating whether the crackle occurs during inhalation or exhalation helps with diagnostic categorization.

Wheezes are caused by the faster movement of turbulent air through narrowed passageways that may also contain secretions (mucus). Narrowed passageways with secretions lead to airway obstruction and trapping of air in the distal portions of the lung. Airway obstruction can be classically found with acute conditions such as asthma or chronic obstructive pulmonary disease. Wheezes are considered a continuous adventitious

sound that usually occur on exhalation and can be monophonic (single-frequency musical note) or polyphonic (multiple musical notes).

Pleural friction rub, as the name implies, occurs when the visceral and parietal layers of the pleural sac become inflamed (pleuritis) or thickened and rub against one another during movement of the chest wall. The friction between inflamed pleural tissues produces a lower pitched sound (compared with crackles) and may be heard during inhalation and exhalation.

Examination of lung sounds should follow a standardized procedure designed to compare the sounds heard from one lung with sounds heard from the other. The procedure should include examination of apical, mid, and lower lobes anteriorly and posteriorly. Examination results should be classified into major categories; their interpretation is shown in Figure 11-12. See Table 11-7 for a description of terms appropriate for documenting sounds and the interpretation of various sounds. Examples of normal and abnormal breath sounds may be found at http://www.wilkes.med.ucla.edu/lungintro.htm and http://www.rale.ca.

Common Conditions Related to Heart and Breath Sounds and the Physical Therapist's Role

Approximately 5 million Americans have CHF. The pharmacotherapeutic approach to managing this condition involves administration of iatrogenic agents that improve heart function, vasodilating agents that reduce the resistance to blood flow, and diuretics that reduce blood volume. Proper medical management can lead to a reduction of signs and symptoms of CHF. Physical activity is recommended for patients with all levels of CHF from mild to severe. CHF is a commonly seen comorbidity in the physical therapy clinic because it often accompanies the primary movement-related disorders for which patients are seen. Competent physical therapy management of patients with CHF requires knowledge of the condition, including signs and symptoms that the condition is becoming worse. If a patient with CHF reports increasing dyspnea, auscultation of the lungs may reveal crackles, and auscultation of the heart may reveal S_3 heart sound. Depending on the practice setting, either of these sounds may warrant a medical referral. If the sounds become worse, this may signal a medical emergency if signs and symptoms of cardiopulmonary compromise occur (see Box 11-8).

Summary

Physiologic measures of the cardiovascular and respiratory systems and measures of body composition are important because they reflect the patient's general health and wellness. BP, HR, and ventilatory rate provide a basic physiologic profile of the cardiovascular and pulmonary systems. Heart and lung sounds can help differentiate individuals with normal function from individuals with disease. BMI has been shown to be related to the risk of developing many of the diseases commonly seen in the physical therapy clinic—osteoarthritis, DM, myocardial infarction, stroke, and certain types of cancer.

Normal values and ranges have been established for these physiologic measures at rest and during activity for various age groups. Significant deviations from these norms may indicate an abnormal condition and are valuable in assessing the patient's risk of developing a disease or disorder. Establishing baseline measurements of vital signs and body composition is a central component of competent health care management. These measurements can be used to help ensure the safety of initiating an exercise program, establish intervention goals, assist in developing an intervention plan, and assess the individual's response to intervention (establish treatment effectiveness). The PT's ability to assess and interpret measures of these important physiologic parameters (vital signs) accurately at rest and during activity and recovery is an important clinical competency in an environment of increasingly independent physical therapy practice.

REFERENCES

1. ACSM guidelines for exercise testing and prescription. 8th ed. Philadelphia: American College of Sports Medicine, Lippincott Williams & Wilkins; 2009.
2. American Physical Therapy Association. Guide to physical therapy practice. 2nd ed. Phys Ther 2001;81:9–744.
2a. APTA House of Delegates. Physical fitness, wellness, and health definitions (BOD Y11-05-15-37). In: Guidelines, Policies, Procedures: Operational and Administrative. November 2009.
3. Bailey RH, Bauer JH. A review of common errors in the indirect measurement of blood pressure: sphygmomanometry. Arch Intern Med 1993;153:2741–8.
4. Bond Brill J, Perry AC, Parker L, et al. Dose-response effect of walking exercise on weight loss: how much is enough? Int J Obes Relat Metab Disord 2002;26:1484–93.
5. Brooks D, Wilson L, Kelsey C. Accuracy and reliability of "specialized" physical therapists in auscultating tape-recorded lung sounds. Physiother Can 1993;45:21–4.
6. Brooks D, Thomas J. Interrater reliability of auscultation of breath sounds among physical therapists. Phys Ther 1995;75:1082–8.
7. Butman SM, Ewy GA, Standen JR, et al. Bedside cardiovascular examination in patients with severe chronic heart failure: importance of rest or inducible jugular venous distension. J Am Coll Cardiol 1993;22:968–74.
8. Campbell NR, Chockalingam A, Fodor JG, et al. Accurate, reproducible measurement of blood pressure. Can Med Assoc J 1990;143:19–24.
9. Campbell NR, McKay DW. Accurate blood pressure measurement: why does it matter? Can Med Assoc J 1999;161:277–8.
10. Chobanian AV, et al. National Heart, Lung, and Blood Institute Joint National Committee on Prevention, Detection, Evaluation, and Treatment of High Blood Pressure; National High Blood Pressure Education Program Coordinating Committee: The seventh report of the Joint National Committee on Prevention, Detection, Evaluation, and Treatment of High Blood Pressure: the JNC 7 report. JAMA 2003;289:2560–72.
11. Christian K, Roberts C, Nosratola D, et al. Effect of diet and exercise intervention on blood pressure, insulin, oxidative stress and nitric oxide availability. Circulation 2002;106:2530.
12. Clinical guidelines on the identification, evaluation, and treatment of overweight and obesity in adults (website), http://www.nhlbi.nih.gov/guidelines/obesity/ob_home.htm. Accessed August 10, 2009.
13. Di Loreto C, Fanelli C, Lucidi P, et al. Make your diabetic patients walk: long-term impact of different amounts of physical activity on type 2 diabetes. Diabetes Care 2005;28:1524–5.
14. Donnelly JE, Blair SN, Jakicic JM, et al. American College of Sports Medicine: American College of Sports Medicine Position Stand. Appropriate physical activity intervention strategies for weight loss and prevention of weight regain for adults. Med Sci Sports Exerc 2009;41:459–71.
15. Eason JM. Cardiopulmonary assessment. Cardiopulmonary Phys Ther J 1999;10:135–42.
16. Freedman DS, Khan LK, Serdula MK, et al. Trends and correlates of class three obesity in the United States from 1990 through 2000. JAMA 2002;288:1758–61.
17. Frese EM, Richter RR, Burlis TV. Self-reported measurement of heart rate and blood pressure in patients by physical therapy clinical instructors. Phys Ther 2002;82:1192–200.
18. Goodman CC, Snyder TE. Differential diagnosis in physical therapy. Philadelphia: Saunders; 1995.
19. Griffin SE, Robergs RA, Heyward VH. Blood pressure measurement during exercise: a review. Med Sci Sports Exerc 1997;29:149–59.
20. Hillegass EA, Sadowsky HS. Essentials of cardiopulmonary physical therapy. Philadelphia: Saunders; 1994.
21. Hollerbach AD, Sneed NV. Accuracy of radial pulse assessment by length of counting interval. Heart Lung 1990;19:258–64.
22. Irwin S, Tecklin JS. Cardiopulmonary physical therapy. 3rd ed. St Louis: Mosby; 1995.
23. Ishmail AA, Wing S, Ferguson J, et al. Interobserver agreement by auscultation in the presence of a third heart sound in patients with congestive heart failure. Chest 1987;91:870–3.
24. Jarvis C. Physical examination and assessment. Philadelphia: Saunders; 1992.
25. Johnson JH, Prins A. Prediction of maximal heart rate during a submaximal work test. J Sports Med Phys Fitness 1991;31:44–7.
26. Jones A, Jones RD, Kwong K, et al. Effect of positioning on recorded lung sound intensities in subjects without pulmonary dysfunction. Phys Ther 1999;79:682–90.
27. Kemper KJ, Benson MS, Bishop MJ. Interobserver variability in assessing pediatric postextubation stridor. Clin Pediatr (Phila) 1992;31:405–8.
28. Kenchaiah S, Evans JC, Levy D, et al. Obesity and the risk of heart failure. N Engl J Med 2002;347:305–13.
29. Kenchaiah S, Sesso HD, Gaziano JM. Body mass index and vigorous physical activity and the risk of heart failure among men. Circulation 2009;119:44–52.
30. Kispert CP. Clinical measurements to assess cardiopulmonary function. Phys Ther 1987;67:1886–90.
31. Knowler WC, Barrett-Connor E, Fowler SE, et al. Diabetes Prevention Program Research Group: Reduction in the incidence of type 2 diabetes with lifestyle intervention or metformin. N Engl J Med 2002;346:393–403.
32. Krieger B, Feinerman D, Zaron A, et al. Continuous noninvasive monitoring of respiratory rate in critically ill patients. Chest 1986;90:632–4.
33. Lehmann R, Spinas GA. Role of physical activity in the therapy and prevention of type II diabetes mellitus. Ther Umsch 1996;53:925–33.
34. Lok CE, Morgan CD, Ranganathan N. The accuracy and interobserver agreement in detecting the "gallop sounds" by cardiac auscultation. Chest 1998;114:1283–8.
35. Mahler DA, Mejia-Alfaro R, Ward J, et al. Continuous measurement of breathlessness during exercise: validity, reliability, and responsiveness. J Appl Physiol 2001;90:2188–96.
36. Mion D, Pierin AMJ. How accurate are sphygmomanometers? Hum Hypertens 1998;12:245–8.
37. National Health and Nutrition Examination Survey: Body measures/obesity (website), http://www.cdc.gov/nchs/nhanes/nhanesmmwrs_obesity.htm. Accessed August 10, 2009.
38. O'Flynn I. Three methods of taking the brachial systolic pressure to measure the ankle/brachial index: which one is best? J Vasc Nurs 1993;11:71–5.
39. Oldridge NB, Haskell WL, Single P. Carotid palpation, coronary heart disease and exercise rehabilitation. Med Sci Sports Exerc 1981;13:6–8.
40. Patel R, Bushnell DL, Sobotka PA. Implications of an audible third heart sound in evaluating cardiac function. West J Med 1993;158:606–9.
41. Perloff D, Grim C, Flack J, et al. Human blood pressure determination by sphygmomanometry. Circulation 1993;88:2460–70.
42. Pescatello LS, Franklin BA, Fagard R, et al. American College of Sports Medicine: American College of Sports Medicine position stand: exercise and hypertension. Med Sci Sports Exerc 2004;36:533–53.
43. Poirier P, Despres JP. Waist circumference, visceral obesity, and cardiovascular risk. J Cardiopulm Rehabil 2003;23:161–9.
44. Pollock ML, Broida J, Kendrick Z. Validity of the palpation technique of heart rate determination and its estimation of training heart rate. Res Q 1972;43:77–81.

45. Racette SB, Deusinger SS, Deusinger RH. Obesity: overview of prevalence, etiology, and treatment. Phys Ther 2003;83:276–88.

46. Roberts CK, Vaziri ND, Barnard RJ. Effect of diet and exercise intervention on blood pressure, insulin, oxidative stress, and nitric oxide availability. Circulation 2002;106:2530–2.

47. Sagiv M, Hanson PG, Ben-Sira D, et al. Direct vs. indirect blood pressure at rest and during isometric exercise in normal subjects. Int J Sports Med 1995;16:514–8.

48. Sagiv M, Ben-Sira D, Goldhammer E. Direct vs. indirect blood pressure measurement at peak anaerobic exercise. Int J Sports Med 1999;20:275–8.

49. Scherer SA, Noteboom JT, Flynn TW. Cardiovascular assessment in the orthopaedic practice setting. J Orthop Sports Phys Ther 2005;35:730–7.

50. Sneed NV, Hollerbach AD. Accuracy of heart rate assessment in atrial fibrillation. Heart Lung 1992;21:427–33.

51. Stoffers HE, Kester AD, Kaiser V, et al. The diagnostic value of the measurement of the ankle-brachial systolic pressure index in primary health care. J Clin Epidemiol 1996;49:1401–5.

52. Turjanmaa VM, Kalli ST, Uusitalo AJ. Blood pressure level changes caused by posture change and physical exercise: can they be determined accurately using a standard cuff method? J Hypertens 1988;6(suppl):S79–81.

53. Yamanouchi K, Shinozaki T, Chikada K, et al. Daily walking combined with diet therapy is a useful means for obese NIDDM patients not only to reduce body weight but also to improve insulin sensitivity. Diabetes Care 1999;22:1754–5.

Upper Quadrant Screening Examination   12

William G . Boissonnault, PT, DPT, DHSc, FAAOMPT

Objectives

After reading this chapter, the reader will be able to:

1. Provide a rationale for use of quadrant screening examinations.
2. Describe the primary objectives of the upper quadrant screening examination related to the differential diagnosis process.
3. Describe the specific examination elements that constitute the upper quadrant screening examination.
4. Explain the relevance of each of the specific examination elements as they relate to the differential diagnosis process, including identification of clinical red flags that would result in a patient referral or consultation.

Sahrmann provides two patient experiences relevant to this chapter and Chapter 13 in her editorial titled, "Are Physical Therapists Fulfilling Their Responsibilities as Diagnosticians?"[10] One patient was diagnosed with hip bursitis, the other was presenting 5 months after total knee replacement; both had seen multiple practitioners over months with no resolution of symptoms. Sahrmann's examinations revealed the debilitating complaints were originating in the lumbar spine, not the knee or hip. She questioned whether physical therapists (PTs) are doing the most basic movement examination to ensure they are targeting the appropriate body region for treatment. Not being fooled by the location of patients' chief complaints is one of the primary goals of quadrant screening examinations.

The history, physical examination, and related tests and measures provide much of the examination data PTs need to meet the clinical decision-making challenges associated with patient management. The clinician's goal is to develop efficiently and quickly an effective plan of care designed to meet the individual patient's needs. Chapters 6 through 9 present a detailed description of the history-taking process as it relates to differential diagnosis and clinical decision making. One of the objectives of the patient history is to help guide the clinician regarding what to prioritize in the physical examination. Chapter 10, which presents physical examination information associated with general patient observation, and Chapter 11, which presents information associated with patient vital signs, are relevant for all patients. Building on this information, the emphasis of most of the initial visit physical examination is on the patient's chief presenting symptom (see Chapters 6 and 7) and associated functional limitations.

If the chief presenting symptom is knee pain associated with prolonged standing and walking, the clinician would spend most of the time examining the knee and related anatomic areas (lumbar spine, pelvis and hip, and foot and ankle regions, with little time spent examining the elbow, wrist, and hand). Broadening the scope of the examination to the trunk and lower extremity can be prohibitive if these areas are examined in detail, considering the initial visit time constraints many clinicians face. Examining these anatomically related areas is essential, however, especially when local trauma has not precipitated the knee pain. The knee pain may be referred from another body region (e.g., hip or lumbar spine), or treating the foot and ankle region may be the key to resolving the local knee condition.

Do clinicians have to complete an extensive and detailed examination of the trunk and entire lower extremity to identify the source of the symptoms and the primary impairments associated with the patient's condition? An exhaustive examination is unnecessary, but the regions need to be adequately screened with a cluster of selected examination tools so that by the end of the initial visit the PT has necessary answers. Figure 12-1 illustrates a general decision-making sequence leading to a differential diagnosis and plan of care, including a possible referral of the patient to another provider.

Physical Examination General Principles

Chapter 5 describes strategies designed to facilitate an effective and efficient patient history. Similar strategies exist to enhance an effective and efficient physical examination, as well. First, an adequate-size space is important for efficiency and safety. Next, preparing the examination environment before the patient's arrival in the room is key, ensuring the appropriate equipment and supplies are available, such as linen for draping, chairs and stools, and reflex hammers and other examination tools. Having to come and go from the room multiple times can severely disrupt the examination process. Having established positive rapport (see Chapter 5) during the history-taking enhances the patient's comfort level as the PT begins the "hands-on" portion of the examination. Providing a general description to the patient of what is going to happen next should help alleviate patient anxiety, especially for a patient who has never seen a PT before. The better the patient understands what is going to happen during the examination and why, the more information the PT will be able to collect efficiently. In addition, proper body mechanics are important to prevent injury to the PT and to perform examination techniques effectively.

Also important to the overall success of the visit is protecting patient modesty, which can be influenced by numerous factors, including cultural issues (see Chapter 3). Adequately exposing body areas is especially important for portions of the examination such as observation, palpation, and assessment of range of motion, but what the PT deems adequate may go beyond the patient's comfort level. Explaining what the PT plans to do and why is part of the process of receiving consent from the patient

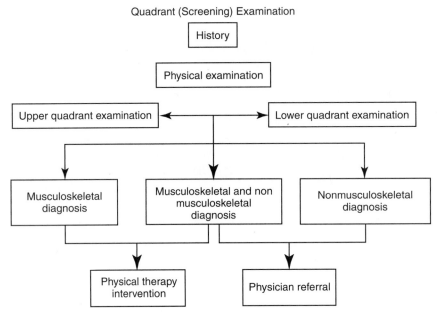

Quadrant (Screening) Examination

FIGURE 12-1 Flow of patient data collection and clinical decision making.

to proceed. If the PT is paying attention to patient nonverbal responses to the initial portions of the examination, he or she may detect signs of discomfort on the patient's part. Important to the patient being comfortable and relaxed is how comfortable and relaxed the clinician is. If the PT is uneasy or nervous about a portion of the examination, the patient is likely to be nervous as well. Finally, it is helpful to plan steps to take next during the examination based on the data already collected.

Although, ultimately, PTs treat impairments related to functional limitations, alteration of symptoms during the examination is key to determining the source of symptoms to whatever level possible and to becoming suspicious of a red flag. As described in Chapter 6, symptoms associated with neuromusculoskeletal impairments are typically related to a change in the patient's posture or movement. In most cases, symptoms can be reproduced or altered during the palpation, active or passive movement, resisted tests, neurologic tests, or special test segments of the physical examination. If the symptoms are not reproduced or altered, the PT should become suspicious of a functional (psychological) or pathologic condition or consider what other body regions to examine.

The fact that symptoms are altered during the examination does not absolutely rule out the presence of a pathologic condition, however. A pathologic fracture can result in low back pain that may vary in intensity with movement and changes in posture as the spine is mechanically loaded and unloaded. In these cases, other information from the history and physical examination should help steer the PT toward the conclusion that the patient's symptoms may not be based on a neuromusculoskeletal impairment. Finally, although PTs should be concerned if they fail to alter a patient's symptomatic presentation, sometimes symptoms associated with impairments are still part of the etiology. The patient's condition may not be "irritable" (as defined by Maitland[8]), meaning considerable activity on the patient's part is necessary to provoke the symptoms, and the PT cannot clinically stress the tissue sufficiently to bring on or alter the symptoms.

Purposes of the Examination

This chapter and the next (Chapter 13) present an upper and a lower quadrant screening examination designed to do the following:

- Narrow the search for the source of symptoms to a specific body region (and the tissue at fault, if possible).
- Identify red flags that, along with the history findings, suggest that the PT initiate a patient referral or consultation.
- Determine which body regions or body systems require a more detailed examination during the initial or subsequent patient visits.
- Identify primary contributing impairments related to the patient's symptoms, functional limitations, and disability.
- Improve rehabilitation outcomes by avoiding inaccurate diagnoses or by the timely referral of patients to other practitioners.
- Provide guidance, along with the history findings, regarding specific interventions that may help the patient or may be contraindicated.

When to Use and Not Use the Examination

Important general guidelines regarding upper and lower quadrant screening examinations described in this chapter and Chapter 13 include the following:

- Quadrant screening should be included as the primary portion of the physical examination at the initial visit.
- The novice practitioner should use the entire quadrant screening examination as presented before using additional special testing procedures, to minimize the chance of misdiagnosis.
- The experienced practitioner, at a minimum, should screen at least one joint or body region above and below the patient's chief complaint. Clinical experience leads to the ability to recognize patient presentation patterns that more quickly identify the diagnostic possibilities that have the highest probability of being correct.

In some situations, the proposed quadrant screening may not be incorporated during the initial visit, as follows:

- If the patient has an obvious acute injury (e.g., sprained ankle with edema, bruising, local pain), or if the visit is postoperative, the emphasis at the initial visit should be on the components of the screening examination most directly related to the involved joint or body region (e.g., ankle/foot). A priority of the physical examination after trauma is ruling out fracture or ligamentous instability and postoperatively screening for infection and deep venous thrombosis. The remainder of the screening examination is appropriate during follow-up visits after the patient begins to recover from the injury or surgery.
- If the patient has symptoms other than pain associated with a medical condition, such as urinary incontinence, much of the proposed screening examination would probably be irrelevant and should be replaced with an examination that has a different clinical focus.

It is important to appreciate that the recommendation is not to cut the body in half, ignoring the lower half. For this chapter, the assumption is that the patient history has provided the clinician with direction that the primary focus should be the upper portion of the body in terms of probable source of symptoms and most likely location where the primary contributing factors (impairments) would be found. Elements of the upper quadrant screening examination include a gross screening of the entire body, including posture and gait assessment.

The quadrant screening examinations are organized by patient position: standing, sitting, supine, and prone. This organization promotes efficiency and minimizes patient position changes, which is especially helpful for patients in acute pain or who are severely impaired. This sequence works well for most patients, but needs to be modified in certain circumstances. Data collected during the history regarding symptom description (see Chapter 6) may identify certain positions (e.g., sitting) or movements that significantly increase the symptom intensity to the degree that the PT alters the sequencing of data collection (seated tests completed last). By ignoring the patient history information and sticking with the examination sequence as listed on paper, the patient's condition may become so aggravated early in the examination that the PT is unable to examine the patient in adequate detail in other positions, and the patient may leave in more pain than before the visit.

The components of both quadrant examinations include the following standard examination categories:

- Inspection/observation
- Palpation
- Active range of motion
- Passive range of motion, including passive overpressures
- Neurologic screening
- Special tests

These categories of patient data assist in identifying the region or source of symptoms and the primary area of impairment associated with the patient's loss of function. The physical examination and the resultant diagnosis are only as good as the PT performing the examination. Careless or faulty testing techniques produce invalid and inappropriate findings and

provide inaccurate diagnosis, treatment plan, and eventual patient outcome.

The upper quadrant screening examination at first glance may appear to be long and cumbersome because it entails performing sample testing of the head, neck, upper thoracic spine (and viscera), and upper extremities; comparing the involved and the uninvolved upper extremity; and screening the nervous and peripheral vascular systems. As noted earlier, however, going directly to the chief complaint area in most cases (exceptions—the obvious acute injured area and postoperative site) can be very misleading and delay appropriate treatment. So in actuality, although this examination scheme may take longer to perform in its entirety, the screening may result in a more quickly established accurate diagnosis and intervention plan. Screening of this scope is necessary to meet the objectives expected of an autonomous practitioner and doctor of physical therapy. Also affecting the length of time needed to complete the proposed screening scheme is that some of it occurs during the history-taking as noted in Chapter 10.

The upper quadrant screening examination, organized by patient position, is presented in Box 12-1.

Description of Examination Elements by Position

Standing

POSTURAL ASSESSMENT. A brief assessment is made of standing posture, primarily focusing on the upper quadrant, but also screening for significant lumbopelvic or lower extremity findings that may affect upper quadrant posture and function. The patient should be viewed from anterior, posterior, and lateral perspectives.

GAIT SCREEN. Although the patient's chief symptoms or functional limitations relate to an upper body region or activity, gathering information regarding the general gait pattern and its influence on upper quadrant posture, movement (or lack of), and symptoms is important. The patient should be instructed to relay information to the examiner regarding at what point during the gait cycle the symptoms are aggravated. As with posture assessment, the gait screening should include viewing the patient from all perspectives (anterior, posterior, and lateral).

Sitting

GENERAL SURVEY. The items listed under "general survey" in Box 12-1 are relevant to all patients. As described in Chapter 10, observing skin, including general color and specific lesions; hair patterns and loss; and nails begins during the patient interview and continues throughout the remainder of the examination. Signs of an inflammatory response (local redness or hyperemia) or ecchymosis indicating bleeding under the skin from injury of underlying tissues may be noted. Scars should also be noted and examined for their state of healing. In addition, a patient may not inform the PT of a surgical procedure or trauma, so observing the scar can prompt the PT to initiate a line of questioning. The presence of keloid, or excessive scarring, may be an indication of the general response of the patient to trauma and potential complications associated with the healing process. Being vigilant for rashes, such as the malar rash associated with systemic lupus erythematosus,

BOX 12-1

Upper Quadrant Screening Examination

STANDING
Posture observation
Gait
Weight/height (see Chapter 11)

SITTING*
General survey
    Skin, nails, hair, surface anatomy (see Chapter 10—starts during the history)
    Vital signs (see Chapter 11)
    Respiratory pattern
    Posture assessment (observe during the history)
Head, face, neck observation (see Chapter 10)
    Eyes (occurs during the history)
        Pupils
        Ptosis
        Visual gaze (strabismus)
    Facial contour (occurs during the history)
        Eyes/mouth (CN VII)
        Cheeks (masseter muscle, CN V)
    Intraoral
        Teeth (dentition and occlusion)
        Gingiva (gums)
        Tongue and other soft tissues
        Anterior neck (trachea and sternal notch—during the history)
Head, face, and neck palpation
    Glands (parotid, submandibular salivary, thyroid)
    Lymph nodes (preauricular and postauricular, suboccipital, tonsillar, submandibular, submental, superficial and posterior cervical, supraclavicular)
    Trachea
    Carotid pulses
    Bony/joint lines including spinous processes, scapula, clavicle, acromioclavicular and sternoclavicular joints
Head, face, and neck neurologic screening (see Chapters 9 and 10)
Physical examination screening (*optional*—dependent on history and observation findings)
    Smell (CN I)
    Visual acuity (CN II): Snellen eye chart
    Pupils: light reaction (CNs II and III)
    Extraocular eye movements (CNs III, IV, and VI)
    Sensory (CNs V, and C2 and C3)
    Motor (CNs V and VII, and C1-C3)
    Motor cervical flexion (C1-C3; CN XI—spinal accessory); extension (C1-C8; CN XI—spinal accessory); lateral flexion (C2-C4; CN XI); rotation
    Facial expression: eyes, mouth (CN VII)
    Hearing: air conduction (CN VIII)
    Hearing: bone conduction (CN VIII)
    Gag reflex (CNs IX and X)
    Shoulder shrug (CN XI)
    Tongue motor response (CN XII)
Active range of motion (with passive overpressure when appropriate)
    Mandibular depression (observe and palpate)
    Cervical spine
        Flexion
        Rotation (be vigilant for signs of vascular compromise)
        Lateral flexion
        Extension (be vigilant for signs of vascular compromise)

Cervical spine vertical compression/distraction
Shoulder girdle/upper extremity
    Observation
    Palpation
        Lymph nodes (clavicular, axillary, and epitrochlear)
        Pulses (radial, ulnar)
        Joint lines and soft tissues
Active range of motion (with passive overpressure when appropriate)
    Shoulder girdle
        Elevation, depression, protraction, retraction
    Shoulder complex
        Hand behind head
        Hand behind back
        Horizontal abduction
    Elbow (may do before shoulder active range of motion screening if history of significant elbow injury or pathology)
        Flexion
        Extension
        Pronation
        Supination
    Wrist
        Flexion
        Extension
        Radial/ulnar deviation
    Thumb
        Flexion/extension
        Opposition
    Fingers
        Flexion/extension
Upper extremity neurologic screening
    Hoffman's reflex
    Cutaneous sensation (light touch, sharp/dull assessment [C4-T6 dermatomes; see Figure 12-19])
    Myotome testing[†]
        Scapular elevation (CN XI, spinal accessory)
        Shoulder abduction (C4-C6, axillary)
        Elbow flexion (**C5**, C6, musculocutaneous)
        Elbow extension (C6, **C7**-C8, radial)
        Wrist extension (**C6**-C8, radial and ulnar)
        Finger flexors (C7, **C8**, median)
        Finger abduction/adduction (C8, **T1**, ulnar)
    Deep tendon reflexes
        Biceps (C5, C6)
        Brachioradialis (C5, C6)
        Triceps (C6, C7)

SUPINE
Upper extremity neurologic screening
    Repeat motor and sensory testings if findings positive in weight-bearing postures
    Neuromobility assessment—upper limb tension testing

---

*All positive neurologic findings in the sitting position should be retested in non–weight-bearing positions.
†Myotome testing—the spinal levels in **bold** are consistent with the Standard Neurological Classification of Spinal Cord Injury. (Savic G, Bergström EM, Frankel HL, et al: Inter-rater reliability of motor and sensory examinations performed according to American Spinal Injury Association Standards, *Spinal Cord* 45:444-451, 2007.)
CN, cranial nerve.

is also important when assessing the head and facial regions. Last, calluses and blisters should be noted, because they are indicative of excessive friction or irritation of the skin.

Assessing vital signs (see Chapter 11) including blood pressure and heart rate, documenting weight and height, and calculating body mass index may identify important health issues that need to be brought to another health care practitioner's attention or become a focus of the PT's intervention plan. These assessments may be done by someone other than the PT, depending on the clinic's staffing model.

Sitting posture should be assessed during the patient history, when the patient is unaware that his or her posture is being examined. Noting head on neck (upper cervical), head and neck on thorax (mid-cervical and lower cervical), shoulder girdle on thorax, and overall trunk position provides direction to the clinician regarding what specific body regions to assess in more detail. Observation of the thorax may reveal structural deformities such as barrel chest, excessive kyphosis, and "pigeon" chest (pectus excavatum). A respiratory screen should also be done at this time, including respiratory pattern (chest versus abdominal versus accessory muscles) and pursed-lip breathing.

HEAD, FACE, AND NECK

Observation. In addition to the aforementioned observations, a close look at the eyes and face begins a general nervous system screening (see Chapters 9 and 10). Observation of the eyes includes assessment of the pupils (size and shape), ptosis, gaze, position of the eye relative to the orbit (e.g., exophthalmus), and color (e.g., abnormal patterns of redness). Abnormal findings may include the following:

- Bulging of the eye(s)—exophthalmus from thyrotoxicosis, hyperthyroidism, Graves' disease, space-occupying mass in the orbit
- Drainage—blockage of nasolacrimal gland, infections
- Ptosis—Horner's syndrome, Pancoast's tumor of the lung, cranial nerve III dysfunction
- Color of sclera—yellow for jaundice, hepatitis, liver disease; redness for ciliary flush, inflammation, infection
- Nystagmus—alcohol abuse, upper motor neuron disease, labyrinth irritability
- Abnormal gaze—strabismus (involvement of cranial nerves III, IV, or VI), orbital fracture, space-occupying mass in the orbit

Observing whether the trachea and associated structures are vertically oriented and whether the sternal notch (bordered by the sternocleidomastoid muscles and the manubrium of the sternum) is present is also important. A space-occupying mass may result in a deviation from the midline of the trachea, and an enlarged thyroid gland or nodules can "fill in" the sternal notch.

Screening intraoral structures includes identifying how many teeth are present, the condition of the teeth, the occlusal pattern, and the condition of associated soft tissue structures. There can be eight teeth in each of the four quadrants starting medially and going laterally:

- Central incisor
- Lateral incisor
- Canine
- Bicuspids ("premolars") (two)
- Molars (three)

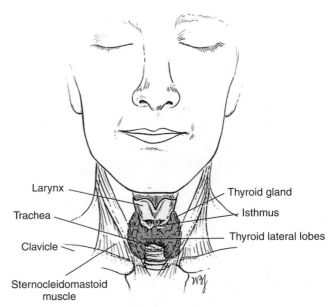

FIGURE 12-2 Anatomic location of thyroid gland. (From Swartz MH: *Textbook of physical diagnosis: history and examination,* 5th ed, Philadelphia, 2006, Saunders, p 196.)

Absent, chipped, or cracked teeth indicate that an assessment by a dentist is warranted, and shiny, worn spots on teeth may indicate bruxism. The relationship of the maxillary to the mandibular incisors when the teeth are in contact may also identify malocclusive or temporomandibular disorders, which suggest the patient should be referred to a dentist. The maxillary incisors should vertically overlap the mandibular incisors (overbite) by approximately 30%, with minimal distance noted in the anterior/posterior direction (overjet if excessive). Inflammation or irritation of soft tissues or intraoral bleeding may indicate serious disease or conditions (gingivitis) that require dental intervention. This type of observational screening includes looking at the back of the throat (e.g., soft palate, uvula) for masses and abnormal tissue conditions.

Palpation. The principles of palpation apply to this body region as in all others. The "layer palpation" approach is recommended, going from superficial to deeper structures as different structures are assessed and identified. General instructions to the patient are also standard, including requesting feedback regarding whether more than just pressure is felt and whether symptoms change, for better or worse, as the area is assessed. General observation of surface anatomy (see Chapter 10) may reveal abnormalities that lead the practitioner to detailed palpation of a region.

Any lump or bump felt should not be assumed to lie within a muscle belly or fascial layer. Numerous glands and lymph nodes are located in the head, face, and neck region (Figures 12-2 and 12-3).

Feeling a lump or bump does not automatically indicate a pathologic condition because many of these structures are superficially located. A hard lump or nodule, whether it is tender or not, should lead to questioning the patient about the finding:

- Have you noticed this lump?
- Has a physician checked this spot and told you what the lump is?
- If the physician is aware of the lump, has it changed in size, shape, or consistency since the last visit?

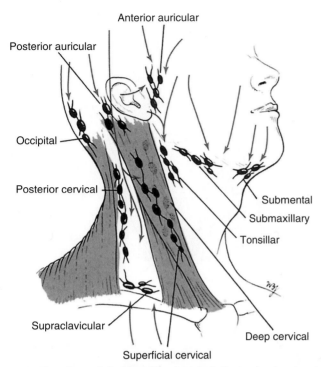

FIGURE 12-3 Anatomic location of lymph nodes in the head and neck region. (From Swartz MH: *Textbook of physical diagnosis: history and examination,* 5th ed, Philadelphia, 2006, Saunders, p 197.)

The same abnormal criteria apply to assessment of these nodes as discussed in Chapter 10, including the following:
- More than 1.5 cm in diameter
- Hard consistency
- Tender, painful node or nontender with hard consistency
- Immobile

A lump that has not been checked by a physician or has changed since the last physician assessment should direct the PT to encourage the patient to make an appointment. Finally, palpating along the trachea is important for noting any abnormal anatomy (e.g., deviation from the midline) or abnormal response (e.g., provocation of symptoms) to the pressure applied to the area, and each carotid artery can be palpated near the level of the cricoid cartilage, just medial to the sternocleidomastoid muscles. The carotid assessment is primarily for intensity and symmetry of pulsations and potentially localized pain provocation.

Neurologic Screening. Relevant screening questions and tests should be included when the following occur:
- The PT observes any of the abnormal anatomic findings described earlier in this chapter or in Chapters 9 and 10.
- The patient describes local head or facial symptoms (see Chapter 6) or a pattern of numbness, paresthesia, or weakness that does not fit a peripheral nerve entrapment or a spinal nerve root pattern.
- The patient has a history of a primary neurologic condition such as multiple sclerosis or a history of a stroke or head injury.
- The patient describes direct trauma to the head and neck region or a whiplash type of incident.

The focus of the screening questions should be to identify findings that are unusual or atypical, representing a change from the norm for the patient:
- Sense of smell (cranial nerve I)
- Visual acuity (cranial nerve II)
- Diplopia (double vision) (cranial nerves III, IV, VI)
- Sense of taste (cranial nerves VII, IX)
- Difficulties with swallowing (cranial nerves IX, X)
- Hearing loss (cranial nerve VIII)
- Numbness or paresthesia (cranial nerve V, upper cervical spine)
- Balance or gait difficulties (cranial nerve VIII)
- Mentation, orientation, or behavioral abnormalities

The questions complement screening tests (Table 12-1) that can be organized in sequential order of the cranial nerves (I through XII) or by anatomic region (recommended).

CRANIAL NERVE ASSESSMENT BY REGION

Face

Sensation (Cranial Nerve V). Light touch, including sharp/dull at a minimum, should be assessed over the forehead (ophthalmic branch), the cheeks (maxillary branch), and the jaw (mandibular branch). It is often helpful to perform this first over an area of skin that is not within the area of symptoms and is thought to be of normal sensation. The patient should be asked to close the eyes as the face is examined and to report if something is felt and where it is felt. A loss of sensation in this region suggests a lesion of either the trigeminal nerve or higher sensory pathways.

Motor (Cranial Nerves V and VII). The motor status of the trigeminal nerve is assessed by asking the patient to bite down hard and hold while the PT palpates the masseter and temporalis muscles bilaterally, noting strength of contraction (degree of tissue resistance during palpation). Subtle asymmetry may be detected in patients with temporomandibular joint or dental occlusion conditions. Next, the status of the facial nerve is assessed by the PT observing for facial symmetry as the patient is asked to perform the following activities:
- Raise both eyebrows
- Frown
- Close both eyes tightly
- Show both the upper and the lower teeth
- Smile
- Puff out both cheeks with mouth closed

Cranial nerve VII is also involved in taste sensation of the anterior two thirds of the tongue, so a lesion of this nerve may also have symptoms of altered taste.

Eyes

Visual Acuity (Cranial Nerve II). Symptoms of having difficulty seeing should lead to additional screening to determine whether to refer the patient to another practitioner. Visual acuity can be checked with a Snellen eye chart (Figure 12-4). With the patient positioned 20 feet from the chart, using glasses or contact lenses if needed, the patient is asked to cover one eye at a time and read the smallest line of print possible. Visual acuity for each eye is recorded and compared with what the patient knows to be his or her normal vision when checked. If the patient can read at best the 20/200 line, this is interpreted as the ability to read at 20 feet what a person with normal vision can see at 200 feet. If the patient

TABLE 12-1

Evaluating the Cranial Nerves

Nerves	Function	Location	Tests	Significant Findings
I—olfactory	Smell	Olfactory bulb and tract	Odor recognition (unilaterally)	Lack of odor perception on one or both sides
II—optic	Vision	Optic nerve, chiasm, and tracts	Visual acuity; peripheral vision; pupillary light reflex	Reduced vision
III—oculomotor	Eye movement; pupil contraction and accommodation; eyelid elevation	Midbrain	Extraocular eye movements; pupillary light reflex	Impairment of one or more eye movements or dysconjugate gaze; pupillary dilation; ptosis
IV—trochlear	Eye movement	Midbrain	Extraocular eye movements	Impairment of one or more eye movements or dysconjugate gaze
V—trigeminal	Facial sensation; muscles of mastication	Pons	Sensation above eye, between eye and mouth, below mouth to angle of jaw; palpation of contraction of masseter and temporalis muscles	Reduced sensation in one or more divisions of fifth nerve; impaired jaw reflex; reduced strength in masseter and temporalis muscles
VI—abducens	Ocular movement	Pons	Extraocular eye movements	Reduced eye abduction
VII—facial	Facial expression; secretions; taste; visceral and cutaneous sensibility	Pons	Facial expression; taste of anterior two thirds of tongue	Weakness of upper or lower face or eye closure; reduced taste perception (salty, sweet, bitter, sour)
VIII—acoustic	Hearing; equilibrium	Pons	Auditory and vestibular	Reduced hearing; impaired balance
IX—glossopharyngeal	Taste; glandular secretions; swallowing; visceral sensibility (pharynx, tongue, tonsils)	Medulla	Gag reflex; speech (phonation); swallowing	Impaired reflex; dysarthria; dysphagia
X—vagus	Involuntary muscle and gland control (pharynx, larynx, trachea, bronchi, lungs, digestive tract, heart); swallowing and phonation; visceral and cutaneous sensibility; taste	Medulla	Phonation; coughing; gag reflex	Hoarseness; weak cough; impaired reflex
XI—accessory	Movement of head and shoulders	Cervical	Resisted head; shoulder shrug	Weakness of trapezius and sternocleidomastoid
XII—hypoglossal	Movement of tongue	Medulla	Tongue protrusion	Deviation, atrophy, or fasciculations of tongue

is unable to read any of the lines, the patient is asked to state how many fingers the clinician is holding up in front of the patient's face.

Peripheral Vision (Cranial Nerve II). The patient's temporal or peripheral vision is checked with the patient sitting and the PT in front of and facing the patient. The patient covers one eye while looking straight ahead (as does the PT). The PT places his or her hand several feet lateral to the patient on the side of the eye to be tested and slowly brings a finger or object (e.g., pen) toward the midline until the patient states he or she sees it; this is grossly compared with the opposite eye's ability when it is tested. This test can be repeated, moving the finger or object medially in from an upper and lower visual quadrant.

Pupils (Cranial Nerves II and III). After inspecting the pupils for size and symmetry (see Chapter 10), the pupillary reaction test (Figure 12-5) should be performed. In a darkened room, a penlight is aimed into one eye at a time (the examiner placing a hand at the bridge of the nose to divide the visual field in two). The patient is asked to focus on an object 6 to 10 feet

behind the PT and not directly on the light or the PT's hand. Normal response should be twofold: immediate, mild constriction of the ipsilateral pupil (the direct response) and constriction of the pupil of the opposite eye (the consensual response).

Extraocular Movements (Cranial Nerves III, IV, and VI). The patient is asked to focus attention on an object (the PT's finger or a pen) directly in front of him or her at a comfortable distance (approximately 12 inches). The patient is then asked to follow the object with his or her eyes as it is moved in an "H" pattern, while holding the head still. The examiner notes the eyes' ability to track the object and symmetry of movement into all quadrants (Figure 12-6), with the expectation that the eyes will move smoothly together and track symmetrically.

Ears

Acuity. The first recommended auditory acuity screening test is the "whisper test." Standing behind the patient at a 45-degree angle (to ensure the patient cannot read the PT's lips), the PT whispers familiar words, numbers, or letters (e.g., weather,

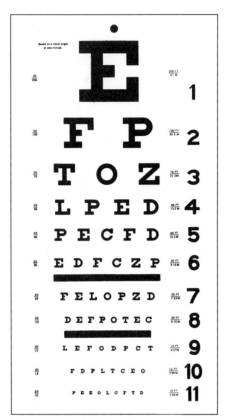

FIGURE 12-4 Snellen chart, which is used to assess visual acuity. (From American Academy of Ophthalmology, San Francisco, CA, 1993, p 8.)

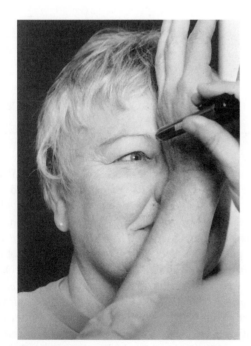

FIGURE 12-5 Pupillary light reaction test should be performed in a dimly lit room with the patient looking at a distant object. The PT's hand divides the patient's visual field and the PT shines the light into one eye, watching that pupil for a direct response. The PT then shines the light in the same eye, watching the opposite pupil for a response (consensual response). This process is repeated by shining the light in the other eye.

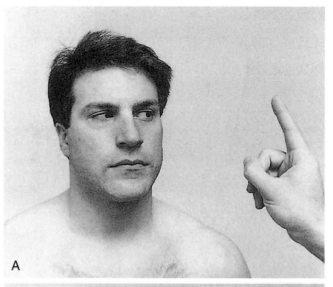

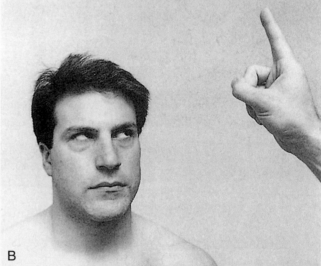

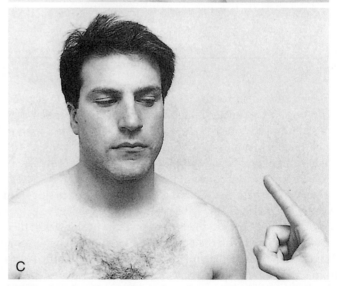

FIGURE 12-6 Assessment of gaze into all quadrants. **A,** Eyes following the target to the right (lateral gaze). **B,** Eyes following the target laterally and superiorly. **C,** Eyes following the target laterally and inferiorly. (From Boissonnault W: *Examination in physical therapy practice: screening for medical disease,* 2nd ed, New York, 1995, Churchill Livingstone, p 216.)

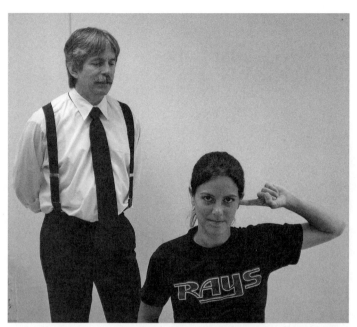

FIGURE 12-7 The "whispered voice" screening test for hearing impairment. The PT stands at arm's length behind the patient off to one side. The patient places the index finger into the ear not being tested and moves/rubs the finger tip inside the ear. The PT then whispers three to four words and asks the patient to repeat the words.

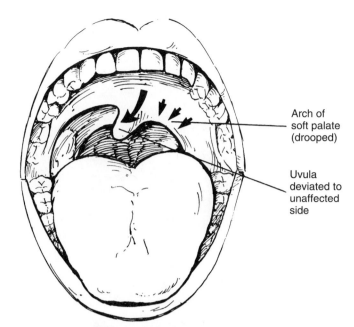

Arch of soft palate (drooped)

Uvula deviated to unaffected side

FIGURE 12-8 Lower motor neuron lesion of the vagus nerve may be noted during testing of the gag reflex or when the patient says "ahh." (From Wilson-Pauwels L, Akesson EJ, Stewart PA: *Cranial nerves: anatomy and clinical comments,* Philadelphia, 1988, Decker.)

thirteen, hot dog) and asks the patient to repeat what has been whispered. To test one ear at a time, the patient should cover the ear not being tested with his or her hand (Figure 12-7). If a unilateral or bilateral deficit is noted, or if the findings are equivocal, follow-up testing with a tuning fork can be performed.

Balance (Including Vestibular) Testing. If the patient subjectively reports dizziness or balance problems (see Chapters 7 and 9), balance testing is in order. The degree of balance problem the patient describes dictates where the PT begins with the screening. The lowest level of screening has the patient standing with feet together on a fixed surface (floor) with the eyes open for 20 to 30 seconds. The next level is the same maneuver, but with eyes closed, followed by testing on a soft surface with eyes open, then moving to single-leg stance testing. Balance concerns are noted during the history, and the PT should stand close to the patient for safety reasons. Other tests to consider include the Dix-Hallpike maneuver and cervical vertigo tests (see Chapter 7).

Nose (Cranial Nerve I). If the patient reports difficulty with the sense of smell or if other neurologic deficits are noted during the examination, a follow-up test is in order. To assess the sense of smell, an aromatic stimulus (e.g., orange, coffee, or vanilla), rather than a noxious stimulus, is used. The patient's eyes should be closed during the assessment, and he or she is asked to identify the source of the odor. One side (one nostril) should be tested at a time.

Mouth

Gag Reflex (Cranial Nerves IX and X). PTs should screen for the gag reflex after asking the patient to swallow and noting any difficulties. With the patient's mouth wide open, the PT observes the status of the soft palate and position of the uvula and asks the patient to say "ahh" while observing for symmetric

rise of the soft palate and uvula (cranial nerve X). Any deviation of the uvula or asymmetry of the soft palate position indicates possible cranial nerve involvement (Figure 12-8). Last, the PT places a tongue blade on the back of the tongue (cranial nerve IX innervates the posterior two thirds of the tongue) and watches for the same motor response seen with the "ahh" action. Any deviation of the uvula or asymmetry of the soft palate position indicates possible cranial nerve involvement.

Tongue (Cranial Nerve XII). The patient is asked to protrude the tongue, with the PT observing for fasciculation, symmetry, atrophy, or deviation from the midline. Manual resistance to side-to-side movements of the tongue screens for asymmetry of strength. The PT may ask the patient to push the tongue into the inside of each cheek while providing mild resistance with a tongue blade as the patient holds against the pressure.

Temporomandibular Joint. The joint lines are first palpated (bilaterally) externally over the mandibular condyles, checking for pain provocation, tenderness, and edema. The patient is asked to open the mouth fully as the PT checks for extent of opening (normal active range of motion is approximately 45 to 60 mm), deviation from the sagittal plane, and any alteration of usual condition. Preventing any neck movement during this activity is important because any pain provoked may be referred from the cervical spine.

CERVICAL SPINE

Cervical Active Range of Motion. The patient should be seated upright with the feet supported to promote a reproducible position as cervical flexion, rotation, lateral flexion, and extension are assessed from anterior and lateral views. If symptoms are not altered during active movement assessment, a passive overpressure is applied to exclude the cervical spine as a source of symptoms (Figure 12-9). In addition to assessing quantity and quality of motion, the PT must appreciate that, during cervical

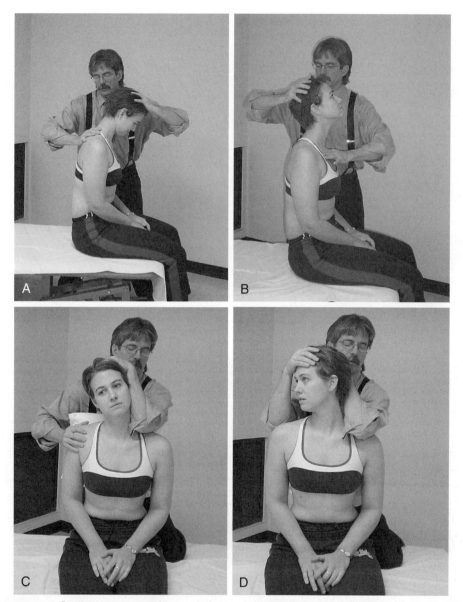

FIGURE 12-9 Passive overpressure of the cervical spine. **A,** Flexion. **B,** Extension. **C,** Side-bending. **D,** Rotation.

rotation, and to some degree extension, the initial gross assessment for vertebrobasilar artery insufficiency has begun. During the assessment of active cervical left and right rotation, the patient is asked to maintain the head and neck at the end of the movement for an additional 10 to 30 seconds while the PT looks for manifestations that may be related to vascular compromise. The most common manifestations include the following:

- Dizziness
- Dysarthria
- Dysphagia
- Nausea
- Visual disturbances
- Extremity sensory changes

Cervical Vertical Compression and Decompression. With the patient sitting with feet supported, the examiner places both hands on top of the patient's head and slowly compresses the head and neck, stopping just shy of producing movement of the cervical region (Figure 12-10). This position is also held for approximately 5 to 8 seconds, with questioning regarding any change in

symptoms. The examiner then places his or her hands around the sides and back of the patient's head ("hooking" the mastoid processes on the heel of the hand between the thenar and hypothenar eminences) and gently lifts straight up—"unweighting" the weight-bearing surfaces of the neck (Figure 12-11). This position is held for approximately 5 to 8 seconds. The patient is asked again whether any change in symptoms is noted. A pillow is placed between the PT and the patient to help maintain an upright patient position. This pillow also allows for the maintenance of "personal space" between the PT and patient.

UPPER EXTREMITY

Observation. The examiner observes for overall size, contour, symmetry, and posturing of the upper extremities. The hands are examined for clubbing of nails (chronic heart, lung, or liver disease; see Chapters 9 and 10); enlargement of joint structures, as in Heberden's nodes (distal interphalangeal joints—osteoarthritis) and Bouchard's nodes (interphalangeal and metacarpophalangeal joints—rheumatoid arthritis); and ulnar drift of the metacarpophalangeal joints. The skin is observed for

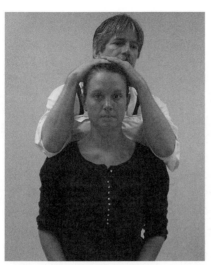

FIGURE 12-10 Vertical cervical compression for symptom alteration. ("Patient, I want to know whether your symptoms get better or worse when I apply this pressure.") PT stands behind the patient and applies light to moderate downward pressure through the cranium in an attempt to load the weight-bearing structures of the cervical spine. The patient's head and neck should be positioned so that with the downward pressure the neck does not move into flexion or extension. Pressure is maintained for 5 to 8 seconds.

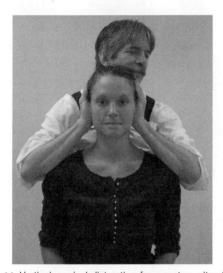

FIGURE 12-11 Vertical cervical distraction for symptom alteration. ("Patient, I want to know whether your symptoms get better or worse when I apply this pressure.") PT stands behind the patient and applies contact under the mastoid processes with hand (between thenar and hypothenar eminences). PT gently unweights the head and neck for 5 to 8 seconds. PT should avoid applying pressure through the mandible.

sores or ulcerations (e.g., psoriasis), red streaks (local infection, usually distal), swelling (edema and effusion), temperature and color (more diffuse, cold, pallor typically associated with venous or lymphatic conditions; increased warmth and redness more commonly associated with arterial problems), skin texture, and scars. See Chapter 10 for more details regarding interpretation of findings.

Palpation. The general principles of layer palpation and instructions to the patient also apply to upper extremity palpation. Structures to be aware of include lymph nodes and arteries for pulse assessment (see Chapter 10). Specific assessment of lymph node

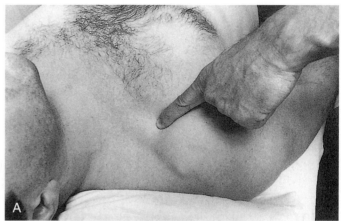

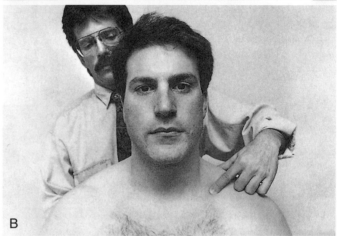

FIGURE 12-12 A, Palpating for infraclavicular lymph nodes between deltoid and pectoralis major muscles. **B,** Palpating for supraclavicular lymph nodes lateral to sternocleidomastoid attachment on clavicle. (From Boissonnault W: *Examination in physical therapy practice: screening for medical disease,* 2nd ed, New York, 1995, Churchill Livingstone, p 404.)

areas is also called for in the presence of diffuse upper extremity swelling; a history of breast cancer (in particular with axillary node involvement); wounds; abrasions; or red streaks noted on the hand, wrist, or forearm regions. An awareness of lymph node location is important so that PTs do not assume that lumps found during palpation lie within a muscle belly or fascial layer. Pulse assessment is also important to screen for vascular compromise. Comparing left with right side for ease or difficulty in finding the pulses and noting general skin temperature and skin trophic changes provide the PT with necessary information.

Clavicular Lymph Nodes. There are nodes in the supraclavicular regions, lateral to the distal attachment of the sternocleidomastoid muscles and inferior to the clavicle in the triangle bordered by the anterior deltoid and pectoralis major muscles and the lateral third of the clavicle (Figure 12-12).

Axillary Lymph Nodes. There are several sets of lymph nodes in the axillary region, which can be viewed as a pyramid with four walls for palpation (Figures 12-13 to 12-16), with lymph nodes present along all four walls: medial (thoracic cage), anterior (posterior surface of pectoralis major), posterior (anterior surface of subscapularis, teres major, and latissimus dorsi), and lateral (upper shaft and neck of the humerus) walls. The same technique is used to palpate these nodes as in the cervical region,

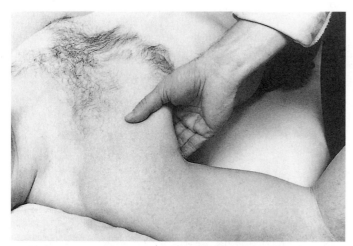

FIGURE 12-13 Palpating for lymph nodes along anterior axillary wall, posterior surface of pectoralis major. (From Boissonnault W: *Examination in physical therapy practice: screening for medical disease,* 2nd ed, New York, 1995, Churchill Livingstone, p 404.)

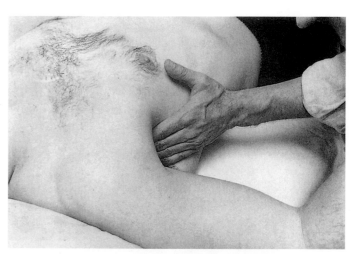

FIGURE 12-16 Palpating for lymph nodes along medial axillary wall, along thorax. (From Boissonnault W: *Examination in physical therapy practice: screening for medical disease,* 2nd ed, New York, 1995, Churchill Livingstone, p 406.)

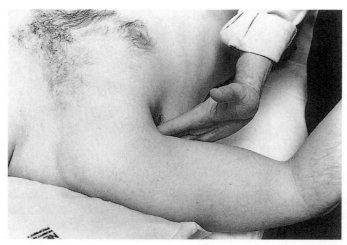

FIGURE 12-14 Palpating for lymph nodes along lateral axillary wall, along shaft of upper humerus. (From Boissonnault W: *Examination in physical therapy practice: screening for medical disease,* 2nd ed, New York, 1995, Churchill Livingstone, p 405.)

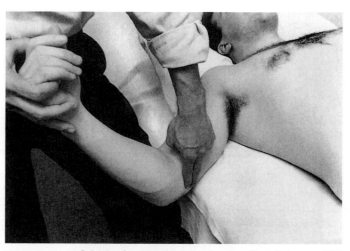

FIGURE 12-17 Palpating for epitrochlear lymph nodes. (From Boissonnault W: *Examination in physical therapy practice: screening for medical disease,* 2nd ed, New York, 1995, Churchill Livingstone, p 406.)

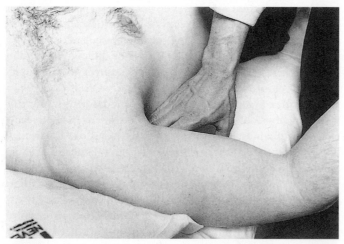

FIGURE 12-15 Palpating for lymph nodes along posterior axillary wall, anterior surface of teres major and latissimus dorsi. (From Boissonnault W: *Examination in physical therapy practice: screening for medical disease,* 2nd ed, New York, 1995, Churchill Livingstone, p 406.)

assessing for the same characteristics. As in the cervical spine, it is common to palpate normal nodes in the axillary regions.

Epitrochlear Lymph Nodes. Epitrochlear lymph nodes are located just above the elbow in the proximity of the medial epicondyle of the humerus (Figure 12-17).

Pulse Assessment. A grading system exists for pulses similar to the system for deep tendon reflexes. Although subjective, this system provides a means to describe pulse amplitude in a manner consistent with physician and nurse assessment and documentation:

   0: Absent
   1: Diminished
   2: Normal
   3: Increased
   4: Bounding

Brachial Artery. The brachial pulse is assessed at the medial upper arm at the middle to distal third of the humerus, medial to the biceps tendon (Figure 12-18).

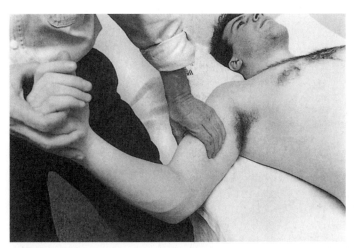

FIGURE 12-18 Assessing pulse at brachial artery along medial shaft of humerus. (From Boissonnault W: *Examination in physical therapy practice: screening for medical disease,* 2nd ed, New York, 1995, Churchill Livingstone, p 407.)

Radial/Ulnar Artery. The radial/ulnar pulse is assessed at the volar aspect of the distal forearm, with the radial artery classically used for assessment of heart rate in beats per minute (see Chapter 11).

UPPER EXTREMITY ACTIVE RANGE OF MOTION WITH PASSIVE OVERPRESSURE

Shoulder Girdle. The movements of elevation (cranial nerve XI when manual resistance is applied), depression, protraction, and retraction all should be assessed while monitoring head and neck posture and movement and glenohumeral motion. Muscle imbalances or joint dysfunction in the shoulder girdle region could lead to multiple compensations throughout this body region.

Shoulder Complex. In lieu of local trauma to the shoulder or a surgical procedure, the movement screening can begin with combined movements, including having the patient put the hand behind the head and hand behind the back, and horizontal abduction. If movement abnormalities are noted, a cardinal plane assessment can be performed and measured because a more detailed shoulder examination is warranted. If the active movement findings do not provide definitive guidance, passive overpressure should be performed to allow the PT to say with confidence whether the shoulder complex is an area that needs to be screened in more detail.

Elbow. As noted in Box 12-1, there may be times when the elbow should be screened before the shoulder is passively examined, such as in patients with a history of significant past or recent trauma to the elbow region. Passive overpressure for many of the shoulder movements mechanically stresses the elbow to the point of potentially exacerbating an underlying condition. To screen the elbow/forearm complex, flexion, extension, pronation, and supination all should be assessed actively and passively if indicated. To save time, these active motions can be assessed bilaterally.

Wrist and Hand. The wrist/hand complex can be assessed actively and passively, if indicated, including wrist flexion and extension and radial/ulnar deviation. As with the elbow, these active movements can be assessed bilaterally. For screening the hand, the thumb should be assessed separately from the fingers with flexion, extension, and opposition. All the fingers can be actively assessed simultaneously with flexion and extension, followed by passive overpressure if indicated.

UPPER EXTREMITY NEUROLOGIC SCREENING EXAMINATION

For consistency and reproducibility, the patient should be sitting upright with the feet supported. Controlling head and neck position is essential because certain postures "open" the cervical foramen and others "close" them. The patient should be looking straight ahead as the testing is being performed.

Myotomes. Selected muscles have been identified (see Box 12-1) to assess the motor status of cervical spinal nerve roots and upper extremity peripheral nerves.

Dermatomes. See the description under head, face, and neck sensory assessment, which notes that the patient's eyes should be closed during the assessment. If an alteration in sensation is noted, the examiner takes additional time testing to map the area and make a determination regarding nerve root versus peripheral nerve involvement (Figure 12-19).

Deep Tendon Reflexes. For the upper quadrant examination, three deep tendon reflexes are assessed: biceps, brachioradialis, and triceps. In each case, the tendon in question should be placed slightly stretched from a mid-position; it is helpful to support the limb to gain additional feedback by palpation in addition to visual assessment of the reflex. This action should be repeated three to five times to ensure a valid response. Grading the reflex response is accomplished by determining the response on a 0 to 4+ scale (Table 12-2). If no response is noted, a Jendrassik maneuver may be used by asking for a contraction of other muscles not involved in the reflex.

Finally, Hoffmann's reflex is analogous to Babinski's reflex. Hoffmann's reflex assists in the screening for upper motor neuron involvement. While the PT supports the proximal phalanges of the second finger, he or she sharply "flicks" the distal phalanx into flexion. A positive finding would be observation of a simultaneous thumb interphalangeal joint flexion.

Supine

UPPER EXTREMITY NEUROLOGIC SCREENING EXAMINATION.

As presented in Chapter 13 on lower quadrant screening, if positive neurologic findings occur, retesting in non–weight-bearing positions can be useful. If findings are present in upright postures but not in non–weight-bearing positions, if possible home exercises should be done in non–weight-bearing formats. Upper limb tension testing should be conducted to assess for symptom alteration and identification of movement abnormalities that may be related to patients' functional limitations and disabilities. The ULTT1, ULTT3, and UTLL4 as described by Magee[7] allow for assessment of the C5, C6, C7, C8, and T1 nerve roots.

Summary

The overall examination of the patient is not finished when the testing maneuvers have been completed. At this point (after the history and upper quadrant screening examination), the PT should have a strong hypothesis regarding the source of symptoms, primary impairments related to functional limitations, and disability and should have identified potential red flags. In many instances, the collected information provides enough guidance so that treatment can be initiated without further examination.

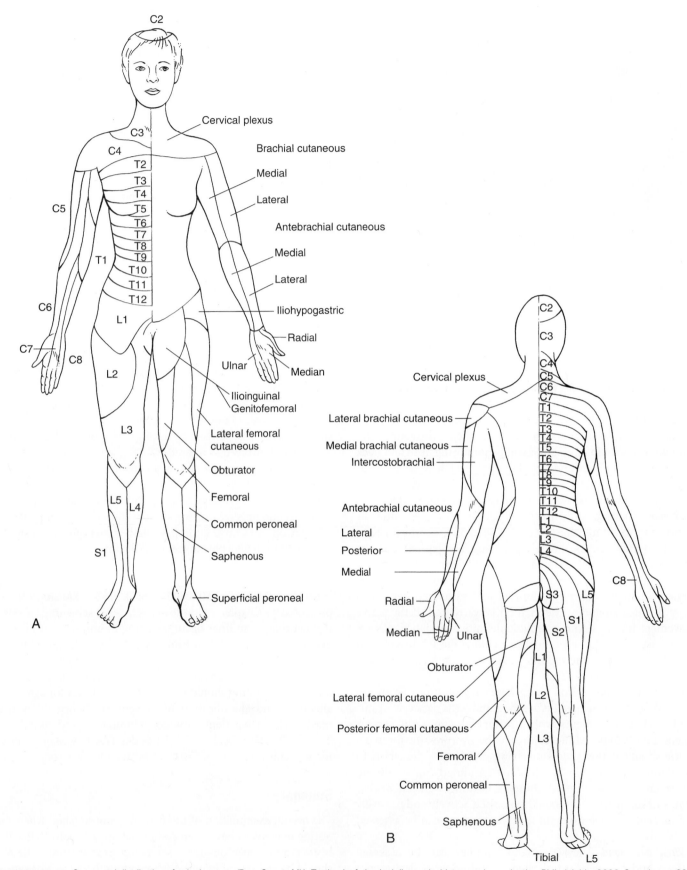

FIGURE 12-19 Segmental distribution of spinal nerves. (From Swartz MH: *Textbook of physical diagnosis: history and examination,* Philadelphia, 2002, Saunders, p 697.)

TABLE 12-2

Tendon Reflex Grading Scale

Grade	Description
0	Absent
1+ or +	Hypoactive
2+ or ++	Normal
3+ or +++	Hyperactive without clonus
4+ or ++++	Hyperactive with clonus

In addition, a determination regarding what joint complexes may require more detailed assessment (which may occur at subsequent visits) would also have been made.

The novice practitioner should complete the screening examination as presented to minimize the chance of a misdiagnosis. Experienced practitioners can recognize patterns of symptoms or signs that would allow them to skip steps in the examination process and initiate effective treatment many times during the examination itself. In this case, careful assessment of treatment outcome is necessary to avoid the clinical scenarios described by Sahrmann that were mentioned at the beginning of this chapter. Finally, when the PT examines a patient after trauma or surgery, the focus of the initial examination should be the involved area.

As healing and recovery occurs, the PT should begin screening other body regions to identify contributing factors related to the injury itself or to help prevent a reinjury. The reader is directed to textbooks listed in the bibliography for additional resources describing a detailed neuromusculoskeletal examination.

BIBLIOGRAPHY

1. Bickley LS. Bates' guide to physical examination and history taking. 10th ed. Philadelphia: Lippincott Williams & Wilkins; 2009.
2. Boissonnault W. Examination in physical therapy practice: screening for medical disease. 2nd ed. New York: Churchill Livingstone; 1995.
3. Cyriax J. Textbook of orthopaedic medicine: diagnosis of soft tissue lesions. 8th ed. London: Bailliere-Tindall; 1982.
4. Donatelli R, Wooden M. Orthopaedic physical therapy. 3rd ed. New York: Churchill Livingstone; 2001.
5. Goodman C, Snyder T. Differential diagnosis for physical therapists: screening for referral. 4th ed. Philadelphia: Saunders; 2000.
6. Goroll AH, Mulley AG. Primary care medicine. 5th ed. Philadelphia: Lippincott Williams & Wilkins; 2006.
7. Magee DJ. Orthopedic physical assessment. 5th ed. Philadelphia: Saunders; 2008.
8. Maitland G, Hengeveld E, Banks K. Maitland's vertebral manipulation. 6th ed. Oxford: Butterworth/Heinemann; 2001.
9. Meadows J. Orthopedic differential diagnosis in physical therapy. New York: McGraw-Hill; 1999.
10. Sahrmann S. Are physical therapists fulfilling their responsibilities as diagnosticians? J Orthop Sports Phys Ther 2005;35:556–8.
11. Swartz MH. Textbook of physical diagnosis: history and examination. 5th ed. Philadelphia: Saunders; 2006.

Lower Quadrant Screening Examination 13

William G. Boissonnault, PT, DPT, DHSc, FAAOMPT

Objectives

After reading this chapter, the reader will be able to:

1. Describe the primary objectives of the lower quadrant screening examination as a part of the differential diagnosis process.
2. Describe the specific examination elements that make up the lower quadrant screening examination.
3. Explain the importance of each specific examination element as part of the differential diagnosis process.
4. Explain the relevance of each of the specific examination elements as they relate to the differential diagnosis process, including identification of clinical red flags that would result in a patient referral or consultation.

Purposes of the Examination

This chapter and Chapter 12 present lower and upper quadrant screening examinations designed to do the following:

- Narrow the search for the source of symptoms to a specific body region (and the tissue at fault, if possible).
- Identify red flags that, along with the history findings, suggest that the physical therapist (PT) initiate a patient referral or consultation.
- Determine which body regions or body systems require a more detailed examination during the initial or subsequent patient visits.
- Identify primary contributing impairments related to the patient's symptoms, functional limitations, and disability.
- Improve rehabilitation outcomes by avoiding inaccurate diagnoses or by the timely referral of patients to other practitioners.
- Provide guidance, in accordance with the history findings, regarding specific interventions that may help the patient or may be contraindicated.

When to Use and Not Use the Examination

Important general guidelines regarding lower and upper quadrant screening examinations described in this chapter and Chapter 12 include the following:

- Quadrant screening should be included as the primary portion of the initial visit physical examination.
- A novice practitioner should use the entire quadrant screening examination as presented before using additional special testing procedures, to minimize the chance of misdiagnosis.
- An experienced practitioner, at a minimum, should screen at least one joint or body region above and below the patient's chief complaint. Clinical experience leads to the ability to recognize patient presentation patterns that more quickly identify the diagnostic possibilities that have the highest probability of being correct.

Following are descriptions of situations in which the proposed quadrant screening may not be incorporated during the initial visit:

- If the patient has an obvious acute injury (e.g., sprained ankle with edema, bruising, local pain), or if the visit is postoperative, the emphasis of the initial visit should be on the screening examination components most directly related to the involved joint or body region (e.g., ankle/foot). A priority of a physical examination after trauma is ruling out fracture or ligamentous instability, and a priority postoperatively is screening for infection and deep venous thrombosis. The remainder of the screening examination is appropriate during follow-up visits after the patient begins to recover from the injury or surgery.
- If the patient has symptoms other than pain associated with a medical condition, such as urinary incontinence, much of the proposed screening examination would probably be irrelevant and should be replaced with an examination that has a different clinical focus.

The lower quadrant screening examination is performed during the initial patient visit in two scenarios: (1) when the patient's primary symptoms are located in the lower half of the body and (2) when symptom fluctuation is related to movements, postures, or activities that involve primarily the lower portion of the trunk and lower extremities, leading one to believe the primary impairments would be found in this region. The upper half of the body is screened during the postural and gait assessment, when a whole-body screening is conducted. In addition, assessment of trunk active range of motion (AROM) includes a close observation of the upper quadrant regions while the patient is moving.

Chapter 10 discusses elements of the physical examination that begin during the history and that are germane to all patients at the initial visit, including the skin assessment and the screen of the general nervous system. Chapter 11 describes the collection of patient vital signs, again germane to all patients. As stated previously, the history-taking process at this point has led the PT to believe that the origin of the chief symptom and the primary impairments lie in the lower half of the body.

As with the upper quadrant, the lower quadrant screening examination is organized by patient position: standing, sitting, supine, and prone. The recommended sequence works well for most patients but must be modified in certain circumstances. A patient with acute low back pain may state that he cannot sit for more than 5 minutes without a significant increase in back and leg symptoms. In such a situation, the PT may choose to perform the sitting portion of the examination last instead of second. If the PT ignores the patient information and strictly adheres to the printed examination procedure, the examination may aggravate the patient's symptoms to the point that the PT cannot examine the patient in sufficient detail in the supine and prone positions, and the patient may leave in more pain than he or she felt before the visit. Box 13-1 presents the lower quadrant screening examination, organized by patient position.

Description of Examination Elements by Position

Standing

POSTURE ASSESSMENT. The PT can begin with a simple request, such as "please stand and look straight ahead." This request describes the task at hand, yet the instruction is open ended enough that the patient, it is hoped, would assume his or her typical posture. The postural assessment should occur with the patient's shoes and socks off, but if the patient's symptoms are primarily influenced by standing and walking or running, the PT should assess the effect of the patient's footwear on posture and movements.

The patient's posture should be assessed from anterior, posterior, and lateral perspectives, noting major deviations and asymmetries of trunk and limb alignment. Is a lateral trunk shift or a pronounced anterior pelvic tilt present? Is the patient bearing minimal weight on one leg with the lower extremity positioned in abduction and external rotation? (This is a position of comfort for patients with femoral head or neck fractures [see Chapter 20]). The PT should also assess skin condition (e.g., skin lesions, rashes, erythema). When this initial assessment is completed and the PT is ready to begin palpation, the patient position (e.g., feet a foot's width apart) should be standardized so that after treatment the PT can reposition the patient and reassess for any resultant changes.

PALPATION. Palpation includes specific bony landmarks to help the PT better understand and interpret the patient's postural presentation. Examples of landmarks useful as references include the following:

- Spinous processes (T6 to S2); palpating for a step that may suggest possible listhesis deformity
- Inferior angle of the scapula (T7)
- Twelfth ribs
- Iliac crests (approximately L4-L5 level)
- Posterior superior iliac spine (approximately S2 level)
- Superior aspect of greater trochanters
- Fibular heads (superior aspect)

Observed deformity or asymmetry of the lower leg, ankle, or foot may lead to palpation of the following:

- Medial malleoli (inferior aspect)
- Calcaneus
- Navicular tuberosities

Regarding palpation of soft tissues, the PT can assess skin temperature, texture, and muscle tone.

GAIT. The PT assesses gait from the anterior, posterior, and lateral perspectives, noting upper and lower quadrant characteristics associated with the patient's gait pattern. The PT notes any gross alterations in the mechanics of gait and any change in symptoms related to the gait cycle.

STANDING SQUAT. With light fingertip pressure on a ledge or table for balance support, the patient is asked to squat down toward the floor as far as possible. The PT observing from the back should note any change in symptoms, the overall extent of the movement, and any difficulty or asymmetry while going down and returning to the upright position. The PT also can observe regional range of motion (ROM) contributions (or lack of ROM) of the lumbar pelvic, knee, and ankle/foot complexes during the movement. The PT should compare the patient's ability to perform this movement with feet flat versus allowing the heels to rise up to screen for length of the gastrocnemius-soleus complex. Finally, the squat maneuver grossly screens for quadriceps (L2 to L4) weakness. If the patient has difficulty performing the squat movement, it should be attempted unilaterally to get a more accurate assessment of strength. If the patient has no change in symptoms and completes the movement fully and easily, it is unlikely that significant structural issues or impairments exist at the hip, knee, foot, and ankle complexes. This conclusion would allow the PT to spend more time examining other body regions during the remainder of the visit.

ACTIVE RANGE OF MOTION: TRUNK AND HIPS. The evaluation of the functional abilities of the spine and hip joints continues with active movements of trunk flexion, extension, and lateral flexion; these movements also help identify the source of the patient's symptoms. The PT should use a standardized and reproducible position by having the patient spread his or her feet apart a specific distance, such as the width of the PT's foot, or the PT can have the patient straddle a tile on the floor.

Patients should be instructed to move as far as possible, reporting any change in symptoms (better or worse) and what stops them from moving any farther. Patients are instructed to keep the knees straight. Viewing the patient from lateral and posterior perspectives provides the most complete assessment of quantity and quality of movement. Trunk flexion is listed as the first motion to be tested, but the history may dictate that the provided sequence be altered. If acute low back pain and radiculopathy are provoked with minimal trunk flexion activities, the PT may want to test forward flexion last to avoid flaring the patient's condition to the point at which everything the patient does is extremely painful. At least a couple of repetitions of each motion are warranted to be able to realize fully the effect that motion has on the patient's symptoms.

Neuromobility assessment begins with active trunk flexion. Comparing trunk flexion ROM and symptom provocation with the head and neck relaxed with head and neck flexion before trunk flexion can provide useful information. If trunk ROM is significantly reduced or lower body symptoms are magnified when head and neck flexion precedes the trunk flexion, neurologic tissues are implicated, requiring more detailed testing in other positions.

Quantity of motion assessment includes overall trunk motion and regional contributions to the motion. Overall quantity of trunk ROM may be excellent (during forward bending of the trunk, the patient may able to touch the floor with the fingertips), yet the patient may present with regional limitations (e.g., incomplete reversal of the lumbar lordosis or reduced hip rotation). When the overall motion is assessed, the regional contributions of the thoracic spine, lumbar spine, pelvis and hips, and lower legs can be compared. This comparison may identify a specific body region to be examined in more detail related to length of tissues. In contrast, some patients are hypermobile at the lumbar spine but are very limited at the pelvis and hips, leading to

---

BOX 13-1

Lower Quadrant Examination Sequence

STANDING

Postural observation

Gait

Palpation, including soft tissues, bony landmarks (iliac crests, posterior superior iliac spine, greater trochanters, popliteal creases/fibular heads, malleoli, anterior superior iliac spine)

Standing squat (general clearing of lumbar, pelvic, hip, knee, foot, and ankle regions)

Balance

Bilateral stance

Unilateral stance

Trunk AROM (with passive overpressures if symptoms not produced during active movements); rotation to be done in sitting position

Flexion (with head and neck relaxed and preceded with head and neck flexion)

Right and left lateral flexion

Extension

Neurologic screening; myotome and dermatome testing

Heel walk (S1, S2) tibial nerve and superficial peroneal nerve

Toe walk (L4, L5) deep peroneal nerve

Sensation of posterior lower extremities (S1, S2; see Figure 13-6)

SITTING

Posture (observe during the history)

Head, face, and neck (observe during history—see Chapter 10)

Eyes

Pupils

Ptosis

Visual gaze (strabismus)

Facial contour

Eyes/mouth (cranial nerve VII)

Cheeks (masseter muscle, cranial nerve V)

Respiratory excursion (thorax versus cervical or shoulder girdle—observe during history)

Palpation of bony landmarks of the pelvis

Active trunk rotation and overpressures

Vertical trunk compression and decompression (spine in neutral position)

Neurologic screening

Sensory

Lower extremities: L1 to S1 (see Figure 13-6)

Myotome*

Hip flexion: L1, **L2**, L3 (femoral nerve)

Knee extension: L2, **L3**, L4 (femoral nerve)

Knee flexion: L4, L5, S1, S2 (sciatic-tibial nerve)

Dorsiflexion: **L4**, L5 (deep peroneal nerve)

Extensor hallucis longus: **L5** to S1 (deep peroneal nerve)

Plantarflexion: **S1**, S2 (tibial nerve)

Note: Test only in sitting if frank weakness noted in standing (S1 and S2, tibial nerve)

Deep tendon reflexes

Patellar tendon: L2, L3, L4

Achilles tendon: S1, S2

SUPINE

Posture

Palpation (compare with standing bony landmark findings)

Thorax and abdomen

Observation and inspection

Palpation of abdominal region

Abdominal aorta (width and strength of pulse); auscultate if concerns about involvement of the aorta

Sensory T7 to T12 anterior aspect

Superficial abdominal reflex (T7 to L1)

Femoral triangle palpation

Pulses: femoral artery auscultation for bruit if indicated

Lymph nodes: inguinal nodes—vertical and horizontal chains

Lower extremity palpation

Pulses (popliteal artery, posterior tibial artery, dorsalis pedis artery)

Sacroiliac tests, compression and gapping, and ileal shear testing

Trunk AROM: double knee to chest (if standing trunk flexion was symptomatic)

Lower extremities AROM and PROM (add overpressures if symptoms not produced during AROM)

Knee flexion and extension

Hip flexion

Hip internal and external rotation

FABER (flexion in abduction and external rotation) and FADIR (flexion in adduction and internal rotation) tests

Ankle dorsiflexion, plantarflexion, inversion and eversion

Toe flexion and extension

Straight-leg raise

Neck flexion dural tension testing

Neurologic screening

Babinski's test

Repeat or include any or all myotome, sensory, and deep tendon reflexes tests that were positive in sitting or standing or that were not conducted previously

PRONE

Postural observation

Palpation of bony landmarks; compare with standing findings

AROM/PROM (add overpressures if symptoms not produced during AROM)

Prone press-up (if standing trunk extension was symptomatic)

Hip extension

Neurologic screening

Sensory testing: S1, S2, if positive in standing (S2, S3, S4: anal region if patient reports any symptoms suggestive of cauda equina)

Femoral nerve tension test

*Myotome testing—the spinal levels in **bold** are consistent with the Standard Neurological Classification of Spinal Cord Injury. (From Savic G, Bergström EM, Frankel HL, et al: Inter-rater reliability of motor and sensory examinations performed according to American Spinal Injury Association Standards, *Spinal Cord* 45:444-451, 2007.)
AROM, active range of motion; *PROM,* passive range of motion.

---

less-than-expected overall trunk forward flexion. Developing a treatment program to increase flexibility focused on the specific area of impairment should provide a better outcome.

Quality of motion assessment is also extremely valuable and includes the following:

- Trunk deviation from the desired plane of movement (e.g., trunk list to the left with forward flexion)
- Aberrant speed of motion

- An increase, decrease, centralization, or peripheralization of symptoms
- Experience of an end-range atypical sensation (e.g., intense stretching sensation noted in the right posterior thigh at end of range of trunk flexion)

If symptoms do not change during the active motion assessment, the PT can apply a passive overpressure to the spine (Figures 13-1 to 13-3) to clear the spine as a source of symptoms.

Another method PTs may prefer that places increased mechanical stresses on the spine and hip complex beyond that of AROM is to have the patient perform repeated active trunk motions. AROM alone is insufficient for clearing a region as a source of symptoms and a site of relevant impairments.

NEUROLOGIC SCREENING. The final tests in the standing position are designed to test the integrity of lumbosacral myotomes, specifically heel walking (L4, L5) and toe walking (S1, S2). These particular myotomes, along with unilateral squatting with balance support (quadriceps L2-L4), are best tested unilaterally and while the patient is weight bearing to detect subtle to moderate weakness. These maneuvers also test a patient's balance mechanisms and proximal stability. The PT can assess these

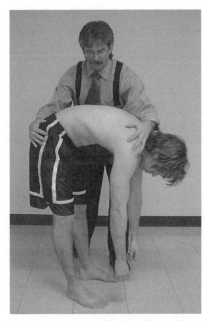

FIGURE 13-1 Passive overpressure with the patient in the position of standing trunk forward flexion.

same myotomes with the patient sitting if symptoms, impaired balance, weakness, or patient anxiety related to the task performance prohibit the tests from being conducted while the patient is standing. Sensation (S1, S2 dermatomes) of the posterior aspect of the lower extremities can also be assessed while the patient is standing.

Sitting

OBSERVATION AND PALPATION. Weight-bearing tests continue with the patient in the sitting position. The PT briefly assesses trunk posture and compares it with the findings in the standing position and with the patient's sitting posture noted during the interview (which may give the most accurate picture of the patient's normal sitting posture). With the feet supported, palpation of iliac crests, posterior superior iliac spine, anterior superior iliac spine (ASIS), sacral sulci, and inferior lateral angles allows for a comparison of findings noted in standing. This assessment may assist in determining the influence of leg length on perceived pelvic and spinal deformities and deviations from the norm.

The PT also performs a brief screening of the lower rib cage ROM by observing whether the patient is breathing from the abdomen or the shoulder girdles and then by palpating laterally around the chest wall while the patient deeply inhales and exhales. The PT should note the amount of rib cage excursion, symmetry, and any change in symptoms. Detection of abnormalities should lead the PT to perform a more extensive examination of this region when the patient is in recumbent positions.

ACTIVE RANGE OF MOTION: TRUNK ROTATION. The patient is asked to cross the arms across the chest and then rotate the trunk to each side. The PT should perform a gross assessment of overall trunk ROM and then, from a posterior viewpoint, specifically observe position changes in the lower thoracic and lumbar spine. If symptoms are not changed with active movements, the PT applies passive overpressure in each direction (Figure 13-4). The hips contribute little movement while the patient is sitting, so a change in symptoms most likely has a spinal origin.

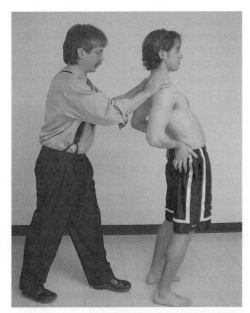

FIGURE 13-2 Passive overpressure with the patient in the position of standing trunk backward bending.

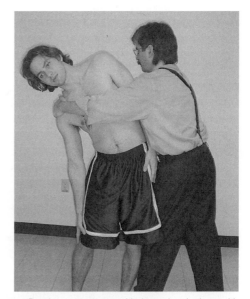

FIGURE 13-3 Passive overpressure with the patient in the position of standing trunk lateral flexion.

VERTICAL TRUNK COMPRESSION AND DECOMPRESSION. Two provocation tests for vertical trunk compression and decompression (Figure 13-5) stress primarily the weight-bearing (vertebral bodies, intervertebral disk, facet joints) and ligamentous structures of the spine. The PT first applies a compression load on the trunk, holding for approximately 5 to 8 seconds and noting any change in symptoms. Next, the PT applies an unloading force, or "decompression," to the trunk for the same amount of time and notes its effect (better or worse) on symptoms. The PT should attempt to avoid producing any movement of the trunk except in the vertical plane. A patient response of increased symptoms with vertical compression and relief with unloading should direct the PT to implement traction and other unloading interventions in the initial plan of care.

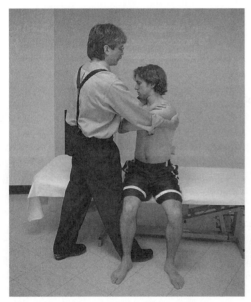

FIGURE 13-4 Passive overpressure for trunk rotation with the patient in the position of seated trunk rotation.

NEUROLOGIC SCREENING: TRUNK AND LOWER EXTREMITIES. Patients should be placed in reproducible positions (an upright posture if tolerated) to help ensure each time these tests are reassessed the results are not influenced by extremes of trunk or spinal positions. Rechecking the patient's posture during testing is prudent because patients may try to see what is being done, placing them in head and neck and trunk flexion—potentially influencing the test results. If the patient has thoracic complaints, myotome, dermatome, and deep tendon reflexes testing must include the trunk and the lower extremities. Myotome testing of the trunk is very general because the innervations of muscles are multisegmental; identifying one particular thoracic nerve root as the source of any weakness is virtually impossible. The PT should instruct the patient to "hold and meet my pressure—don't let me move you" as resistance is applied in anterior, posterior, lateral, and rotary directions. The patient holds this position for 10 seconds, with the PT noting performance as weak or strong, firm or poor quality/inconsistent resistance, and any change in symptoms.

For dermatome testing, as in the upper quadrant screening examination (see Chapter 12), sharp or dull sensation is assessed for the lower body. If symptoms exist in the trunk, the PT needs to assess the T6 through S2 dermatomal areas (Figure 13-6). Abdominal reflexes should also be carried out with the patient supine. If the thoracic region is asymptomatic, the examination can include the L1-S2 spinal levels for all three types of testing.

Supine

As the patient settles into the supine position, the PT notes trunk and lower extremity positions and compares findings with the assessment conducted with the patient standing. The chosen position of comfort itself may provide clues of underlying pathology; examples provided by Swartz[9] include the following:

- Forward lean: Pancreatitis, pericarditis
- Knees flexed: Peritonitis
- Right hip flexion: Appendicitis
- Left hip flexion: Diverticulitis
- Hip abducted and externally rotated: Hip fracture

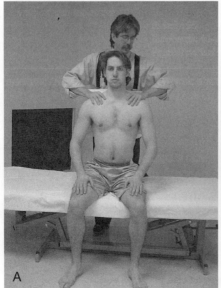
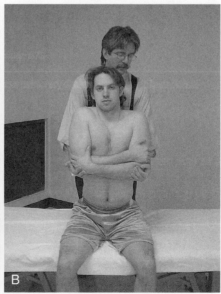

FIGURE 13-5 A, Seated trunk vertical compression test (stressing weight-bearing structures of the spine); **B,** Seated trunk vertical distraction test.

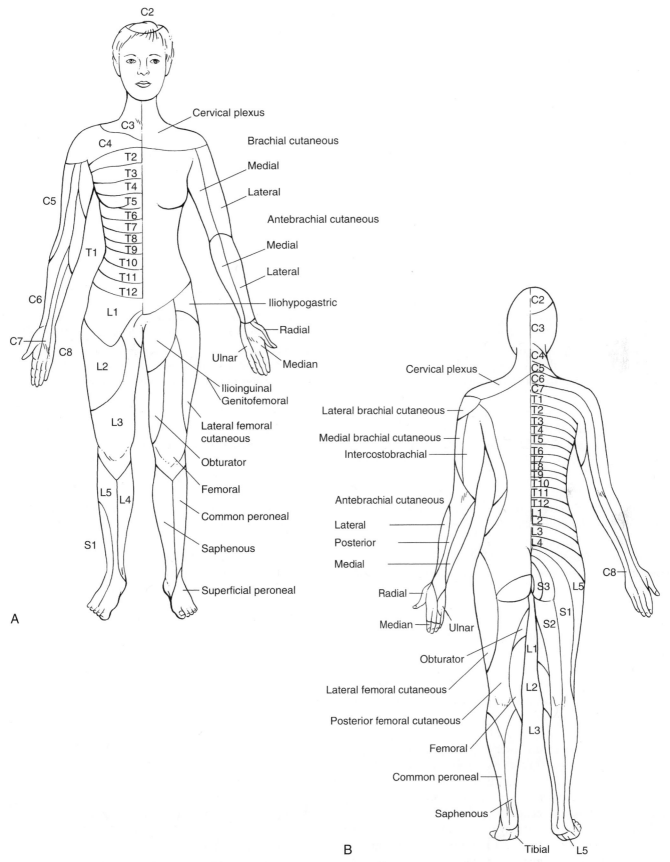

FIGURE 13-6 A and **B,** Segmental distribution of the spinal nerves. (From Swartz MH: *Textbook of physical diagnosis: history and examination,* Philadelphia, 2002, Saunders, p 623.)

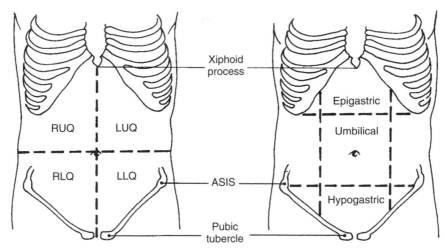

FIGURE 13-7 Terminology used to delineate regions of the abdomen. *ASIS,* anterior superior iliac spine; *LLQ,* left lower abdominal quadrant; *LUQ,* left upper abdominal quadrant; *RLQ,* right lower abdominal quadrant; *RUQ,* right upper abdominal quadrant. (From Boissonnault W: *Examination in physical therapy practice: screening for medical disease,* 2nd ed, New York, 1995, Churchill Livingstone, p 111.)

If the patient assumes any of the aforementioned positions, the PT should have the patient move out of the posture; if abdominal or deep back or pelvic pain is provoked, a more detailed abdominal screening is warranted. After the general observation is completed, if tolerated, the patient should again assume a standard position, which the PT can produce by asking the patient to perform a bridging activity to "reset" trunk position.

ABDOMINAL SCREENING. Figure 13-7 represents two ways to "divide" the abdomen geographically for anatomic reference, documentation purposes, and understanding physician literature and patient notes. For nonmidline findings, the abdomen is divided into right and left and upper and lower quadrants. Dividing the midline into epigastric, umbilical, and hypogastric (or suprapubic) regions is standard for nonmidline findings. The series of screening maneuvers includes observation and inspection, palpation, percussion, and auscultation.

Observation and Inspection. Observations of skin condition, asymmetry in surface contour, and position of the umbilicus all are relevant. Assessment of skin includes noting general skin color (e.g., jaundice), skin lesions with suspicious characteristics (see Chapter 10), scars that may not have been accounted for in the patient history, rashes, and striae (stretch marks). Striae that are flesh-colored or a silverish hue are normal; pink or purple striae may be associated with Cushing's syndrome. A prominent dilated venous plexus is also an unusual finding that may be associated with hepatic cirrhosis or inferior vena cava obstruction. The umbilicus should lie in the midline. If not, an abdominal mass or a neurologic lesion of lower thoracic and upper lumbar nerve roots may be present. In addition to observing the position of the umbilicus, the PT may find the umbilicus to be everted (possible causes include increased abdominal pressure from ascites or a mass, or umbilical hernia) or discolored. A bluish hue of the umbilicus (Cullen's sign) may represent hemoperitoneum.

Associated with skin assessment is noting surface contour, including movements, asymmetry in contour, and masses. A pulsatile mass, although not unusual to observe on a person of thin build, may represent an abdominal aortic aneurysm (see Chapter 20). If such a mass is noted, palpation of this area would be warranted (see later under Palpation). Peristalsis, a

wavelike movement, may also be seen on a person of very thin build but may represent intestinal obstruction. The two upper and lower quadrants should be symmetric in contour. Asymmetry could be associated with a structural deformity of the rib cage or sternum, the presence of a prominent scoliosis, or a soft tissue lesion (a space-occupying mass). Ascites may be a cause of abdominal distention. In the supine position, the fluid tends to "pool" at the flanks—the abdominal periphery. As the patient changes positions, the fluid pools dependently. (With the patient in left side-lying position, the fluid settles into the left abdominal quadrants.) If a hernia is suspected (umbilical and inguinal regions), having the patient cough and noting whether a sudden bulging occurs in the area provides additional evidence supporting concerns.

Palpation. The PT next performs palpation of the abdominal area to assess local anatomy (masses), help rule out nonmusculoskeletal sources of the patient's symptoms, and identify local impairments related to the patient's functional limitations. The palpation is not intended to enable the PT to diagnose a specific visceral problem but to contribute to the overall investigation for potential sources of back, pelvic, and hip symptoms (see Chapter 6). As elsewhere, firm but light pressure is applied first in a circular fashion, comparing one quadrant with the other and asking the patient whether he or she feels more than just pressure and whether the symptoms improve or worsen.

A broad hand contact (flat), not palpating with fingertips, minimizes the sense of ticklishness. If there is no major resistance and no complaint of symptoms, the PT continues with deeper pressure. Although not unusual, areas of tenderness should be noted, especially if associated with other findings, a local mass, area of muscle guarding, and referral of pain from that spot. Local pain complaints, combined with palpatory tenderness and muscle guarding, should raise the suspicion of peritoneal inflammation. If the same pain is provoked with a cough and percussion, the suspicion is supported, with the final test being assessment for rebound tenderness. Firm downward-directed force is applied followed by a quick release of pressure, and the PT notes whether the downward pressure or quick release (more indicative of peritoneal inflammation) was more

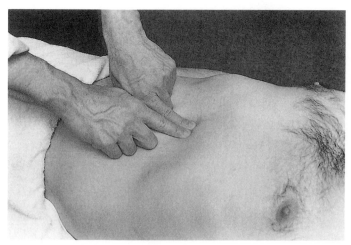

FIGURE 13-8 Palpation over abdominal aortic artery. (From Boissonnault W: *Examination in physical therapy practice: screening for medical disease,* 2nd ed, New York, 1995, Churchill Livingstone, p 412.)

painful. This finding would warrant immediate contact with the patient's physician.

The *abdominal aorta* was mentioned in the section on observation and inspection. Having the patient's hips and knees flexed tends to relax the abdomen and allow for easier palpation. The PT should first locate the pulse (typically along the left parasternal line) and assess it for intensity using the 0 to 4+ arterial scale (0 = absent; 2+ = normal; 4+ = bounding). The PT assesses the width of the aortic pulse by placing the index fingers of both hands side by side over the pulse and then slowly moving them apart until the borders of the pulsation are noted (Figure 13-8). If the PT suspects widening ("lateralization") of the pulse (the normal width of the vessel is approximately 2 to 3 cm), or if back pain is provoked, the PT should auscultate over the blood vessel, assessing for a bruit. If pain is provoked, or if a bruit is noted, physician contact is warranted. See Chapter 20 for details related to screening for abdominal aortic aneurysm.

Percussion. Beyond or in support of abdominal observation and palpation, *manual percussion* can be a valuable tool: as a provocation test (see section on supine palpation), to identify potential abnormal anatomy (a mass)—to be confirmed by a physician—and to help locate thoracic and abdominal structures. For example, the PT has determined that deep soft tissue mobilization is required in the subcostal area, right upper quadrant, secondary to a large scar from an "old" gallbladder procedure. The question is, is the perceived soft tissue restriction solely from the scar, or might the liver be extending below the ribs accounting for part of this finding? Percussion can be used to identify the caudal liver border, and if it extends below the ribs, the soft tissue mobilization pressure should be applied away from the rib cage and not deep "under" the ribs.

The sound produced from manual percussion helps determine whether the underlying structure is air-filled, fluid-filled, or solid, as noted by the presence of the four different sounds or notes produced:

- Flatness: Solid, dense tissues such as that of the anterior thigh
- Dullness: Liver, heart, diaphragm, spleen
- Resonance: Lung
- Tympany: Gastric (stomach) bubble, bowel

Manual percussion is performed as follows: Hyperextend the middle finger of your nondominant hand. Press the distal interphalangeal joint firmly on the surface to be percussed. Avoid contact by any other part of the hand because this could dampen the vibrations. Position your other forearm close to the surface, with the hand cocked upward (wrist extended). The middle finger should be partially flexed and relaxed, and with a quick, sharp, but relaxed wrist motion, strike the interphalangeal joint of the finger in contact with the skin with your middle finger of the dominant hand. You are simply trying to transmit vibrations through the bones of this joint to the underlying chest wall. Use two strikes, then pause, and then either repeat or move on to another location.

This technique can be used over each of the four abdominal quadrants, where the tympanic sound should be noted, and over the thorax, where either a deep resonance (normal lung tissue sound) or a dullness should be noted if over the liver or heart. A couple of specific examples follow for this technique for identifying solid organ location.

- *Liver:* For *percussion,* the PT starts just above the umbilicus along the right mid-clavicular line and progresses cephalad, noting first tympany of bowel until hearing *dullness* of the liver. When the dullness is noted, the PT continues along the mid-clavicular line for an expected 6 to 12 cm (Figure 13-9), when a new sound should be noted, the *resonance* of lung tissue. If the dullness from the liver starts much caudad to the rib cage or extends for much greater than 12 cm, an enlarged liver or possibly a lung mass may be responsible. This can be followed by palpation on the right side, lateral to the rectus abdominis margin, and below the inferior border of the liver dullness noted during percussion. The PT places the left hand under the patient's back, around the T10-T11 region on the right, and lifts gently. The fingers of the right hand apply a moderate pressure slightly cephalad and posteriorly. The patient is asked to hold a deep breath; the PT may note the liver edge as it moves down into the fingers; the PT documents any change or reproduction of symptoms.

- *Spleen:* Percussion starts at the lowest rib interspace along the left anterior axillary line. The sound produced should be abdominal tympany. Moving posteriorly, percussion should produce splenic dullness, normally noted in the mid-axillary line from the left nineth to the eleventh ribs (Figure 13-10). An enlarged spleen would account for the dullness to be noted more medially and caudally. If the PT is concerned, *palpation* in this area would be warranted similar to in the liver. The PT positions one hand posteriorly under the patient's left side and lifts upward. The PT places the other hand at the left upper abdominal region and applies gentle pressure in a cephalad and posterior direction, having the patient take and hold a deep inspiration, noting any change or reproduction of symptoms.

Percussion as strictly a provocation test is performed sometimes as a special test over the kidneys. As described in Chapter 6, patients with kidney disease may complain of pain over the costovertebral angle (ipsilateral thoracolumbar junction) with referral of pain to the iliac crest. The pain may be colicky (see Chapter 6) in nature and often is unchanging with assumption of a different position and movement. If the PT notes this pain pattern, he or

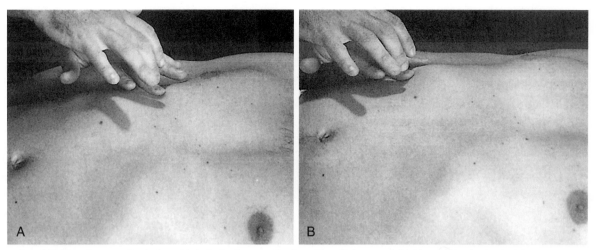

FIGURE 13-9 A and **B,** Manual percussion in the mid-clavicular line over the liver. (From Boissonnault W: *Examination in physical therapy practice: screening for medical disease,* 2nd ed, New York, 1995, Churchill Livingstone, p 111.)

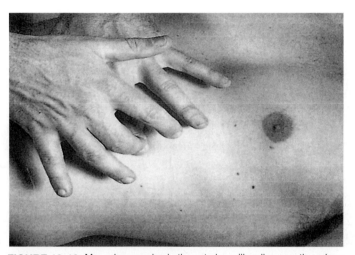

FIGURE 13-10 Manual percussion in the anterior axillary line over the spleen. (From Boissonnault W: *Examination in physical therapy practice: screening for medical disease,* 2nd ed, New York, 1995, Churchill Livingstone, p 112.)

she can perform *percussion* over the kidneys with the patient sitting. A firm "thumping" with the PT's fist over the costovertebral angle, first the left and then the right side, often provokes intense symptoms if the kidneys are inflamed or irritated.

Auscultation. Abdominal auscultation over the four abdominal quadrants may reveal bowel sounds, bruits, or friction rubs. Bowel sounds, consisting of high-pitched clicks and gurgling, are normal and expected sounds—every 5 to 10 seconds, or 5 to 34 times per minute. A "rush" of high-pitched bowel sounds associated with complaints of abdominal cramping may be indicative of intestinal obstruction—warranting communication with the patient's physician. Bruits are abnormal abdominal sounds—pulsations suggesting turbulent blood flow—indicating arterial disorders including renal arterial stenosis and abdominal aortic aneurysm. Auscultating over the four quadrants and along the left parasternal line to the umbilicus allows for assessment of the renal, aortic, and iliac arteries. If concerns are raised regarding the status of the vascular system, auscultating over the femoral arteries would also be warranted. Finally, noting a friction rub is important because it may indicate an inflammatory process of the peritoneum or a liver or splenic disorder.

Neurologic Screening: Abdomen

Sensory Testing. Sharp and dull testing over the abdominal region from the xiphoid process to just above the inguinal ligament (see Figure 13-6) assesses the sensory status of the T7 through T12 dermatomes.

Superficial Abdominal Reflex. With the PT using an object such as the end of a reflex hammer, each of the four abdominal quadrants is lightly stroked, moving the stimulus across the "outer" edges of each quadrant (Figure 13-11). A normal response includes the umbilicus moving in the direction of the stimulus.

MUSCULOSKELETAL TRUNK AND LOWER EXTREMITY SCREENING

Trunk Active Range of Motion (Double Knee to Chest). If standing trunk forward flexion provokes symptoms (of the back or lower extremity), the PT should assess this movement with the patient in a non–weight-bearing position. The PT may find that although standing forward flexion worsens the symptoms, *double-knee-to-chest* movement produces only a sensation of "good stretch" in the low back region. This finding would give the PT a method of working on improving this important trunk movement.

Sacroiliac Joint Stress Tests. Two tests help in implicating or ruling out the sacroiliac joint as a source of symptoms. For the compression and gapping test, the PT first makes contact just lateral to the ASIS of the iliac crests and applies pressure with both hands slowly in a medial direction. The PT should hold this pressure for approximately 5 seconds. Next, the PT's arms are crossed, the heels of the hands are placed on the medial aspects of the iliac crests (near the ASIS), and pressure is applied in a lateral direction bilaterally, again holding for approximately 5 seconds.

Another useful test is the ileal shear test described by Magee.[6] Stabilizing one ASIS with anteroposterior pressure, the PT applies an anteroposterior shear force to the opposite ASIS. The PT repeats this procedure on the opposite side, holding for approximately 5 seconds each time. The ileal shear test allows the PT to assess end feels, comparing the left side with the right side in addition to noting any change in symptoms.

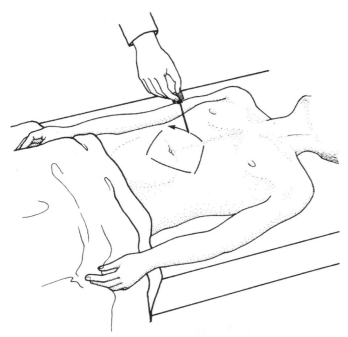

FIGURE 13-11 Superficial abdominal reflex testing. (From Magee DJ: *Orthopedic physical assessment,* 4th ed, Philadelphia, 2002, Saunders, p 530.)

LYMPH NODE PALPATION. The inguinal lymph nodes located in the femoral triangle (bordered by the inguinal ligament and the sartorius and adductor longus muscles) are divided into horizontal and vertical chains. The PT first locates the inguinal ligament, running between the ASIS and the pubic tubercle. Just caudal and running parallel to this ligament is the horizontal chain. In the medial third of the femoral triangle is the vertical chain, running parallel to the adductor longus. See Chapter 10 for normal and abnormal characteristics of lymph nodes.

Arterial Pulse: Lower Extremities. The PT should assess each of the lower extremity pulses for location, intensity, and symmetry, especially in patients presenting with complaints of intermittent claudication, symptoms of cold feet, or trophic or other changes in skin (see Chapter 10). The following landmarks can be used to locate the pulses:

- The femoral pulse is located in the femoral triangle.
- The popliteal pulse is found just cephalad to the popliteal crease. The patient's knee should be flexed to place the posterior soft tissues on slack, facilitating palpation of this deeply set artery. If this artery is difficult to locate with the patient in the supine position, the PT can assess the pulse with the patient in the prone position, again with the knee flexed.
- The posterior tibial pulse is located posterior to the medial malleolus.
- The dorsalis pedis artery is found on the dorsum of the foot over the first and second metatarsal bases.

Clearing the Lower Extremities. Clearing any joint implies examining the joint and related soft tissues to the point that the PT can confidently state that it is, or is not, a source of symptoms and that it is, or is not, involved from an impairment perspective. Clearing of the lower extremities began with the posture and gait screening and the standing-squat maneuver. The following joint clearing uses selected active ROM and passive overpressures in a sequence similar to that used when clearing the upper

extremities (see Chapter 12). Recommended movement tests for the lower extremities include the following:

Hip	Knee	Ankle	Toes
Flexion	Flexion	Dorsiflexion	Flexion
Internal/external rotation	Extension	Plantarflexion	Extension
FABER (flexion in abduction and external rotation) test			
FADIR (flexion in adduction and internal rotation) test			

The PT should clear the knee first because assessment of hip rotation stresses the knee joint. Next, the PT assesses hip flexion, then internal and external rotation, and if symptoms are not altered and the PT does not note significant impairments, the PT should carry out the combined movement tests (FABER and FADIR). After finishing the test of hip ROM, the PT moves to the ankles and feet and completes the movement testing. Performing the active ankle/foot movements bilaterally can save time, as can be done with the wrists and hands during the upper quadrant screening examination.

Neurologic Screening: Lower Extremities including Babinski's Reflex. If the PT noted any positive neurologic findings during myotome or sensory testing with the patient in the weight-bearing positions (standing or sitting), the tests should be repeated now with the patient in the supine or non–weight-bearing positions for comparison. In addition, the PT should routinely assess *Babinski's reflex.* The PT firmly strokes the plantar aspect of the foot, starting at the heel and moving up the lateral side of the sole and eventually across the metatarsal heads medially. The patient often shows a withdrawal response of the hip and knee (flexion), which is normal. An abnormal response or positive Babinski's reflex is extension of the great toe and abduction of the other toes. When this pathologic reflex occurs, it is indicative of upper motor neuron disease.

Neuromobility Testing

Passive Neck Flexion. As the PT passively flexes the head and neck on the thorax, alterations in patient symptoms are noted. A patient with an acute lumbar radiculopathy may experience lumbar and lower extremity pain with the neck flexion maneuver. If the patient experiences acute exacerbation of lumbar and posterior thighs, accompanied by hip and knee flexion, the PT must be suspicious of meningeal irritation.

Straight Leg Raise. After the head and neck flexion test, the straight leg raise should be done. If the patient does not have acute symptoms, he or she first actively performs the movement (with the ankle and foot relaxed) while the PT monitors the ROM and changes in symptoms. Next, the PT fully extends the patient's knee and then slowly flexes the hip passively (again foot and ankle are relaxed) until the patient complains of symptoms. At this point, the patient is instructed to inform the PT when the symptoms begin to subside as the PT lowers the leg. Head and neck flexion followed by ankle passive dorsiflexion can be added to see whether symptoms return; if the symptoms increase again, dural tissue may be implicated as the source of symptoms.

Prone

The PT questions the patient about changes in symptoms during the final position change, as the patient moves into the prone position. The PT observes the trunk and lower extremities in this position, compares results with the results of the standing position, and notes any differences. Having the patient do "reverse" bridging (patient gently lifts trunk off table and returns to the prone position) allows the PT to establish a reproducible position.

ACTIVE RANGE OF MOTION: TRUNK AND LOWER EXTREMITIES. The PT should have the patient perform the *prone press-up* if standing trunk backward bending provokes back or lower extremity symptoms, for the same reasons noted during the supine double-knee-to-chest maneuver. The PT also can assess active hip extension, but the PT is challenged in controlling lumbar spine position and preventing lumbosacral backward bending and rotation during the assessment. Stabilizing over the ipsilateral ischial tuberosity helps localize the movement to the hip.

The patient next performs active knee flexion, followed by passive flexion. This test assesses several structures. It brings the hamstring into play against gravity and places a tensile stress on the femoral nerve and the rectus femoris muscle.

NEUROLOGIC SCREENING: EXTREMITIES. If the PT noted any positive neurologic findings during myotome or sensory testing with the patient standing, the PT should repeat the sensory assessment of the posterior thigh, calf, and plantar aspect of foot regions, as well as motor assessment for S1 and S2 myotomes. As with the comparison of non–weight-bearing assessment of trunk ROM versus weight-bearing trunk ROM, positive neurologic findings may occur only in weight-bearing positions, giving guidance to the PT about body positions to be used in home exercise programs and general patient education.

Summary

As with the upper quadrant screening examination, the overall examination of the patient is not finished when the PT has completed the tests described here. At this point (after the history and lower quadrant screening examination), the PT should have a strong hypothesis about the source of symptoms and the primary impairments related to functional limitations and disability and should have identified red flags. In many instances, the collected information gives the PT sufficient guidance to initiate treatment. In addition, the PT decides which joint complexes may require more detailed assessment at subsequent visits.

As stated previously, when a patient presents with an acute injury, the initial emphasis should be on the injured area and then as the patient begins to recover, the PT should use the lower quadrant screening examination to help identify any contributing factors (impairments) associated with the injury. Systematically proceeding through the screening examination prevents the PT from being fooled by the location of symptoms. The reader is directed to textbooks listed in the bibliography for additional resources describing a detailed neuromusculoskeletal examination.

BIBLIOGRAPHY

1. Bickley LS. Bates' guide to physical examination and history taking. 10th ed. Philadelphia: Lippincott Williams & Wilkins; 2009.
2. Boissonnault W. Examination in physical therapy practice: screening for medical disease. 2nd ed. New York: Churchill Livingstone; 1995.
3. Cyriax J. Textbook of orthopaedic medicine: diagnosis of soft tissue lesions. 8th ed. London: Bailliere-Tindall; 1982.
4. Donatelli R, Wooden M. Orthopaedic physical therapy. 3rd ed. New York: Churchill Livingstone; 2001.
5. Goroll AH, Mulley AG. Primary care medicine. 5th ed. Philadelphia: Lippincott Williams & Wilkins; 2006.
6. Magee DJ. Orthopedic physical assessment. 5th ed. Philadelphia: Saunders; 2008.
7. Maitland G, Hengeveld E, Banks K, et al. Maitland's vertebral manipulation. 6th ed. Oxford: Butterworth/Heinemann; 2001.
8. Meadows J. Orthopedic differential diagnosis in physical therapy. New York: McGraw-Hill; 1999.
9. Swartz MH. Textbook of physical diagnosis: history and examination. 5th ed. Philadelphia: Saunders; 2006.

Diagnostic Imaging 14

Gail D. Deyle, PT, DSc, DPT, OCS, FAAOMPT

Objectives

After reading this chapter, the reader will be able to:

1. Evaluate the details of the patient history, review of systems, and tests and measures to determine whether indications for musculoskeletal diagnostic imaging are present.
2. Apply the known risks, contraindications, and benefits of diagnostic imaging to recommend musculoskeletal imaging only when the diagnostic benefits outweigh the disadvantages.
3. Apply knowledge of the diagnostic utility of the various types of musculoskeletal imaging to select or recommend the appropriate modality for a specific patient presentation.

The role of musculoskeletal imaging in the practice of physical therapy is rapidly evolving. The availability of diagnostic images to physical therapists (PTs) varies greatly depending on the practice setting. PTs in the U.S. Army with primary care physical therapy provider credentials have had privileges for ordering musculoskeletal imaging procedures since the early 1970s (see Chapter 1).[9,33,37,38] In other settings, PTs often practice without the benefit of being able to order or even routinely view diagnostic images. This inability to order diagnostic imaging tests has probably contributed to PTs learning to depend on their clinical examination skills to formulate a clinical diagnosis. Other providers with ready access to imaging procedures may have learned to depend more on diagnostic imaging modalities for making a clinical diagnosis rather than fully developing their physical examination skills. A prospective randomized study comparing PTs and orthopedic surgeons in the primary management of musculoskeletal conditions found that care provided by the PTs was more cost-effective and resulted in higher patient satisfaction, with no difference in patient outcomes. One reason for the cost-effectiveness was that the PTs were less reliant on imaging procedures.[14]

Other studies have found that the use of PTs in a primary care setting reduced the need for diagnostic imaging by 50%.[33,37,38] Studies have confirmed the diagnostic accuracy of PTs for musculoskeletal conditions when compared with the accuracy of other providers. The diagnostic accuracy of PTs before and after magnetic resonance imaging (MRI) studies has been shown to be equal to orthopedic surgeons and superior to other medical and nonmedical health care providers typically involved in the management of patients with musculoskeletal conditions.[56,57]

Regardless of whether PTs can currently order diagnostic imaging studies in their practice setting, they should be familiar with musculoskeletal imaging protocols and standards. PTs are often in a position to provide guidance to other providers for ordering the most appropriate imaging. The type of musculoskeletal imaging modality or the specific views or sequences that would best reveal the suspected pathology, with the least risk to the patient and at a reasonable price, should be recommended. Although most providers who refer to PTs have privileges to order diagnostic imaging, their knowledge and experience associated with musculoskeletal diagnoses may be quite limited.[28,56]

The clinical examination findings from PTs can also provide the appropriate relevance to the pathology identified by the diagnostic imaging tests. This relevance is important considering there are many examples in the published literature of pathology found on images of the spine and extremities in asymptomatic populations.[22,41,54,61,75] Conversely, PTs are also well suited to confirm what may initially seem to be a normal image, a normal variant, or old pathology to the radiologist. Ryder and Deyle[66] reported a case of a patient with breast cancer with acute ankle symptoms that shows the value of combining PT clinical expertise with musculoskeletal image interpretation. The plain films ordered for this patient by the PT because of her severe fracture-quality pain were read by the radiologist as normal without evidence of fracture or bony irregularity. However, the PT was concerned about apparent cortical irregularity in the area of palpation tenderness. A bone scan revealed an active lesion, and subsequent MRI differentiated a near-complete stress fracture from a potential metastatic lesion. In this excellent case example, the PT's careful clinical examination combined with the ability to review and order the appropriate musculoskeletal imaging facilitated discovery and differentiation of important pathology in a timely and cost-efficient manner.

A strong case can be made for making the ordering of diagnostic imaging a routine practice privilege for PTs, within the context of established PT practice guidelines.[4] A comprehensive valid examination scheme and evidence-based intervention strategies are essential to determine the need for diagnostic imaging accurately. Practice guidelines, such as the low back pain (LBP) guidelines presented in this chapter, illustrate the importance of findings from the history and physical examination and the degree of response to physical therapy interventions in making a decision related to the need for musculoskeletal imaging.[10,39]

When there is little likelihood that imaging would reveal anything that would change the course of treatment, musculoskeletal imaging studies should be considered unnecessary. Although imaging may provide evidence of pathology, the mere presence of an abnormality may not change the course of treatment, particularly when there is no evidence for a successful pathology-based

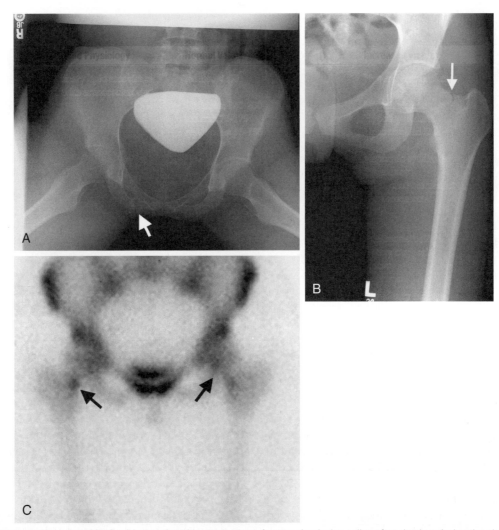

FIGURE 14-1 A, Anteroposterior radiograph of pelvis reveals pubic ramus stress fracture developing callus after simply reducing the physical activity level of the patient. **B,** Anteroposterior radiograph of hip reveals femoral neck stress fracture that requires immediate surgical stabilization to prevent possible consequences of a completed fracture. Although radionuclide bone scans have higher sensitivity than plain radiographs for detecting early femoral neck stress fractures, this antero-posterior film clearly reveals the extent of the fracture line. **C,** Bone scan of a physically active person reveals multiple areas of increased metabolic activity. Increased radiopharmaceutical uptake in femoral necks suggests stress fracture of right femoral neck and stress-related changes of left femoral neck. The stress fracture appears to be primarily on the compression, or inferior, side of the femoral neck and is considered to be more stable than a tension, or superior, side femoral neck fracture.

intervention. A patient may have clinical findings suggesting a particular musculoskeletal pathology. In the absence of evidence that surgery or other strategy based on the pathology would produce a better outcome, musculoskeletal imaging is unnecessary. Similarly, there may be evidence that a surgical procedure could be beneficial for a type of pathology revealed on imaging. If the patient is unwilling to undergo the procedure, or if the patient is an unsuitable candidate for any of the associated risks of surgery, there is no reason to perform the imaging.

Another example of imaging being indicated only when positive findings would change the course of treatment comes from the management of stress fractures. Pubic rami and proximal tibial stress fractures are common injuries in the training military population.[2,5] When appropriately managed, these injuries rarely require medical or surgical intervention. If the patient history, review of systems, and tests and measures do not suggest infection or neoplasm, treatment for these suspected stress fractures may be initiated without imaging. In contrast, stress fractures of

the femoral neck are treated very cautiously and even surgically to prevent the possible catastrophic consequences of a complete displaced femoral neck fracture.[13] Musculoskeletal imaging that reveals the characteristics of a femoral neck stress fracture would alter the conservative treatment course and may dictate the need for surgery. Whenever a PT suspects a femoral neck stress reaction or fracture, imaging that is sensitive for the disorder, such as a bone scan, is promptly indicated (Figure 14-1).

The official interpretation of diagnostic images is the responsibility of the radiologist. In the clinical setting, however, it is not unusual for primary care providers to have access to diagnostic images before the official report. In a situation in which a quick interpretation of imaging is paramount to the disposition of the patient, it may be possible to request a "wet read" (this name originates from when plain film radiographs were hung up wet from developing solution) or less formal opinion from the radiologist as soon as the imaging is completed. At other times, the PT may need to initiate treatment before musculoskeletal images have been read or reviewed by the radiologist. If the images are available, the PT should review them while waiting for the official interpretation by a radiologist, because the images may provide useful information for patient management or clinical decision making.

When ordering a musculoskeletal imaging study, any provider, including the PT, should provide important details of the history (e.g., specific location of symptoms; quality, character, and intensity of pain; mechanism of injury), physical examination, and tests and measures. The radiologist rarely has the opportunity to gather patient information directly. Being able to correlate clinical information with the appearance of the images facilitates the radiologist's interpretation of the study. Guidance on the interpretation of musculoskeletal imaging is beyond the scope of this chapter. PTs may increase their interpretation skills through formal coursework or by independently studying the wealth of material available in textbooks and over the Internet. A recommended resource list is provided at the end of this chapter. Simple search strategies can yield other sites and resources.

Musculoskeletal Imaging as Part of Patient Management

Whenever PTs have privileges for ordering diagnostic imaging or are in a situation in which it is possible to recommend imaging, it is essential that they do not substitute musculoskeletal imaging for the normal comprehensive examination procedures of physical therapy patient management. The imaging results have relevance only in the context of the comprehensive clinical examination. The practice patterns of the expert PT have been previously described. The expert PT uses the history and review of systems for early hypothesis formation, which guides the selection of tests, measures, and intervention strategies. The expert PT also uses cumulative knowledge, clinical experience, and evaluation of movement dysfunction to help determine the need for musculoskeletal imaging.[23,40,41,64]

Physical examination principles that are crucial to appropriate clinical decisions regarding musculoskeletal imaging include palpating all possible injured structures, examining body regions above and below the area of symptoms, and examining the cervical spine for upper extremity symptoms and the lumbar spine for lower extremity symptoms. PTs must also remain vigilant for the possibility of referred pain from proximal structures of the musculoskeletal system and from structures in other systems, such as the cardiovascular, genitourinary, and gastrointestinal systems. Failure to identify the true source of pain may result in images that do not reveal the true area of pathology. Hip problems commonly cause referred symptoms to the knee, particularly in younger patients.[26,51] The initial symptom of slipped capital femoral epiphysis and Legg-Calvé-Perthes disease is commonly pain around the knee. A wide variety of conditions of the cervical spine cause referred symptoms to the upper extremity, and many conditions of the lumbar spine are known to cause referred symptoms to the pelvis and lower extremity.[50,52,72] The following case overview dramatically underscores the importance of examining proximal body regions and structures to determine the true source of distal pain.

An 18-year-old man presented to a military treatment facility with a primary symptom of hip and knee pain for the prior 2 weeks. The patient was uncertain of the origin of his symptoms, although he had been participating in physical training daily. The initial examination by the primary care physician revealed tenderness over the iliac crest, anterior superior iliac spine, and mid-quadriceps. A diagnosis of a quadriceps strain was made, and the patient was prescribed anti-inflammatory medication, activity was restricted, and a referral was written to physical therapy.

By the time the patient was seen in physical therapy 1 week later, his primary symptom was knee pain. Over the next few months, this patient had waxing and waning of his symptoms with physical therapy and medical treatment. His primary symptom was always knee pain, but the painful areas were variable enough to prompt other diagnoses, such as retropatellar pain syndrome and iliotibial band syndrome.

Eventually, a PT who was not previously involved in the patient's care recognized several patient interview red flags, exposed the hip region for examination, and observed and palpated a large mass protruding from the patient's right iliac wing. After completing the examination, the PT ordered radiographs of the hip and pelvis. The radiologist's differential diagnosis based on the radiographic findings was osteogenic sarcoma versus chondrosarcoma. Osteogenic sarcoma became the definitive diagnosis. Despite the large size of this primary malignant tumor, the patient and several providers were misled into thinking this was primary knee pain. Prior radiographs of the patient's knee based solely on the location of symptoms were normal (Figure 14-2).

Significant disease processes or injuries may be obscured in ways other than referred pain. The primary injury in an emergent situation may mask a less symptomatic injury until the primary injury is treated and the acute symptoms are reduced. Injuries associated with alcohol or other drug use or a loss of consciousness require a particularly thorough review of systems and physical examination, because patients are likely to be limited in their ability to guide the diagnostic process during the patient history.

Consistent with the principles of evidence-based medicine, diagnostic test results must be viewed in the context of the pretest probability of the disorder.[31] For diagnostic imaging, the pretest probability may be determined by many factors. Consider the example of an elderly patient with diabetes who exhibits increasing back pain, spasm, fever, and malaise 2 weeks after a surgical procedure for the lumbar spine. This patient history and the clinical signs establish a strong pretest probability of an infection. Normal radiographs viewed in the context of the high pretest likelihood of systemic illness should be regarded with some suspicion. A more sensitive imaging procedure for infection, such as MRI or bone scan, and the appropriate laboratory tests must be ordered to rule out an infection with confidence. In comparison, a patient who is not diabetic and has a postoperative transient increase in back pain without constitutional symptoms of fever or malaise (Chapter 9) may require only a decrease in the intensity of the rehabilitation program. The probability of an infection in the second example is so low that diagnostic imaging in this instance is unlikely to contribute to patient management, and

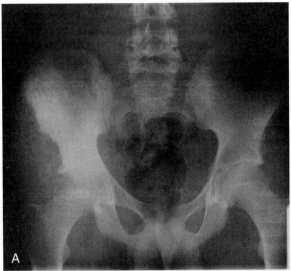

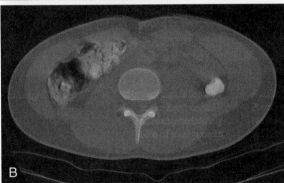

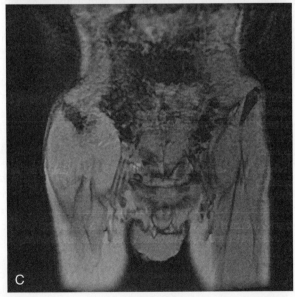

FIGURE 14-2 Despite the significant size of this primary malignant tumor located in the ilium, the patient had a primary symptom of knee pain. This case example highlights the importance of examining the joints and areas proximal to the painful area to rule out referred pain and to image the proper area. (See Chapters 12 and 13.) **A,** Radiograph initially identified lesion. **B,** CT scan reveals bony structure of osteogenic sarcoma. **C,** MRI delineates extent of soft tissue involvement, including the integrity of fascial planes.

imaging findings may reveal only irrelevant pathology. The following case example also reinforces the importance of using the pretest probability to guide the pursuit of diagnostic imaging.

A 64-year-old woman was referred to physical therapy for treatment of progressively intense hip pain. During the history taking, the patient related that she had been limited in her ability to squat or move her hip for approximately 8 months. Her pain had reached a peak approximately 3 months earlier; it then lessened, although her ability to move her hip had correspondingly deteriorated. The patient denied any injury, although she related that she had been active most of her life and that her current occupation was housekeeping for several patients. She had progressively become more limited in her ability to perform her normal cleaning activities, which required squatting, kneeling, and bending. The patient indicated that her primary care physician had ordered radiographs of her hip, but she had not been informed of the results.

Tests and measures revealed a grossly asymmetric gait with the patient weight bearing on her forefoot on the affected lower extremity. Active and passive range of motion of the involved hip was dramatically limited in all directions, and there was an apparent total leg shortening of approximately 2 inches.

The patient's radiographs were unavailable for review, and there was no official reading in the system. The patient stated that the imaging studies were performed 2 weeks earlier after her appointment with her physician. The referring physician was contacted, and the relevant examination findings were detailed. The physician agreed that it would be appropriate to repeat the studies because it seemed likely that the films were misplaced or lost. The new images revealed severe osteoarthritis of the hip with a collapse of the acetabulum and penetration of the femoral head into the pelvic cavity (acetabular protrusion). The patient was subsequently given a referral to orthopedic surgery.

In this example, the diagnostic imaging was repeated because the results of the initial study were unknown. Even if the original films had been read and the reported results were negative, the strong pretest probability of hip pathology in this case requires careful further investigation, including repeating the test when the test results are unknown or the test is reportedly negative.[31] Other possible sources of musculoskeletal imaging test error include imaging the wrong body region or side, imaging the area of referred pain, confusing one set of images with the images of another patient, incorrectly interpreting the images,[30] or selecting an imaging procedure that is not sensitive for the likely pathology.

Common Musculoskeletal Imaging Modalities

Radiography

Conventional radiographs use ionizing radiation to produce high-resolution analog images on specialized film. Radiographs are usually easy to obtain with comparatively minimal associated expense. They provide a means to distinguish air, bone, calcification, fat, soft tissue, and fluids.[34] Radiographs produce superior resolution for fine cortical and trabecular detail in bone. Conventional radiographs are typically used to identify fractures, ranging from stress fractures to avulsion fractures and complex fractures. Radiographs are not useful to distinguish differences in soft tissue contrast for the evaluation of muscle, ligament, or tendon injuries.[24,55,62] Because a film represents a two-dimensional picture of the anatomy, the minimal radiographic examination typically includes two views of the imaged body part at right angles to each other. Specialized views may be required in addition to standard views for adequately assessing the local anatomy and differentiating specific injuries.

Limiting exposure to ionizing radiation is an important aspect of diagnostic radiology. As low as reasonably allowable (ALARA) standards[62] govern the use of ionizing radiation. In radiography, the intensity of the beam of ionizing radiation, the length of time that the beam is on, the distance of the patient from the beam, patient shielding, and the number and type of images taken all determine the patient's exposure to ionizing radiation. Body parts that would be exposed to radiation but are of no interest regarding the differential diagnosis should be adequately shielded with lead garments. Selection of the appropriate view can also help limit radiation exposure. Posterior to anterior, rather than anterior to posterior, views have been recommended for use in patients with scoliosis to limit radiation exposure of the breasts and thyroid gland.[47,48] Oblique views of the lumbar spine have traditionally been used to visualize defects of the pars articularis found in spondylolysis and spondylolisthesis. Because of the high levels of gonadal radiation associated with these views and the evolution of computed tomography (CT) as the diagnostic standard, oblique views of the lumbar spine should not be routinely obtained.

Radiographs may be more specific than MRI in differentiating potential causes of bony lesions because of the proven ability to characterize specific calcification patterns and periosteal reactions. An important limitation of plain radiographs is that they are not considered sensitive to the early changes associated with tumors, infections, and some fractures.[34] The following case example highlights the lack of sensitivity of plain radiographs for certain types of fractures.

An obese 55-year-old man sought physical therapy care for LBP after slipping and landing on his buttocks in a local department store. The patient had been seen in the emergency department after the fall, and anteroposterior and lateral radiographs had been taken of the lumbar spine. The images were interpreted as normal by one of the hospital radiologists. The PT reviewed the lumbar images from the hospital's networked imaging system, and no pathologic findings other than minor degenerative changes were apparent.

The physical examination by the PT revealed severe pain with active range of motion and palpation of the lumbar spine, although the morbid obesity was a limiting factor in performing a typical examination. The neurologic screening examination was unremarkable.

Treatment was initiated consisting of gentle range of motion exercises and walking in the therapeutic pool. After 3 weeks, the patient was concerned about his lack of progress, and he went to a local Veterans Administration hospital for further evaluation. The same radiographic procedure was repeated, this time revealing a 30% compression fracture of the fifth lumbar vertebrae.

The structural elements of the lumbar vertebrae had probably been disrupted by the fall, although there was no initial radiographic evidence. The patient's size may have contributed to the extent of the eventual compression and collapse of the vertebral body. CT, MRI, and a bone scan would have been more sensitive to the bone pathology in this case, and these modalities should be considered when patients with normal radiographs have pain consistent with a fracture or do not respond to treatment.[24,25,31]

Table 14-1 provides typical radiographic views, imaged structures, and commonly revealed pathologic findings. Conventional radiographs are being replaced by digitalized radiographic procedures. Advantages of digitalized radiographic studies include almost immediate access to the images and, in general, less ionizing radiation exposure for the patient.

GUIDELINES FOR SELECTIVE USE OF RADIOGRAPHS. Overuse of radiologic studies has become a significant economic problem in the United States. Although radiographic procedures are relatively inexpensive, the economic impact of high-volume, low-cost procedures can be equal to low-volume, high-cost imaging procedures.[86] Because of the overuse of radiographs, clinical decision rules (CDRs) indicating a need for radiography for specific types of injuries at certain areas of the body have been developed.[60] A CDR is a clinical tool that can quantify individual contributions from the components of the examination to determine the diagnosis, prognosis, or treatment for a given patient. CDRs attempt formally to test, simplify, and increase the accuracy of clinicians' diagnostic and prognostic assessments. Attempts have been made to categorize a CDR based on the criteria of the method of derivation, the validation of the CDR to ensure that its repeated use leads to consistent results, and its predictive value.[53]

Radiographic images of the knee are frequently ordered, although fractures are present in only 6% of cases and, in general, are clinically detectable. The Ottawa knee rules are guidelines for the selective use of radiographs in knee trauma. Application of these rules may lead to a more efficient evaluation of knee injuries and a reduction in health costs without an increase in adverse outcomes.[86] The Ottawa knee CDR summarized in Table 14-2 indicates when radiographic studies are appropriate to consider. Exclusion criteria for these rules are age younger than 18 years; isolated superficial skin injuries; injuries greater than 7 days old; recent injuries being re-evaluated; and patients with altered levels of consciousness, paraplegia, or multiple injuries.[44,50] The Ottawa knee rules have been shown to have almost 100% sensitivity for knee fractures and to reduce the need for knee radiographs by 28% when used by emergency physicians.[67,80,82]

The Pittsburgh CDR for the knee indicating the need for radiographic studies is summarized in Table 14-3. The Pittsburgh rules are not applicable in patients with knee injuries sustained more than 6 days before presentation, in patients with only superficial lacerations and abrasions or a history of previous surgeries or fractures on the affected knee, and in patients being reassessed for the same injury.[68] In a multicenter convenience sample of 934 patients comparing the Pittsburgh CDR and the Ottawa knee rules, the Pittsburgh CDR was determined to be 99% sensitive and 60% specific for knee fractures. The positive predictive value was 24.1, indicating that 24.1% of patients actually had a fracture when positive on the rule. The negative predictive value was 99.8, indicating that 99.8% of the time when the rules indicated that no fracture was present, the patient did

TABLE 14-1

Radiographic Views, Structures Imaged, and Typical Pathologic Condition by Body Region

Region	Radiographic View	Structures Imaged	Common Pathologic Condition
Cervical spine	AP open mouth	Odontoid process, body of axis, lateral masses of atlas and atlantoaxial joint	Fractures of upper cervical spine, asymmetric location of dens between lateral masses indicating ligamentous stretching or injury
	AP	C3-C7 spinous processes and vertebral bodies	Fractures of C3-C7; disk space changes and pathology of the uncovertebral joints
	Lateral (standing, seated, or supine cross-table)	Occiput to C7	Fractures, dislocations, postural curves and contour lines, alignment changes, spondylitic changes
	Lateral flexion/extension	Occiput to C7 in active flexion and active extension	Unstable joint segments from ligamentous injury
	Obliques	Intervertebral foramina, facet joints, pedicles, and uncovertebral joints	Narrowing and degenerative changes of intervertebral foramina and apophyseal joint
	Swimmer's view	Best view of C7-T2, prevents obstruction by shoulders	Fractures of C7-T2
Shoulder	AP	Proximal humerus, lateral clavicle, AC joint, superior lateral aspect of scapula	Fractures of proximal humerus and glenoid; changes in humeral head position from rotator cuff tears or glenohumeral dislocations; osteoarthritis, calcific tendinitis, or bursitis
	AP standing with arm in internal rotation	Humeral head in relation to glenoid	Hill-Sachs lesion
	AP standing with arm in external rotation	Humeral head in relation to glenoid and anteroinferior rim of glenoid	Compression fracture of humeral head usually associated with posterior dislocation
	Axillary, oblique		Anterior and posterior glenohumeral dislocations; fractures of proximal humerus and scapula
	West Point view		Anterior and posterior glenohumeral dislocations; pathology of anterior inferior glenoid
AC joint	AP bilateral with and without weight	Both AC joints, both sternoclavicular joints, clavicles	Ligamentous instability of AC or SC joint; fractures of clavicle
Scapula	AP, lateral scapula	Entire scapula, body of scapula	Fractures of scapula
	Transcapular or Y view	Entire scapula; best view for comminuted and displaced fractures of scapula	Fractures of scapula
Humerus	AP, lateral humerus	Entire humerus	Fractures of humerus; myositis ossificans of anterior compartment
	Transthoracic lateral view	True lateral view of proximal humerus	Fractures of proximal humerus
Elbow	AP	Distal humerus, proximal radius and ulna	Fractures of distal humerus and proximal radius and ulna; dislocations of elbow; ligamentous avulsions with bony attachments; varus and valgus deformities; heterotopic bone formations
	Lateral	Distal humerus, proximal radius and ulna	Supracondylar fractures of distal humerus, radial head fractures; fat pad sign; elbow dislocations
	Internal oblique	Best view of coronoid process	Fractures of coronoid process and medial epicondyle
	External oblique	Best view of radial head, neck, and tuberosity	Fractures of radial head, neck, tuberosity, and lateral epicondyle
	Radial head–capitellum	Best view of radial head, capitellum, and coronoid process	Fractures of radial head, capitellum, coronoid process; joint abnormalities
Forearm	AP, lateral	Entire radius and ulna, wrist, elbow	Fractures of radius, ulna, wrist, and elbow
Hand	PA or dorsal volar, oblique, lateral	Distal radius and ulna to phalanges	Fractures of wrist and hand; rheumatoid arthritis and osteoarthritis; avascular necrosis of lunate or scaphoid; carpal instabilities
Thoracic spine	AP	T1-T12 vertebral end plates, pedicles, and spinous processes; intervertebral disk spaces; costovertebral joints; medial aspect of posterior ribs	Fractures of vertebral bodies, posterior elements, and ribs; pneumothorax
	Lateral	T1-T12 vertebral bodies, pedicles, and spinous processes; intervertebral disk spaces and foramina	Fractures of vertebral bodies and posterior elements; changes in postural alignment from scoliosis, fractures, and ligamentous disruptions; pedicle obliteration from tumors
	PO	Facet joints, pedicles, and pars interarticularis	Fractures of lamina and facets
	AO (right)	Sternum, axillary portion of ribs	Fractures of sternum and ribs; costosternal disruptions

TABLE 14-1

Radiographic Views, Structures Imaged, and Typical Pathologic Condition by Body Region—cont'd

Region	Radiographic View	Structures Imaged	Common Pathologic Condition
Ribs	AP, PA, AO, PO, PA chest	Anterior and posterior aspects of ribs	Fractures of ribs
Lumbar spine	AP	Vertebral bodies and end plates, transverse processes, intervertebral disk spaces, pedicles, and spinous processes	Fractures of vertebral bodies, end plates, and posterior elements; disk space abnormalities
	Lateral	Vertebral bodies, end plates, and posterior elements; intervertebral disk spaces	Fractures of vertebral bodies, end plates, and posterior elements; vertebral alignment; disk space abnormalities
	Coned-down lateral spot	Vertebral bodies, end plates, and posterior elements of L5 and S1; L5-S1 intervertebral disk space	Fractures of vertebral bodies, end plates, and posterior elements; vertebral alignment; disk space abnormalities
	Obliques	Facet joints, lamina	Fractures and defects in pars interarticularis and articular facets
Sacroiliac joint	AP axial, obliques	AP axial images bilateral SI joints; obliques image unilateral SI joint	Degenerative changes, ankylosis
Hip and pelvis	AP unilateral or entire pelvis	Acetabulum, femoral head and neck, greater trochanter, angle of inclination of femoral neck to shaft of femur	Fractures of proximal femur, acetabulum, pubic rami, and ischial tuberosities; hip joint dislocations; slipped capital femoral epiphysis; Legg-Calvé-Perthes disease; osteoarthritis
	Frog-leg lateral	Femoral head and neck, proximal third of femur, acetabulum	Fractures of femoral head and neck, greater and lesser trochanters
Knee	AP	Distal femur, proximal tibia, head of fibula, tibiofemoral joint space	Fractures of patella, tibial plateau, femoral condyles, distal femur, and proximal fibula; osteochondral fragments; osteoarthritis and rheumatoid arthritis; varus and valgus alignment
	AP with valgus or varus stress	Relation of distal femur to proximal tibia	Ligamentous instability; changes in articular cartilage thickness
	Lateral with AP or PA stress	Relation of distal femur to proximal tibia	Ligamentous instability
	Lateral	Relation of patella to femur; length of patella to patellar ligament	Osteochondral fractures, tibial apophysitis, quadriceps tendon ruptures, patellar ligament tears
	Notch or tunnel	Intercondylar fossa, notch of popliteal tendon, tibial spines, intercondylar eminence, posterior aspects of distal femur and proximal tibia, intercondylar eminence of tibia	Osteochondral defects and loose bodies, fractures of tibial spines
	Sunrise axial	Patella, femoral condyles	Relation of patella to femoral condyles, subluxation and dislocation of patella, patellar fractures
	Merchant axial	Patella, femoral condyles	Preferred view of articular surface of patella, subtle dislocations
Lower leg	AP, lateral	Shaft of tibia and fibula	Fractures and dislocations of tibia and fibula
Ankle	AP	Distal tibia and fibula, body of talus, tibiotalar joint	Fractures of distal tibia, fibula, and talus; dislocations and subluxations of tibiotalar joint; osteoarthritis
	AP mortise	Joint space between distal fibula and talus, ankle mortise	Fractures of distal tibia and fibula; fractures of talus
	AP with inversion or eversion stress	Ankle mortise	Fractures and subluxations, mortise instability
	Lateral	Distal tibia and fibula, calcaneus, tibiotalar and subtalar articulations	Fractures and dislocations of distal tibia and fibula, talus, and calcaneus; osteoarthritis
	External oblique	Lateral malleolus, anterior tibial tubercle, distal tibiofibular syndesmosis, talofibular joint	Fractures of lateral malleolus, talus, and tuberosity of calcaneus; disruptions of distal tibiofibular syndesmosis
	Internal oblique	Medial and lateral malleoli, tibial plafond, dome of talus, tibiotalar joint, tibiofibular syndesmosis	Best view of pathology of tibial plafond; fractures of medial malleolus
Foot	AP	Talus, navicular, cuboid, cuneiforms, metatarsals, phalanges	Fractures and dislocations of foot
	Lateral	Calcaneocuboid and talonavicular articulations, calcaneus, talus, subtalar joint	Fractures and dislocations of foot, heel spurs, osteoarthritis
	Oblique	Mid-tarsal joints to phalanges	Fractures of foot

AC, acromioclavicular; *AO,* anterior oblique; *AP,* anteroposterior; *PA,* posteroanterior; *PO,* posterior oblique; *SC,* sternoclavicular; *SI,* sacroiliac.

TABLE 14-2
Ottawa Knee Rules for Radiography

Indications for Radiography, if Any	Exclusion Criteria
Patient >55 years old	Age <18 years
Tenderness at head of fibula	Isolated superficial skin injuries
Isolated tenderness of patella	Injuries >7 days old
Inability to flex to 90 degrees	Recent injuries being re-evaluated
Inability to weight bear 4 steps immediately after injury and in emergency department	Patients with altered levels of consciousness
	Paraplegia or multiple injuries

The rules are 97% sensitive and 27% specific for knee fractures.
From Seaberg D, Yealy M, Lukens T, et al: Multicenter comparison of two clinical decision rules for the use of radiography in acute, high-risk knee injuries, *Ann Emerg Med* 32:8-13, 1998.

TABLE 14-3
Pittsburgh Decision Rules for Radiography

Indications for Radiography if the Mechanism of Injury Is Blunt Trauma or a Fall and Either	Exclusion Criteria
1. Patient <12 or >50 years old	Knee injuries sustained >6 days before presentation
2. Injury causes inability to walk >4 weight-bearing steps in emergency department	Patients with only superficial lacerations and abrasions
	History of previous surgeries or fractures on affected knee
	Patients being reassessed for same injury

The rules are 99% sensitive and 60% specific for knee fractures.
From Seaberg D, Yealy M, Lukens T, et al: Multicenter comparison of two clinical decision rules for the use of radiography in acute, high-risk knee injuries, *Ann Emerg Med* 32:8-13, 1998.

BOX 14-1
Ottawa Ankle Rules for Radiography

INDICATIONS FOR RADIOGRAPHY IF ANY OF THE FOLLOWING ARE PRESENT
1. Bone tenderness at posterior edge or tip of lateral malleolus
2. Bone tenderness at posterior edge or tip of medial malleolus
3. Inability to bear weight immediately and in emergency department

The rules are 100% sensitive and 40% specific for ankle fractures.
Adapted from Stiell I, Greenberg G, McKnight R, et al: Decision rules for the use of radiography in acute ankle injuries: refinement and prospective validation, *JAMA* 269:1127-1132, 1993.

BOX 14-2
Ottawa Foot Rules for Radiography

INDICATIONS FOR RADIOGRAPHY IF ANY OF THE FOLLOWING ARE PRESENT
1. Bone tenderness at base of fifth metatarsal
2. Bone tenderness at navicular
3. Inability to bear weight immediately and in emergency department

Adapted from Stiell I, Greenberg G, McKnight R, et al: Decision rules for the use of radiography in acute ankle injuries: refinement and prospective validation, *JAMA* 269:1127-1132, 1993.

presented in Box 14-3. By using the three questions, the rules had 100% sensitivity and 43% specificity for identifying important cervical spine injuries. The expected radiography ordering rate when using these guidelines is 58% as opposed to the current ordering rates of more than 90% for cervical spine injuries.[52]

Because aspects of the knee, foot, and ankle rules depend on the patient's response to pain-producing stimulus, there is potential for a false-negative response in an extremely stoic patient. Clinical judgment is required. In addition to the aforementioned rules, guidelines exist for the lumbar spine. Because these guidelines are tightly interwoven into decision making regarding the ordering of laboratory tests, they are presented later in this chapter. Beyond the cervical spine, knee, ankle, and foot CDRs and the lumbar spine practice guidelines, similar CDRs or guidelines for other frequently injured and imaged areas of the body are notably lacking.

Scintigraphy

Scintigraphy, or bone scan, reveals pathology through the uptake and subsequent detection of a radiopharmaceutical substance (e.g., radiolabeled phosphate) into areas of reactive bone. Patients who undergo a bone scan receive an intravenous injection with the radiopharmaceutical substance. Hours after the injection, the skeletal system is scanned by a detector for areas of increased radionuclide uptake. Although all living bone absorbs some of the radiopharmaceutical substance, areas of the greatest osteoclastic and osteoblastic activity absorb the most and are revealed as black, or *hot,* areas on the scan. Bone scans are considered sensitive for changes in bone associated with fractures (including stress fractures), infections, and tumors.* Some types of bony lesions, such as lesions associated with multiple myeloma, may not be reactive enough or have enough osteoblastic activity for

not have a fracture. In comparison, the Ottawa knee rules were 97% sensitive and 27% specific for knee fractures, with three missed fractures.[68] The authors concluded that both rules were equally useful for the diagnosis of knee fractures with no significant difference in sensitivity.

The Ottawa ankle (Box 14-1) and foot (Box 14-2) CDRs were developed to help predict fractures in patients with ankle and foot injuries. In general, the Ottawa foot and ankle rules are considered to be 100% sensitive but not specific. The ankle rules have been shown to reduce the need for emergency department ankle radiographs by 36% in some settings.[6,7,78,79,81] Commonly overlooked foot fractures with ankle sprains are shown in Figure 14-3.

CDRs for the evaluation of cervical spine injuries remain controversial, although consensus exists that cervical radiographic studies are overused in the emergency department.[77] Stiell[77] prospectively evaluated outcomes from 8924 adults presenting to the emergency department with head and neck injuries; 1.7% were found to have important cervical spine injuries. Analysis of the data resulted in the Canadian C-Spine Rule. The three questions of the Canadian C-Spine Rule and the important responses are

---

*References 21, 24, 34, 44, 55, 94.

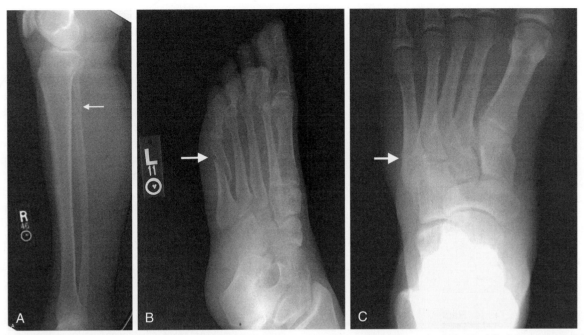

FIGURE 14-3 Radiographs revealing fractures that can be overlooked in the examination of an acute ankle sprain. **A,** Proximal fibula fracture. **B,** Oblique displaced mid-shaft fifth metatarsal fracture. **C,** Nondisplaced base of fifth metatarsal fracture.

BOX 14-3

Canadian C-Spine Rule

INDICATIONS FOR RADIOGRAPHY ARE PRESENT IF ANSWER TO QUESTION 1 IS POSITIVE, OR ANSWER TO QUESTION 2 IS NEGATIVE, OR ANSWER TO QUESTION 3 IS NEGATIVE

1. Is there any high-risk factor present that mandates radiography (e.g., age >65 years, dangerous mechanism of injury, or paresthesias in the extremities)?
2. Is there any low-risk factor that allows safe assessment of range of motion (e.g., simple rear-end motor vehicle accident, normal sitting posture in emergency department, ambulatory at any time since injury, delayed onset of neck pain, and absence of midline tenderness)?
3. Is the patient able to rotate the neck actively 45 degrees to the right and to the left?

Adapted from Stiell I, Wells G, Vandemheen KL: The Canadian c-spine rule for radiography in alert and stable trauma patients, *JAMA* 286:1841-1848, 2001.

---

the bone scan to be positive. These types of lesions are referred to as *cold lesions* and are best revealed by other types of diagnostic imaging such as MRI or CT. Radiographs also eventually reveal the typical osteopenic and radiolucent areas associated with myelomatosis.

Although bone scans are considered sensitive, they are not specific with many of the mentioned processes producing similar appearances on bone scan. Bone scans are important for evaluating the presence and distribution of lesions[24] (Figure 14-4). Bone scans are commonly used by PTs in the U.S. Army to detect stress fractures among training soldiers. Although radiographs may also eventually reveal stress fractures when gross changes or healing are evident, they are not considered sensitive enough to be a reliable screening tool.

Radionuclide bone scan is useful in localizing the extent of multifocal bone disease but is less sensitive than MRI in detecting metastases and does not have the spatial resolution to detail the extent and anatomic association of disease processes often

necessary for optimal clinical decision making.[67] Old and well-healed fractures, degenerative joint disease, open growth plates, and the sacroiliac joints all may have areas of increased uptake and need to be differentiated for relevance during the patient examination.

Tomography

Tomography is radiography of a body section that permits more accurate visualization of lesions too small (1 mm) to be noted on conventional radiographs. Tomography also shows anatomic detail obscured by overlying structures.[34] Conventional tomograms and computed axial tomography (CT scans) use ionizing radiation. Radiation doses to imaged areas may be higher than the radiation doses of plain radiographs. However, the dose to areas outside the areas imaged is greatly reduced and considered negligible.[55] In plain radiographs, the beam of ionizing radiation and the film cassette are positioned and stationary, and the film and the body part are exposed to the radiation. In conventional tomograms, the radiographic film and the tube producing the radiographic image move simultaneously so that only a specific area of the body is not blurred and becomes sharply outlined in a single plane of focus. The radiographer can control the thickness of the imaged area. Images are usually sequentially taken through parallel planes until the desired area has been adequately imaged. Technologic advances have resulted in the ability of the radiographic tube to move in complex angles and arcs, resulting in even greater imaging detail.

The advantage of conventional tomography over conventional radiography includes the improved visualization of subtle fractures, fracture lines, and the presence and extent of fracture healing. Conventional tomograms are particularly useful to evaluate small tumors and cystic and sclerotic lesions. Tomograms and radiographs are often interpreted together for the purpose of comparison.[34]

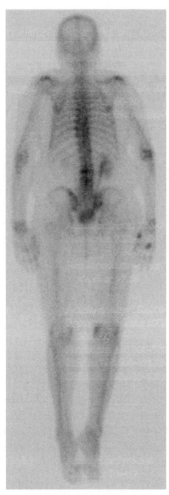

FIGURE 14-4 Although bone scans do not reveal the intricate details of fractures or bony lesions, they are useful to screen for the presence of lesions in the skeletal system. In this case, the areas of relative increased radiopharmaceutical uptake in L4 and L5 are consistent with metastatic prostate cancer. The other areas of increased uptake in this study, such as the elbows, wrists, hands, and knees, are more consistent with degenerative arthritic changes.

COMPUTED TOMOGRAPHY. CT is a radiologic modality containing a source of ionizing radiation, detectors, and a computer data processing system. A CT system includes a circular scanning gantry that houses the radiographic tube image sensors, a table for the patient to lie on, an x-ray generator, and a computerized data processing unit. The patient lies on the table and is placed inside the gantry. The x-ray tube is rotated 360 degrees around the patient and administers multiple x-ray beams projected at different angles; the computer collects the data and formulates axial cross-sectional images of the body, referred to as *slices*.[34] After determining the relative impedance of the body tissues to the x-rays, the computer assigns values of relative density to each point in the body and constructs images in relative shades of gray. The most striking differences are between bone and soft tissue, but differences between the various types of soft tissue are subtle. CT produces excellent detail of bone, but this modality is much less useful for imaging tendons and ligaments. CT also has the capability to provide images in the transverse plane (axial views) and to produce multiplanar reconstructions.

CT provides excellent cortical and trabecular definition that allows for detection and characterization of the complex geometry of triplane fractures and fractures with suspected intraarticular extension.[55] CT is useful to probe further for fractures when radiographic results are normal and the pretest probability strongly suggests fracture (Figure 14-5). High-resolution MRI is also considered valuable in evaluating these types of injuries because of the excellent soft tissue detail. The combination of CT and high-definition MRI reveals combinations of bony and soft tissue injuries, such as a tibial plateau fracture and a meniscal tear.

Other uses for CT include investigating suspected visceral organ injuries, spine and extremity imaging, and investigating suspected head injuries. Soft tissue mineral deposition and destructive humeral head amyloidomas associated with end-stage renal disease are shown by CT. Kinematic CT with slip ring technology has been used to show patellar tracking in chondromalacia and degenerative joint disease. Slip ring technology allows continuous rotation of the x-ray sources and detectors during patient movement. Dupuy and colleagues[20] used slip ring technology and continuous 10-second exposures to show patellar tracking from 45 degrees of knee flexion to full extension. Slip ring technology is also combined with arthrography to reveal additional joint detail and has been particularly useful in the imaging of articular cartilage.[24]

CT is useful to image spinal conditions such as degenerative spondylosis and intervertebral disk disease. MRI scans are considered more useful in evaluating disk herniations, whereas CT is more useful to show the details of spinal osteophytes. Greater understanding of spinal fracture patterns ranging from stress fractures of the pars interarticularis to the complex burst fractures of the intervertebral bodies can be gained from CT. CT allows for the reconstruction of thin axial images from the spinal segment into images in the sagittal, coronal, or oblique planes. The use of contrast material in the subarachnoid space provides even greater detail and contrast of the nerve roots and subarachnoid spaces to spinal images, although this introduces the additional risk associated with invasive procedures. In general, CT is considered to be less complex and expensive than MRI. The main variable in CT is the thickness of the slice. Slices only 1 mm thick may be required to produce good reformations. Finally, CT accurately analyzes bone mineral content, providing valuable information for the diagnosis and treatment of metabolic bone diseases. Disadvantages of CT include the higher radiation dose and cost compared with conventional radiography.[55]

Magnetic Resonance Imaging

The ability of MRI to image bone and soft tissue structures and reveal pathologic conditions in three dimensions has made it a powerful and popular form of imaging. MRI is the primary imaging method for detailed evaluation of a broad spectrum of musculoskeletal disease processes.[25,44,58,59,67] MRI scans use magnetic fields to produce computer-generated axial and sagittal cross-sectional images of the body. Numerous texts provide excellent and detailed descriptions of the complex physics principles involved in MRI.[34,42]

In brief, MRI uses the magnetic characteristics of the body's tissues, rather than ionizing radiation, to produce an image. Patients are positioned in the scanner within a strong magnetic

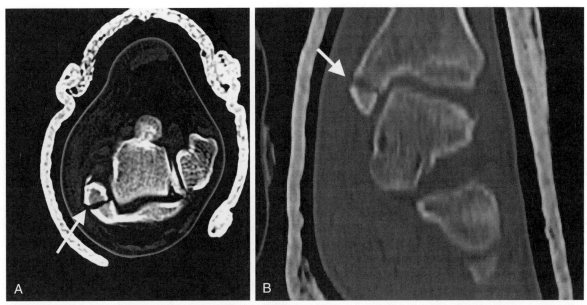

FIGURE 14-5 CT can reveal fractures that may otherwise not be apparent on plain radiographs. **A** and **B,** In this case, medial malleolar fracture was not revealed on plain films but is clearly identified with CT images in transverse **(A)** and frontal **(B)** planes.

field that produces changes in the body's atoms. The ability of MRI to image various parts of the body depends on the intrinsic spin of atoms with an odd number of neutrons or protons, producing a magnetic moment. The atomic nuclei of tissues placed within the field align along the direction of the magnetic field. In general, stronger magnets are associated with better images, although there are some exceptions. Images obtained with these atoms are subjected to the additional influence of magnetic coils and subsequently register the atomic response.

Radiofrequency (RF) pulses from the coils cause the nuclei to absorb energy and produce resonance. When the RF pulse is removed, the energy absorbed is released as an electric signal from which digital images are derived. The signal intensity refers to the strength of the radio wave that a tissue emits after removal of the RF pulse. The strength of the radio wave produces either bright (high) signal intensity or dark (low) signal intensity images. Signal intensity in a specific tissue depends on the concentration of hydrogen ions and the T1 and T2 relaxation times.

MRI scans are subsequently referred to as *T1* or *T2 weighted*. T1 images are obtained with RF pulses that have a short repetition time and a short echo time. The T1 image, or longitudinal relaxation, is used to describe the return of protons back to equilibrium after the application and removal of the RF pulse. T2 images are obtained with a long repetition time and a long echo time. The T2 image, or transverse relaxation time, is used to describe the associated loss of coherence or phase between individual protons immediately after the application of the RF pulse. The necessary imaging contrast between tissues is produced by varying the RF pulse sequences to increase the differences in T1 and T2. Repetition time is defined by the recovery time of the transverse and longitudinal orientation of protons after being subjected to the RF pulse. T1 is typically 8 to 10 times larger than T2. If T1 is the focus, the RF is kept relatively short, allowing tissues of various composition to recover to distinct levels, producing tissue contrast.

The rapid application of a second RF pulse produces a spin echo effect. A spin echo is used to cause magnetization vectors to come back into phase and create an echo of the original signal. Conventional spin echo pulse sequences include T1-weighted, T2-weighted, and proton density–weighted images. Fast spin echo acquisition of images can reduce the required acquisition time and lessen the potential for loss of image quality because of patient movement.

T1-weighted images show subacute hemorrhage and fat as a bright intensity. Fluids contained in abscesses or cysts that contain high levels of protein also have a bright appearance. Other soft tissues have characteristic low signal intensity. T1-weighted images are useful for delineating the architecture of soft tissues such as marrow, fascia, and anatomic planes.[34,42] Bone has a characteristic bright signal in T1-weighted images because of the high fat content. T2-weighted images reveal fluids as high signal intensity images. Kaplan and colleagues[42] suggested remembering the "2" in water (H_2O) to help remember that fluids are bright in T2-weighted images. Fluid-containing structures, such as bursae, inflamed tendons, tumors, and abscesses, have a bright appearance on T2-weighted images.

In certain situations, the high signal intensity of fat should be suppressed to reveal the signal differences between fat and fluid or between fat and contrast material. Fast spin echo T2-weighted images produce particularly bright fat images. Fat suppression or fat saturation is used to produce a dull appearance of fat for a better contrast with fluids. Proton density–weighted images combine the properties of T1-weighted and T2-weighted images and produce good anatomic detail with little tissue contrast.

The magnetic field of the MRI scanner is very powerful. Loud banging noises associated with image acquisition are caused by torque to the structure of the MRI scanner from the powerful magnetic impulses. Ferromagnetic metal implants, such as cerebral aneurysm clips and pacemakers, or metal foreign bodies, such as the fine slivers a machinist may unknowingly have

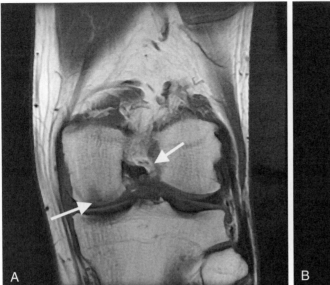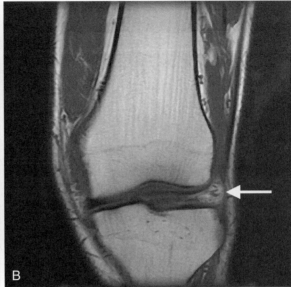

FIGURE 14-6 MRI provides excellent detail of soft tissue injuries. **A,** Coronal section reveals complete anterior cruciate ligament tear with articular cartilage damage to medial femoral condyle. **B,** Coronal section reveals complex degenerative lateral meniscus tear.

lodged in the eye, may be displaced during MRI and are contraindications. Claustrophobia may be a relative contraindication. Although some MRI scanners have a more open design, there is debate whether the quality of the images produced with such devices is comparable with the quality of the images produced in scanners of traditional design.

Advances in technology and design have enabled MRI to produce high-quality images of small joints; fine soft tissue structures; and large joint components such as fibrocartilage, ligaments, capsules, and synovium (Figure 14-6). The ability to provide the appropriate detail largely depends on the use of the appropriate coils and pulse sequences. Joints should be imaged in three orthogonal planes, one of which suppresses the characteristic bright signal of fat for better contrast (fat suppressed). One sequence such as fast spin echo or gradient echo to evaluate articular cartilage should be included in each joint study. Intraarticular contrast material may be used to evaluate the shoulder or hip for rotator cuff tears, labral lesions, or articular cartilage injuries (Figure 14-7).

CT and MRI are capable of producing high-resolution scans, but the ability of MRI to differentiate the different types of tissue based on their signal intensities (soft tissue contrast) sets it apart. A CT image is based on x-ray attenuation properties of tissues, whereas the soft tissue contrast in MRI is related to the differing proton resonances in the tissues.[42] MRI has proven to be superior to CT in simultaneously delineating multiple soft tissue and osseous insults.[24] The gold standard for the evaluation of anterior cruciate ligament injuries is arthroscopy. Compared with this standard, MRI has a diagnostic accuracy of more than 90%. MRI is considered the imaging modality of choice to show acute and chronic stages of muscle damage caused by infarcts from sickle cell disease, diabetes, primary or metastatic tumors, and trauma. MRI is considered more useful than CT in showing bone marrow abnormalities; specific types of MRI sequences can also distinguish benign from malignant spinal lesions.[24] MRI may be more accurate in defining the extent of

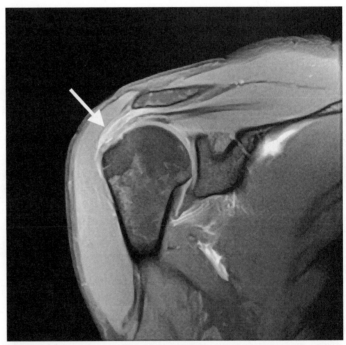

FIGURE 14-7 Magnetic resonance arthrogram reveals complete supraspinatus and partial infraspinatus tear.

tumors and their relationship to neighboring tissues, and functional MRI to measure blood flow may aid in the diagnosis of musculoskeletal neoplasms.

Finally, high field strength magnets have provided a level of detail that surpasses arthrography, CT arthrography, and ultrasonography for depicting changes in articular cartilage.[35] Under routine clinical parameters, MRI provides limited detail within the small tendons and images the coarse detail of muscle. Contrast agents may improve the definition of detail and reveal significant lesions and normal variants.[24,91] Feldman and associates[25] described 30 patients with normal radiographs, bone scans, and

CT scans and determined that MRI allowed identification of acute fractures in the emergency department and subtle subacute or chronic fractures in the context of strong clinical suspicions. They also concluded that MRI is the most sensitive method of simultaneously documenting the earliest changes in traumatized osseous and soft tissue structures. These investigators provided a case example of an elderly patient seen in the emergency department after a fall. The initial radiographs and conventional tomograms were normal, but a T1-weighted MRI scan obtained the same day revealed an intertrochanteric fracture.

Several factors can alter the quality of MRI. Motion from voluntary movements, restlessness, involuntary spasms, respiratory movements of the rib cage, and peristaltic movements of the gastrointestinal system all can reduce the quality of the acquired images. Images that are acquired too close to each other can produce interference. Disadvantages of MRI include intolerance of the procedure by claustrophobic patients, the requirement for patients to be motionless during the procedure, and cost.

ARTHROGRAPHY. Arthrography entails the introduction of a positive contrast agent, such as iodide, or a negative contrast agent, such as air, or a combination of both into the joint space.[34] This procedure is not considered to be technically difficult, and the results are easy to interpret. Arthrography is most often performed in the wrist, shoulder, elbow, and ankle regions. In general, plain film radiographs are obtained before arthrography because of the possibility of obscuring certain radiographic findings after the contrast agent is applied. In some settings, the role of arthrography has become increasingly limited because of the increased use of MRI. Arthrography is primarily used when MRI is contraindicated or when details of intra-articular pathologic conditions, such as labral and articular cartilage lesions, are sought. In addition, arthrography is particularly useful to detect rotator cuff tears of the shoulder and triangular fibrocartilage lesions of the wrist.[34] Finally, the combination of CT and arthrography is frequently used.[55,93]

MYELOGRAPHY. Plain myelography includes plain film radiographs taken after a nonionic water-soluble contrast medium is injected into the subarachnoid space by a puncture needle to produce images of the borders and contents of the dural sac. The contrast medium mixes with the cerebrospinal fluid and travels up or down the thecal sac as the patient's position is altered by tilting the bed or table. CT myelography uses a CT scan, taken after a contrast medium has been injected into the dural sac, in the same manner as for plain myelography. This modality produces axial cross-sectional images of the spine that enhance the distinction between the dural sac and its surrounding structures. For examination of the lumbar segment, a puncture site at L2-L3 or L3-L4 is used, whereas for the cervical segment, a puncture site at C1-C2 is used. Myelographic examination has been almost entirely replaced by high-resolution CT and high-quality MRI.[34]

DISKOGRAPHY. Diskography is an imaging procedure that involves injection of contrast material into the nucleus pulposus of the intervertebral disk. It is typically combined with CT. Diskography has been used less frequently in recent years, but under certain conditions, such as determining the source of a patient's LBP, it may be of some diagnostic benefit. The symptoms produced with the injection of the contrast material may be of even greater diagnostic value than the images produced. Diskography

may be indicated for evaluation of unremitting spinal pain that is unresponsive to conservative treatment.[34]

ULTRASOUND. Ultrasound imaging is a fast and inexpensive tool for excellent images of the musculoskeletal system. Ultrasound is useful for imaging ligaments, tendons, nerves, muscles, tumors, and foreign bodies. Real-time imaging allows for the imaging of muscles as they contract and tendons as they glide. Ultrasound creates an image by sending sound waves into the tissues under the sound head and then imaging the sound waves as they return. Substances that reflect sound, such as bone and metal, cannot be adequately imaged. It is thought that ultrasonography is more useful in thin than in obese patients. Ultrasound is an excellent modality for imaging the rotator cuff of the shoulder, but it is typically unable to image some aspects of the glenoid labrum and certain structures within the knee, such as the menisci, articular cartilage, and cruciate ligaments. Ultrasound has also been shown to be useful in the evaluation of a traumatic hemarthrosis of the knee.[86]

Ultrasound has the advantage of requiring direct operator interaction with the patient. In a fashion, the operator is performing a physical examination and palpating deeply with the aid of ultrasound as guided by the patient description of the symptom location. Operator skill is a major factor in the diagnostic utility of ultrasound images. Power Doppler ultrasound produces detailed images of intramuscular and intratendinous structures and shows hyperemia in the rotator cuff and biceps tendon and other soft tissue shoulder pathologic conditions. Depending on operator skill, power Doppler ultrasound may be as sensitive as MRI and may be particularly useful in distinguishing chronic tendinitis from acute tendinitis and rotator cuff tears. In contrast, MRI performed within routine clinical parameters shows coarse intramuscular structure and poorer detail within small tendons.[91] Ultrasound images are currently used in PT practice to study musculotendinous function, including the quality of muscle contraction, and to detect and quantify the presence of muscle atrophy.[69,88]

Combined Modalities

In certain situations, a combination of diagnostic modalities may be more valuable than a single type of imaging. Feldman[24] described the advantages of a combination of imaging modalities in the case of a patient with hyperparathyroidism. MRI or CT shows the extensive detail of the pathologic condition, whereas radiographs effectively show the classic characteristics of the underlying disease, such as osteopenia, bone resorption, and soft tissue calcification. Radiographs and CT may provide details of a specific lesion, whereas a bone scan may be useful to screen for multiple lesions throughout the skeletal system. An astute PT keeps in mind the diagnostic utility and limitations of each type of imaging modality.

Advances in Musculoskeletal Imaging

Advances in imaging over the last few decades have had a significant effect on patient care largely because of progress in diagnostic capability. The introduction and evolution of digital cross-sectional imaging with CT and the subsequent development of MRI have changed concepts of musculoskeletal imaging. Conventional radiology has evolved from analog images on standard radiographic film to digital datasets produced by laser scanning and "dry processed," or sent through wire or fiber-optic cables to computerized workstation displays.

Technology has progressed to the point of allowing computer-assisted interpretation of certain types of images. Because of increasing demands for more timely distribution of radiographic information and because of space constraints, many departments or practice settings are becoming completely digital. High-speed networks transfer images from acquisition workstation to interpretation workstation. These image transfer systems are called *picture archiving and communication systems.*

Technology of CT and MRI is still evolving, and efforts are focused on improving portability, speed of acquisition, and image quality. Medical facilities of the future may have designs that conveniently locate imaging technology within emergency departments, intensive care units, and high-volume outpatient clinics. Beds from the intensive care unit or emergency department may evolve from being merely portable to being integral, with imaging devices for quick and easy docking, reducing the need for patient transfer. Improved facility design may allow transport of the smaller, but still significantly sized imaging devices.

Progress in imaging technology and the ease of access to diagnostic imaging is likely to drive many changes in use of imaging modalities. As these changes occur in settings where PTs are contributing to the management of patients with musculoskeletal problems, planners would want to provide input whenever possible to improve PT access for viewing and ordering images. Appropriate advance planning of imaging resources is a necessary step to allow all PTs to practice according to published evidence describing musculoskeletal imaging in physical therapy practice.

Risks Associated with Musculoskeletal Imaging

The risks reported with musculoskeletal imaging include exposure to ionizing radiation and procedural complications from invasive procedures, including infection, reaction to contrast materials, interference with mechanical devices such as pacemakers, and dislodging of embedded or implanted metal objects. The risk to special populations, such as patients with scoliosis, for developing cancer caused by radiation exposure has been formally studied.[47,48] A retrospective study of patient cohorts with adolescent idiopathic scoliosis was used to determine the cancer risks associated with the typical radiographic studies. The researchers found that an average of 10 to 12 radiographic procedures over the life span of a typical patient with scoliosis increased the risk of developing cancer of the breast and thyroid gland. The radiation exposure in patients with scoliosis typically occurs during the highest periods of adolescent growth. Cumulative x-ray doses were also found to be higher in patients who were diagnosed at a younger age and with more severe curves. Posteroanterior views reduce radiation exposure to the breast and thyroid by 94% to 96%. By simply ensuring that all radiographs in these patients are posteroanterior views rather than anteroposterior views, the risk of developing breast cancer is reduced threefold to fourfold, and the lifetime risk of developing thyroid cancer is reduced by half.[47,48]

Ordering Musculoskeletal Imaging

Whenever the decision is made that musculoskeletal imaging is necessary, a description of the mechanism of injury and the results of the clinical examination, including the exact location of significant findings, and sites of significant palpation tenderness, are essential information for the radiologist. The radiologist is not likely to have access to the patient when interpreting the image. The description of the presentation and key clinical findings becomes critical to accurate and relevant image interpretation.[55]

It is also crucial to examine for related injuries and image appropriately all areas that could have sustained significant injury or that could be the source of referred symptoms. Clinical examples of commonly missed injuries from incomplete physical examination and imaging include fifth metatarsal fractures accompanying ankle sprains, proximal fibula fractures accompanying malleolar fractures and ankle sprains, compression fractures at thoracic and upper lumbar levels with symptoms or injury to the lower lumbar levels or the lower extremities, proximal radius injuries accompanying distal radius and wrist injuries, and referred pain to the knee from injuries and conditions that exist at the hip and pelvis.[51,55]

It has been my clinical experience that radiologists appreciate the quality of the information provided by PTs when the PT orders musculoskeletal images. Remembering that the PT is essentially the hands, eyes, and ears of the radiologist for the clinical examination helps guide what information to provide when ordering diagnostic imaging. The following clinical example of a diagnostic imaging order provides insight into the value of information supplied by the ordering provider.

The desired study comprised anteroposterior and lateral radiographs of right elbow. The patient was a 13-year-old middle school student who fell directly onto her right elbow while in-line skating 3 days ago at a school retreat. Physical examination revealed moderate ecchymosis and swelling of the proximal lateral forearm and distal upper arm. Pain was present with all active motions of the elbow and forearm, and there was a partial loss of elbow flexion, extension, supination, and pronation. Effusion and tenderness were present over the radial head. The proximal shoulder, distal forearm, wrist, and hand were without significant findings or palpation tenderness.

This brief but comprehensive overview of the clinical presentation helps guide the radiologist to be alert for pathologic conditions from trauma at the elbow. Particular emphasis would be placed on looking for signs associated with fractures or ligamentous injuries of the elbow. Diagnostic imaging findings not associated with the injury or location of symptoms would be kept in the appropriate perspective in the subsequent radiographic report.

Musculoskeletal Imaging Results

There must be consistency between the results of the musculoskeletal imaging and the comprehensive clinical examination. In evidence-based medicine, the clinical examination helps establish the pretest likelihood of the pathologic condition.[84] When the signs and symptoms of a significant injury are present from the clinical examination, a negative diagnostic imaging procedure must be repeated, or an imaging procedure with increased sensitivity must be used. The following case examples reinforce the need to proceed with caution when the history indicates potential or a high pretest likelihood for a significant injury, but the diagnostic imaging is negative.

A 25-year-old male rugby player was referred to physical therapy for treatment of a cervical sprain after an injury sustained in a rugby match 2 days earlier. The consulting physician requested cervical traction for the injury. During the history-taking and review of systems, the patient indicated that he had sustained one of the hardest hits that he had ever received in a sporting event. The patient stated that he attempted to continue to play, but the pain was particularly sharp, and it was difficult to turn his head. Of particular concern to the patient was his ability to participate in the upcoming championship game. The patient was carrying his radiographs, and he stated that they had been read as normal in the emergency department. He denied loss of consciousness, numbness, tingling, or weakness of the extremities. He also denied any previous history of neck injuries despite playing football and rugby for many years.

The tests and measures were carefully performed because the patient was in obvious distress. An upper and lower motor neuron screening examination was normal. Cervical active range of motion was severely restricted in all directions, and gentle palpation performed in the seated position revealed local tenderness at the level of C5 with surrounding muscular spasm.

Based on the examination results, the PT took the films to the radiology reading room and reviewed them with the radiologist on duty. By focusing on the area of the palpation findings from the PT's examination, an abnormality in the lamina of C5 was visualized. The patient's neck was immediately immobilized in a collar and a subsequent CT examination clearly revealed a laminar fracture.

Correspondingly, in the absence of appropriate clinical findings, pathology on imaging may not be significant. Artifacts, overlapping cortices, clothing, and normal variants all can be mistaken for subtle fractures or other pathologic conditions (Figure 14-8). When pathology and symptoms are present in the same region of the body, a common pitfall is to assume that the visualized pathologic condition is the reason the patient is symptomatic. Careful palpation and precise examination skills are required to determine the correlation between pathology and symptoms. Incorrect conclusions may be particularly dangerous when the pathologic condition would not require surgical treatment if the patient was not symptomatic. This teaching point is reinforced with the following case example of an active duty soldier with severe LBP.

An 18-year-old soldier was sent to a regional U.S. Army medical center for further evaluation of LBP. The soldier's pain was particularly severe whenever he tried to run or perform sit-ups. No relief had been achieved with conservative treatment, including rest, medication, physical therapy modalities, and exercise.

The soldier had a grade II spondylolisthesis at the fifth lumbar level identified on plain radiographs and confirmed by CT. The radiologist and neurosurgeon agreed that the images represented a nonunion of a relatively recent injury, although a specific incident could not be identified. The patient was placed

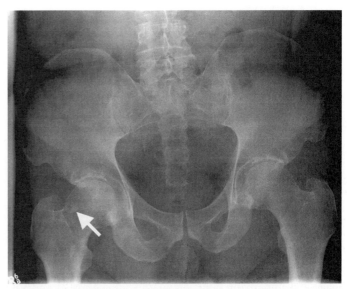

FIGURE 14-8 Significant and insignificant pathologic conditions can be strikingly similar. The radiologist needs the important clinical examination findings to help make the radiographic diagnosis. In this case, the differential diagnosis of the small sclerotic lesions is either benign bone islands or metastatic cancer. The arthritic changes in this hip may produce symptoms and reinforce the importance of a careful clinical examination to distinguish new pathologic conditions, such as metastatic cancer, from other conditions, such as osteoarthritis.

in a body cast to immobilize the "symptomatic" vertebra. The patient's response to this treatment was unanticipated. He had a dramatic increase in LBP, and the cast had to be removed in the emergency department. Surgical fusion of the segment was planned because of the failure of the immobilization to relieve his symptoms. Shortly before the planned surgery, the soldier contracted an acute respiratory infection. He went to the outpatient clinic at the medical center for treatment. On hearing the patient's story about his respiratory ailment and his LBP, a physician's assistant referred the patient to a PT with manual therapy expertise at the medical center.

The physical examination performed by the PT reproduced the soldier's LBP with unilateral segmental palpation at the first and second lumbar levels. After three sessions of joint mobilization reinforced with self range of motion and hip flexor stretching exercises, the patient's symptoms were dramatically reduced, and he was subsequently able to return to full duty and physical training without surgery.

This brief case example is an excellent illustration of how the results of imaging are meaningful only in the context of the larger comprehensive examination. The temptation is to draw conclusions relative to the identification of specific pathologic conditions on diagnostic imaging. The musculoskeletal imaging literature provides many examples of pathologic conditions in asymptomatic individuals.[*] This evidence places a high burden on the clinician to provide clinical relevance to pathology identified by the radiologist.

*References 15, 22, 41, 54, 70, 75, 87.

Specialized Areas of Imaging

Osteochondral Injuries

The diagnosis of articular cartilage injuries depends on a careful clinical examination and the appropriate diagnostic imaging modality. Osteochondral injuries require specialized imaging, and although radiographs are typically the standard for imaging joint abnormalities, they are not sensitive to early articular cartilage changes.[35] The detection of articular cartilage defects is important to facilitate the timely and appropriate management of the injury, and these defects must be differentiated from other common injuries to the involved joint. The PT must be alert for articular cartilage injury in acute injuries and in chronic injuries with persistent pain or mechanical dysfunction.

Osteochondral injuries can accompany other acute injuries such as sprains of the ligaments of the knee or ankle. Acute injuries may produce fragments of pure articular cartilage or cartilage and underlying bone. Standard spin echo MRI and spin echo MRI with fat suppression have proved to be inadequate for evaluating articular cartilage. Spoiled gradient echo sequence MRI with fat suppression is advocated to evaluate articular cartilage changes because it uses the advantages of the reduced imaging time associated with gradient echo pulse sequences and eliminates select frequencies to enhance the contrast of articular cartilage. The technique is useful to evaluate cartilage degeneration, showing signal loss in the superficial bright layer, and can illustrate varying degrees of loss of signal in intermediate and deep layers within the cartilage.[35,49] The water content of these layers of cartilage varies with fibrillation and inflammation, producing variations in the signal intensity.

A trabecular microfracture or bone bruise is the first stage of an osteochondral fracture. Although the injury may not be revealed by conventional radiography, bone contusions have typical appearances on T1-weighted and T2-weighted MRI. Osteochondral fractures resulting from significant impaction and shearing forces may also be missed by conventional radiography. MRI scans may reveal osteochondral fractures as curvilinear fracture lines, irregularities of the cartilage, bone bruises, or loose bodies. MRI with the addition of a contrast agent, conventional arthrography, and CT arthrography all have been advocated for imaging the details of lesions associated with osteochondritis dissecans.[35,49] The lesions of osteochondritis dissecans are commonly found on the capitellum, talus, patella, and femoral condyles.

Advanced degenerative changes in articular cartilage may be revealed by a loss of joint space in the weight-bearing compartment in standing radiographic images. Weight-bearing joint spaces may also be altered by meniscus injuries and subsequent surgical procedures. Additional evidence of degenerative changes on standard radiographs includes subchondral sclerosis and cysts, bone eburnation, articular surface collapse, and bony spurs. Historically, stress radiographs have been used to obtain the same information from the non–weight-bearing joint compartment by using mechanically imposed stress.[85]

Osteoarthritis of the knee is a good example of a condition for which conservative treatment should not be based on the results of musculoskeletal imaging. Clinical diagnostic criteria developed by Altman[3] (Box 14-4) have been found to be 89%

BOX 14-4

Clinical Criteria for the Diagnosis of Osteoarthritis of the Knee

1. Knee pain, age 38 years or younger, and bony enlargement
2. Knee pain, age 39 years or older, morning stiffness more than 30 minutes, and bony enlargement
3. Knee pain, crepitus on active motion, morning stiffness more than 30 minutes, and bony enlargement
4. Knee pain, crepitus on active motion, morning stiffness 30 minutes or less, and age 38 years or older

From Altman R, Bloch D, Bole G Jr, et al: Development of clinical criteria for osteoarthritis, J Rheumatol 14:3-6, 1987.

---

sensitive and 88% specific for knee osteoarthritis. Physical therapy based on clinical findings and not radiographic findings has been shown to be of high benefit, low cost, and no known risk to the patient.[16,17,71] Decisions for surgery are typically based on intolerable pain, progressive loss of function, or a progressive clinically apparent varus or valgus deformity.

Sports-Related Injuries

Imaging in the management of sport injuries, as in other types of injuries, should be focused on the situations in which positive findings on imaging would alter the course of treatment. Relevant questions for the PT may include the following: Does the patient's clinical presentation suggest the presence of a fracture, arthritis, sprain, or strain? Is there evidence that management by musculoskeletal imaging findings is likely to improve the outcome for this patient? Does this patient require rest, immobilization, vigorous rehabilitation, or a consultation for medical or surgical management?[55]

The spectrum of sports injuries ranges from injuries that do not need imaging, to suspected fractures that require imaging, and to injuries that do not normally require imaging but do not respond to treatment and eventually require imaging as part of the plan of care process. An example provided by Mintz[55] is a back injury that does not respond to conservative therapy within the normal time frame and requires appropriate imaging to rule out a pars fracture. The types of injuries seen in different athletic populations vary depending on where the athlete is in his or her life cycle. Children are more susceptible to bony avulsion injuries because of their strong ligament support and relatively weaker bone structure. Pain in proximity to a long bone may herald a bone bruise or muscle injury but may also signal the presence of a pathologic fracture from a bone cyst or neoplasm. See Chapters 16, 17, and 18 for more details regarding the adolescent, obstetric, and geriatric populations.

Fractures and Dislocations

The diagnosis of fractures and dislocations is probably the most recognized use of plain radiographs. Fractures and dislocations are the most common traumatic conditions encountered by radiologists. Fractures are classified as either complete or incomplete depending on whether any of the bony trabeculae are left intact. Dislocations are considered complete when the joint surfaces are no longer in contact. Subluxations represent changes in

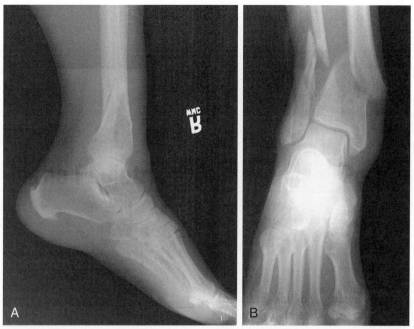

FIGURE 14-9 Two views at 90 degrees to each other are the minimum to reveal the characteristics of a fracture or dislocation on radiograph. **A,** Lateral view of distal tibia and fibula fracture suggests that it is oblique and minimally displaced. **B,** Anteroposterior view reveals true degree of displacement and angulation.

relationship of the articular surfaces when the structures are still in contact.[34]

Plain radiographs taken in at least two planes are required to rule out fractures, to judge the degree of displacement of fracture, and to rule out joint dislocation (Figure 14-9). The evaluation and description of noted fractures should include the site and extent of the fracture; whether the fracture is complete or incomplete; and the alignment of the fragments regarding distraction, foreshortening, angulation, rotation, and displacement (see the Evolve website for color images). The diagnosis of an open fracture (a fracture segment that communicates directly with the outside environment) is based on the clinical examination. Fractures are also described according to the characteristics of the fracture line, such as longitudinal, spiral, transverse, and oblique (see the Evolve website for color images). Special types of fractures include stress or fatigue fractures and pathologic fractures that are typically caused by metabolic changes in bone or tumors.

FRACTURE IN CHILDREN. Fractures in children may be especially challenging to recognize because of difficulties encountered with obtaining the history and performing the review of systems and tests and measures, as well as the often-subtle presentation clinically and on imaging. The PT may have to use various strategies of distracting the child and involving him or her in play while observing the child's willingness to use the injured extremity. Initially palpating well away from the injured area may help the examiner distinguish response to palpation. In an older child, allowing the child to point with one finger to where it hurts the most may be useful. Additional strategies include asking the child to rate the pain as a "big pain" or "little pain" while palpating. The examiner may be able to differentiate the areas for diagnostic imaging and help guide the radiographic interpretation by asking the child, "which hurts the most—when I push here on A, or when I push here on B?" Distracting the child and then palpating

areas of suspected fractures again may provide insight regarding whether the severity of the pain consistently suggests a fracture.

Fractures in children have the potential to interfere with the growth plate and represent a possible danger to the future growth of the involved bone (see Chapter 16). The Salter-Harris classification system is commonly used to classify growth plate injuries (see the Evolve website for color images). Comparison views of the uninvolved extremity or repeating the radiographs after allowing time for cortical reaction may be necessary to reveal a growth plate injury in children.

STRESS FRACTURES. Stress fractures are common injuries in athletes or training soldiers. Stress fractures are multifactorial injuries with contributing factors of gender, hormonal influences, diet, training regimen, footwear, and running surfaces.[2,5,27] Stress fractures are thought to constitute 10% of all sports injuries. They have been described in tennis, football, basketball, and hockey players; aerobic and ballet dancers; runners; gymnasts; kayakers; golfers; and throwing athletes.[63] Stress fractures are thought to be the result of cyclic overloading of bone that exceeds the ability of bony tissue to strengthen and repair itself. High-repetition, low-load cyclic stress and low-repetition, high-load stress may result in the development of stress fractures.

Initial radiographs of early-stage stress fractures may be read as normal. Plain film diagnosis of stress fractures depends on many factors. The site of injury and the timing of the films related to the stage of the osteoclastic resorption, the osteoblastic repair, periosteal reaction, and new bone formation have an effect on the appearance of the injury on plain films. In general, because of the lack of sensitivity to early bone change, there must be significant bone response to the imposed stresses before the changes become apparent on plain film radiographs. Radiographs typically require 2 to 3 weeks to reveal new stress fractures and may be normal for 3 months after the onset of symptoms.

TABLE 14-4

Grading of Stress Fractures from Typical Appearance on Bone Scan and Magnetic Resonance Imaging (MRI)

Grade of Stress Fracture	Bone Scan Appearance	MRI Appearance
1	Relatively small, poorly defined cortical area of moderately increased activity	Mild to moderate periosteal edema on T2-weighted images
2	More defined area of moderately increased cortical activity	Moderate to severe periosteal edema with marrow edema on T2-weighted images
3	Wide to spindle-shaped area of highly increased cortico-medullary activity	Moderate to severe periosteal edema with marrow edema on T2-weighted and T1-weighted images
4	Transcortical area of intensely increased activity	Moderate to severe periosteal edema with marrow edema on T2-weighted and T1-weighted images; fracture line obvious

Adapted from Fredericson M, Bergman A, Hoffman K, et al: Tibial stress reaction in runners: correlation of clinical symptoms and scintigraphy with a new MRI grading system, *Am J Sports Med* 23:472-481, 1995.

Bone scintigraphy is considered a more sensitive but nonspecific modality for diagnosing stress fractures. Bone scans can become positive within 6 to 72 hours of the initial onset of the fracture. Because of the lack of specificity of bone scans, the differential diagnosis process in the presence of a positive bone scan must include ruling out benign and malignant neoplasms and osteomyelitis. Zwas and associates[94] described a system for grading stress fractures based on bone scan images. Grade 1 is described as mildly increased activity in a small, ill-defined area. Grade 2 is a larger, more defined, and elongated cortical area. Grade 3 fractures have highly increased activity in a fusiform corticomedullary pattern. Grade 4 lesions have intensely increased transcortical activity. Typical appearances of stress fractures on MRI and bone scans are summarized in Table 14-4.

Some clinicians may prefer MRI studies for grading stress fractures because of the risk associated with the ionizing radiation exposure from bone scans, the excellent MRI anatomic detail unavailable through bone scan imaging, and the reduced time to complete MRI.[1,27,43,44] Although bone scans remain the gold standard for detecting stress fractures, T1-weighted and T2-weighted MRI reveals the tissue damage associated with a stress fracture. Typical tissue changes seen on MRI include periosteal and bone marrow edema. MRI scans may be more useful than bone scans as an aid in designing rehabilitation programs based on the extent of the injury.

Shoulder and Rotator Cuff Tears

Ultrasound has been shown to be a sensitive and specific diagnostic tool for imaging complete and partial rotator cuff tears.[12,36,89,90] The primary difficulty reported with using ultrasound for shoulder imaging is the apparent long learning curve for mastery of the technique. Ultrasound can detect abnormal amounts of fluid or synovial changes and can provide dynamic assessment of the shoulder region, revealing acromial impingement on subacromial structures. Van Holsbeeck and colleagues[90] studied the diagnostic utility of ultrasound used by a single trained examiner for partial bursal side rotator cuff tears compared with arthroscopic findings. Ultrasound was found to be 93% sensitive and 94% specific, with a positive predictive value of 82% and a negative predictive value of 98%, although the surgeons were not blinded to the preoperative ultrasound results.

MRI has a similar diagnostic utility as CT arthrography in the shoulder, and both modalities have the primary advantage of being noninvasive. Reported sensitivity for detection of labral tears with high-resolution MRI ranges from 74% to 100%, with specificity of 95% to 100%.[8] Magnetic resonance arthrography (MRA) is considered by some authors to be superior to other imaging techniques in evaluating the glenohumeral joint.[8] Pathologic conditions associated with instability and anterior inferior dislocation of the glenohumeral joint are readily identified with MRA. These pathologic conditions include anterior inferior labral tears, classic and osseous Bankart lesions, fracture and sclerosis of the glenoid, Hill-Sachs lesions, and superior labral anterior to posterior (SLAP) lesions. Some normal variants reported to cause diagnostic difficulty are anterosuperior sublabral foramen, Buford's complex, and hyaline cartilage under the labrum.[8] MRA has been found to have a moderate to good correlation to anatomic dissection for determining the size and morphologic features of the glenohumeral ligaments.

Spinal Injuries

Imaging in the event of spinal trauma must be fully evaluated consistent with the forces involved and the metabolic bone health of the patient. Less force is required to produce fractures in the presence of osteoporosis and advanced age. Signs and symptoms such as pain that is not relieved by rest or changes in position, pain that is sharply increased with movement, unremitting paraspinous musculature spasm, and an unwillingness to move the spine all suggest a spinal fracture. Facet and intervertebral disk pathologic conditions are best revealed with CT and MRI. Plain radiographs can adequately reveal spinal fractures, but CT scan remains the imaging modality of choice to reveal the intricate details of spinal fractures (Figure 14-10).

Conventional radiographs are the initial imaging modality of choice for most cervical spine injuries. A typical cervical radiographic series includes anteroposterior, lateral, and open-mouth odontoid views. Flexion and extension views may aid in evaluating suspected cervical instability. It has been reported that 20% of cervical fractures are undetected on plain radiographs. Although some missed cervical fractures and dislocations are the result of misinterpretation, the most common cause of an overlooked injury is an inadequate film series. It is crucial for the

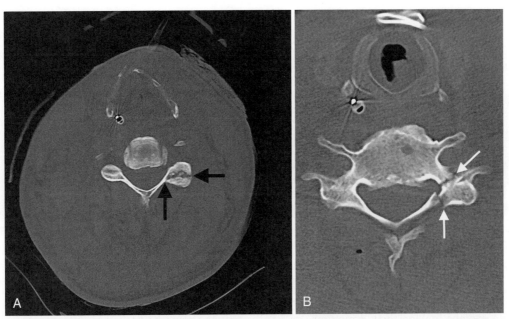

FIGURE 14-10 CT can reveal subtle fractures not apparent on plain films. Two fractures were found in the cervical spine of a patient after a motor vehicle accident. The presence of fractures at different spinal levels underscores the importance of the complete examination. **A,** Facet fracture at C4-C5 level *(arrows)*. **B,** C6 pedicle and lamina fracture *(arrows)*.

lateral view to include all seven cervical vertebrae and the interspace between the last cervical and first thoracic vertebrae.[32]

Significant cervical injury is unlikely in adults with normal mental status; not under the influence of drugs or alcohol; and in the absence of findings such as neck pain, palpation tenderness, loss of consciousness, concurrent distracting injury, or neurologic signs such as numbness or weakness of the upper extremities. Children may have spinal cord injury without radiographic evidence of damage to the cervical spine. Careful examination for neurologic findings is required after any head and neck trauma in these patients. Emergent spinal cord treatment is indicated in the presence of positive neurologic findings. Cervical spinal stenosis can be initially evaluated by plain radiographs with examination for adequate anteroposterior diameter on the lateral view. Normal anteroposterior diameter of the cervical spinal canal is 13 mm. Suspected cases can be evaluated further with myelography, MRI, or CT.

The following brief case example highlights a situation in which the clinical examination and initial radiographs suggest a possible significant injury. Guided by the pretest probability and the inconclusive radiographs, a more sensitive study was ultimately performed with a subsequent diagnosis.

A 21-year-old man was referred to physical therapy for treatment of neck and upper trapezius pain. The patient related a history of passing out at work and striking the back of his head on the desk. The injury had occurred approximately 2 weeks before the physical therapy appointment. The patient stated that shortly after the event it was very difficult for him to move his neck, but this was improving. The patient also related that immediately after the injury there had been numbness and tingling on the top of his head, and he had experienced difficulty swallowing, but those signs and symptoms had also resolved. He denied any significant medical history, including seizures, but stated that he had been out late drinking the night before he passed out at work.

The patient had not undergone diagnostic imaging before seeing the PT. Based on the history findings, the PT decided that it would be inappropriate to perform a physical examination before a radiographic examination was obtained. The PT ordered a cervical series, and the radiologist on duty was contacted to review the study. The radiologist noted an apparent obliquity of the dens and potentially an abnormal position of C1 in relation to C2. The radiologist also thought there was a subtle lucency across the base of the dens. In view of these findings, the radiologist recommended an immediate CT scan. The patient's neck was immobilized, and he was transported by ambulance to the hospital for the CT scan.

CT confirmed the radiologist's suspicions. There was an oblique comminuted dens fracture, with a fracture line involving the right lateral mass of C2. The fracture line extended into the foramen transversarium on the right side. Minimal to mild anterior displacement of C1 was also noted. The patient was subsequently taken to the operating room and stabilized with a halo collar (Figure 14-11). The patient's report of initial difficulty with swallowing was most likely related to retropharyngeal bleeding from the upper cervical fracture.

LOW BACK PAIN. Low back problems are the most common cause of disability in individuals younger than 45 years.[46] Classification of LBP that is useful for imaging decisions has been proposed as follows: (1) LBP from potentially serious underlying conditions, including infections, fractures, neoplasms, aortic abdominal aneurysms, inflammatory conditions of the kidneys, and cauda equina syndrome; (2) LBP with sciatica from irritation or impingement of lumbosacral nerve roots; and (3) LBP with nonspecific symptoms thought to be from the spectrum of musculoligamentous and degenerative conditions. Most LBP falls into the third category and can improve significantly with proper treatment within 4 weeks and does not require diagnostic imaging.[76] Although patients may occasionally request imaging

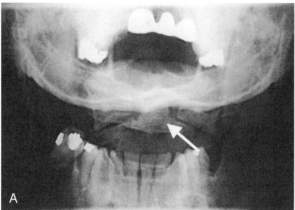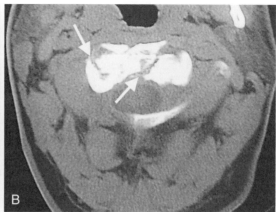

FIGURE 14-11 A, Open-mouth anteroposterior radiograph suggests abnormality of position of the dens with subtle fracture line at the base. **B,** Fracture of the lateral mass and dens of C2 is confirmed by CT scan.

to satisfy their fears regarding the source of LBP, patients who receive an adequate explanation for their symptoms are less likely to want additional diagnostic tests.[18,19,39]

Lower back radiographs are commonly described as overprescribed diagnostic imaging procedures. Plain radiographs are ineffective for diagnosing lumbar nerve root impingement from a herniated disk or spinal stenosis or for ruling out cancer or infection. Only 1 in 2500 radiographs detects something not suspected on the medical history and examination that has an effect on patient care.[76] Overuse of lumbar spine films can result in increased cost, excessive gonadal radiation exposure, and irrelevant findings that lead to inappropriate diagnoses and treatment. Of great concern is the fact that pathologic conditions shown on plain film radiographs and advanced musculoskeletal imaging may not even be relevant to the patient's symptoms.

Studies have shown degenerative changes, bulging disks, and herniated disks at one or more levels in 25% to 50% of asymptomatic people.[41,75] Studies have also shown that patients with LBP who undergo advanced imaging earlier in their presentation and not consistent with best practice guidelines are more likely to enter a management pathway of greater risk that includes surgery and other invasive procedures and greater use of medications.[14,39,47,48] Specific guidelines have been developed to help reduce ordering of lumbar plain films that are of minimal diagnostic value.[10]

In 1994, the Agency on Health Related Quality and Research (formerly the Agency for Health Care Policy and Research) published guidelines on the management of acute LBP in adults.[10] Although these guidelines are now officially archived and not considered to be the current standard for evidence-based practice, the imaging recommendations for acute LBP remain pertinent.[39] According to the guidelines, routine testing such as laboratory tests, radiographs, and other imaging studies is not recommended during the first month of acute LBP management. Most patients, even with symptoms of nerve root impingement, improve within 4 to 6 weeks and do not require diagnostic imaging. The exception is when red flags are noted during the examination that raise suspicions of a dangerous low back or nonspinal condition.[18,39]

When diagnostic imaging is indicated, the initial radiographs should be limited to anteroposterior and lateral views. The additional diagnostic value of coned anteroposterior or lateral views (historically used for a close-up view of the lumbosacral junction region) and oblique radiographs is generally not worth the additional radiation exposure, particularly to women. Oblique lumbar radiographs, usually taken to screen for spondylolysis, rarely add useful clinical information in adults and double the x-ray dose to the patient. Patients with spondylolisthesis can be safely treated in the same fashion as patients with other types of acute low back problems. Radiographs performed specifically to screen for spondylolisthesis are unnecessary for the first 3 months of symptoms. Although oblique radiographs do provide visualization of the pars interarticularis, CT provides the best details of a suspected acute pars fracture. In select circumstances, flexion/extension films may be useful to identify spondylolisthesis with associated instability.[83]

In the case of red flags or key findings (Chapters 6 to 9) that suggest the presence of a serious underlying spinal condition, such as fracture, tumor, infection, or cauda equina syndrome (Chapter 20), more extensive diagnostic evaluation including advanced musculoskeletal imaging such as bone scans, MRI, and CT is often in order even if the initial radiographic findings are negative. Certain diagnoses can be effectively ruled out by using evidence-based screening strategies. In the absence of age older than 50 years, personal history of a primary cancer, unexplained loss of weight, or failure to respond to conservative therapy, cancer can be ruled out in patients with LBP with 100% sensitivity.[39] After 4 weeks of nonresponse to physical therapy, basic laboratory studies including a complete blood cell count and erythrocyte sedimentation rate (ESR) combined with anteroposterior and lateral radiographs help identify patients with conditions such as osteomyelitis and occult neoplasms. The combination of radiographs and ESR is a very sensitive method to screen for occult neoplasms. Deyo and Diehl[18] reported that all cases of occult neoplasms in 1975 screened patients with back pain had either an abnormal film or an elevated ESR.

In the event of signs or symptoms suggesting cauda equina syndrome or progressive major motor weakness, advanced diagnostic imaging, such as MRI, CT, myelography, or CT myelography, in addition to plain film radiographs, is recommended. Facet and intervertebral disk pathologies are best revealed with CT and MRI. Although spinal fractures may be adequately revealed by plain radiographs, CT remains the imaging modality of choice to reveal the intricate details of spinal fractures. Bone scans are considered to be more sensitive than plain films for detecting infections or neoplasms of the spine. MRI provides more anatomic detail and greater sensitivity and specificity at approximately twice the cost of a bone scan.

Particularly in patients with a history of a malignant process, metastatic disease must be ruled out as a cause of LBP. The spine, and the lumbar spine in particular, is considered the most common site for metastasis to musculoskeletal tissues from primary cancers. Common primary cancers that metastasize to the axial skeleton are prostate, thyroid, breast, lung, and kidney. Constitutional symptoms, unexplained weight loss, age older than 50 years, and symptoms that are not relieved with the typical changes in posture or position are cause for concern and must be determined during the history-taking. Plain films without an associated ESR have the least sensitivity for detecting metastasis, whereas bone scans are 74% to 98% sensitive, and MRI is 83% to 93% sensitive.[39]

Equally sensitive combinations of history questions for spinal infections and fractures have not yet been determined.[39] The presence of fever in a patient with acute, increasingly severe LBP is thought to be a specific, but not sensitive finding. In a patient presenting with acute severe LBP, the presence of a fever needs further investigation, but the absence of a fever in a patient likely to have a spinal infection cannot rule out the condition. Spinal infections are associated with intravenous drug use, recent urinary tract infections, pelvic inflammatory conditions, surgery, and immunocompromised status. Patients with immunocompromised status include patients with a history of prolonged corticosteroid therapy, patients who are human immunodeficiency virus positive, organ transplant recipients, patients receiving chemotherapy and radiation, diabetic patients, and elderly patients.[11] Plain films have poor sensitivity in detecting spinal infections because radiographic abnormalities may not be apparent for 2 to 8 weeks.[73,74] MRI has 96% sensitivity and 92% specificity in the diagnosis of spinal infection and has been found to be equally sensitive to spinal infections as CT myelography. In addition, MRI provides better imaging of the vertebral bodies, intervertebral disks, and paravertebral tissues. T1-weighted MRI scans provide more details of the anatomic limits of the abscess, the degree of the cord compression, and paraspinal and vertebral involvement than CT myelography.[73,76]

The physical therapy examination should also assess for red flags of nonspinal conditions, such as vascular, abdominal, urinary, or pelvic pathologic conditions capable of referring symptoms to the lower back (see Chapter 6). If multiple red flags are present, radiographs and laboratory studies are indicated at the initial visit. Clinical judgment is necessary to determine whether plain radiographs or laboratory tests are required at the initial visit because of the presence of a single red flag.[39]

For patients limited by sciatica for more than 4 weeks without clear evidence on physical examination of nerve root compromise, electromyography and Hoffman's reflex tests of the lower limb may provide evidence of suspected neurologic dysfunction. The clinical examination for patients with sciatica should include straight leg raising and neurologic testing. A positive straight leg raise is sensitive, but not specific for disk herniation.[65] A neurologic baseline established by the examination at the first clinical visit can reveal neurologic conditions that require immediate referral and conditions that do not respond to treatment over time. Sensory evoked potentials may be a useful adjunct for assessment of suspected spinal stenosis or spinal cord myelopathy. For patients limited by sciatica for more than 4 weeks with physiologic evidence of neurologic dysfunction, MRI or CT should be considered to provide anatomic detail of a possible herniated disk before surgery.

Most PTs are familiar with the clinical presentation and typical intolerance to upright activities associated with spinal stenosis. A diagnostic strategy for spinal stenosis using an inclined treadmill, which may provide additional insight to the functional implications of the disorder, has been described in the physical therapy literature.[29] There is also evidence for successful physical therapy management of spinal stenosis.[92] Conservative therapy is appropriate for the first few months before surgical consideration, at which time advanced imaging such as MRI and CT may be warranted.

Prompt emergency consultation is reserved for patients with findings of bowel or bladder dysfunction or progressive or severe neurologic impairment. Table 14-5 summarizes the red flags indicating a need for diagnostic imaging and the imaging modality considered to have the greatest diagnostic utility for each condition. Primary care provider education regarding the evidence for the management of LBP has been shown to reduce the use of diagnostic imaging, specialty referrals, and surgery.[45]

Summary

Available Resources for Physical Therapists

Several excellent resources exist that are particularly useful in daily practice. A Suggested Readings list follows the References of this chapter, and complete reference lists may be found on the Evolve site. A wealth of information on imaging of the musculoskeletal system is available on the Internet. The key words *musculoskeletal imaging* and *diagnostic imaging of the musculoskeletal system* produce numerous sites. The sites range from single case teaching examples, to university-based diagnostic image libraries, to central listings of radiology sites with teaching libraries. Focusing on the sites intended for PTs and other primary care providers may initially be more clinically useful for the practicing PT.

Evidence

PTs working in primary care settings with privileges to order musculoskeletal imaging have been shown to be diagnostically accurate and, in general, to reduce the need for musculoskeletal imaging while decreasing episodes of care and the associated costs of many musculoskeletal injuries and conditions. Considering the spiraling cost for the management of musculoskeletal disorders such as LBP, primary access to PTs with the ability to order musculoskeletal imaging as appropriate and consistent with evidence-based guidelines should be appealing to consumers, insurance companies, and legislators. Patients often must undergo one or more medical examinations and perhaps be

TABLE 14-5

Summary of Low Back Pain Red Flags and Appropriate Diagnostic Imaging

Potentially Serious Conditions	History and Review of Systems Red Flags	Diagnostic Testing Indicated
Possible tumor	Age >50 or <20 years; history of cancer; pain that increases when supine or at night	AP and lateral radiographs; CBC, ESR, UA; if radiographs are negative or laboratory tests are positive, bone scan, MRI or CT
Possible infection	Fevers, chills, or unexplained weight loss; recent bacterial infection; intravenous drug use; immunosuppressed from HIV, steroids, or transplantation	Bone scan, MRI, or CT; CBC, ESR, UA
Possible cauda equina syndrome	Saddle anesthesia; recent-onset bladder dysfunction such as urinary retention, overflow, and incontinence; symptoms of severe or progressive neurologic deficit	Emergent surgical consultation when supported by physical findings of unexpected laxity of anal sphincter; perianal/perineal sensory loss; major motor weakness of knee extensors, ankle plantar flexors, ankle dorsiflexors, or ankle evertors; appropriate imaging is MRI or CT or myelography or CT myelography
Possible spinal fracture	History of significant trauma such as a fall from a height, motor vehicle accident, or direct blow to the back for young adult; minor fall or moderate lift in elderly or osteoporotic individual; prolonged use of steroids; age >70 years	AP and lateral radiographs; if negative then MRI or CT

AP, anteroposterior; *CBC,* complete blood count; *CT,* computed tomography; *ESR,* erythrocyte sedimentation rate; *HIV,* human immunodeficiency virus; *MRI,* magnetic resonance imaging; *UA,* urinalysis.

Data from Staiger T, Paauw D, Deyo R, et al: Imaging studies for acute low back pain: when and when not to order them, *Imaging* 105:161-172, 1999.

subjected to unnecessary musculoskeletal imaging before finally arriving at the PT, who provides the definitive treatment for the condition. Evidence exists against such practices, and other evidence suggests patients who are forced into such pathways may be the recipients of unnecessary high-risk procedures.

If during the physical therapy examination or treatment, it becomes obvious that musculoskeletal imaging is required, the patient may be forced to repeat the same time-consuming and costly path to obtain the necessary imaging. Many patients arrive at the initial appointment for physical therapy after advanced imaging has been obtained by the referring provider. In most of these cases, the patients were not surgical candidates, and there were no red flags. Many of these patients have been told that the reason their shoulder, neck, or lower back hurts is because of imaged pathology that may not even correspond with the patient's presentation. Management of these patients can be particularly difficult because the seed has been planted that this pathology somehow needs to be addressed.

Whenever providers are not trained in musculoskeletal medicine, or the provider stands to profit financially from the imaging procedures, the patient may be exposed to the documented risks of unnecessary ionizing radiation and enter an expensive management pathway with higher associated risk to the patient. All PTs must be ready to articulate the research that supports their role in primary care and shows their appropriate and sparing use of musculoskeletal imaging. A streamlined, user-friendly process that directly connects evidence-based diagnostic and screening strategies with expert treatment is the goal.

PTs are likely to continue to establish themselves as medical professionals and user-friendly, low associated risk, providers of choice for the conservative care of neuromusculoskeletal conditions. PTs may soon be able to order diagnostic imaging outside the U.S. military health care system. With such compelling evidence from perspectives of quality of care and cost of care, PTs are likely to achieve wider access to the diagnostic imaging, laboratory tests, and medications that would enable them to care for patients efficiently and effectively within an interdisciplinary health care delivery model.

REFERENCES

1. Ahovuo JA, Kiuru MJ, Kinnunen JJ, et al. MR imaging of fatigue stress injuries to bones: intra- and interobserver agreement. Magn Reson Imaging 2002;20:401–6.
2. Almeida SA, Williams KM, Shaffer RA, et al. Epidemiological patterns of musculoskeletal injuries and physical training. Med Sci Sports Exerc 1999;31:1176–82.
3. Altman RD. Criteria for the classification of osteoarthritis of the knee and hip. Scand J Rheumatol Suppl 1987;65:31–9.
4. American Physical Therapy Association. Guide to physical therapy practice, 2nd ed. Phys Ther 2001;81:9–744.
5. Armstrong 3rd DW, Rue JP, Wilckens JH, et al. Stress fracture injury in young military men and women. Bone 2004;35:806–16.
6. Bachmann LM, Kolb E, Koller MT, et al. Accuracy of Ottawa ankle rules to exclude fractures of the ankle and mid-foot: systematic review. BMJ 2003;326:417.
7. Bachmann LM, Terriet G. The Ottawa rules for ankle sprains. Hosp Med 2004;65:132–3.
8. Beltran J, Rosenberg ZS, Chandnani VP, et al. Glenohumeral instability: evaluation with MR arthrography. RadioGraphics 1997;17:657–73.
9. Benson CJ, Schreck RC, Underwood FB, et al. The role of Army physical therapists as nonphysician health care providers who prescribe certain medications: observations and experiences. Phys Ther 1995;75:380–6.
10. Bigos SJ. Acute low back problems in adults. US Department of Health and Human Services, Public Health Service, Agency for Health Care Policy and Research clinical practice guidelines no. 14, ACHPR publication no. 95-0642; 1994.
11. Carragee EJ. Pyogenic vertebral osteomyelitis. J Bone Joint Surg Am 1997;79:874–80.
12. Chang CY, Wang SF, Chiou HJ, et al. Comparison of shoulder ultrasound and MR imaging in diagnosing full-thickness rotator cuff tears. Clin Imaging 2002;26:50–4.
13. Clough TM. Femoral neck stress fracture: the importance of clinical suspicion and early review. Br J Sports Med 2002;36:308–9.

14. Daker-White G, Carr AJ, Harvey I, et al. A randomised controlled trial: shifting boundaries of doctors and physiotherapists in orthopaedic outpatient departments. J Epidemiol Community Health 1999;53:643–50.

15. Deyle GD. Musculoskeletal imaging in physical therapist practice. J Orthop Sports Phys Ther 2005;35:708–21.

16. Deyle GD, Allison SC, Matekel RL, et al. Physical therapy treatment effectiveness for osteoarthritis of the knee: a randomized comparison of supervised clinical exercise and manual therapy procedures versus a home exercise program. Phys Ther 2005;85:1301–17.

17. Deyle GD, Henderson NE, Matekel RL, et al. Effectiveness of manual physical therapy and exercise in osteoarthritis of the knee: a randomized, controlled trial. Ann Intern Med 2000;132:173–81.

18. Deyo RA, Diehl AK. Cancer as a cause of back pain: frequency, clinical presentation, and diagnostic strategies. J Gen Intern Med 1988;3:230–8.

19. Deyo RA, Rainville J, Kent DL. What can the history and physical examination tell us about low back pain? JAMA 1992;268:760–5.

20. Dupuy DE, Hangen DH, Zachazewski JE. Kinematic CT of the patellofemoral joint. AJR Am J Roentgenol 1997;169:211–5.

21. Dutton J, Bromhead SE, Speed CA, et al. Clinical value of grading the scintigraphic appearances of tibial stress fractures in military recruits. Clin Nucl Med 2002;27:18–21.

22. Ebenbichler GR, Erdogmus CB, Resch KL, et al. Ultrasound therapy for calcific tendinitis of the shoulder. N Engl J Med 1999;340:1533–8.

23. Edwards I, Jones M, Carr J, et al. Clinical reasoning strategies in physical therapy. Phys Ther 2004;84:312–30; discussion 331-315.

24. Feldman F. Musculoskeletal radiology: then and now. Radiology 2000;216:309–16.

25. Feldman F, Staron R, Zwass A, et al. MR imaging: its role in detecting occult fractures. Skeletal Radiol 1994;23:439–44.

26. Flatman JG. Hip diseases with referred pain to the knee. JAMA 1975;234:967–8.

27. Fredericson M, Jennings F, Beaulieu C, et al. Stress fractures in athletes. Top Magn Reson Imaging 2006;17:309–25.

28. Freedman KB, Bernstein J. Educational deficiencies in musculoskeletal medicine. J Bone Joint Surg Am 2002;84:604–8.

29. Fritz JM, Erhard RE, Delitto A, et al. Preliminary results of the use of a two-stage treadmill test as a clinical diagnostic tool in the differential diagnosis of lumbar spinal stenosis. J Spinal Disord 1997;10:410–6.

30. Goddard P, Leslie A, Jones A, et al. Error in radiology. Br J Radiol 2001;74:949–51.

31. Gordon G. Users' guide to the medical literature: essentials of evidence-based clinical practice. Chicago: AMA Press; 2002.

32. Graber MA, Kathol M. Cervical spine radiographs in the trauma patient. Am Fam Physician 1999;59:331–42.

33. Greathouse DG, Schreck RC, Benson CJ. The United States Army physical therapy experience: evaluation and treatment of patients with neuromusculoskeletal disorders. J Orthop Sports Phys Ther 1994;19:261–6.

34. Greenspan A. Orthopaedic radiology: a practical approach. Philadelphia: Lippincott Williams & Wilkins; 2000.

35. Hodler J, Resnick D. Current status of imaging of articular cartilage. Skeletal Radiol 1996;25:703–9.

36. Iannotti JP, Ciccone J, Buss DD, et al. Accuracy of office-based ultrasonography of the shoulder for the diagnosis of rotator cuff tears. J Bone Joint Surg Am 2005;87:1305–11.

37. James JJ, Abshier JD. The primary evaluation of musculoskeletal disorders by the physical therapist. Milit Med 1981;146:496–9.

38. James JJ, Stuart RB. Expanded role for the physical therapist: screening musculoskeletal disorders. Phys Ther 1975;55:121–31.

39. Jarvik JG, Deyo RA. Diagnostic evaluation of low back pain with emphasis on imaging. Ann Intern Med 2002;137:586–97.

40. Jensen GM, Gwyer J, Shepard KF. Expert practice in physical therapy. Phys Ther 2000;80:28–43; discussion 44-52.

41. Jensen MC, Brant-Zawadzki MN, Obuchowski N, et al. Magnetic resonance imaging of the lumbar spine in people without back pain. N Engl J Med 1994;331:69–73.

42. Kaplan PH, Helms C, Dussault R, et al. Musculoskeletal MRI. Philadelphia: Saunders; 2001.

43. Kiuru MJ, Mantysaari MJ, Pihlajamaki HK, et al. Evaluation of stress-related anterior lower leg pain with magnetic resonance imaging and intracompartmental pressure measurement. Milit Med 2003;168:48–52.

44. Kiuru MJ, Pihlajamaki HK, Hietanen HJ, et al. MR imaging, bone scintigraphy, and radiography in bone stress injuries of the pelvis and the lower extremity. Acta Radiol 2002;43:207–12.

45. Klein BJ, Radecki RT, Foris MP, et al. Bridging the gap between science and practice in managing low back pain: a comprehensive spine care system in a health maintenance organization setting. Spine 2000;25:738–40.

46. Kovacs FM, Abraira V, Zamora J, et al. Correlation between pain, disability, and quality of life in patients with common low back pain. Spine 2004;29:206–10.

47. Levy AR, Goldberg MS, Hanley JA, et al. Projecting the lifetime risk of cancer from exposure to diagnostic ionizing radiation for adolescent idiopathic scoliosis. Health Phys 1994;66:621–33.

48. Levy AR, Goldberg MS, Mayo NE, et al. Reducing the lifetime risk of cancer from spinal radiographs among people with adolescent idiopathic scoliosis. Spine 1996;21:1540–7; discussion 1548.

49. Loredo R, Sanders TG. Imaging of osteochondral injuries. Clin Sports Med 2001;20:249–78.

50. Marks R. Distribution of pain provoked from lumbar facet joints and related structures during diagnostic spinal infiltration. Pain 1989;39:37–40.

51. Matava MJ, Patton CM, Luhmann S, et al. Knee pain as the initial symptom of slipped capital femoral epiphysis: an analysis of initial presentation and treatment. J Pediatr Orthop 1999;19:455–60.

52. McCall IW, Park WM, O'Brien JP. Induced pain referral from posterior lumbar elements in normal subjects. Spine 1979;4:441–6.

53. McGinn TG, Guyatt GH, Wyer PC, et al. Users' guides to the medical literature, XXII: how to use articles about clinical decision rules—evidence-based medicine working group. JAMA 2000;284:79–84.

54. Milgrom C, Schaffler M, Gilbert S, et al. Rotator-cuff changes in asymptomatic adults: the effect of age, hand dominance and gender. J Bone Joint Surg Br 1995;77:296–8.

55. Mintz DN. Imaging of sports injuries. Phys Med Rehabil Clin N Am 2000;11:435–69.

56. Moore JH, McMillian D, Rosenthal M, Weishaar M. Risk determination for patients with direct access to physical therapy in military health care facilities. J Orthop Sports Phys Ther 2005;35:674–8.

57. Moore JH, Goss DL, Baxter RE, et al. Clinical diagnostic accuracy and magnetic resonance imaging of patients referred by physical therapists, orthopaedic surgeons, and nonorthopaedic providers. J Orthop Sports Phys Ther 2005;35:67–71.

58. Ohashi K, Brandser EA, el-Khoury GY. Role of MR imaging in acute injuries to the appendicular skeleton. Radiol Clin North Am 1997;35:591–613.

59. Pandey R, McNally E, Ali A, et al. The role of MRI in the diagnosis of occult hip fractures. Injury 1998;29:61–3.

60. Perry JJ, Stiell IG. Impact of clinical decision rules on clinical care of traumatic injuries to the foot and ankle, knee, cervical spine, and head. Injury 2006;37:1157–65.

61. Petren-Mallmin M, Linder J. MRI cervical spine findings in asymptomatic fighter pilots. Aviat Space Environ Med 1999;70:1183–8.

62. Reed MH. Imaging utilization commentary: a radiology perspective. Pediatr Radiol 2008;38(Suppl 4):s660–3.

63. Reeder MT, Dick BH, Atkins JK. Stress fractures: current concepts of diagnosis and treatment. Sports Med 1996;22:198–212.

64. Resnik L, Jensen GM. Using clinical outcomes to explore the theory of expert practice in physical therapy. Phys Ther 2003;83:1090–106.

65. Rubinstein SM, Van Tulder M. A best-evidence review of diagnostic procedures for neck and low-back pain. Best Pract Res Clin Rheumatol 2008;22:471–82.

66. Ryder M, Deyle GD. Differential diagnosis of fibular pain in a patient with a history of breast cancer. J Orthop Sports Phys Ther 2009;39:230.

67. Sartoris D. Musculoskeletal imaging, the requisites. Philadelphia: Mosby; 1996.

68. Seaberg DC, Yealy DM, Lukens T, et al. Multicenter comparison of two clinical decision rules for the use of radiography in acute, high-risk knee injuries. Ann Emerg Med 1998;32:8–13.

69. Segal RL. Use of imaging to assess normal and adaptive muscle function. Phys Ther 2007;87:704–18.

70. Siivola SM, Levoska S, Tervonen O, et al. MRI changes of cervical spine in asymptomatic and symptomatic young adults. Eur Spine J 2002;11:358–63.

71. Silva LE, Valim V, Pessanha AP, et al. Hydrotherapy versus conventional land-based exercise for the management of patients with osteoarthritis of the knee: a randomized clinical trial. Phys Ther 2008;88:12–21.

72. Slipman CW, Plastaras C, Patel R, et al. Provocative cervical discography symptom mapping. Spine J 2005;5:381–8.

73. Smith AS, Blaser SI. Infectious and inflammatory processes of the spine. Radiol Clin North Am 1991;29:809–27.

74. Smith AS, Blaser SI. MR of infectious and inflammatory diseases of the spine. Crit Rev Diagn Imaging 1991;32:165–89.

75. Stadnik TW, Lee RR, Coen HL, et al. Annular tears and disk herniation: prevalence and contrast enhancement on mr images in the absence of low back pain or sciatica. Radiology 1998;206:49–55.

76. Staiger TO, Paauw DS, Deyo RA, et al. Imaging studies for acute low back pain: when and when not to order them. Postgrad Med 1999;105:161–2, 165-66, 171–162.

77. Stiell IG. Clinical decision rules in the emergency department. Can Med Assoc J 2000;163:1465–6.

78. Stiell IG, Greenberg GH, McKnight RD, et al. Decision rules for the use of radiography in acute ankle injuries: refinement and prospective validation. JAMA 1993;269:1127–32.

79. Stiell IG, Greenberg GH, McKnight RD, et al. A study to develop clinical decision rules for the use of radiography in acute ankle injuries. Ann Emerg Med 1992;21:384–90.

80. Stiell IG, Greenberg GH, Wells GA, et al. Prospective validation of a decision rule for the use of radiography in acute knee injuries. JAMA 1996;275:611–5.

81. Stiell IG, McKnight RD, Greenberg GH, et al. Implementation of the Ottawa ankle rules. JAMA 1994;271:827–32.

82. Stiell IG, Wells GA, Hoag RH, et al. Implementation of the Ottawa knee rule for the use of radiography in acute knee injuries. JAMA 1997;278:2075–9.

83. Stillerman CB, Schneider JH, Gruen JP. Evaluation and management of spondylolysis and spondylolisthesis. Clin Neurosurg 1993;40:384–415.

84. Straus SR. Evidence-based medicine: how to practice and teach EBM. 3rd ed. Edinburgh: Elsevier; 2005.

85. Tallroth K, Lindholm TS. Stress radiographs in the evaluation of degenerative femorotibial joint disease. Skeletal Radiol 1987;16:617–20.

86. Tandeter HB, Shvartzman P. Acute knee injuries: use of decision rules for selective radiograph ordering. Am Fam Physician 1999;60:2599–608.

87. Tehranzadeh J, Andrews C, Wong E. Lumbar spine imaging: normal variants, imaging pitfalls, and artifacts. Radiol Clin North Am 2000;38:1207–53, v-vi.

88. Teyhen DS, Gill NW, Whittaker JL, et al. Rehabilitative ultrasound imaging of the abdominal muscles. J Orthop Sports Phys Ther 2007;37:450–66.

89. Thain LM, Adler RS. Sonography of the rotator cuff and biceps tendon: technique, normal anatomy, and pathology. J Clin Ultrasound 1999;27:446–58.

90. Van Holsbeeck MT, Kolowich PA, Eyler WR, et al. US depiction of partial-thickness tear of the rotator cuff. Radiology 1995;197:443–6.

91. Verstraete KL, Van Der Woude HJ, Hogendoorn PC, et al. Dynamic contrast-enhanced MR imaging of musculoskeletal tumors: basic principles and clinical applications. J Magn Reson Imaging 1996;6:311–21.

92. Whitman JM, Flynn TW, Childs JD, et al. A comparison between two physical therapy treatment programs for patients with lumbar spinal stenosis: a randomized clinical trial. Spine 2006;31:2541–9.

93. Yeh L, Kwak S, Kim YS, et al. Anterior labroligamentous structures of the glenohumeral joint: correlation of MR arthrography and anatomic dissection in cadavers. AJR Am J Roentgenol 1998;171:1229–36.

94. Zwas ST, Elkanovitch R, Frank G. Interpretation and classification of bone scintigraphic findings in stress fractures. J Nucl Med 1987;28:452–7.

SUGGESTED READINGS

Bullough PG. Orthopaedic pathology. 3rd ed. London: Mosby-Wolfe; 1997.

Greenspan A. Orthopaedic radiology. 3rd ed. Philadelphia: Lippincott Williams & Wilkins; 2000.

Kaplan P. Musculoskeletal MRI. Philadelphia: Saunders; 2001.

Keats T. Atlas of normal roentgen variants that may simulate disease. St Louis: Mosby; 2001.

Manaster BJ. Musculoskeletal imaging: the requisites. 2nd ed. Philadelphia: Mosby; 2002.

McKinnis LN. Fundamentals of musculoskeletal imaging, 3rd ed. Philadelphia: FA Davis; 2010.

Stoeller D. Magnetic resonance imaging in orthopaedics and sports medicine. Philadelphia: Lippincott Raven; 1997.

WEB RESOURCES

Approaches to differential diagnosis in musculoskeletal imaging, Michael L. Richardson, MD, University of Washington School of Medicine. http://www.rad.washington.edu/mskbook/.

CHORUS: Collaborative hypertext of radiology, Medical College of Wisconsin. http://chorus.rad.mcw.edu/.

Diagnostic imaging for the physical therapist, Darryl Hosford and Ken Hurd. http://www.ptcentral.com/radiology/.

Finding-the-path: a problem-based guide to diagnostic imaging strategies in the emergency room, Leyla Azmoun, MD, Piran Aliabadi MD, B. Leonard Holman, MD, Brigham and Women's Hospital, Harvard Medical School. http://brighamrad.harvard.edu/education/online/ftp/FTP.html.

Radiology teaching files on the Internet with musculoskeletal cases, Amilcare Gentili, MD, Society of Skeletal Radiology. http://www.gentili.net.

Standardized guidelines for reporting of musculoskeletal imaging studies, Lawrence Yao, MD, Amilcare Gentili, MD, UCLA Department of Radiological Sciences. http://www.radsci.ucla.edu:8000/ms/y1/.

Laboratory Tests and Values 15

Connie J. Kittleson, PT, DPT
Sandra Baatz, PT

Objectives

After reading this chapter, the reader will be able to:

1. Provide an overview of the role of laboratory tests and reported values in patient management.
2. Describe the clinical practice implications for the results of commonly used laboratory tests.
3. Describe the rehabilitation exercise precautions and contraindications associated with various laboratory values.
4. Describe the laboratory values associated with certain disease states and the associated clinical practice implications.
5. Describe testing standards and methods.
6. Describe clinical laboratory personnel and testing sites.

Numerous laboratory tests are used in the medical evaluation, diagnosis, and management of patients. The results of these tests can have profound implications for patients and their appropriateness for and tolerance of rehabilitation exercise. It is incumbent on physical therapists (PTs) across the continuum of care to understand laboratory tests, the normal values associated with these tests, and the physical therapy implications associated with abnormal values. The PT first must identify what laboratory test values would be important to know for the provision of physical therapy assessment and treatment of a patient. The PT then must be able to interpret the clinical importance of these results. Finally, the PT must be able to correlate this information with all other data and findings to make sound clinical judgments in providing care for the individual patient.

This chapter first discusses the clinical uses of laboratory tests and issues involved with testing. Most of the material presented in this chapter focuses on individual laboratory tests offered within subgroups of tests. Normal and abnormal values are discussed along with implications for the PT. Integration of laboratory tests into the clinical decision-making process is presented through case scenarios throughout the chapter. Laboratory personnel are discussed, including educational background and regulatory requirements. Finally, laboratory panels, shorthand notations, and cumulative case scenarios are presented. Information provided by the examination of body tissues and cells with histology and cytology is not within the scope of this discussion.

It is important to understand that the implications for physical therapy practice presented in this chapter are general guidelines, not rigid rules. Individual PTs may practice differently based on multiple factors, including educational background, clinical experiences, practice setting, and individual practice style.

PTs need to incorporate abnormal test results into the clinical decision-making process with consideration for facility-specific guidelines, physician-specific guidelines, and patient-specific information. Some facilities have adopted guidelines for physical therapy practice with regards to laboratory values. PTs practicing in such facilities need to understand the guidelines and communicate effectively with other members of the health care team when the guidelines do not seem to apply to a particular patient. Physicians may have standard guidelines for their patients, or they may write specific guidelines in a patient's chart (i.e., "Bed rest if INR >5.0"). Direct communication with the physician is required to modify any such guidelines.

Each patient's medical history and current status guide a PT's interpretation of clinical laboratory values as they relate to rehabilitation exercise. It is important to incorporate the patient's overall presentation, primary diagnosis, past medical history, comorbidities, laboratory value and vital sign trends, and results of prior physical examinations into the clinical decision-making process. The patient's presentation may include such things as level of alertness, anxiety, and presence of pain and other symptoms. When concerns arise, direct communication with the referring physician (or in the case of direct referrals, the patient's primary care physician) is indicated. Other members of the health care team, including laboratory personnel, all are valuable resources for understanding laboratory tests and values. See Table 15-1 for a description of laboratory personnel.[2]

This chapter also serves to dispel the myth that laboratory values are of concern to the practice of physical therapy only in the acute care setting. Patients across the continuum of care may have diseases or disorders that affect laboratory values. The prevalence of hypertension, chronic kidney disease, and diabetes is increasing (Box 15-1). A PT may encounter patients with these disorders in various levels of care. In addition, patients in any practice setting may be receiving medications that require routine laboratory tests. Individuals taking warfarin (Coumadin) have routine laboratory tests for international normalized ratio (INR) values, and individuals taking any of the various statin drugs have laboratory tests to assess liver function. Regardless of practice setting, the PT may have patients who have laboratory values that need to be followed because these values may affect clinical decisions in rehabilitation.

Access to laboratory test values is easiest in acute or critical care. Home care, inpatient intensive rehabilitation, subacute care, and long-term care are areas of care in which these data are fairly accessible. In the outpatient setting, accessing these data can be more difficult. If relationships are cultivated, however, the PT can use physicians' offices for obtaining this information.

TABLE 15-1

Individuals Involved in a Clinical Laboratory Setting

Role	Title	Benchmark Training	Certification
Laboratory scientist	Clinical Laboratory Scientist (CLS) or Medical Technologist (MT)	Bachelor's degree and completion of clinical laboratory scientist program	Certified by American Society for Clinical Pathology (ASCP) or National Credentialing Agency for Laboratory Personnel (NCA)
Laboratory technician	Clinical Laboratory Technician (CLT) or Medical Laboratory Technician (MLT)	Associate's degree and completion of clinical laboratory science technician program	Same as above
Phlebotomist		Completion of formal education program that includes clinical component in phlebotomy	None
Medical director	Usually a pathologist	Doctor of Medicine	Certification by American Board of Pathology

---

BOX 15-1

Prevalence of Hypertension, Chronic Kidney Disease, and Diabetes

A more recent study showed that high blood pressure and prehypertension are increasing in children and adolescents, with this increase lagging 10 years behind increases in obesity.[9] Analysis of data for U.S. adults 20 years or older showed an increase in the prevalence rate of chronic kidney disease from 10% (1988-1994) to 13.1% (1999-2004).[6] The prevalence of diabetes in the United States in 1999-2002 was 9.3% (19.3 million, 2002 U.S. population), of which 2.8% (5.8 million) was undiagnosed.[7] An additional 26% (54 million) of the population had impaired fasting glucose.[7] There are even professional athletes with diabetes.

Laboratory test values are accessible to PTs via electronic links in hospital systems. As the electronic health record becomes more prevalent, PTs must continue to insist on security clearance to access information related to laboratory test values.

Clinical Uses Of Laboratory Tests

Laboratory tests assist physicians in screening, diagnosing, and managing patient health and disease. Screening tests are usually relatively inexpensive, easily performed, and designed to discern the possibility of the presence of disease. Examples of screening tests commonly used today are prostate-specific antigen (PSA) to assess the possibility of prostate cancer and cholesterol level to assist in ascertaining cardiac disease risk. PSA is not specific for prostate cancer, but elevated levels may indicate the presence of cancer. Additional diagnostic work may need to be performed when PSA levels are elevated. Similarly, an elevated cholesterol level signifies the possibility of a lipid disorder or increased risk of coronary artery disease (CAD), signaling the need for additional diagnostic investigations.

Diagnostic tests are designed to be specific in the information they provide and are used to confirm a clinical impression or rule out a disease. Examples include tests for human immunodeficiency virus (HIV), thyroid function, and anemia.

Other laboratory tests are performed to assist the physician in managing the patient's condition. Drug assays help manage therapeutic drug levels to prevent toxicity and ensure efficacy. Liver function tests (LFTs) help monitor side effects of drugs

intended to reduce lipid levels. Some tests provide a prognostic guide; the prothrombin time test provides a guide regarding the anticoagulation effect of warfarin drugs.

Testing Standards

Quality clinical laboratory testing is performing the correct test on the right patient at the right time and producing accurate test results with the best outcome in the most cost-effective manner.[19] The practice of clinical laboratory science requires the development and implementation of a comprehensive quality management system that includes quality control and quality assurance of testing services. The system must also include competency assessment of personnel and continuous process improvement to maximize human resources.

Quality assurance in testing includes internal and external programs. Internal systems include the use of standards, calibrators, controls, and blind samples coupled with statistical analysis of the findings. External efforts include participation in proficiency testing programs, accreditation of laboratories, laboratory inspections, and compliance with Clinical Laboratory Improvement Amendments (CLIA) regulations.

Proficiency testing consists of periodic samples received as a subscription. The analytes in the sample are of unknown concentration. The job of the clinical laboratory is to assay the samples, report concentrations, and show proficiency in performance by reporting the correct results.

CLIA specifies quality standards for proficiency testing, patient test management, quality control, personnel qualifications, and quality assurance for laboratories performing tests of moderate to high complexity. Patient test management includes sample integrity and positive patient identification throughout the testing process.

Testing Considerations

The goal of laboratory testing is to provide the most accurate results possible. This goal can best be achieved through knowledge of and attention to factors that influence test results. These factors are categorized into three areas: preanalytic, analytic, and postanalytic. Many of the preanalytic factors are outside the

TABLE 15-2

Factors Influencing Test Results

Preanalytic Factors: Biologic and Methodologic	Analytic Factors	Postanalytic Factors
Appropriate test ordered	Instrument performance	Recording data
Patient status regarding nutrition, drugs, smoking, stress, sleep, posture	Reagent quality and status	Transmitting and storing data
Specimen collection, labeling, transport, preparation, storage	Standards, calibrators, controls	Providing interpretive information
	Analyst expertise	Clinician interpretation

TABLE 15-3

Testing Sites and Examples of Tests Performed at Each Site

Home	Point of Care	Physician Office	Centralized Laboratory
Blood glucose	Blood glucose	Blood glucose	Blood glucose
Pregnancy status	Electrolytes	Blood counts	Transfusion services
Urine protein	Clotting times	Streptococci detection	Therapeutic drug assays
Drug screens		Urinalysis	Toxicologic studies
Prothrombin times		Sedimentation rates	Enzyme assays

laboratory. An attempt is made to control these factors through the use of procedure manuals for health care team members regarding patient preparation, sample collection, and specimen transport for specific tests. Analytic factors relate to the actual analysis of samples and are addressed within the laboratory. Postanalytic factors occur after analysis is completed and are largely controlled by the use of computer applications and interpretation of results by clinicians (Table 15-2).

Testing Sites

Laboratory tests are performed in the home by patients, at the point of care, in physician office laboratories, and in centralized laboratories. Instruments and methods of detection have been designed specifically for use in different settings by operators with varying levels of expertise. The reliability of test results tends to increase with the use of moderately to highly complex methods, increased analyst expertise, and the use of quality assurance plans. Centralized laboratories have traditionally provided the highest level of reliability.

Home, point-of-care, and physician office tests provide greater access and shorter turnaround times. The challenge at these sites is to have methods that provide useful and reliable information. More recent advances in technology address many of these concerns. In addition, clinical laboratory personnel now commonly organize, implement, and oversee point-of-care quality programs in health care settings.

Table 15-3 lists examples of the tests performed at each site. Blood glucose levels may be performed at all sites of testing, but different methods of determining the glucose level are used at different sites.

Methods

Many test methods and detection systems are used in clinical laboratory assays. Methods that are selected for use in clinical laboratories depend on what has been researched and developed for possible use, technical information about the methods, and managerial aspects of the methods. Information about methods is collected from manufacturers, sales representatives, colleagues, scientific presentations, and scientific literature. The

managerial aspects for consideration are costs, including cost per test; test throughput; sample volume and type; personnel requirements, space, environment, and utility requirements. The technical aspects include the following:

- Analytic sensitivity—the smallest concentration that can be accurately measured
- Analytic specificity—the ability to measure only the analyte of interest
- Linear range—the concentration range over which the measured concentration is equal to the actual concentration
- Interfering substances as they relate to analytic specificity
- Estimates of imprecision and inaccuracy

When a method for a specific assay is selected and implemented, it is continuously monitored by the quality assurance program.[4]

Reported Values and Interpretation

Each laboratory test ordered by a physician and performed by the laboratory is reported and becomes a part of the medical record for the given patient. The report identifies the patient, the test, the findings of the test, and information to use in the interpretation of the test findings. Test findings are most often quantities. In the United States, mass per unit volume, expressed in milligrams per deciliter (mg/dL), is the typical expression of quantity. Much of the rest of the world uses Systeme Internationale (SI) units, or moles per unit volume (the gram molecular weight of a substance per liter of solution). Mass per mole varies with the gram molecular weight of the analyte, making conversion from one system to the other cumbersome. Some test results are expressed in units of activity per unit of volume.

The interpretation of laboratory test results is a comparative decision-making process. The results of a test for a given patient are compared with a reference range to make a medical diagnosis, manage therapy, or provide other physiologic assessment.[25] The reference range is the interval between and including the lower and upper reference limits. The interval is determined statistically by the assay of the analyte of interest in a selected population. The range reflects the selected population only. The traditional reference range for quantitative tests is the range of values of the central 95% of the healthy population.

HEMATOLOGY

Procedure:	WBC	HBG	HCT	PLT	MPV	RBC
Units:	K/UL	GM/DL	%	K/UL	M/UL	M/UL
Ref. range:	(4.0-10.0)	(12.0-16.0)	(36.0-48.0)	(150-400)	(9.0-13.0)	(4.00-5.30)
1/21/09 2152	13.5 H	13.0	39.4	265	11.0	4.40
1/22/09 0715	12.2 H	11.6 L	34.4 L	248	10.8	3.76 L
1/23/09 0525	9.9	10.7 L	32.1 L	234	11.1	3.54 L

Indices data

Procedure:	MCV	MCH	MCHC	RDW
Units:	FL	PG	GM/L	FL
Ref. range:	(79.0-99.0)	(26.0-34.0)	(32.0-36.0)	(38.0-50.0)
1/21/09 2152	89.5	29.5	33.0	44.9
1/22/09 0715	91.5	30.9	33.7	45.0
1/23/09 0525	90.7	30.2	33.3	44.3

FIGURE 15-1 Example of partial laboratory report.

Reference ranges are commonly established for adult populations but also are studied for patients by age, by gender, and in specific populations (e.g., hemoglobin variants in individuals of Mediterranean descent). All reference ranges reported in this chapter are for the healthy population. These are generally not applicable to other patient populations and may vary by laboratory method.

When physicians, PTs, or other members of the health care team see laboratory results as a part of a patient's medical record, they see the result of the test and the reference range appropriate for the age and sex of the patient, the methods used, and any other considerations essential to help make an interpretation in light of the patient's history and physical findings.

A partial laboratory report is shown in Figure 15-1. Reports vary greatly from laboratory to laboratory. References ranges may or may not be included in the report. When included, reference ranges are reported in the same units as the test result and vary depending on the method used. There can be multiple reference ranges for the same analyte because there are multiple methods to assay the same analyte. With experience, clinicians develop a working knowledge of commonly assayed analytes and their reference ranges. Because of reference range variations caused by methods used, it is important to note the reference range information that accompanies test results, however. A caution to this interpretive information is in order: A given specimen from a healthy individual is unlikely to have all analytes within the reference range. Laboratory test findings need clinical correlates to substantiate their significance.[30] Today, some reference limits may be based on the risk of disease as determined from outcome studies.[10] Cholesterol reference limits are an example of the application of outcome studies. In addition, reference ranges are specific to the sex and age of the population. Other considerations reported may include ethnic origin, pregnancy, height, weight, body surface area, nutritional status, time of day, time of last drug dose and type of drug administered, time of last meal, and smoking status.

Laboratory reports may also differ with regard to the identification of abnormal results. These results may be flagged as seen in Figure 15-1, where an *H* next to a result indicates an abnormally high value, and an *L* indicates an abnormally low value. Other characters, such as an asterisk (*), may be used to identify abnormal values.

Additional statistical concepts related to test interpretation are sensitivity, specificity, and predictive value. There is overlap between test results in healthy and unhealthy individuals. Evaluating the test results in terms of sensitivity, specificity, and the likelihood of disease is a pragmatic approach in discerning overlap. Sensitivity is the ability of a test to detect disease; results are positive when the disease is present. Specificity is the ability of a test to give normal results in patients without a particular disease. The mathematical likelihood that a test result correctly identifies a patient as normal or abnormal is the predictive value.[10]

Other interpretive assistance is available. Laboratories may add statements to test reports that are interpretive or that provide considerations for interpretation. Flowcharts and pathways exist for reference. Centralized laboratories may offer online reporting of current and past test results. Some services provide secure electronic clinical laboratory reporting systems for physicians. Such laboratory services focus on providing patient-centered diagnostic testing.

Critical Values for Laboratory Tests

Critical values for laboratory tests indicate the need for an immediate medical interpretation. What constitutes a critical value is often established by consensus of the medical staff of critical care and emergency care units of hospitals and may be related to specific medical conditions. When a critical value is identified in the clinical laboratory, the laboratory should immediately contact the ordering provider or patient care area with the test results.

Common Laboratory Tests and Implications for Physical Therapy

For the purposes of facilitating learning, laboratory tests have been categorized into the following subgroups:

- Cellular components
- Fluid and electrolyte balance
- Kidney function
- Carbohydrate metabolism
- Acid-base balance
- Hemostasis
- Cardiac status
- Inflammatory markers
- Cardiovascular disease risk
- Hepatic function
- Miscellaneous tests

Cellular Components

Cellular components are often ordered as a panel (see Tables 15-4 and 15-19) known as the *complete blood count* (CBC). Table 15-4 presents normal values for cellular components.

HEMOGLOBIN. Hemoglobin is the red, iron-based, oxygen-carrying pigment of the erythrocyte, or red blood cell (RBC). Erythrocytes are made in the bone marrow. Hemoglobin concentration measures the total amount of hemoglobin in the peripheral blood and is a reflection of the number of RBCs in the blood. Hemoglobin composes approximately one third of each RBC. Because oxygen binds to hemoglobin, oxygen saturation as measured by pulse oximetry (SaO_2) is a measure of the percentage of hemoglobin binding sites that are occupied by oxygen molecules. Normal SaO_2 is 95% or more. Individuals are considered to be hypoxemic when SpO_2 is less than 90%. Oxygen saturation is discussed in detail in the section on acid-base balance considering arterial blood gases.

Hemoglobin levels can be increased in various physiologic and pathophysiologic states (see Table 15-4). People living at higher altitudes normally have a higher hemoglobin compared with people living at lower elevations because of physiologic polycythemia, in which the body produces more RBCs. This condition can also occur in a pathologic condition known as *polycythemia vera*, in which there is an excess of RBCs produced by the bone marrow. Hemoconcentration also increases hemoglobin values; this occurs in individuals who are significantly dehydrated or volume depleted. Hemoglobin values return to baseline when fluid hemostasis is achieved. In addition, in patients who are early in the course of disease states such as congestive heart failure (CHF) and chronic obstructive pulmonary disease (COPD), the body attempts to build more binding sites for oxygen to use, and hemoglobin values may be elevated.

Hemoglobin values can also be decreased in various physiologic and pathophysiologic states (see Table 15-4). Values may be decreased because of dilutional effects, such as by taking in (orally or intravenously) or retaining excess fluid that is held within the vasculature. Hemoglobin values are artificially decreased in these individuals and returns to the patient's baseline when fluid hemostasis is achieved. Cirrhosis can cause decreased hemoglobin because of RBC destruction in the liver. Patients with sickle cell anemia also have decreased hemoglobin because of abnormal RBCs. Women who are pregnant may have decreased hemoglobin because of increased blood volume. Patients with severe burns may have decreased hemoglobin because of bone marrow stress and blood loss. Patients with various cancers may have decreased hemoglobin levels because of the pathologic process itself or as a consequence of treatment. Patients with systemic lupus erythematosus can have low hemoglobin levels because of an abnormal immune response leading to hemolytic anemia.

Various anemias also lead to decreased hemoglobin values, including iron deficiency anemia and anemias secondary to vitamin B_{12} and folate deficiencies, all of which cause decreased RBC production. Anemias may also be due to RBC destruction or blood loss. If the workup for anemia is negative for a causative factor, and the patient has multiple medical problems, it is assumed to be anemia of chronic disease.

Physical Therapy Implications for Hemoglobin Values. When the hemoglobin value is known, the PT needs to determine whether the intended physical therapy intervention for the patient is appropriate. Remembering that this information is not taken in isolation from all of the other data obtained regarding the patient, there are some general guidelines to consider.

The most important thing to consider is the patient's oxygen supply versus demand. If oxygen supply is diminished because of decreased hemoglobin levels (fewer binding sites for oxygen to be carried to the tissue level), one can expect that endurance would be low. Depending on the hemoglobin trends for the patient, low hemoglobin levels may be tolerated well at rest and with activity. If the low hemoglobin levels are acute or below levels that the patient can compensate for, symptoms of low oxygen supply to the tissue occur, however. When considering symptoms, the PT must think of the major organs first: the brain, heart, and kidneys. These organs are the most susceptible to relative low oxygen supply, or *hypoxia*. Signs and symptoms of low oxygen supply to the brain include dizziness, lightheadedness, presyncope and syncope, symptoms of transient ischemic attack or cerebrovascular accident (CVA), and seizure. Signs and symptoms of cardiac hypoxia include any and all anginal symptoms, myocardial infarction (MI), sudden and slow onset of CHF, and arrhythmias. Signs and symptoms of low oxygen supply to the kidney include low urine output, increased creatinine and blood urea nitrogen (BUN), and potential fluid retention. For these reasons, some physicians believe that patients with active underlying cerebrovascular, cardiac, and renal disease should be closely monitored when hemoglobin is less than 9 g/dL.

The PT can expect lower endurance levels when hemoglobin levels decrease acutely to less than 10 g/dL. Monitoring of tolerance and potential alteration in the therapeutic plan may be indicated. When hemoglobin levels are greater than 10 g/dL, resistive exercise should be tolerated well from a hemodynamic standpoint. In an acute postoperative patient, hemoglobin levels and blood volume levels may be compromised, causing decreased tolerance to activity. Monitoring of orthostatic blood pressure and pulse is indicated on initial assessment at least. Traditionally, a decrease in systolic blood pressure more than 20 mm Hg with a corresponding increase in heart rate defines a positive orthostatic decrease. The PT must compare the data

TABLE 15-4

Tests for Cellular Components (Complete Blood Count)

Laboratory Test (units)	Related Physiology	Normal Values	Increased in	Decreased in
Hemoglobin (Hgb) (g/dL)	Iron-based, oxygen-carrying pigment of RBC	Adults	Congenital heart disease	Anemia
		Men: 14-18	Polycythemia vera	Hemorrhage
		Women: 12-16	Dehydration/ hemoconcentration	Hemolysis
		Pregnant women: >11	COPD	Hemoglobinopathy
		Elderly: values are slightly decreased	CHF	Nutritional deficiency
		Children	High altitude	Lymphoma
		Newborn: 14-24	Severe burns	SLE
		0-2 wk: 12-20		Sarcoidosis
		2-6 mo: 10-17		Kidney disease
		6 mo–6 yr: 9.5-14		Splenomegaly
		6-18 yr: 10-15.5		Neoplasia
		Possible critical values: <5 or >20		
Hematocrit (Hct) (%)	Measure of ratio of RBCs to whole blood volume	Adults	Congenital heart disease	Anemia
		Men: 42-52	Polycythemia vera	Hyperthyroidism
		Women: 37-47	Severe dehydration	Cirrhosis
		Pregnant women: >33	Erythrocytosis	Hemolytic reaction
		Elderly: values may be slightly decreased	Eclampsia	Hemorrhage
		Children	Burns	Dietary deficiency
		Newborn: 44-64	COPD	Bone marrow failure
		2-8 wk: 39-59		Normal pregnancy
		2-6 mo: 35-50		Rheumatoid arthritis
		6 mo–1 yr: 29-43		Multiple myeloma
		1-6 yr: 30-40		Leukemia
		6-18 yr: 32-44		Hemoglobinopathy
		Possible critical values: <15 or >60		
Red blood cell (RBC) count ($RBC \times 10^6/\mu L$ or $RBC \times 10^{12}/L$ [SI units])	Produced in bone marrow; responsible for transport of oxygen to tissues and carbon dioxide from tissues	Adult/elderly	High altitude	Hemorrhage
		Men: 4.7-6.1	Congenital heart disease	Hemolysis
		Women: 4.2-5.4	Polycythemia vera	Anemia
		Newborn: 4.8-7.1	Dehydration/ hemoconcentration	Hemoglobinopathy
		2-8 wk: 4-60	Cor pulmonale	Advanced cancer
		2-6 mo: 3.5-5.5	Pulmonary fibrosis	Bone marrow fibrosis
		6 mo–1 yr: 3.5-5.2	Thalassemia	Leukemia
		1-6 yr: 4-5.5		Antineoplastic chemotherapy
		6-18 yr: 4-5.5		Chronic illness
				Renal failure
				Overhydration
				Multiple myeloma
				Pernicious anemia
				Rheumatoid disease
				Subacute endocarditis
				Pregnancy

USED TO CATEGORIZE ANEMIAS BY SIZE AND HEMOGLOBIN CONCENTRATION OF RBCs

Laboratory Test (units)	Related Physiology	Normal Values	Increased in	Decreased in
Mean corpuscular volume (MCV) (μm^3)	Average volume (size) of single RBC	Adults/elderly/children: 80-95	Liver disease	Iron deficiency anemia
		Newborn: 96-108	Antimetabolite therapy	Thalassemia
			Alcoholism	Anemia caused by chronic illness
			Pernicious anemia (vitamin B_{12} deficiency)	
			Folic acid deficiency	

TABLE 15-4

Tests for Cellular Components (Complete Blood Count)—cont'd

Laboratory Test (units)	Related Physiology	Normal Values	Increased in	Decreased in
Mean corpuscular hemoglobin (MCH) (pg)	Average amount of hemoglobin in RBC (weight)	Adults/elderly/children: 27-31	Macrocytic anemia	Microcytic anemia
		Newborn: 32-34		Hypochromic anemia
Mean corpuscular hemoglobin concentration (MCHC) (g/dL)	Average concentration of hemoglobin in single RBC	Adults/elderly/children: 32-36	Spherocytosis	Iron deficiency anemia
		Newborn: 32-33	Intravascular hemorrhage Cold agglutinins	Thalassemia
White blood cell (WBC) count (per mm^3)	Produced in bone marrow; provide defense against foreign agents/organisms	Adults/children >2 yr: 5000-10,000	Infection	Drug toxicity
		Children ≤2 yr: 6200-17,000 Newborns: 9000-30,000	Leukemic neoplasia Trauma	Bone marrow failure Overwhelming infections
		Possible critical values: <2500 or >30,000	Stress	Dietary deficiency
			Tissue necrosis Inflammation	Autoimmune disease Bone marrow infiltration Congenital marrow aplasia
Platelet count (Plt) (per mm^3)	Primary function is to initiate clotting sequence; also cause local vasoconstriction and chemotaxis for fibroblasts, smooth muscle cells, and white cells	Adults/elderly: 150,000-400,000	Malignant disorder	Hypersplenism
		Premature infants: 100,000-300,000	Polycythemia vera	Hemorrhage
		Newborns: 150,000-300,000	Postsplenectomy syndrome	Immune thrombocytopenia
		Infants: 200,000-475,000	Rheumatoid arthritis	Leukemia and other myelofibrosis disorders
		Children: 150,000-400,000	Iron deficiency anemia	Thrombotic thrombocytopenia Inherited thrombocytopenia disorders DIC SLE Pernicious anemia Hemolytic anemia Cancer chemotherapy Infection

CHF, congestive heart failure; *COPD,* chronic obstructive pulmonary disease; *DIC,* disseminated intravascular coagulopathy; *SLE,* systemic lupus erythematosus.

from orthostatic checks with other data to determine the efficacy of therapy. Baseline blood pressures must be considered in this decision-making process.

More recent research suggests that transfusion of packed red blood cells (PRBCs) is not indicated for most patients with a hemoglobin greater than 7 g/dL.[18,23] There are situations in which transfusion beyond this level is indicated. It may be disconcerting for the PT to work with patients with significantly low hemoglobin levels. However, one must look at the entire clinical picture in making decisions regarding therapy treatment.

HEMATOCRIT. Hematocrit is a measure of the ratio of PRBC volume to whole blood volume. It is represented as a percentile and is usually approximately three times the value of hemoglobin. Similar to hemoglobin, hematocrit levels vary based on gender. The pathologic conditions that increase or decrease hematocrit levels are the same as the conditions for hemoglobin and are not repeated here.

Physical Therapy Implications for Hematocrit Values. Traditional thought has been that light exercise is permitted with hematocrit levels greater than 25%, and resistive exercise is permitted with hematocrit levels greater than 30%. Exercise often can be and is appropriate at much lower levels, however. Comorbidities are a large factor in determining what level of therapy is appropriate and what precautions should be taken. Drugs such as erythropoietin can be used in some anemias to stimulate bone marrow production of RBCs. Clinical scenarios involving hemoglobin and hematocrit follow.

CLINICAL SCENARIO: HEMOGLOBIN/HEMATOCRIT

SETTING

Inpatient hospital—acute care

REFERRAL

Evaluate and treat for functional mobility

DIAGNOSIS

Right total hip replacement

PAST MEDICAL HISTORY

A history of osteoarthritis and CAD in a 62-year-old woman

PHYSICAL THERAPY MANAGEMENT

The patient was evaluated on postoperative day (POD) #0 and tolerated standing at bedside and initiation of an exercise program. On POD #1, the PT performed a chart review, including review of the most recent laboratory values, which showed the patient's hemoglobin/hematocrit to be 8.2 g/dL/24.7%. The PT decided to proceed with the treatment with caution and to monitor the patient for orthostatic hypotension.

In supine, the patient appeared pale but denied any lightheadedness. Vital sign testing revealed her blood pressure to be 112/65 mm Hg with a heart rate of 102 beats/min. The patient was able to move from supine to sit with moderate assistance and denied any lightheadedness with this positional change. After 2 minutes of sitting, vital sign testing revealed a decrease in blood pressure to 89/52 mm Hg with a heart rate of 122 beats/min. The patient denied any lightheadedness or dizziness but did complain of nausea. The PT determined that the patient displayed orthostatic hypotension (>20–mm Hg decrease in systolic blood pressure) and returned the patient to supine, providing moderate assistance. The PT continued to instruct the patient in exercises, while closely monitoring her blood pressure. At the end of the session, the PT notified the nursing staff of the patient's response to positional change and documented all findings including vital signs.

In the afternoon of the same day, the patient displayed a similar response to positional change, experiencing symptoms related to her orthostatic hypotension. The PT again documented these findings and discussed them with the medical team. Despite a hemoglobin level greater than 7g/dL, the physician decided to have 2 U of PRBCs transfused, elevating the patient's hemoglobin/hematocrit to 10 g/dL/30.2%. On POD #2, the patient tolerated physical therapy interventions, including transfers and ambulation, without signs or symptoms of orthostatic hypotension.

DISCUSSION

If the PT had not monitored the patient's blood pressure in this scenario, the patient may not have become symptomatic until she had already transferred to a bedside chair or possibly until she had walked with assistance away from the bed. Under those circumstances, the transition back to supine would take longer and the patient could possibly lose consciousness. Although a hemoglobin value of 8.2 g/dL does not always indicate the need for transfusion, the PT's documentation and communication with the medical team factored into the physician's decision to transfuse, which enabled the patient to participate in functional mobility more quickly and discharge per the clinical pathway outcome.

CLINICAL SCENARIO: HEMOGLOBIN/HEMATOCRIT

SETTING

Inpatient hospital—acute care

REFERRAL

Evaluate and treat for functional mobility

DIAGNOSIS

Multiple sclerosis exacerbation

PAST MEDICAL HISTORY

A history of multiple sclerosis and idiopathic pancytopenia in a 47-year-old woman

PHYSICAL THERAPY MANAGEMENT

On initial review of the patient's chart, the PT noted that the patient's hemoglobin/hematocrit was 6.7 g/dL/20.2% and that there was a physician's order for transfusion of 2 U of PRBCs. The PT confirmed with the nursing staff that the patient had not yet received the PRBCs, and the decision was made to postpone the evaluation until the following day.

DISCUSSION

If the PT had not looked at the patient's laboratory values, he or she may not have understood why the physician ordered a transfusion.

CONTINUED PHYSICAL THERAPY MANAGEMENT

The next day, the PT returned to find that the transfusion initially increased the patient's hemoglobin/hematocrit levels to 8.1 g/dL/24%, but the values decreased again to 6.9 g/dL/21.1%. The PT discussed the case with the nursing staff, who related that the physician was aware of the patient's current laboratory values and that there were no new orders to transfuse the patient. Because of the patient's pancytopenia, historically transfusions have elevated her hemoglobin/hematocrit only temporarily. Given the patient's lack of any cerebrovascular, cardiac, or renal disease, the PT decided to proceed cautiously, monitoring vital signs throughout the evaluation. The patient was able to tolerate a functional evaluation, including bed mobility, transfers, and ambulation 150 feet, without adverse signs or symptoms.

DISCUSSION

Although a hemoglobin value of 6.9 g/dL generally indicates that physical therapy evaluation and interventions should be postponed, this patient's laboratory values were interpreted with consideration for what was normal for her. Because of her history of pancytopenia, she was able to tolerate

TABLE 15-5

Classification of Anemias

Type of Anemia	Red Blood Cell Morphology	Examples/Causes
Normocytic, normochromic anemia	Normal size, normal color*	Iron deficiency (detected early), chronic illness, acute blood loss, aplastic anemia, acquired hemolytic anemia
Microcytic, normochromic anemia	Small size, normal color*	Renal disease
Microcytic, hypochromic anemia	Small size, decreased color[†]	Iron deficiency (detected late), thalassemia, lead poisoning
Macrocytic, normochromic anemia	Large size, normal color*	Vitamin B_{12} or folic acid deficiency, hydantoin ingestion, chemotherapy, some myelodysplastic syndromes, myeloid leukemia, ethanol toxicity, thyroid dysfunction

*Normal color = normal hemoglobin content.
[†]Decreased color = decreased hemoglobin content.
From Pagana KD, Pagana TJ: *Mosby's diagnostic and laboratory test reference,* 9th ed, St Louis, 2009, Mosby.

---

much lower hemoglobin/hematocrit values than the general population. If the PT had postponed the evaluation until the patient's laboratory values returned to normal, the patient likely would never have received physical therapy intervention.

RED BLOOD CELL COUNT. The RBC count is the pure number of RBCs in 1 µL of blood. Within the RBC are molecules of hemoglobin that allow transport and exchange of oxygen to the tissues and carbon dioxide from the tissues.[26] This value is rarely used in physical therapy as a clinical indicator of appropriateness of rehabilitation exercise because hemoglobin and hematocrit can be ordered separately and are more widely used in making clinical decisions. Because the RBC count actually looks at how many RBCs are in the whole blood, hemoglobin and hematocrit are critically linked to this value.

RED BLOOD CELL INDICES. RBC indices are used by physicians to diagnose and classify types of anemia. The mean corpuscular volume describes RBCs in terms of size and classifies macrocytic, normocytic, and microcytic anemias. Mean corpuscular hemoglobin and mean corpuscular hemoglobin concentration detect hypochromic or normochromic anemias. These indices are not significant in therapy intervention, but it is helpful for the PT to be familiar with the tests to know whether the information is critical for making decisions. Table 15-5 provides a description of various anemias.

WHITE BLOOD CELL COUNT. The white blood cell (WBC) count is the measure of mature and immature WBCs in 1 µL of blood. In general, WBCs increase with infection, inflammation, or tissue damage; this is called *leukocytosis.* Specific pathologic causes of leukocytosis are parasitic or bacterial infection, inflammation or necrosis of tissue, some blood-borne cancers, allergic reactions, and acute hemorrhage.

The WBC count may also be abnormally low—a condition called *leukopenia.* Leukopenia occurs in some viral infections, some blood-borne cancers (leukemias and lymphomas), or with bone marrow suppression (chemotherapy, radiation, HIV/acquired immunodeficiency syndrome [AIDS], and post–bone marrow transplant). Leukopenia may also be seen late in the course of alcoholism and diabetes mellitus.

Physical Therapy Implications for White Blood Cell Count Values. Leukocytosis, in the presence of infection, is a relative issue for the PT. One must consider the patient's overall medical condition

with the infection in determining efficacy of treatment. In the presence of sepsis or septicemia, more caution is in order. If there is hemodynamic compromise, therapy may be contraindicated until the infection is controlled.

There may be more specific precautions for a leukopenic patient, especially with an absolute neutrophil count that is extremely low—*neutropenia.* Usually, when the patient has a WBC count of less than 5000/mm³ and has a fever greater than 100° F, exercise may be contraindicated. This precaution is patient and physician specific, however. If the patient has an absolute neutrophil count of less than 1000/mm³, the patient may be in "reverse isolation" or in "neutropenic precautions" to protect the patient from risk of infection. In this patient population, following the isolation precautions, particularly in regard to hand washing, is crucial. A clinical scenario involving WBC count follows.

CLINICAL SCENARIO: WHITE BLOOD CELL COUNT

SETTING

Inpatient acute

REFERRAL

Evaluate and treat for functional mobility

DIAGNOSIS

Pneumonia, acute renal failure, sepsis, weakness, frequent falls

PAST MEDICAL HISTORY

A history of hypertension, CAD, diabetes mellitus, and COPD in a 74-year-old woman

PHYSICAL THERAPY MANAGEMENT

On review of the patient's medical record, the PT noted her WBC count to be 22,000. The patient's temperature taken approximately 30 minutes previously was 102.7° F. The PT decided to postpone the physical therapy evaluation at this time.

DISCUSSION

The PT's decision to postpone the physical therapy evaluation was not based solely on an elevated WBC count. That finding alone was not surprising considering the patient's diagnoses of pneumonia and sepsis. There

is no specific contraindication to rehabilitation exercise based on a specific number given an elevated WBC count. The PT's decision to postpone the evaluation included consideration of the presence of multiple comorbidities including sepsis and the fact that the patient's temperature was elevated. Exercise can elevate body temperature. Also, fever can increase a patient's metabolic rate. Such patients may experience fever-related fatigue or rigors or both.

WHITE BLOOD CELL DIFFERENTIAL. Physicians can order a WBC differential to be performed automatically as part of the CBC if the WBC count is elevated or can order this test separately as "WBC count with differential." This test identifies and counts the different types of WBCs. Although this test is not of great importance to the PT, it helps to understand what the physician may be looking for with an individual patient. There are two main types of WBCs: granulocytes and agranulocytes. Granulocytes include basophils, eosinophils, and neutrophils. Agranulocytes include lymphocytes (T and B cells) and monocytes. Usually the total WBC count is distributed as follows: neutrophils (55% to 77%), lymphocytes (20% to 40%), monocytes (2% to 8%), eosinophils (1% to 4%), and basophils (0.5% to 1%).[26]

Polymorphonuclear neutrophils are important in fighting bacterial infections. Mature neutrophils are "segs," whereas "bands" are immature neutrophils that may be called up from the bone marrow to help fight severe infections. If a patient has what is termed a *left shift,* there has been increased production of immature neutrophils, and the patient has either a severe or an acute bacterial infection. This information would indicate to the PT that the patient is more acutely ill. This and other information would assist the PT in determining the efficacy of treatment.

Eosinophils are elevated with allergic or parasitic infections. Basophils are increased with parasitic infections and hypersensitivity or allergic reactions. This is part of a cascade in allergic reactions with the release of histamine, which causes vasodilation and bronchoconstriction. Physical therapy would not be indicated in acute, severe allergic reactions because of this response.

B-cell lymphocytes are important in humoral immunity because they produce antibodies. T-cell lymphocytes are also called *killer T cells* and are important in cell-mediated immunity. They also respond to viral infection.

Monocytes are increased whenever the body has identified something as foreign and has mounted an inflammatory response. Monocytes clean up debris from this response. The most common monocyte is the macrophage.

PLATELETS. The platelet count is a count of the number of platelets or thrombocytes per cubic milliliter of blood.[26] Platelets are structures formed in megakaryocytes and released from their cytoplasm. The primary function of platelets is to initiate the clotting sequence. They also cause local vasoconstriction and chemotaxis for fibroblasts, smooth muscle cells, and WBCs.

Increased values of platelets, or *thrombocytosis,* can be seen pathologically in myeloproliferative diseases, collagen disorders, chronic pancreatitis, and acute infections. Decreased platelets,

or *thrombocytopenia,* can be pathologically seen in some cancers (lymphomas and leukemias), postchemotherapy, pancytopenia from various causes, idiopathic thrombocytopenia purpura, and a serious condition seen in critical care called *disseminated intravascular coagulopathy.*

Physical Therapy Implications for Platelet Values. Resistive exercise can continue until platelets are less than 50,000. Discussion with the physician should occur before therapy when platelet counts are less than 20,000 because spontaneous bleeding is a serious danger.[26] The PT must be cautious with handling patients who have low platelet counts to avoid bruising. Spontaneous bleeding rarely occurs with a platelet count greater than 40,000, but prolonged bleeding from surgery or trauma may occur.[26] A clinical scenario involving platelets follows.

CLINICAL SCENARIO: PLATELETS

SETTING

Home care

REFERRAL

Evaluate and treat for range of motion, strengthening, mobility, and home safety

DIAGNOSIS

COPD exacerbation, weakness

PAST MEDICAL HISTORY

A history of COPD and idiopathic thrombocytopenia purpura in a 63-year-old man

PHYSICAL THERAPY MANAGEMENT

The PT had available the patient's most recent hemogram indicating a platelet count of 88,000 (reference range 150,000 to 400,000). The PT proceeded with the patient's evaluation with particular attention paid to removing obstacles throughout the home.

DISCUSSION

This patient's low platelet count was appropriate given his history of idiopathic thrombocytopenia purpura. Although this is likely his baseline for platelet count and not a contraindication to proceeding with rehabilitation, his thrombocytopenia places him at increased risk of bleeding. Falls or bumping into obstacles can result in significant bruising or bleeding.

SUMMARY STATEMENTS FOR COMPLETE BLOOD COUNT VALUES. Guidelines for therapy precautions with CBC values vary depending on the setting in which the PT practices. CBC results should never be taken in isolation in clinical decision making regarding physical therapy intervention. Some subsets of patients may show bone marrow suppression as a result of medications (i.e., chemotherapy and various medications used to treat autoimmune disorders). The clinical result is a relative pancytopenia, which includes anemia, thrombocytopenia, and leukopenia. In patients receiving chemotherapy, the relative myelosuppression is more severe than in other drug regimens used to treat autoimmune disorders, with the lowest counts being at the nadir, which is usually 10 to 14 days postchemotherapy.

Fluid and Electrolyte Balance

Tests commonly used with the assessment of fluid and electrolyte balance include sodium, potassium, chloride, calcium, and carbon dioxide. Many of these electrolyte tests are often ordered as part of a panel (see Tables 15-6 and 15-19) known as the *basic metabolic panel* (BMP or PBM). The normal values for these analytes are listed in Table 15-6.

SODIUM. Sodium (Na^+) is the major extracellular cation, which serves to regulate serum osmolality, fluid, and acid-base balance. It influences blood volume and pressure through the retention or loss of interstitial fluid. Sodium also maintains the transmembrane electric potential for neuromuscular functioning. Abnormally elevated levels of sodium, *hypernatremia,* can be caused by various conditions, including increased dietary or intravenous intake of sodium, conditions that cause decreased sodium loss, or conditions that case excessive water loss. An excess of adrenocortical hormones, such as seen in Cushing's disease and Conn's syndrome (primary hyperaldosteronism), can cause hypernatremia through a decrease in the normal loss of sodium. Aldosterone is responsible for sodium retention and potassium excretion; excess aldosterone causes increased sodium retention and hypernatremia. Excessive water loss can cause a hemoconcentration effect and can be seen with excessive sweating, diabetes insipidus, extensive thermal burns, and antidiuretic hormone insufficiency.

Abnormally decreased levels of sodium, *hyponatremia,* can be the result of inadequate sodium intake, an increase in the loss of sodium, increased retention of water, and third spacing of fluids accompanied by sodium. The dilutional effect of increased water retention can be seen with excessive oral or intravenous water intake, chronic renal failure (CRF), and syndrome of inappropriate antidiuretic hormone secretion. Patients with CRF may be unable to excrete adequate amounts of free water, whereas patients with CHF may be hyponatremic because of the dilutional factor of increased circulating blood volume or because of the loss of sodium caused by diuretic management of CHF. In addition, levels may be decreased by excessive water loss accompanied by electrolyte loss (as seen with vomiting, suctioning, trauma, severe diarrhea, and diuretic therapy) or by excessive loss of sodium as seen in Addison's disease (adrenal gland insufficiency resulting in decreased aldosterone production).

Physical Therapy Implications for Sodium Values. The brain is very susceptible to fluid changes. Mental status changes may manifest when sodium values are abnormal. The PT should monitor for symptoms of low sodium levels, including weakness, confusion, stupor, hypotension, seizures, edema, and weight gain.[15]

POTASSIUM. Potassium (K^+) is the major intracellular cation responsible for maintaining hydration and osmotic pressure. It is critical for maintenance of the sodium-potassium pump needed for normal skeletal muscle contraction and relaxation and normal muscle activity of the heart, intestines, and respiratory tract. Abnormally elevated levels of potassium, *hyperkalemia,*

can be caused by excessive intake of potassium, conditions that alter kidney function, adrenal gland insufficiency, long-term heparin therapy (which causes suppression of aldosterone), lead poisoning, acidosis, and trauma such as crush injuries and burns. Abnormally decreased levels of potassium, *hypokalemia,* can be caused by increased intestinal or urinary losses of potassium as seen with prolonged vomiting or diarrhea, trauma, and medications such as steroids and potassium-wasting diuretics (i.e., thiazides and loop diuretics).

Physical Therapy Implications for Potassium Values. Potassium is critical for normal neuromuscular function. Hyperkalemia can result in electrocardiogram changes, irritability, nausea, and diarrhea. The myocardium is most susceptible to potassium abnormalities. Hypokalemia may result in cardiac dysrhythmias, dizziness, and hypotension.[15,26] Recent and current cardiac status should always be considered when making decisions regarding a patient's appropriateness for rehabilitation exercise. Cardiac status should also be monitored closely before, during, and after exercise. Caution should be taken with potassium levels less than 3.2 mmol/L or more than 5.1 mmol/L because of the risk for arrhythmia. Discussion with other members of the health care team may be indicated for the individual patient. Individuals with CRF may have chronically elevated levels of potassium and tolerate levels of 5.5 mmol/L.[12]

CHLORIDE. Chloride (Cl^-) is an extracellular cation that maintains the electrical neutrality of the extracellular fluid. Increased chloride levels, *hyperchloremia,* can be caused by dehydration, renal dysfunction, and hyperventilation. Decreased levels, *hypochloremia,* can be caused by dilutional factors as seen with overhydration and CHF. Hypochloremia may also be the result of excess loss of chloride such as with prolonged vomiting, gastrointestinal suctioning, and diuretic therapy.

Physical Therapy Implications for Chloride Values. There are no specific activity guidelines related to abnormal chloride levels. Detection of an electrolyte imbalance may lead to further testing.[15]

CALCIUM. Calcium (Ca^{++}) is a mineral that is important for the strength of teeth and bones. It is also critical for the regulation of neuromuscular activity because it is involved in the transmission of neural impulses and muscle contractility. Calcium also serves as a cofactor in enzyme reactions and in blood clotting. Elevated levels of circulating calcium, *hypercalcemia,* can be caused by such things as hyperparathyroidism, hyperthyroidism, adrenal insufficiency, tumors (especially tumors of bone), osteoporosis, immobility, multiple myeloma, and excess intake of calcium or vitamin D. Abnormally low levels of circulating calcium, *hypocalcemia,* can be caused by inadequate dietary intake of calcium, vitamin D deficiency, impaired absorption from the intestinal tract, severe infections or burns, renal failure, pancreatic insufficiency, hypoparathyroidism, and administration of enemas containing phosphate.

Physical Therapy Implications for Calcium Values. Individuals with hypocalcemia can develop tetany. Trousseau's sign and Chvostek's sign are two clinical indicators of latent tetany. Trousseau's sign is an induced carpal spasm seen when compression is applied to the upper arm (Figure 15-2). Clinically, a PT can check for a positive Trousseau's sign by inflating a

TABLE 15-6

Fluid and Electrolyte Tests

Laboratory Test (unit)	Related Physiology	Normal Values	Increased in	Decreased in
Sodium (Na$^+$) (mEq/L)	Major extracellular cation	Adults/elderly: 136-145 Children: 136-145 Infants: 134-150 Newborns: 134-144 *Possible critical values:* <120 or >160	Excessive intake Cushing's syndrome Hyperaldosteronism Excessive sweating Extensive thermal burns Diabetes insipidus Osmotic diuresis	Deficient intake Addison's disease Diarrhea Vomiting Diuretic administration Chronic renal insufficiency Overhydration CHF SIADH Osmotic dilution Ascites Peripheral edema Pleural effusion Intraluminal bowel loss

Potassium (K$^+$) (mEq/L)	Major intracellular cation	Adults/elderly: 3.5-4
		Children: 3.4-4.7
		Infants: 4.1-5.3
		Newborns: 3.9-5.9
		
		Possible critical values:
		Adults: <2.5 or >6.5
		Newborns: <2.5 or >8
			Excessive intake
			Acute/CRF
			Hypoaldosteronism
			Aldosterone-inhibiting
			  diuretics
			Crush injury to tissues
			Hemolysis
			Transfusion of hemolyzed
			  blood
			Infection
			Acidosis
			Dehydration
				Deficient intake
				Burns
				Gastrointestinal disorders
				Diuretics
				
				Hyperaldosteronism
				Cushing's syndrome
				Renal tubular acidosis
				
				Licorice ingestion
				Insulin administration
				Glucose administration
				Ascites
				Renal artery stenosis
				Cystic fibrosis
				Trauma
				Surgery

Chloride (Cl$^-$) (mEq/L)	Indicator of acid-base balance and hydration	Adults: 98-106
		
		Children: 90-110
		Newborns: 96-106
		
		Premature infants: 95-110
		Possible critical values:
		  <80 or >115
			Dehydration
			
			Renal tubular acidosis
			Excessive infusion of
			  normal saline
			Cushing's syndrome
			Eclampsia
			
			Multiple myeloma
			
			Kidney dysfunction
			Metabolic acidosis
			Hyperventilation
			Anemia
			Respiratory alkalosis
			Hyperparathyroidism
				Overhydration
				
				CHF
				SIADH
				
				Vomiting
				Chronic gastric suction
				
				Chronic respiratory
				  acidosis
				Salt-losing nephritis
				Addison's disease
				Burns
				Metabolic acidosis
				Diuretic therapy
				Hypokalemia
				Aldosteronism
				Respiratory acidosis

Calcium, total (Ca^{++}) (mg/dL)	Measure of parathyroid function and calcium metabolism	Adults: 9-10.5
		
		Elderly: values tend to
		  decrease
		Children >2 yr: 8.8-10.8
		
		Infants 10 days–2 yr: 9-10.6
			Hyperparathyroidism
			
			Nonparathyroid
			  PTH-producing tumor
			Metastatic tumor to bone
			
			Paget's disease of bone
				Hypoparathyroidism
				
				Renal failure
				
				Hyperphosphatemia
				  secondary to renal
				  disease
				Rickets

TABLE 15-6

Fluid and Electrolyte Tests—cont'd

Laboratory Test (unit)	Related Physiology	Normal Values	Increased in	Decreased in
Calcium, total (Ca⁺⁺) (mg/dL)—cont'd		Newborns <10 days: 7.6-10.4 *Possible critical values:* <6 or >13	Prolonged immobilization Milk-alkali syndrome Vitamin D intoxication Lymphoma Granulomatous infection Addison's disease Acromegaly Hyperthyroidism	Vitamin D deficiency Osteomalacia Malabsorption Pancreatitis Fat embolism Alkalosis Hypoalbuminemia

CHF, congestive heart failure; *CRF,* chronic renal failure; *PTH,* parathyroid hormone; *SIADH,* syndrome of inappropriate antidiuretic hormone secretion.

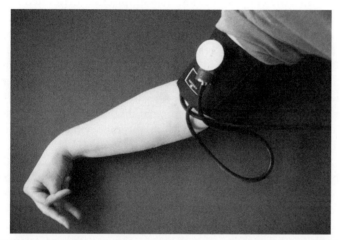

FIGURE 15-2 Trousseau's sign is a clinical indicator of latent tetany associated with hypocalcemia. This sign can be tested for by inflating a blood pressure cuff on the upper arm to a level between diastolic and systolic blood pressure and maintaining this inflation for 3 minutes. A positive test results in the carpal spasm shown here. (From Ignatavicius DD, Workman ML: *Medical-surgical nursing: critical thinking for collaborative care,* 5th ed, Philadelphia, 2006, Saunders.)

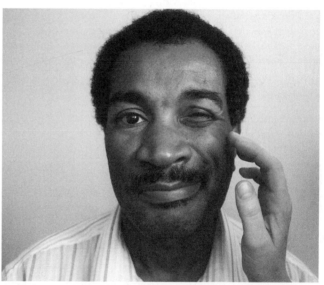

FIGURE 15-3 Chvostek's sign is another clinical indicator of latent tetany associated with hypocalcemia. This sign can be tested for by tapping the facial nerve above the mandibular angle, adjacent to the ear lobe. A facial muscle spasm that causes the person's eye and upper lip to twitch, as shown, is a positive sign. (From Ignatavicius DD, Workman ML: *Medical-surgical nursing: critical thinking for collaborative care,* 5th ed, Philadelphia, 2006, Saunders.)

blood pressure cuff placed around the arm to between systolic and diastolic blood pressure and maintaining the pressure for several minutes. Chvostek's sign is a unilateral contraction of the oris muscle (seen as a lip curl) induced by tapping of the facial nerve anterior to the external auditory canal (Figure 15-3).

SUMMARY OF CLINICAL MANIFESTATIONS OF FLUID AND ELECTRO-LYTE IMBALANCE. If intravascular volume is elevated, additional strain is placed on the heart, and the patient may experience acute CHF. In some cases, there may also be extravasation of fluid by osmotic pressure into the extracellular spaces, commonly referred to as *third spacing of fluid.* If blood volume is decreased, there may be a resultant decrease in blood pressure. The PT should monitor for orthostasis. The body's normal response to a decrease in blood pressure is a reflexive tachycardia. In addition, if blood volume is decreased, the patient may experience alterations in respiration, as well. A clinical scenario involving fluid and electrolyte imbalance follows.

CLINICAL SCENARIO: FLUID AND ELECTROLYTE IMBALANCE

SETTING

Inpatient acute care

REFERRAL

Evaluate and treat for functional mobility, deconditioning

DIAGNOSIS

Altered mental status

PAST MEDICAL HISTORY

A history of hypertension, degenerative joint disease, and osteoporosis in an 87-year-old woman. The patient lives alone and was independent with all functional activities before admission.

PHYSICAL THERAPY MANAGEMENT

On review of the patient's chart on day #1 of admission, the PT noted that the patient is reportedly confused and has bed alarms in place to prevent self-mobilization. She is receiving intravenous normal saline at 100 mL/hr. A computed tomography (CT) scan of the patient's head was negative for abnormalities. A review of laboratory values showed a sodium value of 112 mEq/L. The PT proceeded with a physical therapy evaluation, which revealed no functional focal deficits despite the patient's significant confusion and inability to follow directions well. The patient showed a need for physical therapy interventions for functional mobility related to safety. The PT documented all findings and developed a plan of care with concern for the patient's ability to return safely to living independently. On the second day of admission, the PT noted the patient's sodium value to have increased to 137 mEq/L. The patient was alert and oriented with no functional deficits or safety concerns. The PT again documented all findings and promptly notified the health care team of the patient's lack of need for physical therapy interventions.

DISCUSSION

In this scenario, the PT was able to attribute the patient's initial confusion and subsequent rapid return to cognitive baseline to her change in sodium values. Prompt discussion of findings with the health care team facilitated appropriate discharge planning and prevention of delivery of unnecessary services.

Kidney Function

Tests commonly used with the assessment of renal function include creatinine and BUN. These tests are often ordered as part of the basic metabolic panel (see Tables 15-7 and 15-9). The normal values for these analytes are listed in Table 15-7.

CREATININE. Creatinine is a waste product of muscle metabolism that is cleared by the kidneys. An individual's muscle mass is relatively constant, and an increase in serum creatinine is generally directly related to renal function. Creatinine levels are not affected by protein intake. Creatinine levels may be increased in the presence of renal disease, in which case the increase in serum creatinine directly correlates to the amount of nephron loss. Creatinine levels can be used as an approximation of glomerular filtration rate.[26] Increased creatinine levels can also be seen with acromegaly, muscle degeneration (as may be seen with extreme physical exercise, rhabdomyolysis, and increased corticosteroid dosage), and kidney impairment from drugs. Creatinine levels may be mildly elevated with dehydration. Creatinine levels may be decreased in the presence of decreased muscle mass as seen with debilitation, protein starvation, liver disease, and conditions such as muscular dystrophy and myasthenia gravis.

BLOOD UREA NITROGEN. BUN is an amino acid waste product of protein metabolism that is formed in the liver and excreted by the kidneys. BUN levels are affected by protein intake. Increased levels may indicate renal failure, increased protein intake or catabolism, severe burns, gastrointestinal bleeding, dehydration, starvation, and heart failure. Decreased BUN levels may indicate

hepatic damage or disease. Low BUN levels may also be seen with pregnancy, negative nitrogen balance (malnutrition or malabsorption), and overhydration.

BLOOD UREA NITROGEN/CREATININE RATIO. The BUN/creatinine ratio is used as an assessment of kidney and liver function. This ratio may be increased with dehydration, acute obstruction, and acute glomerulonephritis. Decreased ratio values may indicate the presence of severe skeletal muscle injury, liver disease, malnutrition, or renal dialysis. Patients with burns are especially likely to have elevated BUN levels.[12]

Physical Therapy Implications for Renal Function Indicators

Implications Related to Abnormal Values. In general, abnormal creatinine or BUN values do not contraindicate participation in rehabilitation exercise. In severe cases, however, the patient may be too lethargic or confused to participate in therapy. Understanding the cause of the abnormal values factors into the clinical decision-making process. If elevated creatinine/BUN levels result from dehydration, the patient may experience dizziness or lightheadedness. The PT should monitor the patient's blood pressure and symptoms during treatment. If elevated creatinine and BUN values are the presence of renal disease, the patient may have a range of other symptoms that would influence a result of his or her tolerance for therapy. Individuals with CRF or end-stage renal disease (ESRD) may also have uremia, anemia, hypertension, thrombocytopenia, general deconditioning, and low endurance.[32]

Implications Related to Renal Dialysis. Individuals with renal failure often receive dialysis. The PT must consider the type of dialysis the patient is receiving when planning physical therapy interventions. In severe acute cases of renal failure, patients may receive continuous renal replacement therapy. If these patients are not hemodynamically stable, they are inappropriate candidates for rehabilitation exercise. When hemodynamically stable, they may participate in rehabilitation exercise, but technologic issues with equipment may limit treatment. Individuals with CRF or ESRD may perform peritoneal dialysis at home through a peritoneal dialysis catheter. This type of dialysis occurs many times per day in an attempt to mimic kidney function closely. Peritoneal dialysis is time intensive and requires dedication from the patient. Most individuals with CRF undergo hemodialysis. These patients have either a dialysis catheter placed in a central vein or an arteriovenous fistula placed peripherally through which the patient is connected to a dialysis machine multiple times per week for approximately 3 to 4 hours at a time. Hemodialysis results in a dramatic shift of blood constituents and is generally an exhausting process for the patient. The timing of rehabilitation exercise can be challenging for patients receiving hemodialysis. The PT must involve the patient in decisions regarding the scheduling of therapy.

Implications Related to Kidney and Liver Disease. If abnormal creatinine or BUN values indicate the presence of kidney or liver disease, consideration should be given to any increased effects of medications not being properly metabolized by the liver or cleared by the kidneys.

Carbohydrate Metabolism

Tests commonly used with the assessment of carbohydrate metabolism include measurements of blood glucose and glycosylated hemoglobin. The normal values for these tests are listed

TABLE 15-7
Renal Function Indicators

Laboratory Test (units)	Related Physiology	Normal Values	Increased in	Decreased in
Creatinine (Cr) (mg/dL)	Waste product of muscle metabolism that is cleared by kidneys	Adults	Glomerulonephritis	Debilitation
		Men: 0.6-1.2	Pyelonephritis	Decreased muscle mass
		Women: 0.5-1.1	Acute tubular necrosis	
		Elderly: decrease in muscle mass may cause decrease in values	Urinary tract obstruction	
		Adolescents: 0.5-1	Reduced renal blood flow	
		Children: 0.3-0.7	Diabetic nephropathy	
		Infants: 0.2-0.4	Nephritis	
		Newborns: 0.3-1.2	Rhabdomyolysis	
		Possible critical values: >4 (serious renal impairment)	Acromegaly	
			Gigantism	
			Dehydration	
Blood urea nitrogen (BUN) (mg/dL)	Waste product of protein metabolism that is formed in the liver and cleared by kidneys	Adults: 10-20	Renal disease/impairment	Liver failure
		Elderly: may be slightly higher than in adults	Hypovolemia	Overhydration caused by fluid overload or SIADH
		Children: 5-18	Shock	Negative nitrogen balance—malnutrition/malabsorption
		Infants: 5-18	Burns	Pregnancy
		Newborns: 3-12	Dehydration	Nephrotic syndrome
		Cord: 21-40	CHF	
		Possible critical values: >100	MI	
			Gastrointestinal bleeding	
			Excessive protein ingestion	
			Alimentary tube feeding	
			Excessive protein catabolism	
			Starvation	
			Sepsis	
			Ureteral obstruction	
			Bladder outlet obstruction	

CHF, congestive heart failure; *MI*, myocardial infarction; *SIADH*, syndrome of inappropriate antidiuretic hormone secretion.

in Table 15-8. Blood glucose is often ordered as part of the basic metabolic panel (see Table 15-19).

GLUCOSE. Glucose is a simple six-carbon sugar molecule that serves as the primary energy source for all of the body's cellular functions. Increased blood glucose levels, *hyperglycemia,* may be indicative of a postprandial state (the individual just ate); diabetes mellitus; pancreatitis; or Cushing's syndrome, in which there is increased cortisol production because of an increase in adrenocorticotropic hormone. The administration of intravenous glucose and high-dose steroids can also increase blood glucose levels. Decreased blood glucose levels, *hypoglycemia,* may be indicative of an excess of insulin, pituitary deficiency, Addison's disease, or the presence of a benign insulin-producing tumor (insulinoma). Glucose testing is used most often for screening, diagnosing, and monitoring of individuals with diabetes mellitus.

GLYCOSYLATED HEMOGLOBIN. Glycosylated hemoglobin is a test that is used as an indicator of long-term blood glucose levels. When blood glucose levels are elevated, glucose can become attached to hemoglobin via the process of glycosylation. When bound to hemoglobin, the glucose generally remains there for the life cycle of the RBC, which is approximately 120 days. Glycosylated hemoglobin provides information regarding average blood glucose levels over the past 2 to 3 months. Increased values indicate poorly controlled blood glucose levels (uncontrolled diabetes mellitus).

Physical Therapy Implications for Blood Glucose Values. In general, rehabilitation exercise is generally contraindicated in individuals with a blood glucose level less than 60 mg/dL or greater than 350 mg/dL.[15] In an acute care setting, caution should be exercised with levels greater than 250 mg/dL. In the critical care setting, blood glucose levels are closely monitored and treated to maintain levels 80 to 120 mg/dL. PTs should understand and monitor for the signs and symptoms of hypoglycemia and hyperglycemia (Box 15-2).

In patients with diabetes, hypoglycemia may result from an overdose of insulin, late or skipped meals, or strenuous exercise.

TABLE 15-8

Carbohydrate Metabolism

Laboratory Test (units)	Related Physiology	Normal Values	Increased in	Decreased in
Glucose (mg/dL)	Reflects status of carbohydrate metabolism	Adults (and children >2 yr)	DM	Insulinoma
		Fasting: 70-110	Acute stress response	Hypothyroidism
		Casual: ≤200	Cushing's syndrome	Hypopituitarism
		Children <2 yr: 60-100	Pheochromocytoma	Addison's disease
		Infants: 40-90	CRF	Extensive liver disease
		Neonates: 30-60	Glucagonoma	Insulin overdose
		Premature infants: 20-60	Acute pancreatitis	Starvation
		Cord: 45-96	Diuretic therapy	
		Possible critical values:	Corticosteroid therapy	
		Men: <50 or >400	Acromegaly	
		Women: <40 or >400		
		Infants: <40		
		Newborns: <30 or >300		
Glycosylated hemoglobin (GHb, GHB, HbA$_{1c}$) (%)	Used to monitor average blood glucose levels over previous 2-3 mo	Nondiabetic adults/children: 4-5.9	Newly diagnosed diabetic patient	Hemolytic anemia
		Good diabetic control: <7	Poorly controlled diabetes	Chronic blood loss
		Fair diabetic control: 8-9	Nondiabetic hyperglycemia	CRF
		Poor diabetic control: >9	Asplenic patients	
			Pregnancy	

CRF, chronic renal failure; *DM*, diabetes mellitus.

BOX 15-2

Signs and Symptoms of Hyperglycemia and Hypoglycemia

HYPERGLYCEMIA
- Extreme thirst
- Hunger
- Frequent urination
- Dry skin
- Nausea
- Drowsiness
- Blurred vision
  Onset is *gradual* and may progress to diabetic coma.

HYPOGLYCEMIA
- Headache
- Nervousness and shakiness
- Sleepiness
- Feeling anxious or weak
- Confusion
- Difficulty speaking
- Perspiration
- Dizziness/lightheadedness
- Hunger
- Neuromuscular incoordination
  Onset can be *sudden* and may progress to insulin shock.

The individual may complain of a headache, weakness, nervousness and shakiness, irritability, sleepiness, confusion, dizziness or lightheadedness, or difficulty speaking. The individual may perspire and appear to have a lack of muscular coordination (similar to someone with alcohol intoxication). Hypoglycemia can appear with a very sudden onset and may progress to insulin shock (diabetic coma), a rare but life-threatening medical emergency in which the individual becomes unconscious and may experience seizures, respiratory arrest, or cardiac arrest. Individuals may experience signs and symptoms of hypoglycemia when their blood glucose levels appear normal or elevated. This condition occurs when there is a rapid decline in blood glucose levels (i.e., 400 to 200 mg/dL).[12] The rapidity of the decrease is the stimulus for sympathetic activity–based symptoms. Usually people become symptomatic at blood glucose levels of 60 mg/dL or less.

Hyperglycemia may result in frequent urination, extreme thirst, dry skin, hunger, blurred vision, drowsiness, and nausea. In general, the onset of hyperglycemia is gradual, and it may progress to diabetic ketoacidosis. Diabetic ketoacidosis is a condition in which there is a severe insulin deficit. Without insulin, glucose is unable to pass from the blood into the cells. Cells turn to an alternative fuel, fat. The beta-oxidation of free fatty acids results in the production of ketone bodies, which have a fruity, acetone odor. Individuals with diabetic ketoacidosis may have acetone breath, dehydration, a weak and rapid pulse, and Kussmaul's respirations (deep labored respirations as the individual attempts to blow off more carbon dioxide). Diabetic ketoacidosis represents a medical emergency, and immediate care is required.

In addition to monitoring for signs and symptoms of hypoglycemia and hyperglycemia (including diabetic ketoacidosis), the PT should monitor patients' blood glucose levels before and after exercise. This monitoring is especially important when initiating a new strenuous activity, such as may be implemented in outpatient sports rehabilitation. Monitoring should continue until a patient's response to a certain activity is known and predictable in maintaining stable blood glucose levels. The PT should also instruct the patient in continued monitoring of blood glucose levels because the effect of exercise can be felt 12 to 24 hours after exercise.

To monitor and respond to a patient with diabetes mellitus properly, the PT must have on hand a means of testing blood glucose levels (outpatients should be instructed to bring their testing device to exercise sessions), a fast-acting glucose source (e.g., glucose tablets, glucose gels, nondiet soda, fruit juice), and a long-acting glucose source (e.g., graham crackers). In the event of hypoglycemia, fast-acting glucose rapidly elevates an individual's blood glucose to normal. The long-acting glucose maintains normal blood glucose values. If a clinician is uncertain whether a patient is hypoglycemic or hyperglycemic, fruit juice or honey should be administered; this would not harm the hyperglycemic patient, and it may potentially save a patient who is hypoglycemic.[12] A clinical scenario involving glucose follows.

CLINICAL SCENARIO: GLUCOSE

SETTING

Outpatient clinic

REFERRAL

Evaluate and treat for gait, strengthening, and range of motion

DIAGNOSIS

Right total knee replacement

PAST MEDICAL HISTORY

A history of hypertension, insulin-dependent diabetes mellitus, and supraventricular tachycardia in a 65-year-old man

PHYSICAL THERAPY MANAGEMENT

The patient presented to the clinic for his third physical therapy treatment after having total knee replacement surgery 10 days ago. The PT began working with the patient on a stationary bicycle for the first time. Vitals signs before activity were as follows: heart rate 78 beats/min and blood pressure 134/72 mm Hg. The patient tested his own blood glucose at the beginning of the therapy session and reported his glucose reading to be 110 mg/dL. After cycling for 15 minutes, the patient became diaphoretic and dizzy. Exercise was stopped immediately. Testing revealed heart rate 107 beats/min, blood pressure 140/74 mm Hg, and glucose 60 mg/dL. As instructed by the PT, the patient had a fast-acting and a long-acting glucose source readily available, which relieved the patient's symptoms and returned his blood glucose to normal.

DISCUSSION

As a result of diligent monitoring by the PT, the source of the patient's dizziness was quickly determined to be hypoglycemia, which was treated immediately. Vital sign monitoring helped rule out orthostatic hypotension and supraventricular tachycardia.

Acid-Base Balance

ARTERIAL BLOOD GASES. Arterial blood gases are used to assess the patient's oxygenation, ventilation, and metabolic acid-base hemostasis. Oxygenation is the exchange of oxygen (and carbon dioxide) at the alveolar-capillary interface. Ventilation is the movement of gas (oxygen and carbon dioxide) in and out

of the lung. To some extent, the acid-base balance also assesses the kidney's ability to function. Measurements included in the arterial blood gas panel include pH, partial pressure of carbon dioxide dissolved in the plasma (PCO_2), bicarbonate (HCO_3^-), partial pressure of oxygen dissolved in the plasma (PO_2), and oxygen saturation (SaO_2). Normal values for arterial blood gases are shown in Table 15-9 (see also Table 15-19).

pH. pH is inversely proportional to the actual hydrogen ion concentration in the blood. As the pH decreases, the blood is more acidic, and as it increases, the blood is more basic. Normal pH values are 7.35 to 7.45. Increases in pH are associated with respiratory or metabolic alkalosis. Decreases in pH are associated with respiratory or metabolic acidosis.

PARTIAL PRESSURE OF CARBON DIOXIDE. PCO_2 is the measure of the partial pressure of carbon dioxide in the blood. It is a measure of ventilatory capability.[26] As one breathes faster and deeper, more carbon dioxide is blown off in exhaled gas, and the PCO_2 decreases. PCO_2 is known as the respiratory component of the acid-base determination because it is primarily controlled by the lungs. As PCO_2 levels decrease, pH levels increase, so there is an inverse relationship between PCO_2 and pH.

PCO_2 level in blood and cerebrospinal fluid is a major stimulant to the breathing centers of the brainstem. As PCO_2 levels increase, the breathing center is stimulated. If PCO_2 levels continue to increase acutely, breathing cannot keep up with demand to blow off carbon dioxide, the brain is depressed, and coma occurs.[26] If the increase in PCO_2 is slow, the brain accommodates to this change. The patient's drive to breathe may switch from the need to blow off carbon dioxide to a hypoxic drive to breathe, sensed in the carotid bodies.

PCO_2 values increase with hypoventilation, acute respiratory acidosis, compensated metabolic alkalosis, and carbon dioxide retention with some cases of pulmonary disease. PCO_2 values decrease with respiratory alkalosis, compensated metabolic acidosis, and hyperventilation.

BICARBONATE. HCO_3^- is a measure of the metabolic (renal) component of the acid-base equilibrium.[26] HCO_3^- is regulated in the kidneys. As HCO_3^- increases, pH also increases; their relationship is directly proportional. Increases in HCO_3^- are seen in metabolic alkalosis and compensated respiratory acidosis. Decreases are seen in metabolic acidosis and compensated respiratory alkalosis.

PARTIAL PRESSURE OF OXYGEN. PO_2 is an indirect measure of the oxygen content in the blood obtained by measuring the tension (pressure) of oxygen dissolved in the plasma. PO_2 increases with hyperoxygenation using supplemental oxygen and can be very high with mechanical ventilation. PO_2 decreases with conditions causing hypoxemia, such as anemia, atelectasis, pulmonary edema, pneumothorax, and severe hypoventilation. PO_2 is rarely used by PTs except in critical care because blood gases are rarely available.

OXYGEN SATURATION. The PT uses SaO_2 more frequently in clinical practice. SaO_2 is the measure of the percentage of hemoglobin molecules saturated with oxygen. When the SaO_2 is equal to or greater than 92%, tissues are adequately oxygenated assuming a normal oxygen dissociation. As PO_2 decreases, SaO_2 also decreases per the oxyhemoglobin dissociation curve. If PO_2 becomes less than 60 mm Hg, small changes in PO_2 cause large

TABLE 15-9

Arterial Blood Gases

Laboratory Test (units)	Related Physiology	Normal Values	Increased in	Decreased in
pH	Measure of alkalinity and acidity	Adults/children: 7.35-7.45	Metabolic alkalosis	Metabolic acidosis
		Newborns: 7.32-7.49 2 mo–2 yr: 7.34-7.46 *Possible critical values:* *<7.25 or >7.55*	Respiratory alkalosis	Respiratory acidosis
Partial pressure of carbon dioxide (Pco_2) (mm Hg)	Measure of partial pressure of CO_2 in blood. Measure of respiratory component (ventilation capability) of acid-base equilibrium	Adults/children: 35-45	Respiratory acidosis	Respiratory alkalosis
		Children <2 yr: 26-41 *Possible critical values: <20 or >60*	COPD Oversedation Head trauma Pickwickian syndrome	Hypoxemia Pulmonary emboli Anxiety Pain Pregnancy
Bicarbonate (HCO_3^-) (mEq/L)	Measure of metabolic (renal function) component of acid-base equilibrium	Adults/children: 21-28	Metabolic alkalosis	Metabolic acidosis
		Newborns/infants: 16-24 *Possible critical values:* *<15 or >40*	Chronic vomiting Chronic high-volume gastric suction Aldosteronism Mercurial diuretics COPD	Chronic and severe diarrhea Long-term use of loop diuretics Starvation DKA ARF
Partial pressure of oxygen (Po_2) (mm Hg)	Measure of partial pressure of O_2 in blood	Adults/children: 80-100	Polycythemia	Anemias
		Newborns: 60-70 *Possible critical values: <40*	Increased inspired O_2 Hyperventilation	Mucous plug Bronchospasm Atelectasis Pneumothorax Pulmonary edema ARDS Restrictive lung disease Cardiac septal defects Emboli Inadequate O_2 inspired air Severe hypoventilation
Oxygen saturation (Sao_2) (%)	Indication of percentage of hemoglobin saturated with oxygen molecules	Adults/children: 95-100		Anything that lowers Po_2 levels—although this is not a linear relationship
		Elderly: 95 Newborns: 40-90 *Possible critical values: ≤75*		

ARDS, acute respiratory distress syndrome; *ARF*, acute renal failure; *COPD*, chronic obstructive pulmonary disease; *DKA*, diabetic ketoacidosis.

changes in Sao_2. When Sao_2 becomes less than 70%, tissues cannot extract enough oxygen from the bloodstream to function adequately.[26]

INTERPRETING ARTERIAL BLOOD GASES

Step 1. Determine whether the patient is acidotic or alkalotic by looking at the pH (Table 15-10).

Low pH (<7.35) = acidosis.

High pH (>7.45) = alkalosis.

Step 2. Determine what is causing the abnormal pH by looking at the Pco_2 and HCO_3^-.

High levels of Pco_2 (>45 mm Hg) or low levels of HCO_3^- (<22 mEq/L) cause acidosis.

Low levels of Pco_2 (<35 mm Hg) or high levels of HCO_3^- (>26 mEq/L) cause alkalosis.

Step 3. Determine whether the disorder is respiratory or metabolic in nature.

Pco_2 levels are regulated by the lungs by either decreased respirations (retaining carbon dioxide) or hyperventilation (blowing off carbon dioxide). If pH irregularity is caused by abnormal Pco_2 levels, the acidosis or alkalosis is respiratory in nature.

TABLE 15-10

Interpreting Arterial Blood Gases

pH	CO$_2$	HCO$_3^-$	Organ Affecting Change in pH		Disorder
High	Normal	High	Kidneys	Decompensated	Metabolic alkalosis
Low	Normal	Low	Kidneys	Decompensated	Metabolic acidosis
High	Low	Normal	Lungs	Decompensated	Respiratory alkalosis
Low	High	Normal	Lungs	Decompensated	Respiratory acidosis
High	High	High	Kidneys	Compensated	Metabolic alkalosis
Low	Low	Low	Kidneys	Compensated	Metabolic acidosis
High	Low	Low	Lungs	Compensated	Respiratory alkalosis
Low	High	High	Lungs	Compensated	Respiratory acidosis

HCO$_3^-$ levels are regulated by the kidneys through retention or excretion. If the pH irregularity is caused by abnormal HCO$_3^-$ levels, the acidosis or alkalosis is metabolic in nature.

Step 4. Determine whether there is an effort being made to compensate for pH irregularity.

When respiratory acidosis or alkalosis is present, the kidneys may attempt to compensate through retention or excretion of HCO$_3^-$. If HCO$_3^-$ levels are normal, the order is decompensated (not compensated for). If HCO$_3^-$ levels are abnormal (<22 or >26 mEq/L), the condition is considered to be a compensated respiratory acidosis or alkalosis.

When metabolic acidosis or alkalosis is present, the lungs may attempt to compensate through retention or exhalation of carbon dioxide. If the Pco_2 levels are normal, the order is decompensated (not compensated for). If Pco_2 levels are abnormal (<35 or >45 mm Hg), the condition is considered to be a compensated metabolic acidosis or alkalosis.

When a compensated respiratory or metabolic acidosis or alkalosis is present, the pH may return to normal or near-normal range.

Physical Therapy Implications for Arterial Blood Gases. Patients should be monitored for hypoxemia at rest or with activity. Physical activity increases the patient's oxygen demand. The rehabilitation prescription may need to be modified when a patient is having difficulty maintaining appropriate Sao_2. When Sao_2 levels decrease below normal or below physician's orders during activity, that activity should be stopped until the patient's levels increase to within the appropriate range. If a patient is unable to maintain appropriate Sao_2 levels at rest, rehabilitation exercise is contraindicated.

Noninvasive oxygen saturation measurements (Spo_2) can be taken with the use of pulse oximetry. The pulse oximeter can be a valuable tool for the PT when working with patients who have underlying acute or chronic cardiac or pulmonary disease. The pulse oximeter can serve as a biofeedback tool to assist in identifying symptomatic activity end points that correlate with relative hypoxia. Various factors may affect the accuracy of the pulse oximeter, including the level of peripheral circulation, the presence of nail polish, probe position and connection, patient movement, and the presence of arrhythmias. The pulse identified on the device should always be accurate to the patient's pulse. The PT should correlate the data from the pulse oximeter with the patient's clinical presentation and other data obtained when making clinical decisions.

The PT should also watch for clinical symptoms of hypoxemia, such as nasal flaring; a change in or dysrhythmic breathing pattern; or dyspnea. Later, as Sao_2 decreases, the PT may notice cyanosis in the nail beds (this may be a chronic change as well), cyanosis in the perioral area, confusion or mental status changes, and cardiac dysrhythmias. Patients should be monitored before, during, and after activity because some patients experience postexertional desaturation with or without breath retraining.

It is crucial that PTs follow the titration orders for supplemental oxygen for a given patient (e.g., supplemental oxygen at 2 to 4 L to maintain Spo_2 >92%). Some patients with COPD retain carbon dioxide. In these patients, increasing the supplemental oxygen can decrease respiratory drive. Normally, a person's drive to breathe is to blow off carbon dioxide because the brain is sensitive to high carbon dioxide levels. In a patient who retains carbon dioxide, the drive to breathe may change to a drive to obtain oxygen (sensed by chemoreceptors in the carotid bodies). Increasing supplemental oxygen beyond that listed in the prescription (titration orders) can cause patients who retain carbon dioxide to stop breathing. Discussion with the patient's physician is warranted in determining Spo_2 precautions.

Some patients with chronic lung disease also have chronic hypoxia. It may be "normal" for these patients to have a significant decrease in Spo_2 into the middle and lower 80th percentile range with activity. Discussion with the patient's pulmonologist or primary physician is recommended to identify specific precautions for the patient.

Any indication of hyperventilation (i.e., decreased carbon dioxide level or increased respiratory rate) should be addressed during physical therapy. Relaxation techniques and breathing exercises, such as pursed-lip or diaphragmatic breathing, can be incorporated into the treatment plan. Hypoventilation, as noted by shallow breathing, can be addressed by deep-breathing activities and upright positioning to improve carbon dioxide removal and optimize oxygenation.

Changes in the metabolic aspects of arterial blood gases may affect other organ systems and affect a patient's tolerance for physical activity. The PT must always monitor the patient's vital signs and tolerance for activity and observe for associated signs and symptoms. In general, physical therapy interventions are not carried out when arterial blood gas results reflect the critical value range.[12]

Hemostasis

The coagulation of blood is an important part of the process of hemostasis, which prevents excessive blood loss when an artery or vein is injured. Platelets are a part of primary hemostasis and are discussed in the section on cellular components. Secondary hemostasis involves the coagulation cascade, consisting of the intrinsic and extrinsic clotting pathways. Abnormalities in hemostasis may be due to liver disease, congenital clotting factor deficiencies, vitamin K deficiencies, disseminated intravascular coagulopathy, and administration of anticoagulation therapy. Test results used to assess hemostasis include prothrombin time, INR, and activated partial thromboplastin time APTT. Table 15-11 presents normal values for these tests.

PROTHROMBIN TIME. Prothrombin time is a blood test that measures the extrinsic clotting pathway, which involves clotting factors V, VII, and X and prothrombin and fibrinogen. This test is used as a screen for clotting deficiencies. It can also be used as a measure of oral anticoagulant therapy (administration of warfarin); however, it may be inaccurate between test reagents and between laboratories.

Prothrombin time results may be decreased when there are insufficient clotting factors. Results may be lower than desired with insufficient anticoagulation therapy. Prothrombin time may be increased with oral anticoagulation therapy (this is a desired response) or pathologically with vitamin K deficiencies and liver disease.

Physical Therapy Implications for Prothrombin Time. The prothrombin time therapeutic range for anticoagulation is 1.5 to 2 times the reference range. The PT should consult with the physician if the prothrombin time is more than 2.5 times the reference range to discuss the potential of spontaneous bleeding.

INTERNATIONAL NORMALIZED RATIO. INR is a ratio of the individual's prothrombin time results to the reference range, corrected for variations in test material. This test result is followed when the patient is taking oral anticoagulants. INR makes the prothrombin time results comparable from laboratory to laboratory, as well.

Physical Therapy Implications for International Normalized Ratio. When patients are given anticoagulation after CVA or deep vein thrombosis, the desired INR value range is 2.0 to 3.0. For patients who have received mechanical heart valves, the desired INR value range is 2.5 to 3.5. For patients who are not anticoagulated, the PT should discuss the case with the physician if the INR is greater than 2.0. INR values exceeding 3.0 may place the patient at risk of hemarthrosis, which requires care during therapy and exercise.[27] Patients who have received anticoagulation are at relative risk for spontaneous bleeding when the INR is more than 5.0. INR values can be increased more rapidly when beginning oral anticoagulation by the concomitant use of low-dose heparin or low-molecular-weight heparin (LMWH) for a short time.

Many pharmacologic agents and foods can affect INR. Patients are counseled when beginning anticoagulation. INR values must

TABLE 15-11

Tests for Homeostasis

Laboratory Test (units)	Related Physiology	Normal Values	Increased in	Decreased in
Prothrombin time (PT) (sec)	Used to assess extrinsic clotting pathway	11-12.5; normal values vary depending on the reagents used	Liver dysfunction	
		Patients receiving anticoagulation therapy: 1.5-2 times reference range	Vitamin K deficiency	
		Possible critical values: >20	Salicylate intoxication	
			Oral anticoagulation therapy	
			DIC	
			Massive blood transfusion	
			Hereditary factor deficiency	
International normalized ratio (INR)	Reflects standardized reporting of prothrombin time so that results are comparable among laboratories	0.8-1.1	See prothrombin time	
		Possible critical values: >5.5		
Activated partial thromboplastin time, partial thromboplastin time (APTT, PTT) (sec)	Used to assess intrinsic clotting pathway and common pathway of clot formation	APTT: 30-40	Clotting factor deficiencies	Early stages of DIC
		PTT: 60-70	Cirrhosis of liver	Extensive cancer
		Patients receiving anticoagulation therapy: 1.5-2.5 times reference range	Vitamin K deficiency	
		Possible critical values:	DIC	
		APTT: >70	Heparin administration	
		PTT: >100		

DIC, disseminated intravascular coagulopathy.

be followed regularly. The PT should be aware of INR values when working with patients who are anticoagulated to make sound clinical judgments regarding relative risk of bleeding or risk of clot formation. A clinical scenario involving INR follows.

CLINICAL SCENARIO: INTERNATIONAL NORMALIZED RATIO

SETTING

Outpatient

REFERRAL

Evaluate and treat for mobility, strengthening, and gait training

DIAGNOSIS

Status post total knee arthroplasty

PAST MEDICAL HISTORY

A history of cardiovascular disease and osteoarthritis in a 78-year-old woman who underwent total knee arthroplasty 5 days ago. The patient was discharged from the hospital on acetaminophen for pain, warfarin for deep vein thrombosis prophylaxis, and aspirin for cardiovascular protection.

PHYSICAL THERAPY MANAGEMENT

The PT was following the patient's INR values through the hospital computer system. Between the second and third visits, the PT noted that the patient's INR had increased to 5.2. The PT called the referring physician to discuss the patient's INR value and the current physical therapy plan of care.

DISCUSSION

In this situation, the PT cannot assume that the physician was aware of the type of interventions the PT uses with rehabilitation and whether or not they are inappropriate in the presence of increased INR values. It is incumbent on the PT to understand the significance of the patient's laboratory test results and their implications for physical therapy interventions.

ACTIVATED PARTIAL THROMBOPLASTIN TIME. The activated PTT or PTT is a blood test that measures the function of the intrinsic clotting pathway. It is also used to screen for hemophilia and to monitor for the effectiveness of intravenous anticoagulant therapy (heparin administration). When anticoagulation is administered intravenously, the values should be 2 to 2.5 times baseline (50 to 70 seconds). PTT values should be normally increased when the patient is receiving intravenous anticoagulation. PTT can also be pathologically increased with liver disease, disseminated intravascular coagulopathy, clotting factor deficiencies, and vitamin K deficiencies.

Physical Therapy Implications for Partial Thromboplastin Time. A significantly elevated PTT may indicate that the patient is at risk for bleeding. In addition, if a patient is receiving intravenous anticoagulation, and the PTT value indicates that the patient is supratherapeutic, discussion with other members of the health care team should occur to determine efficacy of therapy and precautions until ranges return to normal or therapeutic.

ADDITIONAL HEMOSTASIS COMMENTS

End-Stage Liver Disease. Patients with end-stage liver disease may also have decreased and dysfunctional platelets, placing them at additional risk for easy bleeding. INR, activated PTT, and platelet counts may be within reference range margins but collectively put the patient at risk for bleeding.

Low-Molecular-Weight Heparin. Although heparin anti–factor Xa (anti-Xa) concentrations can be used to monitor the effectiveness of LMWH (i.e., enoxaparin [Lovenox]), this is not a commonly used test. LMWH is administered according to body weight, and, in contrast to unfractionated heparin, LMWH binds less strongly to plasma proteins, undergoes less inactivation by platelet factor IV, and is more bioavailable. These factors make the effects of LMWH more predictable and, in general, eliminate the need for monitoring via laboratory tests.[28]

Cardiac Status

Some laboratory tests provide information related to a patient's cardiac status. When cardiac tissue undergoes stress or sustains damage, substances such as enzymes, peptides, and proteins may be released into the bloodstream. Tests that assay for these substances can assist in diagnosis when acute MI or CHF is suspected.

CARDIAC ENZYMES. Cardiac enzymes are substances released from injured myocardial tissue. They are used in one set of tests to assist in diagnosis when acute MI is suspected. Other tests include electrocardiography and imaging studies such as thallium scans and angiography. Historically, various cardiac enzymes have been used for diagnosing acute MI. Currently, the enzymes that provide the most significant information include creatine phosphokinase (CPK), creatine kinase–MB (CK-MB) level, and troponin. Normal values for these enzymes are listed in Table 15-12.

Creatine Phosphokinase and Creatine Kinase–MB Level. CPK is found primarily in skeletal and cardiac muscle and the brain. In the case of a myocardial event, serum CPK levels begin to increase 4 to 6 hours after the event. These levels peak 12 to 24 hours after the event and return to normal in 4 to 5 days. Because CPK can be found in tissues other than cardiac muscle, it is not myocardial specific. Elevated CPK levels may indicate injury to tissues other than cardiac muscle, such as skeletal muscle trauma (as seen in rhabdomyolysis) and cerebral contusion. CPK can be separated into subunits or isoenzymes, however. CK-MB is a cardiac isoenzyme that is specific to the myocardium. CK-MB levels may be elevated with cardiac injury or insult, including acute MI, severe cardiac ischemia, cardiac surgery, myocarditis, ventricular arrhythmias, and cardiac defibrillation. When the percent relative index (CK-MB fraction of total CPK) is greater than 5%, acute MI is probable.

Cardiac Troponin. Troponins are proteins found within muscle. Cardiac troponins are specific to myocardium and can be used to assess for and diagnose the degree of MI. There are two main types of cardiac troponins: I and T (cTnT, cTnI). Serum troponin levels increase 4 to 8 hours after MI. In contrast to CK-MB, troponin levels remain elevated for 5 to 9 days, permitting late diagnosis of MI. The test used for cTnI is more specific to that particular troponin than the test for cTnT (which may also register non–cardiac-related troponins). cTnI is the test commonly used in assessing for acute MI.

TABLE 15-12

Cardiac Indicators

Laboratory Test (units)	Related Physiology	Normal Values	Increased in
Creatine phosphokinase (CPK, CK) (U/L)	Enzyme found in striated muscle (skeletal and heart) and brain	Adults Men: 55-170 Women: 30-135 *Values higher after exercise* Newborns: 68-580	Injury to skeletal muscle, heart muscle, or brain
CK-MB (%)	Isoenzyme of CPK that is more myocardial specific	0	Acute MI Cardiac surgery Cardiac defibrillation Myocarditis Ventricular arrhythmias Cardiac ischemia
Troponin, cardiac (cTnT, cTnI) (ng/mL)	Myocardial-specific proteins released into blood-stream after injury to myocardium	cTnT: <0.2 cTnI: <0.03	Myocardial injury MI
Myoglobin (μg/L)	Protein found in striated muscle (cardiac and skeletal) that is released with muscle damage	<90	Injury to cardiac or skeletal muscle
Brain natriuretic peptide (BNP) (pg/mL)	Substance released by cardiac ventricles when stretched	<100	CHF MI Systemic HTN Cor pulmonale Heart transplant rejection

CHF, congestive heart failure; *HTN,* hypertension; *MI,* myocardial infarction.

Aspartate Aminotransferase and Lactate Dehydrogenase. Historically, other enzymes have been used to assist in the diagnosis of MI, such as aspartate aminotransferase and lactate dehydrogenase. However, these enzymes are not myocardial specific and do not offer time-related windows of diagnosis that are dramatically different from the markers mentioned earlier that are more myocardial specific.

Physical Therapy Implications for Cardiac Enzymes. When CPK and CK-MB levels are elevated, if the percent relative index is greater than 5%, acute MI is probable. cTnI that is above normal is a positive indicator of acute MI. The amount of increase in CK-MB and troponin correlates with the extent of MI. If enzyme testing is positive for acute MI, physical therapy interventions should be held until the enzymes are decreasing. The PT should continue to monitor the patient's vital signs and Spo₂. Most often, cardiac enzymes are ordered in a series of three every 8 hours because of the delay in detectable increase of enzyme levels from onset of event. If the initial one or two sets of enzymes are determined to be normal, the PT must still wait for any pending sets before initiating physical therapy interventions. If any set of enzymes indicates a positive diagnosis of MI, physical therapy interventions can begin when a subsequent set indicates that the cardiac enzyme levels are decreasing. The levels do not need to return to normal for therapy interventions to begin. See Figure 15-4 for a clinical decision algorithm related to cardiac enzymes.

Any patient with significant arrhythmia or myocardial dysfunction, such as angina, hypotension, or CHF, may be excluded from physical therapy. Activity may be increased according to the cardiac rehabilitation protocol in use. The patient should always be monitored for bradycardia or tachycardia, arrhythmias, and associated signs and symptoms of MI (chest pain, unexplained perspiration, nausea, vomiting, shortness of breath, feeling of impending doom).[12]

OTHER CARDIAC INDICATORS RELATED TO ACUTE MYOCARDIAL INFARCTION. Historically, various biochemical markers have been investigated for their usefulness in assisting with cardiac-related diagnoses. Examples of two such markers are myoglobin and ischemia-modified albumin.

Myoglobin. Myoglobin is an oxygen-binding protein found in striated skeletal and cardiac muscle. It is released into the bloodstream when muscle is damaged. Myoglobin can serve as an early marker of acute MI. However, because it is not myocardial specific, it is more often used to rule out acute MI. Serum myoglobin levels begin to increase 2 to 6 hours after acute MI. Levels peak 3 to 9 hours after the event and return to baseline 24 to 36 hours after MI. Normal values for myoglobin are listed in Table 15-12.

Ischemia-Modified Albumin. Free radicals of cardiac ischemia can modify the amino acid sequence of albumin already present in the bloodstream. This ischemia-modified albumin appears within minutes of ischemia onset and returns to baseline in 6 hours. Ischemia-modified albumin may serve as a marker of ischemia before infarction.[34]

NATRIURETIC PEPTIDES. Natriuretic peptides are factors that are involved in various regulatory mechanisms within the body. These include atrial natriuretic peptide, brain natriuretic peptide (BNP), and C-type natriuretic peptide. With regards to assisting in diagnosis of cardiac disorders, only BNP is discussed.

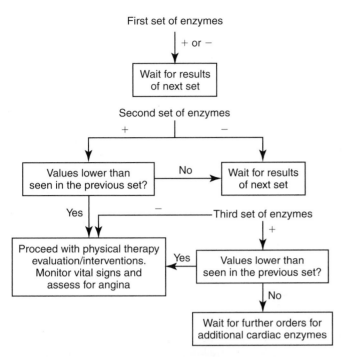

First set of enzymes

Wait for results of next set

Second set of enzymes

Values lower than seen in the previous set? — No → Wait for results of next set

Third set of enzymes

Proceed with physical therapy evaluation/interventions. Monitor vital signs and assess for angina

Values lower than seen in the previous set?

Wait for further orders for additional cardiac enzymes

(+) = Values elevated and indicative of AMI
(−) = Values within normal range, not indicative of AMI

FIGURE 15-4 Algorithm for physical therapy implications related to cardiac enzymes. *AMI*, acute myocardial infarction.

TABLE 15-13

Brain Natriuretic Peptide Values Associated with New York Heart Association Classification of Congestive Heart Failure

NYHA Classification of CHF	BNP (pg/mL)
I	244 ± 286
II	389 ± 374
III	640 ± 447
IV	817 ± 435

BNP, brain natriuretic peptide; *CHF*, congestive heart failure; *NYHA*, New York Heart Association.

Maisel AS, Krishnaswamy P, Nowak RM, et al. Rapid measurement of B-type natriuretic peptide in the emergency diagnosis of heart failure. *N Engl J Med* 2002; 347(3):161-167. Accessed from http://content.nejm.org/cgi/reprint/347/3/161.pdf on February 20, 2009.

Brain Natriuretic Peptide. BNP is a substance that is released primarily by cardiac ventricles when they are stretched as part of the normal process of regulating vascular volume. Normal values are listed in Table 15-12. When the vascular volume is elevated, the ventricles undergo increased stretch during ventricular filling, which results in the release of BNP. Increased serum BNP causes increased renal loss of sodium and water, which decreases the vascular volume, returning the ventricles to their normal size.

Although BNP is part of a normal physiologic process, it can be used in the diagnosis and prognosis of CHF.[21,29] Individuals with CHF have a decreased cardiac ejection fraction; this leads to decreased renal perfusion. Instead of the decreased vascular volume expected with increased BNP levels, there is instead an increased vascular volume because of decreased renal perfusion. There is increased ventricular stretch and increased BNP release. Studies have shown that the mean BNP concentrations increase with increasing New York Heart Association (NYHA) classification of CHF (Table 15-13).[21] Although the typical threshold for a diagnosis of CHF is a serum BNP level of 100 pg/mL or greater, some more recent studies have shown that 10% to 21% of patients with heart failure have BNP levels less than 100 pg/mL.[16,31]

Physical Therapy Implications for Brain Natriuretic Peptide. BNP levels greater than 100 pg/mL indicate active CHF. Patients with CHF may have poor exercise tolerance. The PT should always confirm the current medical status of the patient before initiating examination and intervention. Factors to consider include the following: (1) whether the patient has right-sided heart failure, left-sided heart failure, or both; (2) the current status of diuresis; (3) the patient's heart rate and rhythm and other appropriate vital signs; and (4) the patient's ejection fraction if available.

Inflammatory Markers

Various inflammatory markers exist that may assist physicians in the diagnosis of a particular disease or disorder or in monitoring disease progression. Examples are provided in Table 15-14.

ERYTHROCYTE SEDIMENTATION RATE. Erythrocyte sedimentation rate (ESR) is a measurement of the rate at which RBCs (erythrocytes) settle in plasma over a specific time frame. It is a nonspecific test and is not used frequently in routine study. It can be used as an indicator of the course of a disease and to monitor disease progression.[26] This laboratory result is elevated with inflammation or infection and in some autoimmune disorders and some neoplastic diseases. ESR can be used by the PT as an indicator of what the physician may be looking for based on laboratory and diagnostic tests ordered. Other more specific tests are usually ordered in combination with ESR, such as a vasculitis screen for temporal arteritis in patients who have neurologic symptoms.

C-REACTIVE PROTEIN. C-reactive protein (CRP) is produced primarily by the liver when acute inflammation or infection manifests somewhere in the body. It is a nonspecific indicator of infection or inflammation. High-sensitivity assays for CRP (hsCRP) can detect very low levels of the protein. Current understanding of the role of the inflammatory process in the development of atherosclerosis has led to research involving hsCRP as a potential risk factor for cardiovascular disease. This research has shown hsCRP levels to be an important predictor of first coronary events and future atherosclerotic events.[8,33]

RHEUMATOID FACTOR. Rheumatoid arthritis is a chronic inflammatory disease in which immunoglobulins react with components of abnormal immunoglobulin antibodies to produce immune complexes that activate components of the inflammatory process and cause joint damage. Rheumatoid factor is the reactive immunoglobulin. Although it is present with rheumatoid arthritis, it is not specific to this disease.

ANTINUCLEAR ANTIBODY. Antinuclear antibodies are substances involved in various autoimmune diseases. An antinuclear antibody test is often used to assist in the diagnosis of systemic lupus erythematosus, but it is not specific to this disease.

TABLE 15-14

Inflammatory Markers

Laboratory Test (units)	Related Physiology	Normal Values	Increased in	Decreased in
Erythrocyte sedimentation rate (ESR) (mm/hr)	Nonspecific indicator of infection or inflammation	Adults	CRF	Sickle cell anemia
		Men: ≤15 Women: ≤20 Children: ≤10 Newborns: 0-2	Malignant disease	Spherocytosis
			Bacterial infection Inflammatory diseases Necrotic tissue diseases Hyperfibrinogenemia Macroglobulinemia Severe anemias	Hypofibrinogenemia Polycythemia vera
C-reactive protein (CRP, hsCRP) (mg/dL)	Nonspecific indicator of bacterial infection or inflammation	<1	Arthritis	
	hsCRP used to assess risk for CVD	*Cardiac risk:*	Acute rheumatic fever	
		Low: <1 Average: 1-3 High: 3	Reiter's syndrome Crohn's disease Vasculitis syndrome SLE Tissue infarction or damage Acute MI Pulmonary infarction Kidney transplant rejection Bone marrow transplant rejection Soft tissue trauma Bacterial infection Postoperative wound infection UTI Tuberculosis Malignant disease Bacterial meningitis	
Rheumatoid factor (RF) (U/mL)	Assists in diagnosis of rheumatoid arthritis but is not specific to this inflammatory disease	Negative: <60	Rheumatoid arthritis	
		Elderly patients may have slightly increased values	Other autoimmune diseases (SLE) Chronic viral infection Subacute bacterial endocarditis Tuberculosis Chronic hepatitis Dermatomyositis Scleroderma Infectious mononucleosis Leukemia Cirrhosis Syphilis Renal disease	
Antinuclear antibody (ANA)	Group of antinuclear antibodies used to diagnose SLE	Negative at 1:40 dilution	SLE	
			Rheumatoid arthritis Chronic hepatitis Periarteritis (polyarteritis) nodosa Dermatomyositis Scleroderma Infectious mononucleosis	

Inflammatory Markers—cont'd

Laboratory Test (units)	Related Physiology	Normal Values	Increased in	Decreased in
Antinuclear antibody (ANA)—cont'd			Raynaud's disease Sjögren's syndrome Other immune diseases Leukemia Myasthenia gravis Cirrhosis	

CRF, chronic renal failure; *CVD,* cardiovascular disease; *MI,* myocardial infarction; *SLE,* systemic lupus erythematosus; *UTI,* urinary tract infection.

Cardiovascular Disease Risk

Lipid assays assist physicians in identifying a patient's risk for CAD and CVA because high blood cholesterol levels are a risk factor for the development of atherosclerosis. The American Heart Association endorses the National Cholesterol Education Program (NCEP) guidelines for detection of high cholesterol levels. The Third Report of the Expert Panel on Detection, Evaluation, and Treatment of High Blood Cholesterol in Adults (Adult Treatment Panel III), released in 2001, recommends that everyone age 20 and older have a fasting lipoprotein profile every 5 years. This report also presents the NCEP's current clinical guidelines for cholesterol testing and management. The Adult Treatment Panel III guidelines provide detailed information on topics such as classification of lipids and lipoproteins, CAD risk assessment, lifestyle interventions, drug treatment, specific dyslipidemias, and adherence issues. Recommendations for special populations such as patients with CAD, patients at high risk for developing CAD, patients with diabetes, women, older adults, young adults, and racial and ethnic groups are provided.[1,24]

LIPIDS. Lipids or lipoproteins include total cholesterol, high-density lipoproteins (HDLs), low-density lipoproteins (LDLs), and triglycerides. Cholesterol is the main lipoprotein identified in the formation of atherosclerotic vascular disease. However, cholesterol is necessary for the production of steroids, sex hormones, bile acids, and cellular membranes.[26] Cholesterol is broken down in the liver and transported in the bloodstream by LDLs (75%) and HDLs (25%). LDLs are most directly associated with increased risk of CAD. Normal values for lipids are listed in Table 15-15. Table 15-16 presents risk categories.

CHOLESTEROL. Cholesterol testing is usually done as part of a lipid profile, which tests for total cholesterol, LDL, HDL, and triglycerides. Two elevated total cholesterol results indicate the need to treat for hypercholesterolemia. Low cholesterol levels are associated with severe liver disease.

HIGH-DENSITY LIPOPROTEINS. HDLs are the so-called good cholesterol. HDLs are produced in the liver and are believed to remove cholesterol from peripheral tissue and transport it to the liver for excretion. This function of removing lipids from the endothelium is what is believed to be a protective mechanism against heart disease.[26] Studies have shown that total HDL is an inverse risk factor for CAD. Low levels (<40 mg/dL) are believed to increase risk for CAD, whereas high levels (>60 mg/dL) are

considered protective.[26] The desired range for total cholesterol/HDL ratio is 3:1 to 5:1.

LOW-DENSITY LIPOPROTEINS. LDLs are also known as *bad cholesterol.* Cholesterol carried by LDL can be deposited in the lining of blood vessels and is associated with increased risk of atherosclerotic heart disease and peripheral vascular disease.[26] LDL levels are optimally less than 100 mg/dL; individuals at high risk for heart disease should have levels less than 70 mg/dL.

TRIGLYCERIDES. Triglycerides are fats that are carried in the blood by LDL. They act as a source of energy for the body. When triglyceride levels are elevated in the body, they are stored in fat tissue.

SUMMARY FOR CARDIOVASCULAR DISEASE RISK. The American Heart Association recommends that absolute numbers for total blood cholesterol, HDL, and LDL be used instead of ratios in determining appropriateness for treatment of hypercholesterolemia/hyperlipidemia with cholesterol-lowering agents (i.e., statin drugs). Many physicians treat patients with statin drugs regardless of cholesterol levels in secondary prevention of MI and CVA because of the results of the Oxford Study.[13,14] This study showed that the use of statin drugs after MI and CVA, regardless of cholesterol values, reduces the risk of a second event. The support for this finding was stronger for patients after MI than after CVA.[13]

Physical Therapy Implications Related to Lipid Values. The PT bears responsibility as a health care professional to educate patients regarding heart and vascular disease risk and risk reduction. Knowledge of cholesterol values and relative risk is important. There are also potential side effects of the use of statin drugs that are important for the PT to know. Myopathy is a potential side effect of these drugs. Patients may present to the physical therapy clinic with various muscle complaints that may be side effects of medical regimens.

Hepatic Function

The hepatic function panel, or LFTs, consists of specific blood tests whose values reflect the adequacy of the function of the liver. Physicians use LFTs to detect, evaluate, and monitor liver disease or damage. The results of LFTs are elevated in various primary and secondary hepatic disorders. The components of a hepatic function panel and their related normal values are presented in Table 15-17. In general, the PT is primarily concerned with whether LFTs indicate liver dysfunction. More specifically, the PT may be concerned with the albumin results.

TABLE 15-15

Lipids

Laboratory Test (units)	Related Physiology	Normal Values	Increased in	Decreased in
Cholesterol (mg/dL)	Primary lipid associated with arteriosclerosis	Adults: <200 Children: 120-200 Infants: 70-175 Newborns: 53-135	Hypercholesterolemia Hyperlipidemia Hypothyroidism Uncontrolled DM Nephritic syndrome Pregnancy High-cholesterol diet Xanthomatosis HTN MI Atherosclerosis Biliary cirrhosis Stress Nephrosis	Malabsorption Malnutrition Hyperthyroidism Cholesterol-lowering medication Pernicious anemia Hemolytic anemia Sepsis Stress Liver disease Acute MI
High-density lipoproteins (HDLs) (mg/dL)	"Good" cholesterol	Men: >45 Women: >55	Hereditary factors Excessive exercise	Hereditary factors Metabolic syndrome Liver disease Hypoproteinemia
Low-density lipoproteins (LDLs) (mg/dL)	"Bad" cholesterol	60-180	Hereditary factors Nephrotic syndrome Glycogen storage diseases Hypothyroidism Alcohol consumption Liver disease Cushing's syndrome	Hereditary factors Hypoproteinemia Hyperthyroidism
Triglycerides (TGs) (mg/dL)	Form of fat produced in liver; used as part of assessment for coronary and vascular disease	Adults/elderly Men: 40-60 Women: 35-135 Children 0-5 yr, boys: 30-86; girls: 32-99 6-11 yr, boys: 31-108; girls: 35-114 12-15 yr, boys: 36-138; girls: 41-138 16-19 yr, boys: 40-163; girls: 40-128 *Possible critical values*: >400 mg/dL	Glycogen storage disease Hyperlipidemias Hypothyroidism High-carbohydrate diet Poorly controlled diabetes Risk of arteriosclerotic occlusive coronary disease and peripheral vascular disease Nephrotic syndrome HTN Alcoholic cirrhosis Pregnancy MI	Malabsorption syndrome Malnutrition Hyperthyroidism
Cholesterol/HDL ratio	Used as indicator of risk for coronary heart disease	Optimal ratio 3.5:1 *Risk values:* Men ½ average: 3.4 Women ½ average: 3.3 Men average: 5 Women average: 4.4 Men 2× average: 10 Women 2× average: 7 Men 3× average: 24 Women 3× average: 11		

DM, diabetes mellitus; *HTN*, hypertension; *MI*, myocardial infarction.

TABLE 15-16

Classification of Lipid Values

Category	Total Cholesterol (mg/dL)	HDL (mg/dL)	LDL (mg/dL)	Triglycerides (mg/dL)
Desirable/optimal	<200	≥60	<100	<150
Near-optimal			100-129	
Borderline high	200-239		130-159	150-199
High (risk)	≥240	<40 for men	160-189	200-499
		<50 for women		
Very high			≥190	≥500

Data from American Heart Association Recommendations: *Cholesterol levels* (website). http://www.americanheart.org/presenter.jhtml?identifier=4500. Accessed August 16, 2009.
HDL, high-density lipoprotein; *LDL,* low-density lipoprotein.

TABLE 15-17

Hepatic Function

Laboratory Test (units)	Related Physiology	Normal Values	Increased in	Decreased in
Alanine aminotransferase (ALT) (U/L)	Enzyme found mainly in the liver	Adults/children: 4-36 Elderly: may be slightly higher than in adults Infants: may be twice as high as in adults	Hepatitis Hepatic necrosis Hepatic ischemia Cirrhosis Cholestasis Hepatic tumor Hepatotoxic drugs Obstructive jaundice Severe burns Trauma to striated muscle Myositis Pancreatitis MI Infectious mononucleosis Shock	
Alkaline phosphatase (ALP) (U/L)	Enzyme related to bile ducts	Adults: 30-120 Elderly: slightly higher in than in adults Children/adolescents <2 yr: 85-235 2-8 yr: 65-210 9-15 yr: 60-300 16-21 yr: 30-200	Cirrhosis Intrahepatic or extrahepatic biliary obstruction Primary or metastatic liver disease Intestinal ischemia or infarction Metastatic tumor to bone Healing fracture Hyperparathyroidism Paget's disease of bone Rheumatoid arthritis Sarcoidosis Osteomalacia Rickets	Hypothyroidism Malnutrition Milk-alkali syndrome Pernicious anemia Hypophosphatemia Scurvy—vitamin C deficiency Celiac disease Excess vitamin B ingestion Hypophosphatasia
Aspartate aminotransferase (AST) (U/L)	Enzyme found in liver, heart, and muscles	Adults: 0-35 Children 0-5 days: 35-140 <3 yr: 15-60 3-6 yr: 15-50 6-12 yr: 10-50 12-18 yr: 10-40	Liver disease Skeletal muscle disease Acute hemolytic anemia Acute pancreatitis	Acute renal disease Beriberi DKA Pregnancy

Continued

TABLE 15-17

Hepatic Function—cont'd

Laboratory Test (units)	Related Physiology	Normal Values	Increased in	Decreased in
Gamma-glutamyltransferase (GGT) (U/L)	Enzyme released in cytolysis and necrosis of liver cells; also in kidney tissue	Men/women ≥45 yr: 8-38 Women <45 yr: 5-27 Elderly: slightly higher than adult level Children: similar to adult level Newborns: 5 times higher than adult level	Liver dysfunction MI Alcohol ingestion Pancreatitis Pancreatic cancer Epstein-Barr virus CMV Infection Reye's syndrome	
Total bilirubin (mg/dL)	Bilirubin in blood	Adults: 0.3-1 Newborns: 1-12 *Possible critical values:* Adults: >12 Newborns: >15		
Direct bilirubin (mg/dL)	Bilirubin combined with another compound in liver	Adults: 0.1-0.3	Gallstones Extrahepatic duct obstruction Extensive liver metastasis Cholestasis from drugs Dubin-Johnson syndrome Rotor's syndrome	
Albumin (g/dL)	Protein that is formed in the liver; constitutes approximately 60% of total protein	Adults/elderly: 3.5-5 Premature infants: 3.4-2 Newborns: 3.5-5.4 Infants: 4.4-5.4 Children: 4-5.9	Dehydration	Malnutrition Pregnancy Liver disease Protein-losing enteropathies Protein-losing neuropathies Third-space losses Overhydration Increased capillary permeability Inflammatory disease Familial idiopathic dysproteinemia
Total protein (g/dL)	Albumin plus all other proteins (including antibodies)	Adults/elderly: 6.4-8.3 Premature infants: 4.2-7.6 Newborns: 4.6-7.4 Infant: 6-6.7 Children: 6.2-8		
Ammonia (μg/dL)	Liver converts ammonia from blood to urea	Adults: 10-80 Children: 40-80 Newborns: 90-150	Liver failure	

Note: Other tests related to hepatic function may be ordered in addition to the tests found in this table.
CMV, cytomegalovirus; *DKA,* diabetic ketoacidosis; *MI,* myocardial infarction.

ALBUMIN. Serum albumin is the most important of the LFTs to the PT. Albumin is a serum protein. Proteins are the most significant components of the serum that contribute to maintaining appropriate osmotic pressure within the vasculature. This pressure keeps fluid within the vascular space, minimizing extravasation (third spacing) of fluid.[26]

Albumin is formed in the liver and makes up approximately two thirds of the total protein in the plasma. Other than maintaining colloidal osmotic pressure, albumin transports blood constituents, such as drugs, hormones, and enzymes.[26] When the liver is affected by disease, it loses some of its ability to synthesize albumin.

Normal serum albumin level is 3.5 to 5 g/dL. Decreased albumin levels can be associated with malnutrition, malabsorption, liver disease, kidney disease, burns, and severe trauma. Low serum albumin can result in decreased protein synthesis, increased protein loss (nephritic syndrome), protein malnutrition, and third spacing of fluid (loss of proper osmotic pressure). Increased albumin can be seen in cases of severe dehydration.

Albumin is also a measure of nutrition. Poor nutrition with a serum albumin level less than 3.5 g/dL can lead to impaired wound healing. Maintaining appropriate albumin levels is important in critically ill patients and in surgical patients. Many patients with multiple active medical problems, especially elderly patients, have poor appetites and are at risk for poor nutrition. The PT should educate patients regarding the importance of proper nutrition for wound healing and increasing functional capacity.

PHYSICAL THERAPY IMPLICATIONS RELATED TO LIVER FUNCTION TESTS. When liver dysfunction is indicated, the patient should be monitored for signs and symptoms of hepatic disease, such as right upper quadrant pain and musculoskeletal pain. The patient may also have changes in mental status, especially with an increase in serum ammonia. There may be significant edema with third spacing of fluid in the abdomen, or *ascites,* or throughout the body, *anasarca.* A patient with severe liver dysfunction is at increased risk of coagulopathy and infection and requires careful practice of standard precautions.

The heart tries to compensate for fluid shifts and alterations in vascular status as a result of liver dysfunction, necessitating the monitoring of vital signs. Heart failure can occur when collateral circulation can no longer support body systems.

When liver dysfunction results in increased blood ammonia and urea levels, peripheral nerve function can also be impaired. Asterixis and numbness or tingling (misinterpreted as carpal or tarsal tunnel syndrome) can occur as a result of this ammonia abnormality, causing intrinsic nerve pathology.

Albumin, glucose, hemoglobin, and hematocrit levels can help assess nutritional status and monitor wound healing. Guidelines for impaired nutrition and wound healing from the Agency for Health Care Policy and Research specify an albumin level of less than 3.5 g/dL and total lymphocyte count of 1800/mm³. These considerations must be taken into account in planning interventions.[3,12]

Other Miscellaneous Laboratory Tests

THYROID FUNCTION. In a survey of women in an outpatient orthopedic setting, hypothyroidism was reported by 7%, and hyperthyroidism was reported by 1%.[5] The percentages for the overall physical therapy population are probably equal or greater. Tests used to assess thyroid function include thyroid-stimulating hormone, total thyroxine (T_4), free T_4, and triiodothyronine (T_3). Mitchem[22] provides more complete information on thyroid testing.

PHYSICAL THERAPY IMPLICATIONS FOR THYROID FUNCTION TESTS. With adequate replacement therapy for hypothyroidism, individuals are euthyroid and present no particular problem to the PT. Replacement needs vary over time, however, and these patients may become hyperthyroid or hypothyroid. Signs and symptoms of these conditions include myalgia, arthralgia, and numbness, all symptoms for which the patient may seek physical therapy.

Some forms of fibromyalgia present a "hypothyroid tendency" (symptoms with thyroid function tests within the reference ranges). Compromised conversion of T_4 to T_3 may lead to neuromuscular molecular abnormality exhibited by stiffness, aching, decreased basal body temperature, constipation, and dry skin.[12,17,20]

Skeletal Muscle Pathology

Tests commonly associated with diagnosis of skeletal muscle pathology include CPK, CPK isoenzymes, lactate dehydrogenase, aspartate aminotransferase, myoglobin, and cTnT. All these analytes are found in cardiac and skeletal muscle and increase with skeletal muscle injury. Differentiating the source of increased levels of each in the blood is important.

Physical Therapy Implications of Skeletal Muscle Tests

Skeletal muscle injury is uncommonly assessed with blood tests. These tests are performed most often to assess cardiac muscle injury. There is no group of laboratory tests used clinically that provides cost-effective information to assess skeletal muscle directly. The history and symptoms of the patient are usually the most significant sources of information assisting the PT in the evaluation.

Uric Acid

Uric acid is a waste product of cellular metabolism. It is formed primarily in the liver and excreted mainly by the kidneys, but some is also excreted by the gastrointestinal tract. Elevated uric acid levels, *hyperuricemia,* can be caused by an increase in production or by a decrease in excretion, or both. Uric acid levels are increased in gouty arthritis and in renal failure. Normal adult values for uric acid are 4 to 8.5 mg/dL for men and 2.7 to 7.3 mg/dL for women.[26]

Gouty arthritis is a disorder that is commonly seen by the PT. When a uric acid level is ordered, the PT should consider that the patient may have gouty arthritis. Gout is seen predominantly in men older than 45 years. The risk of gout increases with the degree of hyperuricemia. The pathogenesis of gout is closely related to the solubility of urate crystals in body fluids. Overproduction of uric acid accounts for only 10% of the cases of gout, whereas 90% are accounted for by underexcretion of uric acid.

Summary

In the practice of clinical medicine, health care professionals use laboratory tests to provide insight into the physiologic processes of the human body. This insight is used in conjunction with physical findings and patient history. It is incumbent on the PT to understand the rationale for such tests and the implications of test results on physical therapy practice. When knowledge of tests or the implications of their results are unclear to the PT, learning and consultation are encouraged. Laboratory personnel, attending physicians, nurses, and pathologists are valuable resources for information about such laboratory tests.

The tests discussed in this chapter do not constitute an exhaustive list of tests available. The tests discussed here are some of the more commonly performed clinical laboratory assays. Laboratory test reports provide the results and reference ranges and other information that assists in interpreting the results. The complete report, along with the history and physical findings, assists with clinical decision making.

Knowledge of laboratory tests can help a PT provide more cost-effective care for patients. The PT may observe symptoms in a patient that signal the need for additional medical attention; the PT may observe shortness of breath in an elderly patient and confirm an abnormal Sao_2 by pulse oximetry. The PT would then consult with the patient's primary care physician regarding observations and findings. The physician would pursue additional tests based on medical necessity. In this example, the PT began collecting valuable information via noninvasive pulse oximetry rather than immediately suggesting that the patient be referred for arterial blood gases, which is an invasive test that is much more costly to perform.

Knowledge of laboratory tests and the physical therapy implications of abnormal results assist the PT in making sound clinical judgments regarding the appropriateness of various interventions and the expected response of patients to rehabilitation exercise. As part of the health care team for a patient, the PT must be able to converse intelligently with other health care professionals about such tests and understand and defend clinical decisions made with regard to their results. For a summary of laboratory tests, values, and implications for physical therapy practice, see Table 15-18. A list of common abbreviations and a chapter glossary are located at the end of the chapter.

TABLE 15-18

Summary of Laboratory Tests, Values, and Implications for Physical Therapy Practice*

Test (units)	Normal Values	Found in Text under *HEADING*/Common Causes of Abnormal Values	Physical Therapy Practice Implications
Activated partial thromboplastin time, partial thromboplastin time (APTT, PTT) (sec)	APTT: 30-40 PTT: 60-70 Patients receiving anticoagulation therapy: 2-2.5× reference range *Possible critical values:* APTT: >70 PTT: >100	*HEMOSTASIS* *Increased in* Clotting factor deficiencies Cirrhosis of the liver Vitamin K deficiency DIC Heparin administration *Decreased in* Early stages of DIC Extensive cancer	If significantly elevated, risk for bleeding If patient is receiving intravenous heparin therapy and values indicate that patient is supratherapeutic, health care team should be consulted
Albumin (g/dL)	Adults/elderly: 3.5-5 Premature infants: 3.4-2 Newborns: 3.5-5.4 Infants: 4.4-5.4 Children: 4-5.9	*HEPATIC FUNCTION* *Increased in* Dehydration *Decreased in* Pregnancy Liver disease Third-space losses Overhydration Increased capillary permeability Inflammatory disease	Impaired wound healing with albumin level <3.5 *If results indicate liver dysfunction:* May see change in mental status, edema, RUQ pain Increased risk of infection Heart compensates for fluid shift, monitor vital signs Risk of coagulopathy With increased serum ammonia and urea, can have peripheral nerve dysfunction and CNS dysfunction Prolonged effects of medications normally detoxified by liver
Brain natriuretic peptide (BNP) (pg/mL)	<100	*CARDIAC STATUS* *Increased in* CHF MI Systemic HTN Cor pulmonale Heart transplant rejection	100 is threshold for diagnosis of CHF

TABLE 15-18

Summary of Laboratory Tests, Values, and Implications for Physical Therapy Practice*—cont'd

Test (units)	Normal Values	Found in Text under *HEADING*/Common Causes of Abnormal Values	Physical Therapy Practice Implications
Bicarbonate (HCO₃) (mEq/L)	Adults/children: 21-28 Newborns/infants: 16-24 *Possible critical values:* <15 or >40	*ACID-BASE BALANCE* *Increased in* Metabolic alkalosis Compensated respiratory acidosis *Decreased in* Metabolic acidosis Compensated respiratory alkalosis	Therapy generally contraindicated when ABG values are in critical range
Blood urea nitrogen (BUN) (mg/dL)	Adults: 10-20 Elderly: may be slightly more than adults Children: 5-18 Infants: 5-18 Newborns: 3-12 Cord: 21-40 *Possible critical values:* >100	*KIDNEY FUNCTION* *Increased in* Renal disease/impairment Shock Burns Upper gastrointestinal bleeding *Decreased in* Liver failure Malnutrition/malabsorption	No specific contraindications associated with abnormal values If severe, watch for lethargy or confusion Be aware of complications of renal disease
Calcium (Ca) (mg/dL)	Adults: 9-10.5 Elderly: values tend to decrease Children >2 yr: 8.8-10.8 10 days–2 yr: 9-10.6 <10 days: 7.6-10.4 *Possible critical values:* <6 or >13	*ELECTROLYTES* *Increased in* Hyperparathyroidism Metastasis to bone Prolonged immobilization Addison's disease Hyperthyroidism *Decreased in* Hypoparathyroidism Renal failure Vitamin D deficiency Malabsorption	Watch for signs of tetany
Cholesterol, total (mg/dL)	Adults: <200 Children: 120-200 Infants: 70-175 Newborns: 53-135	*CARDIOVASCULAR DISEASE RISK* See HDLs, LDLs, TGs	Increased values indicate CVD risk
Chloride (Cl) (mEq/L)	Adults: 98-106 Children: 90-110 Newborns: 96-106 Premature infants: 95-110 *Possible critical values:* <80 or >115	*ELECTROLYTES* *Increased in* Cushing's syndrome Kidney dysfunction *Decreased in* SIADH Vomiting Chronic gastric suction Addison's disease Burns	No specific contraindications associated with abnormal values
Creatine kinase–MB (CK-MB)	0%	*CARDIAC STATUS* *Increased in* Cardiac insult/injury including acute MI	When cardiac enzymes are ordered, therapy is contraindicated until all sets are negative for acute MI or until elevated enzymes have been shown to be decreasing
Creatine phosphokinase (CPK, CK) (U/L)	Adults Men: 55-170 Women: 30-135 *Values are higher after exercise* Newborns: 68-580	*CARDIAC STATUS* *Increased in* Injury to skeletal muscle, cardiac muscle, or brain	When cardiac enzymes are ordered, therapy is contraindicated until all sets are negative for acute MI or until elevated enzymes have been shown to be decreasing

Continued

TABLE 15-18

Summary of Laboratory Tests, Values, and Implications for Physical Therapy Practice*—cont'd

Test (units)	Normal Values	Found in Text under *HEADING*/Common Causes of Abnormal Values	Physical Therapy Practice Implications
Creatinine (Cr) (mg/dL)	Adults Men: 0.6-1.2 Women: 0.5-1.1 Adolescents: 0.5-1 Children: 0.3-0.7 Infants: 0.2-0.4 Newborns: 0.3-1.2 *Possible critical values: >4 (serious renal impairment)*	*KIDNEY FUNCTION* *Increased in* Renal disease/impairment Dehydration *Decreased in* Debilitation Decreased muscle mass	No specific contraindications associated with abnormal values If severe, watch for lethargy or confusion Be aware of complications of renal disease
Glucose (mg/dL)	Adults (and children >2 yr) Fasting: 70-110 Casual: ≤200 Children <2 yr: 60-100 Infants: 40-90 Neonates: 30-60 Premature infants: 20-60 Cord: 45-96 *Possible critical values:* Men: <50 or >400 Women: <40 or >400 Infants: <40 Newborns: <30 or >300	*CARBOHYDRATE METABOLISM* *Increased in* DM Acute stress response Cushing's syndrome Acute pancreatitis Corticosteroid therapy *Decreased in* Insulin overdose Starvation	Rehabilitation exercise contraindicated if <60 or >300 In acute care, caution with levels >250 PTs should understand and monitor for signs and symptoms of hyperglycemia and hypoglycemia
Glycosylated hemoglobin (GHb, GHB, HbA$_{1c}$) (%)	Nondiabetic adults/children: 4-5.9 Good diabetic control: <7 Fair diabetic control: 8-9 Poor diabetic control: >9	*CARBOHYDRATE METABOLISM* *Increased in* Poorly controlled DM	No specific contraindications associated with abnormal values
Hemoglobin (Hgb) (g/dL)	Adults Men: 14-18 Women: 12-16 Pregnancy: >11 Elderly: values slightly decreased Children Newborns: 14-24 0-2 wk: 12-20 2-6 mo: 10-17 6 mo–6 yr: 9.5-14 6-18 yr: 10-15.5 *Possible critical values: <5 or >20*	*CELLULAR COMPONENTS* *Increased in* Dehydration/hemoconcentration COPD CHF Severe burns *Decreased in* Anemia Hemorrhage Hemolysis	Resistive exercise if >10 Expect low endurance if <10 In the presence of active cerebrovascular, cardiac, or renal disease, monitor closely if Hgb <9 If low Hgb because of blood loss (i.e., postoperative patients), monitor for orthostatic hypotension Watch for orders for patient to be transfused when Hgb becomes too low (<7)
Hematocrit (Hct) (%)	Adults Men: 42-52 Women: 37-47 Pregnancy: >33 Elderly: values may be slightly decreased Children Newborns: 44-64 2-8 wk: 39-59 2-6 mo: 35-50 6 mo–1 yr: 29-43 1-6 yr: 30-40 6-18 yr: 32-44 *Possible critical values: <15 or >60*	*CELLULAR COMPONENTS* See hemoglobin	Light exercise if >25 Resistive exercise if >30 Depending on comorbidities, exercise may be appropriate at much lower levels

TABLE 15-18

Summary of Laboratory Tests, Values, and Implications for Physical Therapy Practice*—cont'd

Test (units)	Normal Values	Found in Text under *HEADING*/Common Causes of Abnormal Values	Physical Therapy Practice Implications
High-density lipoproteins (HDLs) (mg/dL)	Men: >45 Women: >55	*CARDIOVASCULAR DISEASE RISK* *Increased in* Hereditary factors Excessive exercise *Decreased in* Hereditary factors Metabolic syndrome Liver disease Hypoproteinemia	No specific contraindications associated with abnormal values
International normalized ratio (INR)	0.9-1.1 *Possible critical values: >5.5*	*HEMOSTASIS* *Increased in* Liver dysfunction Vitamin K deficiency DIC Warfarin therapy	*Patients not receiving anticoagulation:* May want to discuss with physician if >2 Watch for signs/symptoms of active bleeding Exercise caution with rehabilitative exercise if INR >3 because patient at risk of hemarthrosis *Patients receiving oral anticoagulation therapy:* Anticoagulated patients are at relative risk for spontaneous bleeding if INR >5 *Therapeutic range:* Post CVA, deep vein thrombosis: 2-3 Post mechanical heart valve: 2.5-3.5
Low-density lipoproteins (LDLs) (mg/dL)	60-180	*CARDIOVASCULAR DISEASE RISK* *Increased in* Hereditary factors Nephrotic syndrome Glycogen storage diseases Hypothyroidism Alcohol consumption Liver disease Cushing's syndrome *Decreased in* Hereditary factors Hypoproteinemia Hyperthyroidism	No specific contraindications associated with abnormal values
Oxygen saturation (Sao_2) (%)	Adults/children: 95-100 Elderly: 95 Newborns: 40-90 *Possible critical values: ≤75*	*ACID-BASE BALANCE* *Decreased in* Any condition that causes decrease in Po_2 levels—although this is not a linear relationship	Activity should stop when Sao_2 falls below appropriate level Activity contraindicated if patient cannot maintain appropriate Sao_2 level at rest *Additionally* Use pulse oximetry when appropriate Watch for hypoxemia at rest or with activity Watch for postexertional desaturation Watch for clinical symptoms Follow titration orders for supplemental O_2
Partial pressure of carbon dioxide (Pco_2) (mEq/L)	Adults/children: 35-45 Children <2 yr: 26-41 *Possible critical values: <20 or >60*	*ACID-BASE BALANCE* *Increased in* Respiratory acidosis Compensated metabolic alkalosis *Decreased in* Respiratory alkalosis Compensated metabolic acidosis	Therapy generally contraindicated when ABG values are in critical range

Continued

TABLE 15-18

Summary of Laboratory Tests, Values, and Implications for Physical Therapy Practice*—cont'd

Test (units)	Normal Values	Found in Text under *HEADING*/Common Causes of Abnormal Values	Physical Therapy Practice Implications
Partial pressure of oxygen (Po_2) (mm Hg)	Adults/children: 80-100 Newborns: 60-70 *Possible critical values: <40*	*ACID-BASE BALANCE* *Increased in* Polycythemia Hyperoxygenation Hyperventilation *Decreased in* Anemias Acute/chronic respiratory or cardiac dysfunction	Therapy generally contraindicated when ABG values are in critical range
pH	Adults/children: 7.35-7.45 Newborns: 7.32-7.49 2 mo–2 yr: 7.34-7.46 *Possible critical values: <7.25 or >7.55*	*ACID-BASE BALANCE* *Increased in* Metabolic or respiratory alkalosis *Decreased in* Metabolic or respiratory acidosis	Therapy generally contraindicated when ABG values are in critical range
Platelet count (Plt) (per mm³)	Adults/elderly: 150,000-400,000 Premature infants: 100,000-300,000 Newborns: 150,000-300,000 Infants: 200,000-475,000 Children: 150,000-400,000	*CELLULAR COMPONENTS* *Increased in* Some hematologic malignancies *Decreased in* Some hematologic malignancies Thrombocytopenia caused by various drug therapies	>50,000—resistive exercise can continue <20,000—discuss with physician because spontaneous bleeding is a serious danger PT must be cautious with handling patients who have low platelet count to avoid bruising >40,000—spontaneous bleeding is rare, but prolonged bleeding from surgery or trauma may occur
Potassium (K^+) (mEq/L)	Adults/elderly: 3.5-4 Children: 3.4-4.7 Infants: 4.1-5.3 Newborns: 3.9-5.9 *Possible critical values:* Adults: <2.5 or >6.5 Newborns: <2.5 or >8	*ELECTROLYTES* *Increased in* Excessive intake Acute CRF Hypoaldosteronism Crush injury to tissues Dehydration *Decreased in* Deficient intake Burns/trauma Gastrointestinal disorders (diarrhea, vomiting) Diuretics Hyperaldosteronism Cushing's syndrome Insulin administration	Cardiac status should be monitored closely before, during, and after exercise <3.2 or >5.1 mmol/L may contraindicate physical therapy because of the risks for arrhythmia Individuals with CRF may tolerate levels of 5.5
Sodium (Na^+) (mEq/L)	Adults/elderly: 136-145 Children: 136-145 Infants: 134-150 Newborns 134-144 *Possible critical values:* <120 or >160	*ELECTROLYTES* *Increased in* Excessive intake Cushing's syndrome Hyperaldosteronism Burns *Decreased in* Deficient intake Addison's disease Diarrhea Vomiting SIADH	Mental status changes may occur when sodium values are abnormal Monitor for symptoms of low sodium levels including weakness, confusion, stupor, hypotension, seizures, edema, and weight gain
Total protein (g/dL)	Adults/elderly: 6.4-8.3 Premature infants: 4.2-7.6 Newborns: 4.6-7.4 Infants: 6-6.7 Children: 6.2-8	*HEPATIC FUNCTION* See albumin	

TABLE 15-18

Summary of Laboratory Tests, Values, and Implications for Physical Therapy Practice*—cont'd

Test (units)	Normal Values	Found in Text under *HEADING*/Common Causes of Abnormal Values	Physical Therapy Practice Implications
Triglycerides (TGs) (mg/dL)	Adults/elderly Men: 40-60 Women: 35-135 Children 0-5 yr, boys: 30-86; girls: 32-99 6-11 yr, boys: 31-108; girls: 35-114 12-15 yr, boys: 36-138; girls: 41-138 16-19 yr, boys: 40-163; girls: 40-128 *Possible critical values: >400*	*CARDIOVASCULAR DISEASE RISK* *Increased in* Glycogen storage disease Hyperlipidemias Hypothyroidism High-carbohydrate diet Nephrotic syndrome Alcoholic cirrhosis *Decreased in* Malnutrition/malabsorption Hyperthyroidism	No specific contraindications associated with abnormal values
Troponin (cTnT, cTnI) (ng/mL)	cTnT: <0.2 cTnI: <0.03	*CARDIAC STATUS* *Increased in* Myocardial injury MI	When cardiac enzymes are ordered, therapy is contraindicated until all sets are negative for MI or until elevated enzymes have been shown to be decreasing
WBC count (WBC) (per mm^3)	Adults/children >2 yr: 5000-10,000 Children ≤2 yr: 6200-17,000 Newborns: 9000-30,000 *Possible critical values:* <2500 or >30,000	*CELLULAR COMPONENTS* *Increased in* Infection Leukemia Trauma Tissue necrosis Inflammation Use of steroid medications *Decreased in* Bone marrow failure Overwhelming infections Autoimmune disease	In the presence of sepsis, caution is in order If there is hemodynamic compromise, therapy may be contraindicated until infection is controlled If <5000/mm^3 and fever >100° F, exercise may be contraindicated If <1000/mm^3, patient may be in reverse isolation or neutropenic precautions—follow isolation precautions

*This chart contains some of the laboratory tests and values important in rehabilitation exercise.
ABG, arterial blood gas; *CHF,* congestive heart failure; *CNS,* central nervous system; *COPD,* chronic obstructive pulmonary disease; *CRF,* chronic renal failure; *CVA,* cerebrovascular accident; *CVD,* cardiovascular disease; *DIC,* disseminated intravascular coagulopathy; *DM,* diabetes mellitus; *HTN,* hypertension; *MI,* myocardial infarction; *RUQ,* right upper quadrant; *SIADH,* syndrome of inappropriate antidiuretic hormone secretion.
Data adapted from Pagana KD, Pagana TJ: *Mosby's diagnostic and laboratory test reference,* 9th ed, St Louis, 2009, Mosby.

TABLE 15-19

Panels and Shorthand Schematics

Panel	Constituents of Panel	Shorthand Schematic
Complete blood count (CBC)	Hemoglobin (Hgb) Hematocrit (Hct) Red blood cell (RBC) count RBC indices White blood cell (WBC) count WBC with differential Platelet (Plt) count	WBC Hgb / Hct Plt
Basic metabolic panel (BMP or MPB)	Sodium (Na$^+$) Potassium (K$^+$) Chloride (Cl$^-$) Calcium (Ca^{++}) Carbon dioxide, predominantly bicarbonate form (HCO$_3^-$) Creatinine (Cr) Blood urea nitrogen (BUN) Glucose	Na$^+$ | Cl$^-$ | BUN / Glucose K$^+$ | HCO$_3^-$ | Cr

Continued

TABLE 15-19

Panels and Shorthand Schematics—cont'd

Panel	Constituents of Panel	Shorthand Schematic
Complete (comprehensive) metabolic panel (CMP)	Constituents of basic metabolic panel (above) and hepatic function panel (below)	
Hepatic function panel	Alkaline phosphatase (ALP) Alanine aminotransferase (ALT) Aspartate aminotransferase (AST) Albumin Total protein Total bilirubin Direct bilirubin	
Arterial blood gases (ABGs)	pH Partial pressure of carbon dioxide dissolved in the plasma (Pco_2) Partial pressure of oxygen dissolved in the plasma (Po_2) Bicarbonate (HCO_3^-) Oxygen saturation (Sao_2)	pH | Pco_2 | HCO_3^- | Po_2 | Sao_2

CUMULATIVE CASE SCENARIOS

Case 1

You have received an inpatient referral to evaluate and treat a 68-year-old woman admitted with a diagnosis of upper gastrointestinal bleed. Her past medical history is significant for insulin-dependent diabetes mellitus, CAD, and ESRD. A portion of the laboratory section of the patient's chart reveals the following information from the last 2 days:

1. How would you correlate the abnormal findings for laboratory values with what you already know about this patient?
2. Based on the laboratory values provided, would this patient be appropriate to participate in rehabilitation exercise?
3. What are some specific things that you would monitor for, given the laboratory findings?
4. Is there a point-of-care test that could provide you with more current information related to this patient's appropriateness for exercise?

Case 2

You have received an inpatient referral to evaluate and treat a 57-year-old man admitted through the emergency department with the diagnosis of chest pain. Significant physician orders are for cTnI every 8 hours × 3.

A portion of the laboratory section of the patient's chart reveals the following from earlier today:

CHEMISTRY	
PROCEDURE:	TROPONIN I
UNITS:	NG/ML
REF. RANGE:	[0.00-0.10]
1/15/09 0812	1.72 H
1/15/09 1130	1.37 H

1. Based on this patient's laboratory values, is he appropriate to participate in the physical therapy evaluation at this time?

CHEMISTRY					
PROCEDURE:	BUN	CREATININE			
UNITS:	MG/DL	MG/DL			
REF. RANGE:	[8-21]	[0.7-1.3]			
1/14/09 0130	50 H	2.4 H			
1/15/09 0943	58 H	2.6 H			
PROCEDURE:	GLUCOSE				
UNITS:	MG/DL				
REF. RANGE:	[70-99]				
1/14/09 0130	367 H				
1/15/09 0452	147 H				
01/15/09 0943	80				

HEMATOLOGY						
PROCEDURE:	WBC	HBG	HCT	PLT	MPV	RBC
UNITS:	K/UL	GM/DL	%	K/UL	M/UL	M/UL
REF. RANGE:	[4.0-1.0]	[12.0-16.0]	[36.0-48.0]	[150-400]	[9.0-13.0]	[4.00-5.30]
1/15/09 0130	7.4	8.5 L	27.4 L	356	11.0	3.32 L

Case 3

You have received an inpatient referral to evaluate and treat (POD #0 through discharge) a 78-year-old man with a history of bilateral knee degenerative joint disease that has failed conservative treatment. The patient had bilateral quadriceps-sparing total knee replacements this morning at your facility. Comorbidities include hypertension, CAD status post angioplasty with stenting 2 years prior, and gastroesophageal reflux disease. At the time of initial evaluation, no postoperative laboratory test results are available.

1. With regard to the patient's laboratory values, what information is important to know before seeing the patient on POD #0?
2. Without a postoperative CBC, what other information might lead you to suspect a change in hemoglobin values?
3. With regard to the patient's laboratory values, what information is important to know before seeing the patient on POD #1?
4. How does this information guide your clinical decision-making process?

Case 4

You have received an outpatient referral to evaluate and treat a 62-year-old woman with COPD and stage IIIB non–small cell lung cancer. She is 1 month post radiation therapy and 2 weeks post chemotherapy. She has "overwhelming" weakness. Her medical oncologist has referred her to therapy.

1. What laboratory values are important to know before seeing this patient for evaluation?
2. What laboratory values would be important to follow during this patient's care?

DISCUSSION OF CUMULATIVE CASE SCENARIOS

Case 1

1. How would you correlate the abnormal findings for laboratory values with what you already know about this patient?

   BUN and creatinine—Elevated values of BUN and creatinine correlate with the patient's history of ESRD.

   Glucose—Elevated glucose values correlate with the patient's history of diabetes mellitus and indicate that her glucose was not under control at the time of admission.

   Hemoglobin/hematocrit, RBC—Decreased hemoglobin/hematocrit and RBC values correlate with the patient's diagnosis of upper gastrointestinal bleed.

2. Based on the laboratory values provided, would this patient be appropriate to participate in rehabilitation exercise?

   BUN and creatinine—Although elevated, these values do not contraindicate participate in rehabilitation exercise.

   Glucose—Although elevated on admission, the last value was well within the normal range and would not contraindicate participate in rehabilitation exercise.

   Hemoglobin/hematocrit, RBC—Although decreased, these values alone may not contraindicate participation in rehabilitation exercise. To assist in your clinical decision, you would check the patient's vital sign record and look for any indication of intention to transfuse the patient or any anginal complaints from the patient.

3. What are some specific things that you would monitor for, given the laboratory findings?

   BUN and creatinine—You should be aware of the complications of renal disease. When BUN and creatinine are extremely elevated, you should monitor for lethargy or confusion or both.

   Glucose—You should monitor the patient for signs and symptoms of hypoglycemia or hyperglycemia.

   Hemoglobin/hematocrit, RBC—You should monitor vital signs with this patient (including assessment for orthostatic hypotension) and assess for any complaints of angina (especially given the patient's history of CAD).

4. Is there a point-of-care test that could provide you with more current information related to this patient's appropriateness for exercise?

   A point-of-care glucose test can give you a current reading of the patient's glucose level, which may have changed since the last charted result, particularly if the patient has eaten or received insulin.

Case 2

1. Based on this patient's laboratory values, is he appropriate to participate in the physical therapy evaluation at this time?

   The latest elevated cTnI value would not contraindicate therapy because the value is decreasing compared with the previous result. It is not necessary to wait for the results of the third test to make a clinical decision. Your decision regarding the patient's appropriateness for physical therapy should not be based on laboratory values alone. Important questions to ask regarding this patient include the following:
   - Anginal symptoms
   - Vital signs
   - Level of alertness
   - Other pending tests/procedures (echocardiogram, cardiac catheterization)

Case 3

1. With regard to the patient's laboratory values, what information is important to know before seeing the patient on POD #0?
   preoperative CBC, especially hemoglobin
2. Without a postoperative CBC, what other information might lead you to suspect a change in hemoglobin values?
   Patients lose blood during surgical procedures. The operative note can provide you with information regarding *surgical blood loss* and *fluid provided* during the procedure.
   Blood loss via drains may also be informative.
3. With regard to the patient's laboratory values, what information is important to know before seeing the patient on POD #1?
   CBC, especially hemoglobin
   Note: You could also look for information related to intravenous fluid volume provided and any blood products. In addition, you would monitor vital signs.
4. How does this information guide your clinical decision-making process?
   In a postoperative patient, this information can provide you with *expectations of orthostasis and activity tolerance*.

Case 4

1. What laboratory values are important to know before seeing this patient for evaluation?
   CBC—You would want to know the most recent CBC results to determine whether the patient is close to her nadir for her chemotherapy dose, at which time you can expect her counts to be low. You need to know how low the counts are to determine the appropriate precautions related to rehabilitation exercise and whether or not communication with the physician is needed.

   ABGs if available—If ABGs are available, you can use them to determine whether this patient is generally hypoxic at baseline or whether this patient is classified as a carbon dioxide retainer. This information would assist in your clinical decisions while monitoring the patient's Sao_2.

2. What laboratory values would be important to follow during this patient's care?

CBC—As discussed previously.

Monitor Sao₂—You cannot follow repeated ABGs for this information. Sao_2 measurements can provide you with a timely reflection of what the patient's Po_2 value is and how it is affected by exercise.

Common Abbreviations

ACTH—adrenocorticotropic hormone
AIDS—acquired immunodeficiency syndrome
ALP—alkaline phosphatase
ALT—alanine aminotransferase
ANA—antinuclear antibody
ANC—absolute neutrophil count
APTT—activated partial thromboplastin time
ARDS—acute respiratory distress syndrome
ARF—acute renal failure
AST—aspartate aminotransferase
BMP—basic metabolic panel
BNP—brain natriuretic peptide
BUN—blood urea nitrogen
Ca^{++}—calcium
CAD—coronary artery disease
CBC—complete blood count
CHF—congestive heart failure
CK—creatine phosphokinase
Cl^-—chloride
CLIA—Clinical Laboratory Improvement Amendments
CMP—complete metabolic panel
CMV—cytomegalovirus
CNS—central nervous system
CO_2—carbon dioxide
COPD—chronic obstructive pulmonary disease
CPK—creatine phosphokinase
Cr—creatinine
CRF—chronic renal failure
CRP—C-reactive protein
CRRT—continuous renal replacement therapy
cTnT, cTnI—cardiac troponins
CVA—cerebrovascular accident
CVD—cardiovascular disease
DIC—disseminated intravascular coagulopathy
DJD—degenerative joint disease
DKA—diabetic ketoacidosis
DM—diabetes mellitus
EF—ejection fraction
ESR—erythrocyte sedimentation rate
ESRD—end-stage renal disease
GERD—gastroesophageal reflux disease
GFR—glomerular filtration rate
GHb, GHB—glycosylated hemoglobin
HbA_{1c}—glycosylated hemoglobin
HCO_3^-—bicarbonate
Hct—hematocrit
HD—hemodialysis
HDLs—high-density lipoproteins

Hg, Hgb—hemoglobin
H/H—hemoglobin and hematocrit
HIV—human immunodeficiency virus
hsCRP—high-sensitivity C-reactive protein
HTN—hypertension
IDDM—insulin-dependent diabetes mellitus
IMA—ischemia-modified albumin
INR—international normalized ratio
ITP—idiopathic thrombocytopenia purpura
K^+—potassium
LDH—lactate dehydrogenase
LDLs—low-density lipoproteins
LFTs—liver function tests
LMWH—low-molecular-weight heparin
MCH—mean corpuscular hemoglobin
MCHC—mean corpuscular hemoglobin concentration
MCV—mean corpuscular volume
MPB—metabolic panel, basic
MS—multiple sclerosis
Na^+—sodium
NCEP—National Cholesterol Education Program
NYHA—New York Heart Association
OA—osteoarthritis
Pco_2—partial pressure of carbon dioxide
PD—peritoneal dialysis
Plt—platelets
PMN—polymorphonuclear neutrophil
Po_2—partial pressure of oxygen
POD—postoperative day
PRBCs—packed red blood cells
PSA—prostate-specific antigen
PT—prothrombin time
PTH—parathyroid hormone
PTT—partial thromboplastin time
RBC—red blood cell
RDW—red blood cell distribution width
RF—rheumatoid factor
RUQ—right upper quadrant
Sao_2—oxygen saturation
SIADH—syndrome of inappropriate antidiuretic hormone secretion
SLE—systemic lupus erythematosus
SVT—supraventricular tachycardia
TGs—triglycerides
TIA—transient ischemic attack
TKR—total knee replacement
WBC—white blood cell

Glossary of Terms Used in Chapter

Analyte—substance of interest within a sample
Anasarca—generalized massive edema
Anemia—decrease (below normal) in number of erythrocytes per mm³ or in quantity of hemoglobin or in volume of packed red blood cells per 100 mL of blood
Ascites—effusion and accumulation of serous fluid in the abdominal cavity
Assay—method of testing or detection

Cirrhosis—liver disease with loss of normal microscopic architecture

Hemoconcentration—decrease of fluid content of the blood, with resulting increase in its concentration

Hypercalcemia—elevated blood levels of calcium (above normal)

Hyperchloremia—elevated blood levels of chloride (above normal)

Hyperglycemia—elevated blood levels of glucose (above normal)

Hyperkalemia—elevated blood levels of potassium (above normal)

Hyperlipidemia—elevated blood lipid levels

Hypernatremia—elevated blood levels of sodium (above normal)

Hypocalcemia—decreased blood levels of calcium (below normal)

Hypochloremia—decreased blood levels of chloride (below normal)

Hypoglycemia—decreased blood levels of glucose (below normal)

Hypokalemia—decreased blood levels of potassium (below normal)

Hyponatremia—decreased blood levels of sodium (below normal)

Hypoxemia—deficient oxygenation of the blood

Hypoxia—reduction of oxygen supply to tissues below physiologic levels

Leukocytosis—increase in total WBC count (>10,000)

Leukopenia—decrease in total WBC count (<4000)

Nadir—lowest point; specifically with regard to patients receiving chemotherapy, it is the point at which cellular blood counts are at their lowest, which is usually 10 to 14 days after dose

Neutropenia—decreased blood levels of neutrophils (below normal)

Pancytopenia—deficiency of all cellular elements in the blood

Polycythemia—increase in total red blood cell mass of the blood

Reliability—reflects accuracy and precision of a test method

Sensitivity—conditional probability that a person having a disease would be correctly identified by a clinical test

Sepsis—presence in the blood or other tissues of pathogenic microorganisms or their toxins

Septicemia—systemic disease associated with presence and persistence of pathogenic microorganisms or their toxins in the blood

Specificity—conditional probability that a person not having a disease would be correctly identified by a clinical test

Thrombocytopenia—decreased blood levels of platelets (below normal)

Thrombocytosis—elevated blood levels of platelets (above normal)

REFERENCES

1. American Heart Association Recommendations: Cholesterol levels (website). http://www.americanheart.org/presenter.jhtml?identifier=4500. Accessed August 16, 2009.
2. American Society for Clinical Laboratory Science: Scope of practice position paper (website). http://www.ascls.org/position/scope_of_practice.asp. Accessed August 16, 2009.
3. Bergstrom N. Treatment of pressure ulcers, clinical practice guideline no. 15. Bethesda, MD: Agency for Health Care Policy and Research; 1994.
4. Bishop ML, Duben-Engelkirk JL, Fody EP. Clinical chemistry: principles, procedures, correlations. Philadelphia: Lippincott; 2000. pp 58–75.
5. Boissonnault WG. Prevalence of co-morbid conditions, surgeries and medication use in a physical therapy outpatient population: a multi-centered study. J Orthop Sports Phys Ther 1999;29:506–19.
6. Coresh J, Selvin E, Stevens LA, et al. Prevalence of chronic kidney disease in the United States. JAMA 2007;298:2038–47.
7. Cowie CC, Rust KF, Byrd-Holt DD, et al. Prevalence of diabetes and impaired fasting glucose in adults in the U.S. population: NHANES 1999-2002. Diabetes Care 2006;29:1263–8.
8. de Ferranti S, Rifai N. C-reactive protein: a nontraditional serum marker of cardiovascular risk. Cardiovasc Pathol 2007;16:14–21.
9. Din-Dzietham R, Liu Y, Bielo M-V, et al. High blood pressure trends in children and adolescents in national surveys, 1963 to 2002. Circulation 2007;116:1488–96.
10. Dufour DR. Clinical use of laboratory data: a practical guide. Baltimore: Williams & Wilkins; 1998. pp 3–13.
11. Dufour DR. Tips from the clinical experts. Medical Laboratory Observer August 2002. p 20.
12. Goodman CC, Fuller KS, Boissonnault WG. Pathology: implications for the physical therapist. 2nd ed. Philadelphia: Saunders; 2003. pp 1174–1197.
13. Heart Protection Study Collaborative Group. Effects of cholesterol-lowering with simvastatin on stroke and other major vascular events in 20536 people with cerebrovascular disease or other high-risk conditions. Lancet 2004;363:757–67.
14. Heart Protection Study Collaborative Group. MRC/BHF Heart Protection Study of cholesterol lowering with simvastatin in 20,536 high-risk individuals: a randomised placebo-controlled trial. Lancet 2002;360:7–22.
15. Hergenroeder AL. Implementation of a competency-based assessment for interpretation of laboratory values. Acute Care Perspectives 2006;15:7–15.
16. Hogenhuis J, Voors AA, Jaarsma T, et al. Lower prevalence of B-type natriuretic levels <100 pg/mL in patient with heart failure at hospital discharge. Am Heart J 2006;151;1012e1–e5.
17. Hulme JA. Fibromyalgia: a handbook for self care and treatment. 3rd ed. Missoula, MT: Phoenix Publishing; 2000.
18. Kleinman S, Addison KM: Indications for red cell transfusion in the adult (website). Last updated August 21, 2008. http://www.uptodate.com/patients/content/topic.do?topicKey=~PUZnAWY5WRgXpZ. Accessed August 16, 2009.
19. Kotlarz V. Tracing our roots: origins of clinical laboratory science. Clin Lab Sci 1998;11:5–7.
20. Lowe J, Reichman A, Yellin J. A case-control study of metabolic therapy for fibromyalgia: long-term follow-up comparison of treated and untreated patients. Clin Bull Myofascial Ther 1998;3:65–79.
21. Maisel AS, Krishnaswamy P, Nowak RM, et al. Rapid measurement of B-type natriuretic peptide in the emergency diagnosis of heart failure. N Engl J Med 2002;347:161–7.
22. Mitchem K. NACB releases updated thyroid testing guidelines. Clinical Laboratory News November 2002. p 18.
23. Murphy MF, Wallington TB, Kelsey P, et al. Guidelines for the clinical use of red cell transfusions. Br J Haematol 2001;113:24–31.
24. National Institutes of Health: The Third Report of the National Cholesterol Education Program (NCEP) Expert Panel on Detection, Evaluation, and Treatment of High Blood Cholesterol in Adults (Adult Treatment Panel III, or ATP III) presents the NCEP's updated clinical guidelines for cholesterol testing and management (website). http://www.nhlbi.nih.gov/guidelines/cholesterol/atp3_rpt.htm. Accessed August 16, 2009.
25. National Committee for Clinical Laboratory Standards. How to define and determine reference intervals in the clinical laboratory: approved guideline. 2nd ed. Wayne, PA: NCCLS; 2000.
26. Pagana KD, Pagana TJ. Mosby's diagnostic and laboratory test reference. 9th ed. St Louis: Mosby; 2009.
27. Pratt DS, Kaplan MM. Laboratory tests. In: Schiff ER, Sorrell MF, Maddrey WC, editors. Schiff's diseases of the liver. 9th ed. Philadelphia: Lippincott; 2003. p 221–56.
28. Rydberg EJ, Westfall JM, Nicholas RA, et al. Low-molecular-weight-heparin in preventing and treating DVT. Am Fam Physician 1999;59:1607–12.
29. Steg PT, Joubin L, McCord J, et al. B-type natriuretic peptide and echocardiographic determination of ejection fraction in the diagnosis of congestive heart failure in patients with acute dyspnea. Chest 2005;128:21–9.
30. Stein PD. Antithrombotic therapy in patients with mechanical and biological prosthetic heart valves. Chest 2001;119:220S–7S.

31. Tang WH, Girod JP, Lee MJ, et al. Plasma B-type natriuretic peptide levels in ambulatory patients with established chronic symptomatic systolic heart failure. Circulation 2003;108:2964–6.

32. Valentine V. The patient with diabetes mellitus. In: Lewis S, Heitkemper M, Dirksen S, editors. Medical-surgical nursing: assessment and management of clinical problems. 5th ed. St Louis: Mosby; 2000. p 1367–405.

33. Woodhouse S. C-reactive protein: from acute phase reactant to cardiovascular disease risk factor. Medical Laboratory Observer 2002;34:12–20.

34. Wu A. The ischemia-modified albumin biomarker for myocardial ischemia. Medical Laboratory Observer 2003;35:6.

The Pediatric and Adolescent Population 16

Kristine M. Hallisy, PT, MS, OCS, CMPT, CTI

Objectives

After reading this chapter, the reader will be able to:

1. Describe how population size, age, and gender affect the socioeconomic challenges our country will face in providing health care to adolescents.
2. Comprehend normal development of the child and adolescent (in utero to adulthood).
3. Explain how the psychosocial issues of the developing adolescent (puberty) may affect the development of an effective therapeutic alliance among the physical therapist, patient, and potential caregivers.
4. Explain the multisystem effects of puberty on the developing individual.
5. Comprehend the elements of the American Physical Therapy Association's model of patient management (evidence-based medicine) as it relates to adolescent patients.
6. Properly screen the adolescent for illnesses and conditions specific to this age group.
7. Select appropriate components of an examination for a child or adolescent with a neuromusculoskeletal injury.
8. Comprehend the special features of bone growth and development in the area of pediatric and adolescent neuromusculoskeletal injuries.
9. Explain the role of, and make appropriate referral for, diagnostic imaging of pediatric or adolescent patients with musculoskeletal injuries.
10. Differentiate common neuromusculoskeletal conditions and injuries seen in children and adolescents.
11. Understand and implement interventions, including health-promotion and wellness strategies, for pediatric or adolescent patients (see later, "Developing Healthy People 2020: The Road Ahead").

If we do not care for the children, who will care for the world when we grow old?

Anonymous

Adolescence (Latin, *adolescere,* to grow) is a transitional state of human physical and mental development comprised of unique psychosocial concerns, preferences, and expectations.[163] The teenager is literally in transition between the dependency of childhood and the responsibilities of adulthood. The onset of adolescence coincides with the onset of puberty (typically age 10 for girls and age 12 for boys) and is influenced by genetic (heredity) and environmental factors. The end of adolescence is culturally defined but inevitably comes with legal independence (age 21 in the United States) and the right and responsibility of self-direction.

This period of development is marked by major physiologic, intellectual, and emotional changes. To manage the adolescent patient effectively, the primary care physical therapist (PT) must comprehend the effects of hormonal changes on growth, structure, and function, as well as understand and respect the effect of motor learning and motor control on function. The state of the injury, disease, or surgical procedure and its potential rate of recovery, complications, precautions, and contraindications also are crucial concerns.

The societal role of the adolescent is to engage in family interactions, school, and community activities and possibly fulfill a role in a workplace. Unlike the stereotypical vision of youth, not all youngsters enjoy the carefree days of childhood. World, community, and family events profoundly affect the developing individual. Given these facts, the PT must consider some unique health needs and psychosocial factors when working with this population. The physical, emotional, and psychological state of the adolescent, along with the influence, or lack thereof, from caregivers or peers, can profoundly affect the therapeutic alliance between the health care provider and the adolescent. Failure to respect the adolescent's unique perspective on the world can damage the treatment outcome.

The size and composition of a population are important, because they reveal a nation's support burden. They indicate challenges that a country will face in providing health care to its children and older adults, education to its youth, employment opportunities to its adults (18 to 65 years of age), and support to its older population.[184] At 307.5 million people (4.53% of the world's 6.812 billion inhabitants), the United States is the third most populated country on Earth (estimate as of September 21, 2009).[265] Approximately one in four (24.7%), or 75.95 million, Americans are younger than 18 years of age, and 13.0% (39.98 million) are older than 65 years.[265] Because of declining birth rates and aging baby boomers, by 2030 an estimated 23.6% of the American population will be younger than 18 years, and approximately 71.5 million (over 20%) will be older than 65 years.

The net influence of this population shift is a declining workforce (ages 18 to 65 years) from 62.9% in 2010 to 56.7% by 2030. These demographic facts, along with the current economic climate in America (and worldwide), the rising number of uninsured Americans, and escalating health care costs, obligate health care practitioners to make conscientious choices when providing health care to patients of all ages.

The care of pediatric and adolescent patients (0 to 20 years) is paramount to the overall health and well-being of our society. Unfortunately, adolescents as a group are the primary users of illicit drugs, tobacco, and alcohol and make up the largest group with unwanted pregnancies, abortions, and sexually transmitted diseases (STDs).[120] Additionally, death and long-term disability from chronic illnesses is often preventable in this age group with adequate safety and prevention measures. Sadly, many teenagers fall through the cracks of the flawed American health care system, especially in the areas of mental health and prevention and educational services. Almost 40% of adolescents' health care is paid out of-pocket. In 2006, 13.8% of adolescents 13 through 18 years of age and 28.4% of older adolescents aged 19 through 21 were uninsured. Adolescents at greatest risk of being uninsured are older, are minorities, and have a low household income.[43]

Given the skyrocketing cost of health care, health care practitioners must empower their young patients to care for themselves by educating them in health promotion and wellness (see Chapter 19). Health promotion is not only the detection and prevention of disease but also the endorsement of well-being in the physical, cognitive, emotional, social, and spiritual domains.[39] With the use of a health promotion and wellness model (Box 16-1), physical therapy has the potential, and the responsibility, to improve the quality of life of all members of our society, including this chapter's vulnerable target population—the youth of America. (See later, "Developing Healthy People 2020: The Road Ahead," for more details.)

Preventive Health Care Across the Life Span

Regular preventive health care visits are integral to patient management (Figure 16-1). The American Academy of Pediatrics (AAP) has published age-appropriate guidelines for preventive health care visits for children (0 to 20 years of age). The partnership among the health care provider, the adolescent, and his or her family (whatever form that family takes) should provide and monitor these key components of pediatric health promotion:

- Age-appropriate developmental achievement of the child (e.g., physical maturation, gross and fine motor skills, cognitive achievements, emotional development, social competence, self-responsibility, integration with family and community)
- Health supervision visits that include periodic assessment of medical and oral health (e.g., regular review of systems, height, weight, head circumference [0 to 24 months],[63] heart rate, respiratory rate, temperature, blood pressure [older than 3 years], vision, hearing, developmental assessment, physical examination, age-appropriate immunizations)[14,71]
- Integration of physical examination findings with healthy lifestyles

---

BOX 16-1
Developing Healthy People

Since 1979, Healthy People has set and monitored national health objectives to meet a broad range of health needs, encourage collaboration across sectors, guide individuals toward making informed health decisions, and measure the impact of our prevention activity.[205] Every 10 years, the U.S. Department of Health and Human Services (HHS) leverages scientific insights and lessons learned from the past decade, along with new knowledge of current data, trends, and innovations.[205] As of March 2009, HHS has begun working on the Developing Healthy People 2020 framework related to our nation's health preparedness and prevention.

In 2000, Healthy People 2010 was designed to achieve two overarching goals:
- Goal 1: Increase Quality and Years of Healthy Life. Help individuals of all ages increase life expectancy and improve their quality of life.
- Goal 2: Eliminate Health Disparities. Eliminate health disparities among different segments of the population.[205]

In the Healthy People project, population-based objectives address health care needs according to variables such as age, race, gender, educational attainment, and socioeconomic status (income). The 10 leading health indicators of the Healthy People 2010 project were:
- Physical activity
- Overweight and obesity
- Tobacco use
- Substance use
- Responsible sexual behavior
- Mental health
- Injury and violence
- Environmental quality
- Immunization[14,70]
- Access to health care[70,205]

Healthy People challenges individuals, communities, and health care professionals, to take specific steps to ensure that all can enjoy good health, as well as long life.

Adapted from U.S. Department of Health and Human Services: *Healthy People 2020: the road ahead* (website). http://www.healthypeople.gov/HP2020; and from U.S. Department of Health and Human Services: *Healthy People 2010* (website). http://www.healthypeople.gov/Default.htm.

- Screening procedures and anticipatory guidance (e.g., emotional and mental health, healthy habits, nutrition, oral health,[23,67] peer relationships, prevention or recognition of illness, prevention of risky behaviors and addictions, safety and prevention of injury, self-responsibility and self-efficacy, sexual development and sexuality, community interactions, school and vocational achievement)[255]

Progression through the Tanner stages of sexual maturation identifies the adolescent as a unique subset of the pediatric population. Somatic, sexual, cognitive, moral, and social (e.g., self-identity and relationship to society) issues central to the developing adolescent are shown in Table 16-1. Relevant issues of development, musculoskeletal (MS) growth, and biomechanics across the pediatric life span follow and are shown in Table 16-2.

Overview: Fetal Development to Birth

Fetal development has three distinct stages—pre-embryonic period (0 to 3 weeks), embryonic period (3 to 8 weeks), and fetal period (8 weeks to full term).[56] The differentiation and proliferation of embryonic and fetal cells directly affect pediatric (0 to 20 years) growth and development. *Nelson Textbook of Pediatrics* is an essential text for information on fetal development, pediatric growth and maturation, and the hormonal cascade that stimulates normal and abnormal adolescent development.[163]

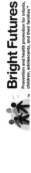

FIGURE 16-1 Recommendations for preventive pediatric health care. (From American Academy of Pediatrics. http://welcomepediatrics.com/visitation.html. Accessed April 8, 2010.)

TABLE 16-1

Central Issues in Early, Middle, and Late Adolescence

Variable	Early Adolescence	Middle Adolescence	Late Adolescence
Age (yr)	10-13	14-16	17-20 and beyond
Sexual maturity rating*	1-2	3-5	5
Somatic	Secondary sex characteristics; beginning of rapid growth; awkward	Height growth peaks; body shape and composition change; acne and odor; menarche; spermarche	Slower growth
Sexual	Sexual interest usually exceeds sexual activity	Sexual drive surges; experimentation; questions of sexual orientation	Consolidation of sexual identity
Cognitive and moral	Concrete operations; conventional morality	Emergence of abstract thought; questioning mores; self-centered	Idealism; absolutism
Self-concept	Preoccupation with changing body; self-consciousness	Concern with attractiveness; increasing introspection	Relatively stable body image
Family	Bids for increased independence; ambivalence	Continued struggle for acceptance of greater autonomy	Practical independence; family remains secure base
Peers	Same-sex groups; conformity; cliques	Dating; peer groups less important	Intimacy; possibly commitment
Relationship to society	Middle-school adjustment	Gauging skills and opportunities	Career decisions (e.g., dropout, college, work)

*Based on Tanner stages of development.
From Klingman RM, Behrman RE, Jenson HB, Stanton BF. *Nelson textbook of pediatrics*, ed 18, Philadelphia, 2007, Saunders Elsevier.

TABLE 16-2

Key Principles of Development Across the Pediatric Life Span

Period	Features
Infancy (0-12 mo)	Physical development is the most rapid of any age. Exploration of the environment is a key component of cognitive and language development. Social and emotional tasks include understanding of self and family, bonding, attachment to caregivers, and trust that physical needs will be met. *Consequences*: Delays in mapping of the sensorimotor cortex are created if physical, nutritional, social, and environmental needs are not met (i.e., the child is unable to appropriately interact with his or her environment).
Early childhood (1-4 yr)	Physical development slows to half the rate of infancy, and growth spurts begin. Gross motor skills, followed by fine motor skills, are acquired via maturation of the neurologic system. Language develops at extraordinary speed. Cognitive development is preoperational and lacks sustained logical thought processes as the child strives toward increased social independence and begins to set personal boundaries. Children either learn to be self-sufficient in many activities, including toileting, feeding, walking, and talking or beginning to doubt their own abilities. *Consequences*: Exposure to human interaction and verbal language exchange (e.g., reading to children) is imperative for language development, psychosocial development, and the attainment of developmental milestones.
Middle childhood (5-10 yr)	Physical growth is steady but at a slower rate than the preschool and adolescent periods. Cognitively, children are concretely operational in their thought processes and begin to display goal-directed exploration of the world. Environmental factors (e.g., family, culture, school) affect learning, self-esteem, social independence, interaction, and the development of self-efficacy. Moral development remains simple, but a child should display a clear knowledge of "right and wrong." *Consequences*: Failure to develop self-esteem in the child's major social structures can lead to guilt and poor self-esteem. Children with physical disabilities and chronic illness begin to face more environmental challenges that may prevent learning and development.
Adolescence (11-20 yr)	Physical transition from childhood to adulthood with extensive endocrine-mediated changes. The adolescent proceeds through the Tanner stages of development. Cognitive development progresses to formal operational thinking; adolescents acquire the ability to reason logically and abstractly, and consider future implications of current actions. Socially and emotionally, this can be a tumultuous time marked by the transition from family-dominated influences to peer influence and increasing autonomy. *Consequences*: The struggle for identity, independence, and intimacy may lead to stress, health-related problems, and often high-risk behaviors. The struggle for self-identity and independence is usually completed by age 20, although for some, full social and emotional maturity takes longer. This struggle also gives the health care professional an important opportunity for health promotion.

In the United States, persons with congenital disorders (i.e., present at birth) and genetic disorders (i.e., hereditary disorders transmitted by the genes that may not manifest at birth but develop over time) typically have entered the health care system before reaching adolescence. Multidisciplinary health care teams that feature pediatric and neurologic PTs most often manage congenital and genetic disorders. As a member of a management team in a medical or educational setting, a PT assists in identifying and ameliorating impairments, functional limitations, and disabilities in pediatric patients (0 to 20 years). Select congenital and genetic conditions that may require interventions that continue into adolescence (and adulthood) and therefore could be seen by the primary care outpatient PT are found in Table 16-3.

Overview: Birth to 4 Years

During the infant and toddler years, the exact rate of growth depends on the individual child. By 2 years of age, a child generally weighs 26 to 28 lb and stands 32 to 33 inches. By 2½ years, a child should quadruple his or her birth weight. Children in this age range require 900 (year 1) to 1400 (age 4) kilocalories (kcal)/day.[7] The child should have developed a complete set of teeth by 3 years of age.[255] Infants and young children develop the ability to sleep through the night and may need only one nap daily (refer to sleep needs by age group in Table 16-4).[198]

Curiosity about the environment motivates the young child to move and learn. The child's acquisition of skills from birth to 4 years (e.g., motor control for crawling, sitting, standing, walking, running, hopping, speaking, communicating with adults, toileting, early cognitive skills) is known as *psychomotor development*.[237] Failure to meet these developmental milestones in early childhood can have deleterious effects on the child's or adolescent's continued cognitive development (including academic achievement), motor function (fine and gross motor tasks), and peer socialization.[56,164,170]

Overview: Preschooler (4 to 6 Years)

The child usually doubles his or her birth height (length) by 4 years of age. At 5 years of age, height and weight are generally the same. Caloric intake becomes gender dependent after age 4 (1200 for girls and 1400 for boys).[117] During the preschool years, the child should begin to thin. The protruding abdomen of the toddler years begins to disappear, and body proportions change as the legs rapidly grow. Posture is more erect, and gait continues to mature. Gross motor tasks of running, hopping, and skipping develop during this period. Control of fine motor skills begins during this time.

Children begin to imitate their adult and older sibling role models, and take initiative in learning. Caregivers should role model proper nutritional habits, adequate fluid intake, and exercise to reinforce lifelong positive health habits. Caregivers should reinforce the child's sleep hygiene, including 9 to 12 hours of sleep per night and possibly a daily nap.[198]

Overview: School Age (6 to 12 Years)

During the early school years, children continue to learn and grow. Weight typically increases by 5 to 7 lb/year, and height increases an average of 3 inches/year. The child may have growth spurts. The intake needed to support growth escalates gradually during the school age years. When puberty starts (age 10 to 12 years), caloric needs vary by gender, typically 1600 calories for girls and 1800 calories for boys.[117] Sleep needs vary from 8 to 12 hours, and these children typically do not require a nap.[198]

The child's gait should be completely normalized to adult patterns by age 7.[201] Vision is 20/20 at 7 years of age. Strength, physical ability, and coordination increase in the school-age child. By 12 years of age, boys typically surpass girls in strength, endurance, and agility, whereas girls exceed boys in flexibility and coordination. In general, both genders should have high energy

levels for gross motor activities. Skills of fine motor manipulation should approximate those of the adult. Children become acutely aware of their physical abilities and interests compared with their peers. Developmental delay in this age group can be a predictor of long-term problems for the child.[56]

Overview: Adolescence (12 to 20 Years)

During puberty, hormones guide the development of the body in conjunction with social systems (e.g., school, church, family, community and cultural programs) designed to foster the transition from childhood to adulthood.[163] Between the ages of 10 and 20 years, children and adolescents undergo rapid changes in body size, shape, physiology, and psychological and social functioning. Except for the first year of life, physical growth is more rapid in adolescence than in any other stage of development.[255]

Children are anatomically and physically different from adults, and there are principles of child development that the PT must heed (see Table 16-2). Caloric requirements during adolescence are 1800 calories (range, 1500 to 2800) for girls and 2200 calories (range, 1800 to 3000) for boys.[117] Proper sleep hygiene for adolescents is 8.5 to 9.25 hours/night, although growth spurts can cause teens to sleep longer.[198] Adequate sleep among adolescents is positively associated with health status and health-related behaviors.[80]

PSYCHOSOCIAL DEVELOPMENT. Key elements of psychosocial development across the life span, as originally outlined by Erik Erikson in 1963, still hold true today.[104] Psychosocial development from birth to the onset of puberty can profoundly affect the adolescent's development of self-esteem. Babies learn at a young age (younger than 12 months) to trust or mistrust that others will care for their basic needs. Infants and toddlers (1 to 3 years) learn to be self-sufficient in many activities, including toileting, feeding, walking, and talking, or to doubt their own abilities (autonomy versus shame or doubt). Psychosocial development in the formative years can sway the cognitive and emotional capabilities of preschool (initiative versus guilt), school-age (industry versus inferiority), and adolescent (identity versus role confusion) youth. If children are made to feel inferior and inadequate before puberty, the development of a stable self-identity in the tumultuous adolescent years can appear to be a monumental task.

Adolescents are trying to answer the age-old question, "Who am I?" Adolescents acquire the cognitive ability to reason logically and abstractly, and consider future implications of their current actions. The rites of passage of adolescence either help teenagers establish ethnic, cultural, gender, sexual, and career identities, or they confuse teenagers about their future roles. Erikson further proposed that after they have passed through adolescence, young adults seek out love and companionship or become isolated from other people.

The ability to learn responsibility for self, others, and society in the teenage years determines whether a child will grow up to be a productive and competent member of society or a burden to society. Health care professionals can help adolescents on this road to maturity by promoting appropriate health behaviors, such as proper nutrition and physical activity, responsible sexual behavior, and intelligent choices about tobacco and alcohol. Given the amount of poverty, crime, and homelessness in America, issues of psychosocial development (i.e., mental

TABLE 16-3

Pediatric Physical Therapy: Congenital, Genetic, and Acquired Pediatric Conditions*

Condition	Features
Achondroplasia (dwarfism)[263] is the most common form of disproportionate short stature.	Persons with achondroplasia typically have delayed motor milestones, hip flexion contractures, bowing of the knees, thoracolumbar gibbus, increased lumbar lordosis, otitis media, obstructive sleep apnea (sweating and snoring at night), speech problems, and abnormal head growth (increased risk for seizures). Physical therapy management of back pain (spinal stenosis) and hip and knee pathology is common.
Cerebral palsy (CP) is a disorder of movement and posture caused by a prenatal, perinatal, or postnatal nonprogressive lesion of the immature brain. LBW (less than 1.5 kg [3.3 lb]) is a significant risk factor for postpartum onset of CP. The incidence of CP in the United States is 1.5 to 4/1000 births.	CP involves one or more of the limbs and often the trunk. It comes in various forms: diplegia (41.5%), hemiplegia (36.4%), dyskinesia or athetosis (10%), quadriplegia (7.3%), and ataxia (5%). The impaired control and coordination of voluntary muscles are often accompanied by mental retardation or learning disabilities (60%), dysarthria (25%), auditory impairments (6%-16%), seizure disorders (20%-30%), visional impairment, usually strabismus or refractory problems (40%-50%), sensory impairments (visual-motor and perceptual deficits); oral-motor, behavioral, social, and family problems may occur secondary to the presence of these primary deficits. Physical therapy interventions include family education, handling techniques, facilitation of optimal sensorimotor development, and orthopedic and neurologic management (ROM, stretching, strengthening, neuromuscular reeducation, positioning, gross motor function, gait, and orthotics). PTs usually are part of a multidisciplinary team involved in the management of the child throughout the life span.
Cystic fibrosis (CF) is the most common life-shortening genetic disease in the white population. It occurs in the United States in about 1/2,500 white, 1/17,000 African American, and 1/90,000 Asian American births. U.S. prevalence is 30,000; 70,000 are affected worldwide. Thirty percent of patients are adults. Median survival is age 35 yr.	CF is an autosomal-recessive disease of the exocrine glands, affecting primarily the GI and respiratory systems, and usually characterized by chronic obstructive pulmonary disease, exocrine pancreatic insufficiency (secondary to blockage), and abnormally high sweat electrolyte levels. Persons with CF often require management by a multidisciplinary team including physicians, nurses, nutritionists, PTs and respiratory therapists (daily chest physical therapy to clear lungs), counselors, and social workers. The goals of therapy are maintenance of adequate nutritional status, prevention of pulmonary and other complications, encouragement of physical activity, and provision of adequate psychosocial support (age-appropriate adjustment at home and school). Despite myriad problems, the occupational and marital successes of patients are impressive. The Cystic Fibrosis Foundation is a significant resource for patients and health care providers alike (http://www.cff.org/).
The incidence of **Down syndrome**[8] **(DS; trisomy 21)** is 1/1000 live births. Maternal age is a key determining variable. There is no association between DS with any culture, ethnic group, socioeconomic status, or geographic region.	Primary impairments include early feeding difficulties, mild to moderate mental retardation, delayed growth and sexual development, hearing loss, hypotonia, low muscle force production, slowed postural reactions, ligamentous laxity (atlantoaxial instability [AAI] in 20% of cases), foot deformities, scoliosis, congenital heart disease, and lung hypoplasia with pulmonary hypertension. Persons with Down syndrome also have a predisposition for immune deficiency, leukemia, and thyroid disease. The exercise prescription for management of Down syndrome obesity includes dietary education, behavioral modification, and increased activity level. AAI tests are required for participation in exercise or Special Olympics. For more information on trisomy 21, see the American Academy of Pediatrics policy statement: Health supervision for children with Down syndrome, *Pediatrics*: 2001;107:442-449.
Hemophilia is an X-linked disorder of blood coagulation present in 1/10,000 males.	Impairment is caused by spontaneous hemorrhaging into any of the tissues of the body: hemarthrosis (hallmark sign)—pain, swelling, limited ROM of affected joint, with elbows, knees, and ankles the joints most often affected; hematoma—bleeding into muscles produces pain, swelling; may produce muscle atrophy; mucous membrane bleeding—gums, nasal passages, and alimentary tract. Hemorrhaging risks include peripheral nerve lesions (compression); intracranial, intraspinal, retropharyngeal, and retroperitoneal bleeds. Joint protection strategies and joint rehabilitation after bleeds or after total joint arthroplasty are common.
Juvenile rheumatoid arthritis (JRA) collectively refers to three forms of childhood arthritis: pauciarticular (few joints) JRA, polyarticular JRA, and systemic-onset JRA (Still's disease). Associated arthritic conditions include systemic lupus erythematosus, dermatomyositis, and scleroderma. The prevalence of JRA varies from 16 to 150/100,000.	Systemic clinical manifestations of Still's disease (systemic-onset JRA) include fever (102° F), rash, anemia, lymphadenopathy, polyarthritis, pericarditis, pleuritis, peptic ulcer disease, and hepatitis. Differential diagnosis includes Lyme disease. Musculoskeletal manifestations include polyarthritis, polyarthralgias, myalgia, myositis, tenosynovitis, and skeletal growth disturbances. Physical therapy interventions for pain control, mobility, strength, endurance (muscular and aerobic), and functional tasks are key for children afflicted by JRA. Loss of joint motion is the strongest indicator of functional disability in children with JRA. Joint protection strategies (e.g., mobility assistive devices, body mechanics education) and daily activity pacing are important to children (and adults) with rheumatoid arthritis; 20% of children with JRA will have moderate to severe joint limitations in adulthood. For more information on JRA, see Ilowite NT: Current treatment of juvenile rheumatoid arthritis, *Pediatrics* 2002;109;109-115.

TABLE 16-3

Pediatric Physical Therapy: Congenital, Genetic, and Acquired Pediatric Conditions*–cont'd

Condition	Features
Neural tube defect (NTD) is a congenital defect in the neural tube that can occur at any level of the spinal cord. Physiologic variations of this condition are many and include sensory or motor loss. NTDs occur in 0.4 to 0.9/1000 live births. Anencephaly (3:1) and thoracolumbar cases have a female preponderance, with equal distribution in the more distal forms of spina bifida.	Three most common NTDs: spina bifida occulta (incomplete fusion of the posterior vertebral arch); meningocele (external protrusion of the meninges); myelodysplasia (protrusion of the meninges and spinal cord). Contributing factors include genetics (chromosomal abnormalities), ethnicity (white > African Americans), teratogens (alcohol), and nutritional deficits (lack of folic acid). Women in their childbearing years are advised to take 0.4 mg of folic acid/day. Folic acid supplementation should begin at least 3 mo before conception. Multivitamins containing folic acid during the first 6 wk of gestation will prevent up to 86% of NTDs. PT responsibilities include mobility and postural alignment via stretching to prevent contractures, orthotic and wheelchair management, skin and wound management, bowel and bladder programs, and functional training. The outpatient orthopedic PT should be aware that 40%-50% of these children develop latex sensitivity because of the high level of medical exposure early in life.
Osteogenesis imperfecta (OA; brittle bone disease) is an inherited connective tissue (type I collagen) disorder with an incidence of 1/20,000 live births. Health care providers should be vigilant to the fact that the most frequent cause of multiple fractures in infants and toddlers is child abuse.[151]	Fracture management includes physical therapy to combat the effects of immobilization. Pain management is via a multidisciplinary approach (physician, PT, and psychologist) to reduce or remove the pain, assist in mental well-being, and improve physiologic function. Physical agents include thermal modalities, transcutaneous electrical nerve stimulation (TENS), gentle myofascial techniques, relaxation training, and biofeedback. Pharmaceutical management includes over-the-counter pain relievers, NSAIDs, topical pain relievers, narcotic medications, antidepressants, and nerve blocks.
Prader-Willi syndrome (PWS) is a chromosomal disorder that can affect people of both genders and of any race or country. Genetic causes include deletion, imprinting error, translocation, or maternal disomy of chromosome 15. It is one of many genetic syndromes affecting movement.	Primary impairments include severe hypotonia and feeding problems in infancy, excessive eating and obesity in childhood, reduced strength, and poor fine and gross motor coordination. Many of these children are involved in birth to three (0-3) rehabilitation programs. The exercise prescription for management of obesity includes diet education, behavioral modification, limited access to food, and increased activity level. Resources available from the PWS Association at www.pwsausa.org. The National Organization for Rare Disorders (NORD) is a federation of voluntary health organizations serving people with rare diseases and their families. They maintain a database of over 1100 rare diseases, many of which are genetic syndromes (e.g., Angelman syndrome, cri-du-chat syndrome, fragile X syndrome, Klinefelter syndrome, neurofibromatosis, PWS Rett syndrome, Smith-Magenis syndrome, Turner syndrome, velocardiofacial syndrome, Williams syndrome, and triple X syndrome (http://www.rarediseases.org/). PTs should be aware of the ethical issues involved with genetic testing in pediatrics. See Nelson RM, Botkjin JR, Kodish ED, et al; Committee on Bioethics: Ethical issues with genetic testing in pediatrics, *Pediatrics* 2001;107:1451-1455.
Sickle cell disease (SCD) is an inherited blood disorder in which normally round red blood cells become distorted and clog vessels. These blockages cause painful episodes known as sickle cell crises. An estimated 1/500 African Americans and 1/1000-1400 Hispanics have this genetic condition, which occurs when a person inherits two copies of a mutated gene for hemoglobin, the oxygen carrier in red blood cells.	Clinical presentation includes jaundice in the first few weeks of life, organomegaly (spleen, liver), moderate to severe anemia, cardiac systolic flow murmur, and musculoskeletal distortion and growth disturbances, particularly in the skull, vertebrae, long bones, and maxilla (may require referral for orthodontics). A multidisciplinary team focus is on caregiver education, including physical assessment skills (vital signs—HR, respiratory rate, temperature), how to treat pain, and when to administer prophylactic antibiotics. Education in stroke prevention is key, because blood transfusions may prevent recurrent stroke in children with SCD. Lung function should be monitored because children with SCD often have abnormal pulmonary function tests (PFTs). Adolescent issues—monitor growth, development, and nutrition. Adolescents and parents should be counseled about potential social problems related to frequent illness, stature, and delayed sexual development. Concern about issues such as body size, sexual dysfunction, pain management, and death often is expressed as rebellion, depression, or refusal to heed treatment plans and medical advice. Adolescents should be advised not to use tobacco, alcohol, and illegal drugs. Postpubertal adolescents should be educated about sexuality, safe sex practices, and the use of condoms to prevent STDs. Girls should be counseled about the risks of pregnancy in women with SCD, safe birth control practices, and the merits of pregnancy at the right age and social circumstances. For more information on SCD, see National Institutes of Health, National Heart, Lung, and Blood Institute: *Management of sickle cell disease,* 4th ed, NIH Publication No. 02-2117. http://www.nhlbi.nih.gov/ health/ prof/blood/sickle/sc_mngt.pdf. (Revised May 28, 2002); Sickle Cell Disease Association (http://www.sicklecelldisease.org); or Section on Hematology/Oncology Committee on Genetics; American Academy of Pediatrics: Health supervision for children with sickle cell disease, *Pediatrics* 2002;109:526-535.

Continued

TABLE 16-3

Pediatric Physical Therapy: Congenital, Genetic, and Acquired Pediatric Conditions*–cont'd

Condition	Features
Spinal muscle atrophy (SMA) is an inherited autosomal-recessive genetic defect of chromosome 5 characterized by loss and degeneration of the large anterior horn cells in the brainstem and spinal cord.	Childhood SMA is divided into four types: Type I, acute infantile onset (0-3 mo) (Werdnig-Hoffmann) causes death by age 18 mo Type II, childhood onset (3 mo-4 yr), Werdnig-Hoffmann (chronic), causes hypotonia, results in shortened life span Type III, juvenile onset (5-10 yr), Kugelberg-Welander, has slower onset, less impairment; patients present with progressive proximal muscle weakness (pelvic girdle and paraspinals), followed by shoulder girdle weakness, bulbar signs; most wheelchair-bound by early adulthood but still potential for normal life expectancy Type IV, adult forms, manifest in the teen years; typically marked by weakness of the distal legs, particularly anterior tibial and peroneal compartments Primary impairment of muscle weakness (lower motor neuron) results from progressive loss of anterior horn cells in the spinal cord. Treatment is directed at minimizing spinal deformity, maintaining joint level mobility, maintaining functional mobility, and preventing contractures. Individuals who maintain ambulation skills have been found to have a lower incidence of scoliosis. For severe scoliosis (curves >45 degrees on the Cobb method), surgical intervention often is required to stabilize the spine, because without it there can be progressive respiratory and swallowing compromise, as well as increased integumentary system stress

*These may be seen during adolescence by a primary care outpatient orthopedic PT.
Adapted from references 1, 8, 56, 120, 151, 163, 200, 263, and 264.

TABLE 16-4

Vital Signs, Caloric Needs, and Sleep Requirements Across the Pediatric Life Span

Age (yr)	HR (beats/min)	HR Limits (beats/min)	RR (breaths/min)	BP (mm Hg)	Caloric Needs*	Sleep Needs (hr)
Newborn	120	70-190	30-40	NA	900-1300	Child develops ability to sleep through the night; may need only one nap/day
1	120	80-160	20-40	NA	1200-1400	
2	110	80-130	25-32	NA	1300-1500	
4	100	80-120	23-30	100-110	1300-1700	
6	100	75-115	21-26	60-70	1300-1700	9-12; may or may not require a nap
8-10	90	70-110	20-26		1400-2000	8-12 hours; does not require a nap
12						
Female	90	70-110	18-22	100-120	1500-2800	
Male	85	65-105		60-80	1800-3000	
14						
Female	85	65-105	18-22		1500-2800	8.5-9
Male	80	60-100			1800-3000	
16						
Female	80	60-100	16-20		1500-2800	
Male	75	55-95			1800-3000	
18						
Female	75	60-100	12-20		1500-2800	
Male	70	55-95			1800-3000	

*Increased physical activity will require additional calories, 0-200 kcal/day if moderately active and 200-400 kcal/day if very physically active.[267]
BP, blood pressure; *HR*, heart rate, *NA*, not applicable; *RR*, respiratory rate.
Adapted from references 120, 149, 198, and 224.

---

health) in our youth should be of paramount concern to every health care professional, parent, and politician.

Puberty: The Approach to Maturity

Puberty and Sexual Maturation

Puberty can be divided into five stages. The PT monitors puberty via sexual maturity ratings (SMRs) based on the Tanner stages of sexual development (Table 16-5). The Tanner stages are used as a guide to the usual progression of male and female sexual maturation.[181,182] The physical changes of puberty include rapid increases in height and weight, changes in body composition (i.e., MS system), growth of pubic hair and axillary hair, changes in thermoregulation (i.e., integumentary system), changes in the circulatory and respiratory systems, and development of sexual organs and secondary sex characteristics.[163,181,182]

The range of normal development among teenagers is wide and varies chronologically by gender, with girls usually proceeding through puberty earlier than boys. On average, girls enter

TABLE 16-5

Tanner Stages of Sexual Development

Female Puberty		
Stage	**Breast Stage**	**Pubic Hair Stage**
1 (preadolescent)	Only papilla are elevated.	Vellus hair only, and hair is similar to development over anterior abdominal wall (i.e., no pubic hair).
2	Breast buds and papilla are elevated, and a small mound is present; areola diameter is enlarged.	There is sparse growth of long, slightly pigmented downy hair or only slightly curled hair, appearing along the labia.
3	Further enlargement of breast mound; increased palpable glandular tissue.	Hair is darker, coarser, more curled, and spreads to the pubic junction.
4	Areola and papilla are elevated to form a second mound above the level of the rest of the breast.	Adult-type hair; area covered is less than that in most adults; there is no spread to the medial surface of thighs.
5 (adult)	Adult mature breast; recession of areola to the mound of breast tissue, rounding of the breast mound, and projection of only the papillae are evident.	Adult-type hair with increased spread to medial surface of thighs; distribution is as an inverted triangle.

Male Puberty		
Stage	**Genital Stage**	**Pubic Hair Stage**
1 (preadolescent)	Testes, scrotum, and penis are approximately the same size and proportion as in early childhood.	Vellus hair over the pubis is no further developed than that over the abdominal wall (i.e., no pubic hair).
2	Scrotum and testes have enlarged, and there is a change in the texture of scrotal skin and some reddening of scrotal skin.	There is sparse growth of long, slightly pigmented, downy hair, straight or only slightly curled, appearing chiefly at base of penis.
3	Growth of the penis has occurred, at first mainly in length but with some increase in breadth. The testes and the scrotum have grown further.	Hair is considerably darker, coarser, and more curled and spreads sparsely over junction of pubes.
4	The penis is further enlarged in length and breadth, with development of glans. The testes and the scrotum are further enlarged. There is also further darkening of scrotal skin.	Hair is now adult in type, but the area it covers is smaller than that in most adults. There is no spread to the medial surface of the thighs.
5 (adult)	Genitalia are adult in size and shape. No further enlargement takes place after stage 5 is reached.	Hair is adult in quantity and type, distributed as an inverted triangle. There is spread to the medial surface of the thighs but not up the linea alba or elsewhere above the base of the inverted triangle.

Data from Marshall WA, Tanner JM: Variations in pattern of pubertal changes in girls, *Arch Dis Child* 44:291-303, 1969; and Marshall WA, Tanner JM: Variations in the pattern of pubertal changes in boys, *Arch Dis Child* 45:13-23, 1970.

puberty at age 10 (range, 8 to 13 years) and boys at age 11 (range, 9.5 to 14 years).[163] Once started, the process of puberty is usually complete in 4.5 years. Girls typically end their pubertal development with a peak velocity growth spurt by age 14 years, compared with age 16 for boys.[255] These growth spurts typically correlate to a Tanner SMR of 3 or 4.

In girls, the first visible sign of puberty is the appearance of breast buds (thelarche), between 8 and 13 years of age.[182] Less obvious changes in the adolescent girl include the following: enlargement of the ovaries, uterus, labia, and clitoris (gonadarche); thickening of the endometrium and vaginal mucosa; and increased vaginal glycogen, predisposing to yeast infections.[163] Menarche, or the first menstrual period, is a significant event (vital sign) in the life of the developing female.[162] There appears to be a critical fat mass (17% of body weight) required for menarche and a higher fat mass (22% of body weight) needed for maintenance of reproductive capacity.[114] Menses typically begins 2 to 2½ years after the development of breast buds (normal range of 9 to 16 years), and around the peak velocity in height growth.[163]

In boys, the first visible sign of puberty is testicular enlargement (gonadarche), which may begin as early as 9½ years.[181] The seminiferous tubules, epididymis, seminal vesicles, and prostate enlarge under the influence of luteinizing hormone (LH) and testosterone. The left testis normally is lower than the right. Gynecomastia (breast hypertrophy) is a common physiologic phenomenon that occurs in 40% to 69% of pubertal boys.[163,176,203] Fewer than 10% of young boys develop gynecomastia sufficient to cause embarrassment and social disability.[163] Breast swelling less than 4 cm in diameter has a 90% chance of spontaneous resolution within 3 years. The presence of gynecomastia could signal endocrine disorders, and a basic panel of hormonal blood tests may guide management. For greater degrees of enlargement, hormonal or surgical treatment may be indicated. Obesity may exacerbate gynecomastia and should be addressed through diet and exercise.[163,176,203]

Parents, caregivers, and health care providers should recognize that pubertal onset is a heritable trait, but that normal progression through the Tanner stages varies widely depending on the individual, his or her nationality or ethnic group, and a host of other environmental and geographic factors.[102,155,163] Children living at lower altitudes and lower latitudes tend to start puberty earlier.[163] Socioeconomic conditions, general health and nutrition, and increased body fat (obesity) and the hormone leptin are environmental triggers for puberty.[102,235] Currently, children in the United States enter puberty somewhat earlier than international norms, perhaps because of increased weight and adiposity.[163]

In the United States, African American girls on average enter puberty first, followed by Mexican American and then white girls. The mean age at onset of pubic hair, breast development, and menarche is 9.5, 9.5, and 12.1 years for African American girls, 10.3, 9.8, and 12.2 years for Mexican American girls, and 10.5, 10.3, and 12.7 years for white girls.[276] These ethnic differences remain even after adjustment for current body mass index (BMI) and several social and economic variables.[276] Non-Hispanic African American boys have an earlier median and mean age for sexual maturity stages than non-Hispanic white and Hispanic American boys.[252]

PRECOCIOUS PUBERTY. Early signs of sexual development, before the age of 8 in girls, and before the age of 9 or 9½ in boys, is known as *precocious puberty*.[163] Precocious puberty currently affects 1 in 5000 children and is 10 times more common in girls.[78] Early prognosticators for precocious puberty include physical changes, such as the appearance of genital hair (pubarche), onset of growth in breast tissue (thelarche), and increased growth rate and skeletal maturity (bone age) relative to chronologic age. Numerous studies have established a relationship among obesity, leptin (hormone that plays a key role in appetite and metabolism),[235] and early puberty and menses in girls, but data linking obesity and early puberty in boys are less convincing.[155]

The child's physician (or other appropriate health care provider) should monitor the child's growth rate compared with sexual maturation using pediatric growth charts.[63] Determining actual bone age as it relates to sexual maturation requires radiographic evaluation of the ossification centers of the hand and wrist and/or iliac crest (Risser sign).[125] Accurate differential diagnosis of precocious puberty requires sensitive hormone screening tests, including testing for gonadotropin-releasing hormone (GnRH) and the gonadotropins (i.e., LH and follicle-stimulating hormone). Because of the underlying disorders that can be associated with precocious puberty (e.g., central nervous system [CNS] disease, trauma, tumors, McCune-Albright syndrome, chronic primary hypothyroidism), suspicion of this condition necessitates referral to an endocrinologist.[163]

A recent study by Ibáñez and colleagues[145] has suggested that low-birth-weight (LBW) female infants with rapid postnatal weight gain (0 to 9 months) tend to have precocious puberty (PP), earlier menarche, earlier growth arrest, shorter stature, and be overweight (visceral fat) and at risk for insulin sensitization. These girls are also at risk for progression to polycystic ovary syndrome (POCS).[102,207] including hyperinsulinemic hyperandrogenism, dyslipidemia, dysadipocytokinemia, and central fat excess.[144] Long-term metformin treatment appears to reduce total and visceral fat in LBW-PP girls and to delay menarche without attenuating linear growth, thereby increasing the likelihood that more appropriate adult height may be reached.[143]

DYSMENORRHEA. A girl who has reached Tanner stage 5 (i.e., the breasts are fully formed and pubic hair resembles adult quantity, texture, and an upside-down triangle form) should have a regular menstrual cycle. Late onset of menarche (after chronologic age 16) is an indication for referral to a gynecologist or an endocrinologist.

Many factors may contribute to a delay in menarche. The evaluating health care practitioner should consider endocrine disorders that cause effects opposite of those of precocious puberty, along with low overall body fat, eating disorders (EDs), and athletic amenorrhea as possible causes. A delay in menarche or menstrual dysfunction is not uncommon among young athletic females, but these delays can have long-term effects on bone metabolism (see later, "Female Athlete Triad").[114,120,163,199]

MALE MILESTONES. Although the cultural significance of menarche has been studied in numerous quantitative and qualitative reports, the male milestones of first orgasm (orgasmarche), first ejaculation (oigarche), and first wet dream (nocturnal emission) have received less attention.[148] The mean age of orgasmarche (age range, 12.2 to 16.2 years) varies by definition (e.g., nocturnal emission, masturbatory, or with a partner) and by country. Internationally, ranges for oigarche have been found to vary from 12 years 8 months to 15 years. Nocturnal emission is a more obscure phenomenon; in one study, almost half of boys did not talk about wet dreams before having them and more than half thought they needed treatment.[148] Male adolescents should be assured that wet dreams are a totally normal function of the body and are not under voluntary control. This phenomenon usually stops when the individual begins masturbating or becomes sexually active.[163]

Puberty and Proper Nutrition

Nutrition is an important regulator of the tempo of human growth, particularly during the adolescent years. Adequate nutrition encompasses proper caloric intake of carbohydrates, proteins, and fats, along with sufficient minerals, vitamins, and fluids. Based on sedentary lifestyle, teenage girls should consume 1600 to 1800 kcal/day, compared with 1800 to 2200 kcal/day for teenage boys. Increased physical activity will require additional calories, 0 to 200 kcal/day for moderate and 200 to 400 kcal/day for strenuous activity.[7] Dietary fat should gradually reduce over the pediatric years from 30% to 40% of total calories in the first year of life to 25% to 35% in the teen years.[117] More than 60% of children and adolescents exceed the daily recommended amounts of saturated fats.[68] Recommended servings by gender (female/male) for foods per day are as follows: lean meat or beans (5/6), fruit (1.5/2), vegetables (2.5/3), and grains (6/7).[117] Only 20% of high school students eat five or more servings of fruit and vegetables per day.[68] Details about nutrition and the Healthy Eating food pyramid can be found at the U.S. Department of Agriculture website (http://www.mypyramid.gov). A nutritional screening checklist is shown in Box 16-2.

Ideally, a sufficient and balanced diet should meet all of a person's micronutrient requirements. Infants, small children, adolescents, and women of childbearing age are the most vulnerable to micronutrient malnutrition.[41] In general, the need for micronutrients increases during the pediatric years, with calcium (1200 to 1500 mg/day), phosphorus (1250 mg/day), and iron (males 11 mg/day; menstruating females 15 mg/day) playing key roles in adolescence. Adolescents should consume 3 cups of milk or dairy products/day to aid in calcium intake. All women capable of becoming pregnant should consume 400 to 800 μg of folic acid daily to reduce the risk of birth defects of the neural tube.[65]

Proper nutrition in adolescence supports not only the cascade of hormonal and biologic systems influencing growth but

BOX 16-2

Nutrition Screening Checklist

Instructions. Check "yes" for each condition that applies, and then total the nutritional score. For total scores of 3 to 5 points (moderate risk) or 6 or more points (high risk), further evaluation is needed (especially for older adults).

I have an illness or condition that made me change the kind and/or amount of food I eat.	Yes (2 points)_____
I eat fewer than 2 meals a day.	Yes (3 points)_____
I eat few fruits or vegetables, or milk products.	Yes (2 points)_____
I have 3 or more drinks of beer, liquor, or wine almost every day.	Yes (2 points)_____
I have tooth or mouth problems that make it hard for me to eat.	Yes (2 points)_____
I don't always have enough money to buy the food I need.	Yes (4 points)_____
I eat alone most of the time.	Yes (1 points)_____
I take 3 or more different prescribed or over-the-counter drugs each day.	Yes (1 points)_____
Without wanting to, I have lost or gained 10 pounds in the last 6 months.	Yes (2 points)_____
I am not always physically able to shop, cook, and/or feed myself.	Yes (2 points)_____
	TOTAL _____

RAPID SCREEN FOR DIETARY INTAKE

Instructions. Ask the patient for a 24-hour dietary recall (perhaps two of these) before completing the form.

Food	Portions Consumed by Patient	Recommended
Grains, cereal, bread group	_____	6-11
Fruit	_____	2-4
Vegetable group	_____	3-5
Meat/meat substitute group	_____	2-3
Dairy group	_____	2-3
Sugar, fats, snack foods	_____	—
Soft drinks	_____	—
Alcoholic beverages	_____	<2

From Bickley LS, Szilagyi PG: *Bates' guide to physical examination and history taking,* 10th ed, Philadelphia, 2008, Lippincott, Williams & Wilkins, p 129.

ongoing bioenergetics (homeostasis) of the body. Bioenergetics, or the flow of energy in a biologic system, is concerned primarily with the conversion of food—large carbohydrates, protein, and fat molecules—into biologically useful forms of energy.[32] Bioenergetics requires proper nutrition and healthy functioning of several large body systems: (1) gastrointestinal tract (including enzymes of digestion and absorption); (2) endocrine system (hormones of metabolism); (3) circulatory and respiratory systems (energy delivery system); (4) musculoskeletal system (the conversion of chemical energy into mechanical energy); and (5) excretory system (management of waste products by sweat mechanisms and kidneys).

BONE HEALTH. Research suggests that 40% of total lifetime bone mass is established during puberty, with the peak calcium accretion rate being attained on average at 12.5 years of age in girls and 14.0 years of age in boys.[124] The most important dietary factor for bone health is calcium (1200 to 1500 mg/day),[120] obtained mainly from dairy foods (45%) and cereal-based foods

(27%).[191] Dietary flaws in childhood and adolescence (e.g., dietary restriction, decreased calcium intake, caffeine use, soft drinks), physical inactivity, or excessive thinness with late menarche or amenorrhea can hasten and intensify the bone loss of aging.[120,199]

FEMALE ATHLETE TRIAD. Athletic endeavors that require high caloric intake, low body fat, or intense weight management can affect the adolescent's metabolism. The female athlete triad refers to the interrelationships among energy availability, menstrual function, and bone mineral density, which may have clinical manifestations, including EDs, functional hypothalamic amenorrhea, and osteoporosis.[199] A 2005 study suggested that most high school athletic programs are not adequately screening girls for components of the female triad, and that schools lack educational programs targeting athletes and coaches.[95] The first aim of treatment is to increase energy availability by increasing energy intake and/or reducing exercise energy expenditure. Nutrition counseling and monitoring are sufficient interventions for many athletes, but EDs warrant psychotherapy.[199]

Poor nutritional guidance by the family, ethnic considerations, and inadequate finances (socioeconomic variables) also can lead to poor food selections by male and female adolescents. In our fast-paced fast food society, the lack of family meal time and the prevalence of vending machines and advertisements for high-fat, high-calorie foods are but a few of the societal influences contributing to poor food choices by Americans. These variables together are more likely to lead to childhood and adolescent obesity, a topic that will be addressed further in the health promotion section of this chapter. See the U.S. Department of Agriculture's web page (www.nal.usda.gov/fnic) for updated gender-specific dietary guidelines across the life span. The AAP also provides numerous guidelines on improving children's nutrition for parents, guardians, caregivers, health care providers, and schools.[117] In recent years, legislation has been drafted to improve nutrition and address the issue of obesity, hypertension (HTN), and hypercholesterolemia in children (e.g., measurement of BMI by school health surveillance staff, restriction of certain foods and beverages available on school grounds, food labeling on portion sizes, regulation of food advertising directed at children).

Puberty and the Musculoskeletal System

The development and health of the musculoskeletal (MS system are a major focus of the primary care PT working with adolescent patients. The MS system is one of four preferred patterns of practice (musculoskeletal, neuromuscular, cardiovascular-pulmonary, and integumentary) for the American Physical Therapy Association.[25] Many connective tissues collectively make up the MS system (e.g., skeleton, ligament, tendon, joint capsule and fascia, fibrocartilage, hyaline [articular] cartilage, striated muscles of the body). A competent nervous system (afferent and efferent peripheral pathways, CNS and autonomic nervous system modulation) is necessary for control of normal patterns of movement, and healthy cardiovascular and pulmonary systems supply the energy to run the human machine.

Skeletal modeling begins in the fifth week of gestation, when the hyaline cartilage skeletal model first appears, and continues until the end of skeletal ossification, as late as age 25 years. Skeletal modeling is the process whereby agents external to a growing tissue affect its growth and direction in ways that fashion its microscopic and gross architecture.[91] Collectively, the skeletal modeling process prepares the growing MS system to endure the demands of adult daily life.

The skeleton of the newborn contains 350 bones that fuse together to form the 206 bones found in the adult skeleton.[228] Symmetry and rate of growth of the axial skeleton (i.e., cranium, spine, thorax) and appendicular skeleton (i.e., pelvic girdle, shoulder girdle, and limbs) should be monitored across the pediatric life span (0 to about 25 years). The major clinical implications of skeletal modeling are the younger the child, the more pliable the skeletal system, and children and adolescents are at risk for traumatic epiphyseal injuries.[91,120,228]

VERTEBRAL COLUMN DEVELOPMENT. The primary (kyphotic) curves of the spine are present at birth. The secondary (lordotic) curves of the cervical and lumbar spine develop as a result of accommodation to upright posture and continue to develop until growth stops in late adolescence or early adulthood. The bipolar neurocentral joints of the vertebral column fuse by age 7 to 8 years; the annular (ring) epiphyses are activated just before puberty (age 7 to 9 years) and close between the ages of 14 and 24 years.[60] Given the natural development of these axial skeleton growth plates, adolescents are susceptible to spinal pathology (tumor, infection) and growth disturbances (e.g., scoliosis, Scheuermann's disease).

Back Pain. Over half of adolescents may have back pain at some point, one third will seek professional help, and one in five (20%) experience a reduced quality of life.[212] Unlike adults, who frequently present with nonspecific back pain, when children or adolescents seek medical care for back pain it is more likely that underlying pathology will be identified. For example, when children and adolescents present to the emergency department for back pain, differential diagnoses include trauma (25%), muscle strain (24%), sickle cell crises (13%), idiopathic cause (13%), urinary tract infection (5%), and viral syndrome (4%).[38] Other items to consider include pyelonephritis, ectopic pregnancy, pelvic inflammatory disease, diskitis, inflammatory spondyloarthropathies, herniated disk, traumatic spondylolysis, and idiopathic scoliosis. As with adults, night pain, fever, malaise, and weight loss are signs of systemic illness that require referral. Diagnostic imaging (plain film radiography, magnetic resonance imaging [MRI], or bone scanning) and laboratory tests (complete blood count, erythrocyte sedimentation rate, and C-reactive protein measurement) are indicated to rule out serious systemic illness.[38,120] It appears that like adults, well-being and self-perception variables are relevant, because low back pain is more common in school-age children with high levels of psychosocial difficulties, conduct problems, and somatic disorders.[38]

THORAX DEVELOPMENT. Babies usually are born with a barrel-shaped chest (i.e., round thorax) and horizontally oriented rib cage. Within a few years of birth, the ribs drop into their normal downwardly sloped position. By 6 years of age, the thorax develops into the more adult-like elliptical shape with an anteroposterior-to-transverse ratio of 1:2 or 5:7.[149] In general, the chest maintains this configuration well into adulthood. Persistence of a barrel-shaped chest after 6 years of age is abnormal and typically

associated with respiratory diseases that cause hyperinflation of the lungs (e.g., asthma, cystic fibrosis).[120,149,177] A widening and flattening of the rib cage is also a normal physiologic and relatively permanent response to pregnancy. Pregnant adolescent females should be educated about changes in the rib cage and the many other physiologic changes associated with pregnancy (see Chapter 17).

Pectus excavatum (funnel chest) and pectus carinatum (pigeon chest) are two abnormal congenital chest configurations that are usually asymptomatic.[149] The latter is less common. Severe depression of the sternum in pectus excavatum can reduce the anteroposterior dimension of the chest, displace the heart, and reduce tidal volume.[177] These configurations may create a negative self-concept and embarrassment for the developing adolescent, particularly during school-related gym activities or sports activities or as he or she begins sexual experimentation.

LONG BONE DEVELOPMENT. The functional divisions of the long bones are displayed in Figure 16-2A. The diaphysis, or the shaft of the long bone, is the portion of bone formed by the primary ossification center. The epiphysis, or the end of the long bone, is formed by the secondary ossification centers. The metaphysis is the wider part of the shaft of a long bone adjacent to the epiphyseal plate. The metaphysis consists of cancellous bone during development; in adulthood, the metaphysis becomes continuous with the epiphysis. The epiphyseal plate represents the bone's growth zone. The two types of epiphyses, pressure and traction, are shown in Figure 16-2B. These regions of growth are common sites of injury in the pediatric patient.

The pubescent MS growth spurt usually begins distally, with enlargement of the hands and feet, and continues with the arms and legs and finally the trunk and chest. Body weight is increased in several ways, including increased height (length of bones), increased bone density, increased lean muscle mass in boys, and a higher fat-to-muscle ratio in girls (breasts, hips, and thighs).[163] Asymmetric growth patterns can give young adolescents a gawky appearance. Akin to the other growth spurts of childhood, adolescence often brings muscle imbalances and issues of coordination or motor control that may predispose to epiphyseal injuries. During periods of adolescent skeletal growth, flexibility exercises should be emphasized to prevent injury to muscles, tendons, joints, and apophyses. Exercise and diet are important to control increased fat mass, whereas strength training will improve bone density and muscle mass, which contributes to overall lean (fat-free) body mass.[60]

Puberty and the Nervous System

The overall function of the nervous system (NS) is well established before adolescence. At puberty, the brain releases hormones, directing other body systems to change. Primary care PTs should be skilled in testing the integrity of the entire NS across the life span because its function can be compromised by a variety of conditions (e.g., space-occupying lesions of the cranium, systemic disease, traumatic brain injuries, peripheral nervous system [PNS] disease, trauma).

At birth, the brain is 25% the weight of the adult brain, whereas the head is already 70% of its adult size.[60] By 6 months of age, the brain has doubled its weight. Glial cell formation is at its peak growth between the ages of 15 and 24 months.[217] The brain

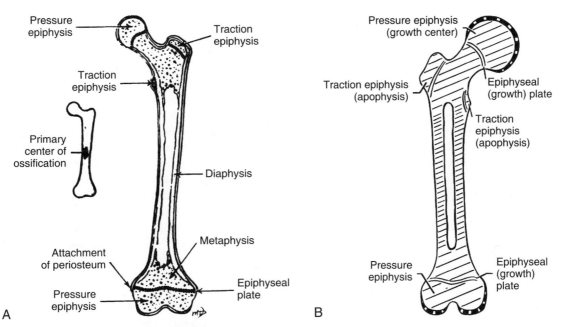

FIGURE 16-2 A, Functional divisions of the long bones (epiphysis, metaphysis, diaphysis, and epiphyeal plates). **B,** Types of epiphyses. (From Salter RB: *Textbook of disorders and injuries of the musculoskeletal system,* 3rd ed, Baltimore, 1999, Williams & Wilkins, p 340.)

reaches 90% of its adult mass by 6 years of age, and at the onset of puberty (age 10 to 12 years), the brain reaches 100% of adult weight. Dendritic branching reaches levels of adult complexity during early and middle adolescence (from 12 to 16 years).[60] Abstract language concepts are possible, and the corticospinal tract is morphologically (but not electrophysiologically) mature. By 13 years of age, low-frequency electroencephalographic rhythms typically change to adult high-frequency rhythms.

Myelination of the PNS is largely complete at birth, giving the newborn sensory access to environmental surroundings (through touch, smell, motion, and taste). All cranial nerves (CNs), with the exception of the optic nerve (CN II), are completely myelinated at birth. Formation of glial cells, unexcitable support tissues of the CNS including astrocytes, oligodendroglial cells, ependymal cells, and microglia continues within the brain into young adulthood. Myelination of association cortices (e.g., frontal, parietal, and temporal lobes, along with reticular formation, internal capsule, and the association fibers) persists into adulthood.[60,218]

Brain metabolism (i.e., utilization of glucose) changes with CNS maturation. Tracking of the brain's glucose utilization via positron emission tomography (PET) is a mechanism for monitoring functional maturation.[60] Glucose utilization is closely linked to synaptogenesis, or synaptic proliferation, which occurs primarily between birth and 4 years of age. Synaptogenesis levels off during middle childhood and then declines in adolescence because of synaptic elimination that occurs within the cortex. The brain further diminishes its energy requirements into adulthood.[84]

A review of the adolescent's dietary history and current nutritional status can lend insight into overall NS and other body systems function. Nutritional habits, environmental quality, socioeconomic variables, and contextual factors (e.g., family, school, and peer group influences) are key determinants of overall health and have been found to correlate to physical dysfunction, disease, and illness behavior.[251] Children who are malnourished before 3 years of age (including the gestational period) reportedly have impaired motor ability.[60] The number of children born to adolescent women who have poor prenatal care, poor nutritional habits, and poor societal support is a significant long-term health and financial concern for the United States (see later, "Responsible Sexual Behavior," for information on teenage pregnancy).

Puberty and the Cardiovascular and Pulmonary Systems

The health of the cardiovascular and pulmonary (CVP) systems affects the amount of oxygen that can be delivered to the various tissues and systems of the body. Whether regarding muscular endurance (peripheral), the cardiovascular pump (central), or the ventilation and gas exchange capabilities of the lungs, the CVP system is literally the engine that allows the body to perform work. There are distinct physiologic issues (e.g., circulation, ventilation, and muscular metabolism) that PTs should consider when managing patients across the life span.

VITAL SIGNS. Heart rate (HR), respiratory rate (RR), and blood pressure (BP) are age dependent (see Table 16-4). The CVP system of the developing child responds differently to metabolic load (exercise), and the atypically developing youngster adds further concern.[33,163,183,268] During the adolescent growth spurt, gender differences in CVP function become apparent.[60] Only the skeletally mature adolescent will have vital signs and cardiopulmonary responses comparable with those of the adult. The fourth vital sign, temperature (98.6° F [37° C]), is influenced by four factors: (1) diurnal cycle (time of day); (2) menstruation cycle in women; (3) exercise; and (4) age. Infants and small children have wider variations in normal body temperature because of less effective heat control systems.[149]

AEROBIC METABOLISM. When maximal aerobic power is expressed as Vo_2 max (mL/kg body weight/min), children are similar to adults. However, absolute Vo_2 max is lower in children because children have smaller bodies and thus smaller hearts, lungs, and lung capacity. Overall, cardiac output (stroke volume × heart rate) is 1 to 3 L/min lower in prepubescent children compared with older adolescents and adults.[170,183]

During adolescence, the peak height velocity of teens leads to a rapid increase in height, allowing for a larger thorax and thus greater potential of the cardiopulmonary system. Between 6 and 12 years of age, the overall physical working capacity of children increases about eightfold.[170] Adolescent males have a greater advantage in height growth, develop larger hearts and lungs, and have higher blood pressure and lower resting heart rates than adolescent females.[163,224]

ANAEROBIC METABOLISM. When adjusted for body weight, young children have about 65% to 70% of the total anaerobic capacity of mature adolescents and adults. Children appear to have equal concentrations of adenosine triphosphate (ATP) and creatine phosphate (CP) compared with adults. However, their ability to use glucose for anaerobic activity is reduced because they have lower concentrations of phosphofructokinase, the rate-limiting enzyme in glycolysis.[170,183,224] As a result of their lower rate of glycolysis, children demonstrate slower production and accumulation of lactate.

At 85% Vo_2 max, adults rapidly begin to show negative side effects of elevated blood levels of lactic acid (e.g., increase in H^+ concentration, decrease in available energy, and decreased muscle contractile force during exercise) and quickly fatigue. Conversely, prepubescent children do not demonstrate elevated levels of lactate accumulation until they reach Vo_2 max of 93%. This literally allows young children to push the anaerobic threshold further, but they have less of an anaerobic reserve compared with adults. This explains why small children are able to go at high levels of intensity but then suddenly fatigue.[170]

The hormonal changes of puberty are so broad that they affect energy utilization systems, literally down to individual cellular metabolism. By late adolescence, a teenager will have an exercise response similar to an adult (i.e., lactate accumulation at 85% Vo_2 max). The adolescent's apparently sudden change in tolerance of anaerobic exercise could be disconcerting to the observer who does not understand the exercise physiology of the developing individual.

According to investigations by the American Academy of Pediatrics, pediatric athletes have superior cardiac functional capacity, greater cardiac volume, and greater chamber size than nonathletes.[16] In general, studies support the theory that the effects of sustained submaximal exercise on cardiac function are similar in children and adults.[16,183,224] Careful assessment of cardiovascular status, including blood pressure and the possible presence of heart murmurs or abnormal rhythms, remains necessary in ongoing medical care of the young person. PTs also should consider thermoregulation when prescribing exercises for patients across the developmental years (see later, "Puberty and the Integumentary System").

CARDIOVASCULAR DISEASE. Assessing for signs and symptoms of cardiovascular disease (CVD) and its risk factors is an essential skill of the PT. As the leading cause of death and morbidity in the United States, CVD is a pediatric disease.[92,157,224] CVD has three periods of development: (1) incubation period (infancy to

adolescence), (2) latent period (adolescence and early adulthood), and (3) clinical manifestation period (adulthood).[224] It is estimated that 75% to 90% of the CVD epidemic is related to dyslipidemia, HTN, diabetes mellitus (DM), tobacco use, physical inactivity, and obesity; the principal causes of these risk factors are adverse behaviors, including poor nutrition.[117]

Risk factors (both nonmodifiable and modifiable) of CVD are indicators of overall health, and several are relevant to teenagers. Nonmodifiable risk factors for CVD include age (women older than 55 and men older than 45 years), male gender, family and genetic determinants, ethnicity, and infection (viral or bacterial). Modifiable risk factors (listed hierarchically according to the efficacy of interventions in reducing the incidence of CVD) include cigarette smoking, high cholesterol, HTN, malnutrition, obesity, physical inactivity, diabetes, altered hormonal status (e.g., oral contraceptives, hysterectomy, or oophorectomy), psychological stress, alcohol consumption (excessive or complete abstinence), and sleep-disordered breathing.[120] Among teens, cigarette smoking remains high (one in five, 20%)[250] and continues to be a major contributor to future CVD in America. Serum cholesterol levels, obesity, physical inactivity, diabetes, and environmental stress are all increasing in American children.[44,224] As many as 40% of school-age children (6 to 12 years) currently display at least one risk factor for heart disease.[224]

An important epidemiologic aspect of CVD risk in children is the tracking of lipid and lipoproteins concentration over time. Data from the Lipid Research Clinics prevalence studies have shown that the concentration of serum lipids and lipoproteins increases during early childhood and reaches concentrations similar to those seen in young adults by approximately 2 years of age.[92] Acceptable, borderline, and high cholesterol levels in children and adolescents 2 to 19 years old are less than 170 mg/dL, 170 to 200 mg/dL and 200 or mg/dL or higher, respectively. Low-density lipoprotein (LDL) cholesterol should be less than 110 mg/dL, with levels of 110 to 129 mg/dL considered borderline, and levels of 130 mg/dL or more are considered high. The American Heart Association also recommends that triglyceride concentrations of greater than 150 mg/dL and high-density lipoprotein (HDL) concentrations of less than 35 mg/dL be considered abnormal for children and adolescents.[92]

Puberty and the Integumentary System

Skin is the largest organ of the body and performs many vital functions. The PT should always assess the skin during observational and palpatory examinations because it can tell us much about the general health of our patients. The integumentary system, which houses hair follicles, apocrine and eccrine units (thermoregulation via perspiration), and sebaceous glands (production of sebum [oil] for lubrication), undergoes significant changes during puberty.

The endocrine system regulates changes in patterns of hair growth and the output of sebaceous and sweat glands. Tanner's stages of sexual development (see Table 16-4) delineate the specific changes in growth of pubic hair. In girls and boys, growth of axillary hair typically begins 2 years after growth of pubic hair. For boys, facial hair also begins 2 years after the onset of puberty.[163] In middle adolescence, activation of hair growth of the sebaceous and sweat glands can lead to issues with acne

TABLE 16-6

Heat Stress Disorders, Clinical Features, and Treatment Recommendations[15,22]

Heat Stress Disorder	Clinical Features	Treatment
Heat illness; weight loss via sweat, less than 5% body weight	Thirst, chills, clammy skin, cramps, nausea, muscle twitches, weakness, and fatigue	Drink a half-cup of water every 15-20 min; during breaks, rest in the shade when possible; remove extra clothes.
Heat exhaustion; weight loss via sweat, 5%-10% body weight	Reduced sweating, dizziness, headaches, shortness of breath, lack of saliva, extreme fatigue, weak and rapid pulse, lack of coordination, thirst	Stop activity and move to a cool place; drink 2 cups of water for every pound lost; remove wet clothes and sit in a chair in a cold shower.
Heat stroke; weight loss via sweat, more than 10% body weight	Lack of sweat, dry, hot skin, lack of urine, hallucinations, swollen tongue, deafness, aggression, ataxia, high temperature, seizures, vomiting, rapid heart rate, diarrhea	**Medical emergency:** Stop activity and move to a cool place; place ice bags on head and back until help arrives; do not attempt to give water (aspiration possible).

Daily water balance depends on the net difference between water gain and water loss. Dehydration (>2% body weight loss from water deficit) can degrade aerobic exercise performance, especially in warm or hot weather. Humidity and temperature, comorbid conditions, age, gender (women), and diet are all critical factors in temperature regulation. Data from American College of Sports Medicine: Position stand: exercise and fluid replacement, *Med Sci Sports Exerc* 39:377-90,2007.

and body odor (i.e., hygiene). Given their stage of psychosocial development, adolescents are naturally concerned with how changes in their integumentary system affect their self-identity and relationships.

ACNE. Acne is a problem of the sebaceous glands, which are stimulated by the hormonal changes of adolescence. It comes in several forms—whiteheads (under the skin), blackheads (at the skin surface), papules (small pink bumps), pustules (red at the bottom and pus on the top), nodules (large, painful, solid pimples), and cysts (deep, painful, pus-filled pimples).[278] In Western cultures, acne affects up to 95% of adolescents and persists into middle age in 12% of women and 3% of men.[129] High-glycemic carbohydrates (e.g., bread, bagels, doughnuts, crackers, candy, cake, chips) that substantially boost blood sugar and insulin levels (which stimulate sebaceous glands) have been linked to acne. Acne is believed to affect young men slightly more than young women, and males are more likely to have severe, longer lasting forms of acne. Hormonal changes associated with the menstrual cycle and the use of cosmetics may make some young women more susceptible to acne problems.[129]

Acne must be treated according to the type of acne, severity, age, and gender. Acne may be a major sign of polycystic ovarian syndrome (females) or adrenal hyperandrogenism (both genders).[108] Most teens manage their acne with over-the-counter treatments, but more than one in three (35%) will consult a physician for treatment.[129] Recalcitrant (unmanageable) acne should be systematically and progressively treated by a variety of pharmaceuticals: topical retinoids, benzoyl peroxide, and topical antibiotics (mild acne); topical agents, oral antibiotics, and hormonal agents (moderate acne); and isotretinoin (Accutane) as a last resort for severe acne.[277] Isotretinoin is an extremely effective treatment for acne, but is a pregnancy teratogen with numerous other side effects (MS, gastrointestinal, neurologic, and hematologic).[277] This drug should never be taken during pregnancy or even 1 month before a planned pregnancy. Unfortunately, approximately 70% of teenage pregnancies are unintended.[136]

THERMOREGULATION. Children (prepubescent), adolescents, and adults differ in their thermoregulatory responses to exercise and heat. There are three reasons why exercising children do not

acclimatize heat as well as adults: (1) children have a greater surface area–to–body mass ratio than adults, (2) children produce more metabolic heat per mass unit than adults, and (3) sweating capacity is considerably lower in children, reducing their ability to dissipate body heat by evaporation.[15] During adolescence, anthropometric (growth) changes influence the surface area–to–body mass ratio, aiding in heat dissipation. Also, pubertal hormones activate apocrine and eccrine units, increasing sweating mechanisms that aid in thermoregulation of the body. Given the fact that pubertal onset varies among individuals, coaches, teachers, caregivers, and young athletes must watch for signs of heat injury and dehydration (more than 2% body weight loss from water deficit).[22] Limiting the time spent playing and training for sports in hot, humid conditions and ensuring adequate fluid intake can prevent heat injury.[22,117] Table 16-6 defines heat stress disorders, their clinical features, and treatment recommendations.

Examination Schema

Adolescent Health Care Issues by Body System

PTs working with the adolescent population should strongly, and appropriately, emphasize examination of the developing neuromusculoskeletal system.[25,251,264] Sullivan and Markos' evaluation model reminds the PT to go beyond the physical systems and examine the other factors (e.g., medical, environmental, social, cultural, and psychological variables) that affect a patient's overall physical capabilities (Figure 16-3A).[251] The interlocking rings (see Figure 16-3B) represent three of the four preferred practice patterns (PPPs) of physical therapy: (1) MS, (2) nervous (i.e., neuromuscular), and (3) cardiovascular-pulmonary systems. The fourth PPP (integumentary system) could be represented by simply encircling the physical systems with a "layer of skin." The development of these four systems and key adolescent issues were previously discussed. Table 16-7 summarizes key adolescent health care issues by body systems. This table highlights normative data, lists signs and symptoms (S/S) of key adolescent diseases, and outlines tests and measures per the *Guide to Physical Therapist Practice*.[25]

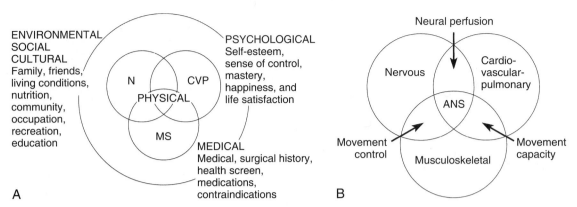

FIGURE 16-3 Examination schema categorizing interaction of many factors influencing physical capability. (From Sullivan PE, Markos PD: *Clinical decision making in therapeutic exercise* Stamford, CT, 1995 Appleton & Lange.)

The examination of the adolescent follows the sequence used with the adult (see Sections One and Two of this text). Communication skills (see Chapter 5) and an appreciation of adolescent culture (see Chapter 3) are critical to the development of a therapeutic alliance between health care provider and the young patient. The cognitive development of the adolescent affects the format of the history and physical examination. Subjective data can be gathered directly from the patient or with the assistance of a primary caregiver, teacher, coach, or employer. This can make subjective interviewing a potentially delicate situation in which health care practitioners must balance individual patient's rights with the caregiver's desire to protect and/or influence the child.

Adolescent health care needs change as the child progresses through puberty (see Tables 16-1 and 16-2). During early adolescence, the physical changes of sexual maturation make modesty during interactions with others paramount. Keep the patient dressed during the subjective history, and leave the room when the patient gowns. Most adolescents prefer to be examined without a parent or caregiver in the room, but this depends on the patient's developmental level, familiarity with the examiner, relationship with the caregiver or parent, and medical issues.[255] For younger adolescents, ask the child and caregiver their preferences. Respectfully allow all adolescents to have control and input into the examination and treatment process. Reassurance and nonjudgmental interaction between the adolescent and health care provider are crucial not only to the development of the youth's social identity but also to the youth's long-term perception of the importance and value of health care.

As with all patients, the initial clinical decision in the patient-management process is to determine whether the adolescent (1) can be safely treated by the PT, (2) can be managed by a PT in consultation with another health care practitioner, or (3) needs medical referral. Because adolescence is a time of unique physical, emotional, and social development, identifying risks to the patient's health (see Chapter 8), investigating presenting symptoms (see Chapter 7), and thoroughly reviewing body systems (see Chapter 9) require a different thought process compared with other age groups. The PT must know the common adolescent health conditions (e.g., respiratory conditions or cancers), relevant teenage lifestyle factors (e.g., illicit drug or alcohol abuse, unsafe sexual practices, or drunk driving), and causes of injury and death (e.g., accidents specific to adolescents).

Mortality and Morbidity in Adolescents

Age, gender, race, ethnicity, and socioeconomic status all play important roles in mortality and development of disease (morbidity).[166] Currently, the top ten leading causes of death (Table 16-8) in the United States are heart disease (26%), malignant neoplasms (23.1%), cerebrovascular conditions (5.7%), chronic lower respiratory diseases (5.1%), unintentional injuries (5%), DM (3%), Alzheimer's disease (3%), influenza and pneumonia (2.3%), nephritis (1.9%), septicemia (1.4%), and all others (23.5%).[77] Among all persons 1 to 44 years of age, unintentional injury is the leading cause of death, whereas heart disease ranks fifth for persons 1 to 34 years of age. For adolescents (10 to 14 years) the leading causes of death are unintentional injuries (35.6%), malignant neoplasms (13.1%), homicide (7.1%), suicide (6.3%), heart disease (4.8%), congenital anomalies (4.7%), chronic lower respiratory disease (1.8%), cerebrovascular conditions (1.5%), septicemia (1.3%), benign neoplasms (1.1%), and all others (22.7 %).[77] For late adolescents (15 to 19 years) and young adults (20 to 24 years), unintentional injuries account for almost half of all deaths (46.5%). Malignant neoplasms (4.7%) drops to number four behind homicide (16.4%) and suicide (12%). Heart disease (3.1%) ranks fifth as a cause of death for persons 15 to 24 years of age, followed by congenital anomalies (1.3%), cerebrovascular conditions (0.6%), and influenza and pneumonia (0.5%). New causes of death for the 15- to 24-year-old age group include human immunodeficiency virus (HIV) at number eight (0.6% of deaths) and complications of pregnancy at number ten (0.5%). Unspecified causes accounts for 13.7% of deaths for persons 15 to 24 years of age.[77]

The unintentional injury death rate (15.0/100,000 children) varies by age: younger than 1 year (24.4), 1 to 4 years (10.8), 5 to 9 years (6.0), 10 to 14 years (7.2), and 15 to 19 years (33.1).[47] The most deaths (56%) occur among adolescents 15 to 19 years, and are chiefly related to motor vehicle accidents (74%), poisoning (7%), and pedestrian accidents (5%). The risk of death by falls is inversely related to age: younger than 1 year (52%), 1 to 4 years (43%), 5 to 9 years (37%), 10 to 14 years (28%), and 15 to 19 years (17%), and falls are the leading cause of non-fatal injury in persons younger than 15 years. Other causes of unintentional death among youths 0 to 19 years of age include drowning (9%), suffocation (8%), fire- and burn-related (5%), poisoning (5%), and bites or stings, which vary by age—14%

TABLE 16-7

Adolescent Health Care Issues by Body System

System	Issues
CIRCULATORY SYSTEM	
Measures of circulation include arterial, venous, and lymphatic circulation and aerobic capacity[*]	This age group is not typically at risk for acquired diseases of the circulatory system (arteriosclerosis, arrhythmias, CAD, PVD). Children, adolescents, and young adults often have an innocent systolic murmur, often called a flow murmur, that is thought to reflect pulmonary blood flow.[39] Murmurs
Examination of the adolescent's circulatory system mirrors the adult physical examination	should be monitored by the adolescent's primary care physician (pediatrician), particularly as part of preparticipation sports physicals.[95]
Examination items include:	*HR norms* (see Table 16-5)
Heart rate	Red flags in adolescents:
Heart rhythm	Bradycardia in a thin adolescent may be caused by anorexia nervosa.
Heart sounds	HR >180-200 beats/min indicates supraventricular tachycardia.
Blood pressure	Bradycardia or tachycardia in a noncooperative patient could be a sign of drug overdose.
Peripheral circulation including skin color, skin texture, skin temperature, hair growth, nails, and distal pulses	Blood pressure (see Table 16-5)
Peripheral edema	Using average (readings on at least three separate occasions) systolic and/or diastolic pressure for age, gender, and height, adolescent blood pressure is defined as follows:
Response of the body to positional changes, movement, and exercise	Normal, <90th percentile
There are currently eight preferred practice patterns (PPPs) specific to the CVP system[*]	High-normal, 90th-95th percentile
	High, ≥95th percentile
	Cholesterol screening: Everyone age 20 and older should have his or her blood cholesterol measured at least once every 5 years. Screening[92] is recommended for persons <20 yr if one parent presents with high blood cholesterol or a parent or grandparent has premature CVD (before age 50). The presence of other risk factors (e.g., diabetes, smoking, high blood pressure, obesity or overweight, a family history of early heart disease, birth control medication [for females]), is an indication to monitor cholesterol levels (mg/dL):
	Total cholesterol < 200 (170 = borderline)
	LDL cholesterol < 110
	HDL cholesterol <35 is low; ≥60 is high
	Triglycerides <150
ENDOCRINE SYSTEM	
Measures of endocrine system include specific questioning in the subjective interview[*]	The functions of the body are regulated by the endocrine and nervous systems.
Examination items include objective tests of the endocrine system—disease-specific	Important glands and hormones of the endocrine system:
	Adrenal cortex (cortisol and aldosterone)
	Anterior pituitary (growth hormone, adrenocorticotropin, thyroid-stimulating hormone, follicle-stimulating hormone, luteinizing hormone, prolactin)
	Islets of Langerhans of the pancreas (insulin, glucagon)
	Ovaries (estrogen, progesterone)
	Parathyroid (parathyroid hormone)
	Placenta (human chorionic gonadotropin, estrogens, progesterone, human somatomammotropin)
	Posterior pituitary (vasopressin, oxytocin)
	Testes (testosterone)
	Thyroid (thyroxine, triiodothyronine, calcitonin)
	Puberty brings extensive physical changes via the endocrine system. Health care providers should monitor adolescents for normal progression through the Tanner stages of sexual development (see puberty discussion, Table 16-6).
	Most common adolescent diseases specific to the endocrine system:
	Cystic fibrosis (see Table 16-4)
	Diabetes (thirst or polydipsia, nocturia)—7% of adolescents aged 12-19 yr have impaired fasting glucose level
	Precocious puberty
	Thyroid disorders (adenoma, cancer hypofunction or hyperfunction)
GASTROINTESTINAL (GI) SYSTEM	
Measures of GI system include specific questioning in the subjective interview[*]	GI signs and symptoms (S/S)—abdominal pain, achalasia, appetite changes, bowel movements (change in control, color, size, and bowel habits), constipation, disordered eating habits, diarrhea, dysphagia, excessive flatulence, excessive flatulence, food intolerance, GI bleeding (hematemesis, hematochezia, and melena), heartburn, hemorrhoids, jaundice, nausea or vomiting.[39,120]
Examination items include objective tests of the GI system; disease-specific but may include height, weight (anthropometrics), inspection, palpation, auscultation, and percussion of organs	Review of systems questioning specific to GI system (see Chapter 9)
	Most common adolescent diseases specific to the GI system:
	Crohn's disease
	Disordered eating patterns (anorexia nervosa, bulimia)
	Gastric ulcer
	Inflammatory bowel disease (IBD)
	Obesity
	Peptic ulcer disease
	Ulcerative colitis

TABLE 16-7

Adolescent Health Care Issues by Body System—cont'd

System	Issues
INTEGUMENTARY SYSTEM	
Inspection and palpation of the integumentary system gives the evaluating therapist insight into the overall health of the adolescent Examination of the adolescent's skin mirrors the adult physical examination Five PPPs currently are dedicated to the integumentary system*	Skin lesions can have various causes.[119] These include physical trauma, contact with injurious agents (e.g., chemical toxins) and infective organisms, reaction to medication, allergens, or radiotherapy; systemic origin (e.g., diseases with cutaneous manifestations; arterial insufficiency), hereditary factors, burns (thermal, electrical, chemical, or inhalation), and neoplasms. Signs and symptoms of skin injury or disease include bleeding, pruritus (itching), urticaria (hives), rash, blisters, and xeroderma (dryness).[120] Specific areas of interest (see puberty discussion): Acne is a key disorder of this age group; sebaceous glands more active with endocrine changes Thermoregulation changes as child enters and advances through puberty Burn injuries, especially to the face, have profound effect on self-esteem, self-identity. Given adolescents' stage of psychosocial development, burns can be psychologically taxing to the adolescent. Delayed wound healing can be a sign of local or systemic disease or even mental illness. Suspicion of self-mutilation (self-injury) should be a red flag for a psychological disorder. Chronic regional pain syndrome (formally reflex sympathetic dystrophy)
MUSCULOSKELETAL (MS) SYSTEM	
Measures of MS system include muscle performance (strength, power, and endurance), joint integrity and mobility, ROM (including muscle length), and functional tasks (e.g., gait and body mechanics)* Examination of the adolescent's MS system mirrors the adult physical examination, with special attention to growth factors There are currently 10 PPPs specific to the MS system*	MS S/S—loss of active or passive ROM, weakness, myofascial pain symptoms (lower back pain, neck pain), joint pain are common MS symptoms. Joint pain is a common symptom in persons seeking health care. Joint pain with systemic symptoms (fever, chills, rash, anorexia, weight loss, or weakness) or other organ symptoms should be referred for medical evaluation. Adolescence is a time marked by skeletal growth, increased muscle mass, and sexual development and maturation. It is not unusual to hear a child complain of growing pains and to require increased sleep. Growth and development produce changes in posture, flexibility, strength, and motor control (neuromuscular coordination). See "Puberty and the Musculoskeletal System" and "Musculoskeletal Disorders of Adolescence".
NERVOUS SYSTEM	
Measures of neuromuscular system include arousal, attention, cognition, cranial and peripheral nerve integrity, motor function, neuromotor development and sensory integration, pain, reflex integrity, and sensory integrity* Examination of the adolescent's nervous system mirrors the adult physical examination Examination items include: CNS, PNS, and ANS Mental status Appearance, behavior Cognitive functions Mood Speech and language Thought and perception There are currently nine PPPs specific to the neuromuscular system*	Nervous system S/S—changes in mood, attention, or speech; changes in orientation, memory, insight or judgment; headache, dizziness, or vertigo; generalized proximal or distal weakness, numbness, abnormal sensation, or loss of sensation; abnormal muscle tone; loss of consciousness; syncope or near-syncope; seizures or tremors Lower motor neuron (LMN) lesion: Ipsilateral flaccid paralysis Reduced tone and deep tendon reflexes; muscle atrophy Sensory disturbances and fasciculation Upper motor neuron (UMN) lesion: Spastic paralysis Increased tone, hyperreflexia, minimal muscle atrophy Possible sensory disturbances Cranial nerve functions (see Chapters 10 and 12 screening) Autonomic nervous system regulates the viscera, overall metabolism, secretions, body temperature, reproduction, blood flow in the viscera, muscle, and periphery. Many chronic pain syndromes (e.g., complex regional pain syndrome [CRPS], fibromyalgia, myofascial trigger points) and mental conditions (e.g., depression, anxiety, attention-deficit/hyperactivity disorder [ADHD]) can be intensified by the influences of the sympathetic nervous system. The treatment approach for these conditions should be multidisciplinary, including patient education; physical, occupational, and behavioral therapy; and pharmacologic treatment with antiepileptic, psychiatric, and/or analgesic drugs. See "Puberty and the Nervous System."
PSYCHOLOGICAL SYSTEM†	
Mental disorders seen in children and adolescents (and adults) The World Health Organization (WHO) predicts that by the year 2020, childhood neuropsychiatric disorders will rise by over 50% internationally to become one of the five most common causes of morbidity, mortality, and disability in youth worldwide	Mental health screening—in addition to screening for NS function, the PT must screen adolescents for behavior changes caused by mental illness, substance abuse (drugs or alcohol), and suicidal tendencies. Up to one third of all primary care visits involve mental health, including depressed mood, anxiety, somatic concerns, and more serious disorders of mood and mental function.[39,120] Risk factors for suicide include psychiatric illness, substance abuse, personality disorder, previous suicide attempt or family history of suicide, gender identity crisis or persecution Most common neuropsychiatric disorders seen in adolescents: ADHD Anxiety disorders (generalized anxiety disorder [GAD], OCD, panic disorder, PTSD, phobias, including specific and/or social phobias, separation anxiety, selective autism) Autism and other pervasive developmental disorders Depressive disorders Disruptive behavior disorders

TABLE 16-7

Adolescent Health Care Issues by Body System—cont'd

System	Issues
PSYCHOLOGICAL SYSTEM†—cont'd	Eating disorders (anorexia nervosa, bulimia nervosa, binge-eating disorder; 35% of those affected are male)
	Learning disabilities
	Manic, bipolar disorder
	Mood disorders
	Schizophrenia
	Tics, Tourette's syndrome
	Current estimates are that 1 in 10 U.S. children and adolescents suffers from mental illness severe enough to impair daily functioning. The National Institute on Mental Health estimates that only 1 in 5 of these youth receives needed treatment.[196]

RESPIRATORY SYSTEM (THORAX AND LUNGS)

Measures specific to the respiratory system include aerobic capacity, ventilation and respiratory gas exchange, joint integrity, and mobility specific to the thorax*

Examination of the adolescent's respiratory system mirrors the adult physical examination

Examination items include:
  Thorax contour
  Respiratory rate
  Respiratory rhythm
  Breathing pattern
  Rib cage expansion
  Joint mobility (thoracic spine and rib cage)
  Percussion auscultation (breath sounds)
  Aerobic capacity

Respiratory S/S—chest pain or discomfort, cough, dyspnea, hemoptysis, sputum (color, quantity), and wheezing could be signs and symptoms of asthma, bronchitis, emphysema, pneumonia, and tuberculosis. This age group is not typically at risk for chronic pulmonary diseases. Smoking in adolescence is a risk factor for future pulmonary and cardiovascular disease.

Examination of this system mirrors the adult physical examination:

Age (yr)	Normal RR of adolescents(breaths/min)
10	20-26
12	18-22
14	18-22
16	16-20
>18	12-20

Common adolescent concerns specific to the respiratory system:
  Asthma: >9.5 million (13.5%) U.S. children <18 yr have been diagnosed with asthma; boys (15%) more affected than girls (11%); Hispanic African American children more likely to have ever been diagnosed with asthma or to still have asthma (20%, 15%) than Hispanic children (13%, 9%) or non-Hispanic white children (11%, 7%). Children in poor families have been diagnosed with or still have asthma (17%, 12%) more frequently than children in families that were not poor (12%, 8%). Children in fair or poor health were 3.5 times as likely to have ever been diagnosed with asthma and 5.5 times as likely to still have asthma (41%, 41%) as children in excellent or very good health (11%, 7%).[193]
  Asthma is a complex disorder involving biochemical, autonomic, immunologic, infectious, endocrine, and psychological factors. It is a long-term, often progressive, disease in which swelling of the lining of the airways and narrowing of the passageways make breathing difficult. It has been described as "arthritis of the airways."
  Allergies—10% of U.S. children <18 yr suffer from hay fever and respiratory allergies. Non-Hispanic white children are more affected by hay fever or respiratory allergies (11%, 10%) than Asian (8%, 7%), Hispanic (8%, 7%) or African American (7%, 7%) children. Children of educated parents (more than a high school diploma) are more likely to have respiratory allergies, hay fever, and other allergies than children of parents with less education. Children in fair or poor health are 3 times more likely to have had respiratory allergies as children in excellent or very good health (24%, 9%).[193]

REPRODUCTIVE SYSTEM (GENITAL SYSTEM)

The reproductive system undergoes significant changes during adolescence (puberty)

Knowledge of normal sexual maturation (Tanner stages) is pertinent to recognizing delayed development or precocious puberty (see discussion of puberty)

Females—age of menarche, menstrual regularity, frequency, duration, and amount of bleeding, dysmenorrhea, amenorrhea, sexual habits, bleeding with or after intercourse, vaginal discharge, sores, itching, exposure to STDs are all part of the reproductive system health history and examination.

Males—hernias, discharges from the penis or sores on the penis, testicular pain or masses, sexual habits, and exposure to STDs are all part of the genital system health history and examination.

Although this system generally is not the domain of the PT, the function of the sacral nerve roots (S2-S4) is part of the lower quarter screening examination.

Common adolescent concerns specific to the reproductive system:
  Sexual habits, preference, interest, and function, sexual satisfaction, birth control methods, condom use, unprotected sex
  Is the adolescent at risk of STDs, pregnancy, or being victimized?
  Issues of confidentiality and privacy laws

Continued

TABLE 16-7

Adolescent Health Care Issues by Body System—cont'd

System	Issues
URINARY SYSTEM Examination of the adolescent's urinary system mirrors the adult physical examination Examination items include: Subjective questions regarding urinary function (e.g., output, control, color) Inspection of external organs (as needed) Palpation of the abdomen Percussion of the kidneys	Urinary and renal S/S—color changes (clear, concentrated yellow, reddish, or brown); dysuria (urgency, frequency, or hesitancy and/or reduced stream); glucuria; hematuria; kidney, flank, or groin pain; nocturia; polyuria; stress incontinence; suprapubic pain or ureteral colic The urogenital system is located primarily within the midline of the abdomen. It has extensive connections to the endocrine system in regard to regulation of overall function. The urinary system consists of the kidneys, ureters, bladder, and urethra. Common adolescent concerns specific to the urinary system: Screening for alcohol or drug abuse Chronic urinary tract infections (UTIs) or bladder infections could be a sign of unsafe sexual practices, putting the adolescent at greater risk for STDs. Untreated pelvic inflammatory disease (PID) can have serious ramifications, including female (more than male) sterility, tubal pregnancies, and congenital infant conditions (e.g., prematurity, eye disease, and pneumonia), and systemic illness (see STD discussion).

*See American Physical Therapy Association: Guide to Physical Therapist Practice. 2nd Edition. American Physical Therapy Association, *Phys Ther* 81:9-746, 2001.
†An extension of the nervous system.

TABLE 16-8

Top Ten Causes of Death (%)

Age (yr)		
All Ages	**10-14**	**15-19**
Heart disease (26)	Unintentional injury (35.6)	Unintentional injury (46.5)
Malignant neoplasms (23.1)	Malignant neoplasms (13.1)	Homicide (16.4)
Cerebrovascular (5.7)	Homicide (7.1)	Suicide (12)
Chronic lower respiratory disease (5.1)	Suicide (6.3)	Malignant neoplasms (4.7)
Unintentional injury (5)	Heart disease (4.8)	Heart disease (3.1)
Diabetes mellitus (3)	Congenital anomalies (4.7)	Congenital anomalies (1.3)
Alzheimer's (3)	Chronic lower respiratory disease (1.8)	Cerebrovascular (0.6)
Influenza an pneumonia (2.3)	Cerebrovascular (1.5)	HIV (0.6)
Nephritis (1.9)	Septicemia (1.3)	Influenza and pneumonia (0.5)
Septicemia (1.4)	Benign neoplasms (1.1)	Complicated pregnancy (0.5)
All others (23.5)	All others (22.7)	All others (13.7)

From Centers for Disease Control and Prevention, National Center for Injury Prevention and Control: *WISQARS leading causes of death reports*, 1999-2006 (website). http://webappa.cdc.gov/sasweb/ncipc/leadcaus10.html. Accessed August 1, 2009.

(younger than 1 year), 9% (1 to 4 years), and 8% (5 to 9 years), respectively.[47]

Geographically, the Northeast has the lowest death rates and southern states rank highest, given a high incidence of transportation-related deaths. Among all racial groups, the unintentional death rate was highest for American Indian and Alaska Native males (29.8/100,000).[47] Among females, only American Indian and Alaska Native females had higher death rates than the national average.[47] Males had higher death rates than females in all age groups (19.3 and 10.4/100,000, respectively).[47] These mortality and morbidity statistics underscore the importance of monitoring geographic, environmental, and lifestyle factors when working with young patients and their caregivers.[166]

CHRONIC CONDITIONS. Observers estimate that there are 11.4 to 13.6 million children (15% to 18%) in the United States with a chronic health condition, but the prevalence of chronic illness ranges from 0.22% to 44% depending on how terms are operationalized.[268] In general, a condition is considered chronic if the following characteristics are met: (1) noncommunicable illness, (2) prolonged duration (longer than 3 months), (3) does not resolve spontaneously, and (4) can rarely be cured completely.[268] Chronic conditions often require extended medical attention across multiple domains of health care practice (e.g., inpatient or outpatient therapies, school-based therapy, home health).[222] PTs are reminded that children with chronic conditions may have limitations in physical performance and exercise tolerance when prevention or rehabilitation programs are undertaken (Table 16-9).[33]

Presently, chronic diseases affect millions of children, almost one in two adults (133 million), accounting for 70% of deaths each year and 75% of annual health care costs ($700 billion).[68] information on chronic conditions by age, gender, race, and

TABLE 16-9

Physiologic Functions that Limit Physical Performance and Exercise Tolerance in Children and Adolescents with Chronic Diseases

Function	Diseases
Low maximal heart rate	Beta blockers, congenital complete atrioventricular block, anorexia nervosa, artificial pacemakers (fixed and variable rate), postsurgical period after Mustard operation for transposition of the great arteries
Low maximal stroke volume	Aortic stenosis, cardiomyopathy, detraining, Ebstein's anomaly of the tricuspid valve (also postoperatively), severe hypohydration, pulmonary stenosis, tetralogy of Fallot (also postoperatively), postsurgical period after Mustard operation for transposition of the great arteries, ventricular septal defect
Low oxygen-carrying capacity of arterial blood	Anemia, cyanotic heart defects, hemoglobinopathies, 2,3-diphosphoglycerate deficiency
Low peripheral oxygen extraction	Detraining, severe malnutrition, muscle atrophies and dystrophies, spina bifida, 2, 3-diphosphoglycerate deficiency
Low lung diffusion capacity	Cystic fibrosis
Low maximal alveolar ventilation	Cystic fibrosis, muscle atrophies and dystrophies, extreme obesity, advanced kyphoscoliosis
High submaximal oxygen cost	Arthritis, cerebral palsy, muscle atrophies and dystrophies, advanced obesity, leg prosthetics (e.g., after amputation)
Low muscle strength	Cerebral palsy, muscle atrophies and dystrophies, storage diseases, Prader-Willi syndrome
Low muscle endurance and peak power	Advanced anorexia, advanced cystic fibrosis, cerebral palsy, McArdle's disease, muscle atrophies and dystrophies

From Bar-Or O: Training considerations for children and adolescents with chronic disease. In Hasson SM, ed: *Clinical exercise physiology*, St. Louis, 1994, Mosby, p 267.

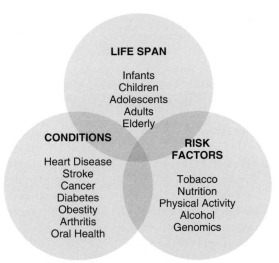

FIGURE 16-4 Framework for preventing chronic disease and promoting health across various health care settings—schools, communities, worksites, health systems. (From National Center for Chronic Disease Prevention and Health Promotion: *Chronic disease: The power to prevent, the call to control. At a glance 2009* (website). http://www.cdc.gov/ nccdphp. Accessed August 1, 2009.)

income can be found at the Centers for Disease Control and Prevention (CDC) National Center for Health Statistics (NCHS) website.[73] Priority chronic conditions and risk factors for promoting health across the life span and in various health care settings are shown in Figure 16-4.

Heart Disease and Stroke. The number of children in the United States with CVD is growing as obesity and physical inactivity grow as societal health care problems.[44,101,205,224] An estimated one in three American adults have HTN, a major risk factor for heart disease and stroke.[68] Evidence suggests a strong familial link for primary childhood HTN (49% to 86%) and secondary childhood HTN (46%).[172] Because arthrosclerosis is an unlikely mechanism of HTN in children as compared with older adults,

once HTN has been confirmed in young patient, an extensive history and careful physical examination should be conducted to identify underlying causes (e.g., renal disease or tumor, systemic lupus erythematosus, Cushing's disease, hyperthyroidism) of the elevated blood pressure and to detect any end-organ damage.[172] PTs should be cognizant that a patient is never too young to have or to be undergoing treatment for HTN. Proper nutrition and exercise is an appropriate tool to combat atherosclerotic HTN in persons of all ages. Parents should be informed that evidence suggests that breast-feeding an infant may have a protective role in preventing childhood HTN.[172]

Diabetes. Of adolescents 12 to 19 years of age, 7% have impaired fasting glucose levels.[68] Approximately 24.3/100,000/year, or 5.5 million children, 0 to 20 years old have been diagnosed with DM. For children, the diagnosis of type 1 DM (15,000/year) is still 4 times more likely than type 2 DM (3,700/year). Among youth under the age of 10 years, most diabetes cases are type 1 DM, regardless of race or ethnicity. The highest rates of type 1 DM is observed in non-Hispanic white youth (18.6, 28.1, and 32.9 for age groups 0 to 4, 5 to 9, and 10 to 14 years, respectively). Although on the rise, the diagnosis of type 2 DM is still relatively infrequent, and the highest rates (17.0 to 49.4/100,000 person-years) were documented among 15- to 19-year-old minority groups.[275] Children with diabetes are 3 times more likely to be hospitalized as their classmates.[101] Diabetes and CVD carry many long-term systemic ramifications (e.g., neuropathy, retinopathy, increased risk of amputation and disability) that will affect the quality of life of these young Americans as they age, as well as increase society's overall economic and health care burdens.

Cancer. Cancer is a leading cause of death worldwide: it accounted for 7.4 million deaths (approximately 13% of all deaths) in 2004.[20] The World Health Organization (WHO) projects that cancer rates could increase to 20 to 26 million new diagnoses and 13 to 17 million deaths by 2030.[274] The use of tobacco, physical inactivity, and obesity in adulthood are known risk factors for several common cancers (lung, esophagus, colorectum, breast in postmenopausal women, endometrium and kidney). A healthy active childhood was the theme of World Cancer Day 2009, recognizing that behavioral changes in regard to tobacco, alcohol diet, and exercise at a young age could do much to curb the growth of cancer worldwide.[274]

Obesity. Physical inactivity and obesity are ubiquitous to the American culture. Being overweight or obese substantially raises the risk of illness from high blood pressure, high cholesterol, type 2 diabetes, heart disease, stroke, gallbladder disease, arthritis, sleep disturbances, breathing problems, and certain types of cancers.[44] Obese individuals, especially children, also may suffer from social stigmatization, discrimination, and lowered self-esteem.[205] (See later, "Physical Activity, Overweight, and Obesity.")

Arthritis. Arthritis has long been a significant chronic health problem among American adults affecting more than 46.4 million (21.6%), disabling 8.6 million more and costing the health care system $300 billion/year.[69] Arthritis comes in many forms, including osteoarthritis (27 million), fibromyalgia (5 million), gout (3 million), rheumatoid arthritis (1.3 million), polymyalgia rheumatics (711,000), Sjögren's syndrome (400,000 to 3.1 million), juvenile arthritis (294,000), lupus 161,000 to 322,000), and giant cell arteritis (228,000).[69,227] In 2007, a CDC benchmark study (first-time national database) estimated that 294,000 children under age 18 (1 in 250) have been diagnosed with arthritis or another rheumatologic condition.[227] This benchmark will allow for assessment of future shifts in the occurrence of arthritis, as well as lay the groundwork for potential interventions, most specifically fighting the childhood obesity epidemic, which is seen as a primary contributor to osteoarthritis.

Oral Health. Approximately 90% of adults have caries (cavities) in their teeth. The average number of retained natural teeth is 24 (of a possible 28) among adults, and 8% of adults are edentulous (toothless).[142] Between 50% and 68% of all U.S. teenagers have untreated caries; this figure is even higher among minorities and those living in poverty.[67] Children and adolescents with special health care needs (SHCNs) are almost twice as likely to have unmet oral health care needs as their peers without SHCNs across all income levels.[239]

Only 43% of adolescents visit the dentist regularly (twice annually). Dental visits for African American and Hispanic teens is even lower (25%). Beyond socioeconomic status, there are other factors that influence the oral health of adolescents, many of which are addressed by the seven tenets of teen oral hygiene.[238] Education on oral hygiene is crucial. PTs can help by learning and advocating the seven tenets of oral hygiene to children, adolescents, and their caregivers in a respectful, comprehensive, and directed way. Health care providers are reminded that high rates of caries, tooth loss, and periodontal disease have been linked to coronary heart disease and the prevalence of the metabolic syndrome.[142]

The seven tenets of teen oral health include the following:
1. Proper basic hygiene (brushing at a minimum of twice daily, and, if possible, after each meal and flossing daily to clean between teeth)[23]
2. Eating a healthy diet
3. Regular dental visits

National Children's Study

The prevalence of chronic diseases in children has increased since the 1980s and will likely increase further unless the epidemics of childhood obesity and physical inactivity are not confronted in a uniform fashion.[268] Prevention of chronic illness in the youth of America is a proactive long-term plan for cutting health costs for the nation.[106] To examine the effects of environmental influences on health and development, the *National Children's Study* (est. 2009), will follow more than 100,000 children across the United States from before birth until age 21. "Environment" is defined broadly to take a number of issues into account: natural and man-made environmental factors, biological and chemical factors, physical surroundings, social factors, behavioral influences and outcomes, genetics, cultural and family influences and differences and geographic locations. The goal of the study is to improve the health and well-being of children by analyzing how these factors interact with each other and what helpful and/or harmful effects they might have on children's health. Similar to the Framingham Heart Study, it is hoped that the National Children's Study will form the basis of child health guidance, interventions, and policy for generations to come. It is anticipated that the preliminary results from the first years of the Study will be available in 2011.

Adapted from National Children's Study Federal Advisory Committee (NCSAC): *National children's study* (website). http://www.nationalchildrensstudy.gov. Accessed March 9, 2010.

4. Fluoride supplementation
5. Oral safety (mouth guards for sports)
6. Avoiding oral piercings because they can chip teeth and facilitate gum recession and periodontal disease
7. Maintaining a healthy lifestyle (no smoking, alcohol, or drugs)[238]

Summary of Chronic Conditions. Our society is currently at war against the ominous enemy of chronic disease,[44] and evaluation and management of disease in children is a proactive way to combat chronic conditions (Box 16-3). The burden of chronic illness has considerable financial and organizational consequences for health care planning and delivery.[268] Recent medical and surgical advances have markedly reduced the mortality rates of children and adolescents with chronic conditions. Given this change in survival, outpatient PTs likely will provide health care to the adolescent who has a specific MS condition and a comorbid chronic illness. Physical therapy interventions should maximize the adolescent's functional abilities and sense of well-being, improve overall health-related quality of life, and facilitate their development into healthy and productive adults. Furthermore, health care providers should be aware that the place where children with complex chronic conditions are cared for and dying may be shifting toward residential homes. This shift is likely caused by the evolving epidemiology of life-threatening childhood conditions, advances in home-based medical technology, and changes in attitudes about pediatric palliative care and hospice services.[109] Racial and ethnic disparities regarding place of death may represent important limitations and opportunities for improvement in the current systems of pediatric chronic and palliative care.[109]

Screening in Childhood and Adolescence

CANCER. Cancers vary across the life span by histology, site of disease origin, gender, race, and ethnicity.[74] Environmental factors also play a role in the development of cancer. The CDC

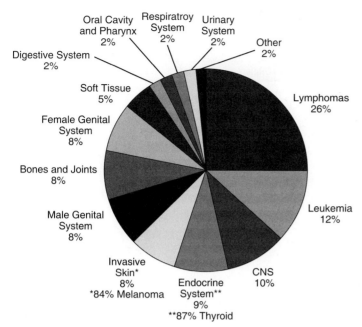

FIGURE 16-5 Cancer in 15- to 19-year olds by primary site. (From Centers for Disease Control and Prevention [CDC]: Trends in childhood cancer mortality—United States, 1990-2004, *MMWR Morb Mortal Wkly Rep* 56:1257-1261, 2007.)

periodically analyzes cancer morbidity and mortality rates for Americans based on type (primary tumor site), temporal (age), and demographic (gender, race, ethnicity) parameters and geographic distribution. The most recent cancer study compiled from the National Vital Statistics System (1990 to 2004) was published in December 2007. Common cancers by primary site for 15- to 19-year old adolescents are shown in Figure 16-5.

Because the spectrum of malignancies in youth is distinct based on age, gender and race, the International Classification of Childhood Cancer (ICCC) categorizes childhood cancers into four distinct 5-year age groups. The most recent classification was published in 2005. The incidence of cancer per million is highest in adolescents age 15 to 19 years (202.2/million), followed by the of those younger than 5 years (199.9/million), the 10 to 14 year age group (117.3/million), and children 5 to 9 years of age (110.2/million).[223] Table 16-10 contains data on specific childhood cancers for all races and by age. Tables 16-11 and 16-12 contain data on gender incidence (male-to-female ratio) and race (white-to-African American ratio), respectively.

The leading risk factors for cancer are advancing age, lifestyle, and personal behaviors (e.g., smoking, poor diet or nutrition, excessive alcohol use, high-risk sexual habits), exposure to viruses, geographic location, environmental variables, gender, ethnicity, socioeconomic status, occupation, heredity, presence of precancerous lesions, and stress.[120,223] Because children and adolescents 0 to 20 years of age have less lifetime exposure to these risk factors, their cancers tend to be more genetic (hereditary) in nature.[74] The adenocarcinomas (e.g., lung, breast, prostate, and colorectal cancers) common in adults are rarely seen in children.[120] The embryonal cancers that predominate among young children younger than 5 years (e.g., neuroblastoma, Wilms' [kidney] tumor, retinoblastoma, hepatoblastoma) are distinctly uncommon among 10- to 19–year olds. Children younger than 14 years also are more

likely to contract acute lymphoblastic leukemia (ALL) and CNS tumors, the more deadly of the childhood cancers.

Cancer is the fourth most common cause of death (after unintentional injury, homicide, and suicide) among persons aged 1 to 19 years in the United States.[74] Each year, one in every 330 children 0 to 20 years of age (over 12,600) is diagnosed with cancer and roughly one in five juveniles (17.6%) succumb to their illness.[223] The type of cancer (primary site) and a high rate of metastatic disease at time of diagnosis (80% in children) compared with adults (20%) are key variables in pediatric death rates.[74] The percentage of childhood cancer deaths by primary cancer site is shown in Figure 16-6. For all cancers combined during 1990 to 2004, per million, boys (33.1) had significantly higher death rates than girls (26.1); adolescents (37.9) had significantly higher death rates than children (26.9); whites (30.1) and African Americans (29.3) had significantly higher death rates than Asians–Pacific Islanders (A-PIs) (26.) and American Indian/Alaska Natives (AI/ANs) (20.0), respectively; and Hispanics (30.3) had significantly higher death rates than non-Hispanics (29.1).[74] Geographically, for all cancers combined, per million, children and adolescents living in the West (31.1) had significantly higher death rates than those living in the Midwest (29.1), the Northeast (28.4), and the South (29.8), respectively.[74]

Over the past several decades, advances in diagnosis and treatment have dramatically improved the 5-year survival rate (percentage of patients alive 5 years after their disease is diagnosed) of pediatric cancer. Currently (2003 to 2006), 79.6% of all children younger than 20 years survive 5 years or more, an increase of 21.5% since 1975 to 1977 (58.1%).[223] Observers currently estimate that 1 in 1000 people between the ages of 20 and 29 is a survivor of childhood or adolescent cancer, and that overall there are more than 270,000 childhood cancer survivors in the United States. One third of them suffer moderate to severe late effects from cancer treatment. Late effects (e.g., cognitive impairments, hearing, vision or tooth loss, changes in growth and development of muscle, bone, and sexual organs, CVP changes) can range from mild to severe, depending on primary cancer type and treatment methodology.[19]

Cancer Prevention Guidelines. Primary care health care providers, including PTs, should teach adolescents to take control of their health at a young age. Teach family members, teens, and the general public to recognize the signs and symptoms of occult disease. Know which cancers are specific to the adolescent population. Of all adult cancers, 50% can be prevented by following seven recommendations outlined in national public health policies.[21,44,205] These seven cancer prevention tips also can lower the long-term risk for heart disease, stroke, and diabetes:

1. Do not smoke.
2. Eat a healthy diet.
3. Maintain a healthy weight.
4. Protect yourself from the sun.
5. Drink less than one alcoholic beverage a day.
6. Get at least 30 minutes of physical activity every day.
7. Protect yourself and your partner(s) from sexually transmitted infections.

INFECTIONS. Clinical manifestations and prognoses for infectious diseases are many and vary with the causative agent (e.g., virus, bacteria, fungus, tuberculosis, parasite) and the body

TABLE 16-10

Childhood Cancer Classifications: Age-Specific Cancer Incidence Rates[*]

Tumor Category	Age (in years) at Diagnosis				Total for 15-19 Age Group (%)
	<5 Rate	5-9 Rate	10-14 Rate	15-19 Rate	
All sites	199.9	110.2	117.3	202.2	100.0
Acute lymphoblastic leukemia (ALL)	58.2	30.3	17.8	12.9	6.4
Acute myeloid leukemia (AML) (Ib)	10.1	4.5	5.7	8.5	4.2
Hodgkin's disease (IIa)	0.8	3.9	11.7	32.5	16.1
Non-Hodgkin's lymphoma (NHL) (IIb, c, e)	5.9	8.9	10.3	15.3	7.6
CNS tumors type III (total))	36.0	31.9	24.6	20.2	10.0
Ependymoma (IIIa)	5.6	1.6	1.3	1.1	0.5
Astrocytoma (IIIb)	15.0	15.9	15.1	12.3	6.1
Medulloblastoma, PNET (IIIc)	9.6	7.3	4.0	2.5	1.2
Neuroblastoma and ganglioneuroblastoma (IVa)	27.4	2.6	0.8	0.5	0.2
Retinoblastoma (V, total)	12.5	0.5	0.0	0.1	0.0
Wilms', rhabdoid, clear cell sarcoma (VIa)	18.0	5.8	0.6	0.4	0.2
Hepatic tumors (VII, total)	4.8	0.4	0.4	1.0	0.5
Hepatoblastoma (VIIa)	4.6	0.2	0.1	0.0	0.0
Osteosarcoma (VIIIa)	0.3	2.8	8.3	9.4	4.6
Ewing's sarcoma (VIIIc)	0.3	1.9	4.1	4.6	2.3
Soft tissue sarcoma (IX, total)	10.9	8.3	10.9	15.9	7.9
Rhabdomyosarcoma and embryonal sarcoma (IXa)	6.5	4.4	3.5	3.9	1.9
Nonrhabdo soft tissue sarcoma (IXb-e)	4.4	4.0	7.4	11.9	5.9
Germ cell, trophoblastic, other gonadal tumors (X, total)	6.9	2.4	6.7	30.8	15.2
Thyroid carcinoma (XIb)	0.1	1.0	4.1	14.6	7.2
Malignant melanoma (XId)	0.8	0.6	2.8	14.1	7.0
Other and unspecified carcinomas (XIf)	0.4	0.8	2.8	10.5	5.2

[*]Age-specific cancer incidence rates per million and percentage of total cases by ICCC category and age group, all races, both sexes SEER, 1986-1995. Adapted from Smith MA, Gurney JG, Gloeckler Ries LA: Cancer among adolescents 15-19 years old, (website). http://seer.cancer.gov/publications/childhood/adolescents.pdf. Accessed March 9, 2010.

TABLE 16-11

Childhood Cancer Classifications: Age-Adjusted Cancer Incidence Rates[*]

Tumor Category	Age (in years) at Diagnosis					
	0-14 Male[*]	0-14 Female[*]	0-14 M/F Ratio	15-19 Male	15-19 Female	15-19 M/F Ratio
All sites	149.5	128.7	1.2	204.3	199.9	1.0
Acute lymphoblastic leukemia	37.1	30.9	1.2	17.5	8.0	2.2
Acute myeloid leukemia (Ib)	6.6	6.5	1.0	8.4	8.5	1.0
Hodgkin's disease (IIa)	6.5	5.0	1.3	28.8	36.5	0.8
Non-Hodgkin's lymphoma (IIb,c,e)	12.3	4.5	2.7	19.4	11.0	1.8
CNS (III)	33.0	27.9	1.2	23.0	17.3	1.3
Osteosarcoma (VIIIa)	3.8	4.3	0.9	11.5	7.1	1.6
Ewing's sarcoma (VIIIc)	2.3	2.2	1.1	5.8	3.3	1.8
Soft tissue sarcomas (IX)	10.9	9.1	1.2	17.4	14.3	1.2
Germ cell tumors (X)	4.3	6.2	0.7	35.2	26.1	1.4
Thyroid carcinoma (XIb)	0.9	2.9	0.3	3.7	26.2	0.1
Melanoma (XId)	1.3	1.6	0.8	10.5	17.9	0.6

[*]Adjusted to the 1970 U.S. standard population, age-adjusted cancer incidence per million by ICCC group, gender, and age, all races, both genders, SEER 1986-1995. Adapted from Smith MA, Gurney JG, Gloeckler Ries LA: Cancer among adolescents 15-19 years old, (website). http://seer.cancer.gov/publications/childhood/adolescents.pdf. Accessed March 9, 2010.

system affected. Systemic symptoms of infectious disease include fever, chills, sweating, malaise, and nausea and vomiting (see Chapter 9). If the infection is specific to the CNS, symptoms also may include the following: focal headache, nausea, vomiting, stiff neck and back; focal neurologic signs, including hemiparesis, aphasia, ataxia, disorders of the limbs, and seizures; temporal lobe disturbances such as memory loss and hallucinations; and a positive Kernig's or Brudzinski's sign (meningeal inflammation). Because the brain (and its network of cerebrospinal fluid) lacks an immune system to fight infection, it is highly susceptible to damage from infection.

TABLE 16-12

Childhood Cancer Classifications: Age-Specific Cancer Incidence*

Tumor Category	White	African American	W/AA Ratio
Total	213.5	144.8	1.5
Acute lymphoblastic leukemia	14.3	6.4	2.2
Acute myeloid leukemia (Ib)	8.3	7.1	1.2
Hodgkin's disease (IIa)	36.5	26.9	1.4
Non-Hodgkin's lymphoma (IIb, c, e)	16.1	9.4	1.7
CNS (III)	21.8	15.8	1.4
Osteosarcoma (VIIIa)	9.2	8.4	1.1
Ewing's sarcoma (VIIIc)	5.4	0.3	18.0
Soft tissue sarcomas (IX)	14.5	20.5	0.7
Germ cell tumors (X)	33.9	13.8	2.5
Thyroid carcinoma (XIb)	15.5	6.7	2.3
Melanoma (XId)	16.1	0.3	53.7

*Rates per million by ICCC group and race, age 15-19 yr, SEER 1986-1995.
Adapted from Smith MA, Gurney JG, Gloeckler Ries LA: *Cancer among adolescents 15-19 years old,* (website). http://seer.cancer.gov/publications/childhood/adolescents.pdf. Accessed March 9, 2010.

Annually, about 1400 to 2800 cases of invasive meningococcal disease occur in the United States. About 20% of cases occur among adolescents and young adults (14 to 24 years).[64] About 10% to 14% die, and another 11% to19% have long-term complications (e.g., deafness, seizures, retardation, loss of limb use).[64] Fever, headache, and a stiff and painful neck are hallmark symptoms of meningitis. A lumbar puncture with bacterial culture is the only absolute means of diagnosing meningitis. Radiographs should be taken to rule out fracture, sinusitis, and mastoiditis; computed tomography (CT) scanning will reveal evidence of brain abscess or infarction.[120]

Encephalitis is an acute inflammatory disease of the brain caused by direct viral invasion. The herpes simplex virus (most often) and mosquito-borne or tickborne virus are the most common infectious agents. Signs and symptoms of viral encephalitis are similar to bacterial CNS infection, but a lumbar puncture will be negative. The brain electroencephalogram (EEG) is always abnormal. Vascular studies and CT or magnetic resonance imaging (MRI) scans will display cerebral edema and vascular damage. A brain biopsy is necessary to diagnose the herpes simplex virus.

Herpes simplex encephalitis (HSE) is responsible for about 10% of all encephalitis cases, with a frequency of about 2 cases/million/year. It is the most common nonepidemic encephalitis. Thirty percent of cases represent new infection; most are reactivation of an earlier infection. HSE caused by herpes simplex type 1 (cold sores) is most common in adolescents (younger than 20 years) and those older than 40 years. With the exception of acyclovir (Zovirax), an antiviral medication for the treatment of a herpes simplex virus, treatment is targeted to prevent complications of cerebral edema and includes surgical decompression, hyperventilation, and mannitol (a diuretic). The use of corticosteroids is controversial because of possible suppression of antibody protection within the CNS.[185]

Brain abscess (local infection of the brain) is an uncommon disorder, accounting for 2% of intracranial mass lesions.[119] It is

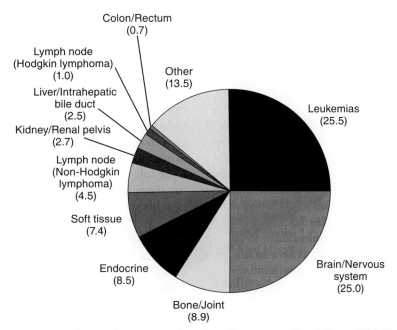

FIGURE 16-6 Percentage of childhood cancer deaths by primary cancer site and leading diagnosis, United States, 2004. (From Centers for Disease Control and Prevention [CDC]: Trends in childhood cancer mortality—United States, 1990-2004, *MMWR Morb Mortal Wkly Rep* 56:1257-1261, 2007.)

more likely to occur with concomitant bacterial, viral, fungal, or parasitic infections. A patient developing a brain abscess will present with fever, chills, headache, and focal neurologic signs that progress with time. These signs and symptoms, along with a recent history of infection or immunosuppression, lead to suspicion of brain abscess or neoplasm. CT and MRI scans are required to differentiate a tumor from an abscess. Treatment of abscess can include antibiotics specific to the infectious agent, corticosteroids to control cerebral edema, and surgical drainage to reduce mass effect. Almost half of all persons with a brain abscess are left with neurologic sequelae (e.g., focal signs, seizure activity).[120]

Although infections of the CNS are rare because of the protection of the blood-brain barrier, they have been noted in the adolescent population. Given the nature of their activities and environment (e.g., frequent exposure to large numbers of people through living in dormitories, by attending school activities and concerts), adolescents are more susceptible to CNS infections than other age groups. Many observers advocate vaccination of adolescents against meningococcal disease, particularly those living in dormitories (see later, "Immunization").[14,16,71]

Given the growth potential of pediatric patients, infections of synovial joints can be particularly harmful to long-term function. There are four types of infectious arthritis: (1) bacterial arthritis (e.g., gonococcal, infectious endocarditis, Lyme disease, septic arthritis, syphilis, tuberculosis; (2) fungal arthritis (e.g., *Candida*); (3) viral arthritis (e.g., Epstein-Barr virus [EBV], hepatitis, HIV, mumps, and rubella; and (4) reactive arthritis (e.g., acute rheumatic fever, chlamydial infections, enteric infections, Reiter's syndrome).[120] Lyme disease has been heralded as the fastest growing infectious disease in the United States after acquired immunodeficiency syndrome (AIDS).[66]

Adolescents also can develop infections from routine orthopedic surgeries (e.g., arthroscopy, peripheral joint ligamentous reconstruction), from open traumatic injuries (e.g., lacerations, abrasions), and occasionally from closed traumatic injury. Olecranon bursitis and prepatellar bursitis resulting from traumatic injury are the closed space conditions most likely to develop an abscess.[171] Spinal infections are particularly rare in adolescents, given that most cases of diskitis are associated with postoperative complications of diskectomy (3% postoperative incidence in the 25- to 45-year-old age group).[120]

Children and adolescents who develop an insidious limp or joint irritability with pain on active or passive motion, numbness, or tingling and weakness should be thoroughly examined (see Chapter 7). Referral for first-order diagnostic imaging (i.e., radiography) is always indicated for the pediatric patient with pain and loss of function about a joint, even in the absence of macrotrauma or prior surgical intervention.[175] Occult disease (e.g., inflammatory condition or infection) may also deem laboratory work necessary for differential diagnosis.

Sexually Transmitted Diseases. The PT must be vigilant for STDs, another source of infection in adolescents. STDs are hidden epidemics of enormous health and economic consequence in the United States. Currently, over 65 million Americans are living with a viral (incurable) STD.[71] Of the 18.9 million new cases of STDs each year, 9.1 million (48%) occur among 15- to 24-year-olds. Although they represent only 25% of the sexually active population, they account for almost half of all new STDs each year.[127] African Americans and Hispanics have higher rates of STDs than whites; this disparity is made worse by a lack of access to health care among socioeconomically disadvantaged minorities.[205]

Teens experimenting with sex are at a high risk for acquiring most STDs. Teenagers and young adults are more likely than any other age group to have multiple sex partners, engage in unprotected sex, and for young women, engage in sexual acts with persons older than themselves. In 2008, the CDC reported that one in four teenage girls had an STD. Women generally suffer more serious STD complications than men, including pelvic inflammatory disease, ectopic pregnancy, infertility, chronic pelvic pain, and cervical cancer caused by the human papilloma virus (HPV).[205] Moreover, teenage women are biologically more susceptible to chlamydia, gonorrhea, and HIV.[72] There is also compelling worldwide evidence that the presence of other STDs increases the likelihood of transmitting and acquiring HIV infection.[2] More than 25 diseases can be spread through sexual activity, but only some (chlamydia, gonorrhea, syphilis, hepatitis A and B, HIV) are required to be reported to state health departments and the CDC. Other commonly tracked STDs include genital herpes, HPV, trichomoniasis, bacterial vaginosis, and chancroid. The American Social Health Association[28] and the CDC[71] provide excellent up to date data on STDs across race, ethnicity, gender, age, and geographic distribution.

Chlamydia. Chlamydia is the most common (370 cases/100,000 persons) curable bacterial STD, caused by *Chlamydia trachomatis*. Over 1 million cases are reported each year to the CDC, but the actual number of cases could be 2 to 3 times higher because most women (75%) and some men (~50%) have no symptoms. If symptomatic, men and women experience proctitis (inflamed rectum), urethritis (inflamed urethra), conjunctivitis (inflamed eyelid), and soreness and redness of the throat or mouth. Occasionally, women will experience vaginal discharge and burning with urination. If the infection spreads to the fallopian tubes, women will have lower back pain, pain with intercourse, bleeding between menstrual cycles, and nausea or fever. Infected females can also pass complications on to infants (e.g., premature birth, eye disease, pneumonia). Men may experience one or more of the following: pus, watery or milky penial discharge, pain or burning with urination, or pain or swelling of the testicles. Among all age groups, teens and young adults have the highest rates of infection. Chlamydia is transmitted during vaginal and anal sex and, on rare occasions, oral sex. Untreated, chlamydia is particularly dangerous to female teens, with almost half (40%) of untreated females developing pelvic inflammatory disease (PID). One in five women with PID become sterile. Females infected with chlamydia are three to 5 times more likely to get HIV.[71]

Gonorrhea. Gonorrhea ("the clap") is a curable bacterial STD (*Neisseria gonorrhea)* transmitted by vaginal, anal, or oral sex (performing or receiving). Currently, gonorrhea has a yearly infection rate of 119 cases/100,000 people, but has a higher rate for female adolescents (200 cases/100,000) and African Americans (800 cases/100,000). The CDC estimates that only about 50% of cases are reported annually. Most men exhibit symptoms within 2 to 5 days of exposure (range, 1 to 30 days), whereas most women remain asymptomatic. The symptoms of gonorrhea are similar to those of chlamydia. About 1% of persons with gonorrhea develop disseminated gonococcal infection (DGI), sometimes known as gonococcal arthritis. Symptoms of DGI include fever, skin lesions, painful swelling of joints (arthritis), myocarditis, and meningitis. Like chlamydia, gonorrhea can be passed from mother to child during birth, and carries significant child morbidity, including blindness from untreated eye infection, arthritis, meningitis, and sepsis (bacterial infection of the blood).[71]

Syphilis. Like chlamydia and gonorrhea, syphilis is a curable bacterial STD (caused by *Treponema pallidum)* with an overall infection rate of 13.7/100,000. Infection rates are further delineated by category of disease, per 100,000: primary and secondary syphilis (3.8), early latent (3.6), late latent (6.1), or congenital (10.5). Syphilis can be spread by sexual contact (vaginal, anal, or oral sex), nonsexual transmission (toilet seats, towels, skin lesions) and mother-to-child transmission during pregnancy or childbirth. It is a genital ulcerative disease with significant complications if untreated, and its presence facilitates the transmission of HIV.

Primary syphilis (10 to 90 days after contact with the bacteria) is marked by the presence of a genital ulcer (chancre). Signs and symptoms of secondary syphilis (17 days to 6.5 months after infection) include a rough, reddish-brown palmar or plantar rash, rashes on other parts of the body, syphilitic "warts," mucosal sores, patchy hair loss, and a general sense of ill health. Symptoms of primary and secondary syphilis will clear up with or without treatment, and the person will enter a latent stage in which there are no signs of the disease 2 to 30 years after infection. The only way to diagnosis syphilis during the latent stage is via blood test. Tertiary syphilis is marked by gummas (small tumors in the skin, bones, liver, or any other organ), problems with the heart and blood vessels, and chronic NS disorders, such as blindness, insanity, and paralysis. With treatment, gummas will disappear, but this cannot repair or reverse the damage that occurred before treatment.[71]

Hepatitis A Virus. Hepatitis A virus (HAV) is a liver disease with the following symptoms: low-grade fever, malaise, fatigue, loss of appetite, nausea, abdominal discomfort, dark-colored urine, and jaundice, typically manifesting 15 to 50 days (average, 28) after exposure. The CDC estimates that there are between 125,000 and 200,000 total infections annually, with 84,000 to 134,000 showing symptoms and approximately 100 people dying annually from HAV. HAV is transmitted primarily through oral-fecal contact via contaminated food or water sources, sexual contact, especially oral-anal sex, and day care environments (e.g., through diapers).[9] Once recovered, an individual is immune and will not get HAV again.[71]

Hepatitis B Virus. In contrast, hepatitis A virus (HBV) is a noncurable viral infection that causes acute and chronic inflammation of the liver, cirrhosis, and an increased risk of liver cancer. One in 20 people will become infected with HBV at some point in their lives. The CDC estimates that 1.25 million people are living with chronic HBV, and another 75,000 new infections occur annually.

This virus is 100 times more infectious than HIV, and is transmitted via several routes—unsafe heterosexual or homosexual sex (over 50% of cases), injecting drugs, household contact, health care employment, and maternal to infant transmission during birth. HBV, along with HAV and HPV, are the only vaccine-preventable STDs. An encouraging trend is that the incidence of acute hepatitis B in the United States declined as much as 80% between 1987 and 2004, attributable to effective vaccination programs and universal precautions in needle use and in health care in general.[160] Current CDC guidelines call for hepatitis vaccination for children and adolescents, and Gardasil vaccination for HPV (cervical cancer) for teenage girls.[71,72]

Genital Herpes. The CDC records up to 1.6 million new cases of genital herpes each year. One in 5 Americans are infected (50 million adults), yet up to 90% of those with herpes are unaware they have it.[28] One in two African America adults already has genital herpes, and the CDC projects that up to 40% of all men and half of all women will be infected by 2025. This lifelong (but manageable) condition requires patient education and counseling when diagnosed.[28]

Genital herpes is caused by the herpes simplex virus, type 1 or 2 (HSV-1 or HSV-2) that travels from the skin to the NS, where it stays in the body. Symptoms of genital herpes may include tingling, itching, sores, bumps, redness, aches and pain in the genital area, or flulike symptoms. The symptoms recur most typically when the immune system is challenged by illness, poor diet, sleep or hygiene, and/or emotional or physical stress. Symptoms usually resolve within 2 to 12 days, and persons should abstain from sexual activity until all symptoms are gone. Because most genital herpes is spread when no symptoms are present, using daily antiviral medication (e.g., U.S Food and Drug Administration [FDA]–approved Valtrex) and condoms can reduce the risk of spreading the infection.[28] Having genital herpes triples the risk of getting HIV from an infected partner, and is believed to play a major role in the heterosexual spread of HIV in the United States.[72] Although it is uncommon for herpes to cause problems with pregnancy, it can still be passed to the baby during childbirth. If a woman first gets herpes in her third trimester, the likelihood of infecting the child is higher. A pregnant woman who does not have herpes should avoid contact with an infected partner during the third trimester.

Human Papillomavirus. Human papillomavirus (HPV) infections account for about half of STDs diagnosed among 15 to 24-year-olds each year.[127] By age 50, at least 80% of women will have acquired genital HPV (6 million new diagnoses/year). Most people with HPV do not develop symptoms, but cervical cancer is linked to the high-risk types of HPV. Regular pap smears are a warranted early detection method to address the risk of cervical cancer. In June 2006, the FDA approved the vaccine Gardasil as safe and effective for use among girls and women aged 9-26. The vaccine prevents infection with the types of HPV most likely to lead to cervical cancer.[127]

HIV and AIDS. HIV is the virus responsible for AIDS. HIV is transmitted via blood or sexual fluid contact or during pregnancy, delivery, or receiving breast milk from a HIV-infected female. The sharing of needles is a means of transmission among drug abusers. Health care workers carry an occupational risk for exposure to infected blood and body fluids (e.g., through needle sticks, sharps injury, inadvertent splash), making the use of standard precautions a benchmark for the industry. Assuming that all persons are potentially infectious, washing hands, using barriers, and safe work practices are safeguards against transmission in the workplace.[213]

Worldwide, the Joint United Nations Programme on HIV/AIDS estimates that there are 42 million people in the world living with HIV, and 3.2 million of those are children younger than 15. Approximately 90% of all children living with HIV acquired the infection from their mothers during pregnancy, birth or breast-feeding,[2] and approximately 850,000 to 950,000 people in the United States are living with HIV.[205] About 50% of all new HIV infections in the United States are in people younger than 25 years and most are infected through sexual behavior.[2] Of all young people, 20% to 25% become infected in their teenage years but do not manifest symptoms until their 20s. During these years, they unwittingly carry and spread the disease each time they engage in unprotected sexual behavior or intravenous drug use.[2,31]

Since the beginning of the global epidemic, 25 million people have died from complications of AIDS.[2] HIV infection is the leading cause of death for African American men aged 25 to 44 years, and the eighth leading cause of death among persons 15 to 24 years of age.[77] Every hour, about 31 young children die as a result of AIDS (mostly in sub-Saharan Africa, the Caribbean, Latin America, and Southeast Asia).[2]

The CDC has reported gender, age, racial, and ethnic disparities in the prevalence of HIV/AIDS. Among adolescents (13 to 19 years of age), 50% of new cases occur in African Americans, 28% in whites, 20% in Hispanics, and 2% in other ethnic or racial groups.[72] African Americans have long been disproportionately affected by the AIDS epidemic (40% of all AIDS-related deaths). Both male and female African Americans are most likely to become infected through sex with a man, with drug abuse (injecting) being the second most frequent cause of infection. Poverty levels, lack of access to health care, and the stigma surrounding men who have sex with men (MSM) influence African American HIV and AIDS death rates.[31]

Geographically, the HIV-AIDS epidemic in the United States was once concentrated mainly in the gay populations on the East (New York City) and West (San Francisco) Coasts, but in recent years, there is an increasing prevalence in African American and Hispanic communities in many southern states.[31] In the last 2 decades, the number of women living with HIV has tripled, and African American and Hispanic teens accounted for 82% of the cumulative HIV-AIDS cases among young women aged 13 to 19 years.[31]

MSM still accounts for approximately two thirds of HIV diagnoses among male adults and adolescents.[31] The HIV prevalence among African American MSM (46%) is twice that of white MSM (21%).[72] In recent years (2001 to 2006), the rates of HIV infection among MSM have increased 8.6%. It is proposed that the availability of antiretroviral treatment has led to complacency in the use of condoms by young MSM.[31]

Historically, injecting drug users (IDUs) have accounted for 25% of all HIV-AIDS diagnoses in the United States. Despite the fact that the CDC reported a 9.5% decline in HIV transmission among IDUs using needle exchange programs between 2001 and 2006, these services are no longer federally funded programs.[31]

Currently, about 13% of all new adult male and adolescent cases of HIV-AIDS cases are IDUs, with another 5% being both MSM and IDUs.[72]

Although declining rates of sexual activity and increased condom use among sexually active youth sound a hopeful note, the HIV-AIDS epidemic among young people of color and MSM underscores the need for more focused, gender-appropriate, and culturally appropriate prevention programs. By the time they reach 19 years of age, 7 in 10 teens have engaged in sexual intercourse,[127] but only 62% of teens (females, 55%; males, 69%) report using a condom.[72] Condom use varies by race, with non-Hispanic African-American teens (67%) being more likely than non-Hispanic white (60%) and Hispanic (61%) youth to report condom use. This pattern holds for males and females.[72] Condom use is higher among younger students with 69% of those in grade 9 reporting condom use compared with those in grades 11 (62%) and 12 (54%). This drop is likely to the result of other forms of birth control in older students, although it is still a concern because condoms are the best form of effective control against STDs for those who are sexually active.[71]

Females who have sex with older male partners are at greater risk for STDs and HIV.[71] Older male sexual partners are more likely to be infected than their younger male counterparts because of increased potential for more sexual partners and more varied sexual and drug experiences. Although the phenomenon of older men engaging in sexual relations with younger women is widespread, a disproportionately high percentage of adult men with minor partners are African American and Hispanic.[127] Overall, the risk of HIV infection is higher among urban African American and Hispanic women who are living in or near poverty because of high rates of injection drug use in these communities.[71] A small proportion of American teens (approximately 1.3%) put themselves and their sexual partners at risk of HIV infection through injection drug use.[154]

Consequences of untreated STDs include PID, sterility (females more than males), systemic illness and death, tubal pregnancies, and congenital conditions in infants (e.g., prematurity, eye disease, pneumonia).[72,120] Although abstaining from sex or having a long-term mutually monogamous partner who is not infected is the only way to protect oneself completely, latex condoms used consistently and correctly are highly effective (98%) in protecting against HIV and other STDs. Consistent condom use provides substantial protection against the acquisition of many STDs, including statistically significant reduction of risk against HIV, chlamydia, gonorrhea, herpes, and syphilis.[71] Using condoms also promotes the regression of HPV lesions in women and men.[71]

The lifetime cost of health care associated with HIV infection, in light of recent advances in HIV diagnostics and therapies, is conservatively estimated at $155,000 or more per person.[205] The 2010 federal budget request ($25.9 billion) for HIV-AIDS includes $19.4 billion designated for domestic spending (75%) and $6.5 billion (25%) for global HIV-AIDs actions. Domestic spending is roughly 51% for patient care, 11% for research, 9% for cash and housing assistance, and only 4% for prevention.[136]

SUBSTANCE ABUSE. Substance abuse is common in U.S. society among people of every age and social, economic, professional, and educational class. Substance abuse includes a wide variety of mood-affecting chemicals—caffeine (e.g., coffee, black tea, chocolate, soft drinks), cannabis (marijuana), depressants (e.g., alcohol, sedatives, tranquilizers), narcotics (e.g., heroin, opium, morphine, codeine), stimulants (e.g., amphetamines, cocaine, crack), anabolic androgenic steroids, and tobacco (e.g., cigarettes, cigars, chewing tobacco).[120] On an individual level, substance abuse can impair judgment, delay wound healing, and slow the rehabilitation process. Its societal ramifications include violence, homicide, assault, accidental injury, suicide, STDs, and 50% of all motor vehicle accidents.

Substance abuse in the formative years has long been a concern of parents, caregivers, teachers, coaches, and health care providers. Athletic associations at all levels of competition prohibit the use of performance-enhancing drugs, and youth associations also ban tobacco, alcohol, and illicit drugs. If ever there was a group of humans susceptible to the traps and pitfalls of substance abuse, it is the adolescent age group. Trial and error learning, questioning of authority, and peer pressure all can lead to physical addiction and psychological craving and dependence.

Monitoring the Future (MTF), a long-term study of licit and illicit drug use, has been scrutinizing substance abuse among U.S. adolescents (grades 8, 10 and 12) since 1975.[154] Over time, this study has monitored trends in the use of drugs, perceived risk, availability, and personal disapproval. According to the latest version of the MTF study, there has been an 7.2%, 11.5% and 7.3% decline in overall drug use in grades 8, 10, and 12 during the first 8 years of the new millennium. This finding generates a more positive picture of American youth than was seen at the end of the last century.[154]

These declines were broad, with only two major classes of drugs, hallucinogens other than lysergic acid diethylamide (LSD; up 0.9%) and narcotics other than heroin (up 2.6%) showing any sign of increase in use. Oxycontin and Vicodin (narcotics other than heroin) were added to the MTF drug list in 2002 for high school seniors. Currently, 1 in every 20 high school seniors has tried these powerful narcotics and the annual prevalence has been holding relatively steady (9.1%) since its peak rate in 2004 (9.5%). Methods whereby adolescents obtain prescription drugs (e.g., narcotics, tranquilizers, amphetamines) include the following: (1) given to teen by friend or relative, (2) bought from a friend or relative, (3) bought from a dealer, (4) stolen from a friend or relative, (5) obtained by medical prescription, or (6) Internet dealing.

In 2008, MTF reported that 19.6% of all eighth graders, 34.1% of all tenth graders, and almost half of all twelfth graders (47.9%) had tried some sort of illicit drug (lifetime prevalence).[154] Drugs on the rise among teenagers in the early years of the new millennium included the club drugs (e.g., LSD, 3,4-methylene-dioxymethamphetamine [MDMA; ecstasy], methamphetamine, ketamine [special K]); use of the date rape drugs (e.g., flunitrazepam [Rohypnol] and GHB [gamma-hydroxybutyrate]) has decreased in recent years. Given their availability, inhalants have historically been the only drug abused more by younger teens (15.8% of eighth graders compared to 12.8 and 9.9% of tenth and twelfth graders, respectively). Heroin use (injected or without a needle) currently remains low and stable across all age groups (approximately 1.3%). Table 16-13 shows the lifetime prevalence rates for key drugs used by adolescents in 2008.

TABLE 16-13

Trends in Lifetime Prevalence of Drugs in Grades 8, 10, and 12

Drug Use*	Grade Level		
	8	10	12
Any illicit drug	19.6	34.1	47.4
Alcohol	38.9	58.3	71.9
Been drunk†	18.0	37.4	54.7
Amphetamines	6.8	9.0	10.5
Cigarettes	20.5	31.7	44.7
Cocaine	3.0	4.5	7.2
Crack	2.0	2.0	2.8
Ecstasy (MDMA)	2.4	4.3	6.2
Hallucinogens (other than LSD)	2.5	4.8	7.8
Heroin	1.4	1.2	1.3
Inhalants	15.7	12.8	9.9
LSD	1.9	2.6	4.0
Marijuana	14.6	15.9	24.9
Methamphetamine	2.3	2.4	2.8
Narcotics other than heroin	—	—	13.2
PCP	—	—	1.8
Sedatives	—	—	8.5
Smokeless tobacco	9.8	12.2	15.6
Steroids	1.4	1.4	2.2
Tranquilizers	3.9	6.8	8.9

*2008 data. Entries listed as percentage of students who have used the substance.
†Subgroup of alcohol users.
Data from Monitoring the Future: *2009 data from in-school surveys of 8th-, 10th-, and 12th-grade students* (website). http://www.monitoringthefuture.org/data/09data .html#2009data-drugs. Accessed March 9, 2010.

Anabolic Androgenic Steroids. Anabolic androgenic steroids (AAS) is the name for synthetic substances related to the male sex hormone, testosterone. Anabolic steroids are abused by 1.4% of eighth graders, 1.4% of tenth graders, and 2.2% of twelfth graders.[154] These drugs have medical uses, such as treating delayed puberty, some types of impotence, and wasting of the body caused by HIV infection or other diseases. However, when abused, AAS can have serious health consequences. In boys and men, the abuse of AAS can reduce sperm production, shrink the testicles, and cause impotence and irreversible breast enlargement. Girls and women can develop more masculine characteristics, such as laryngeal growth, with deepening of the voice and excessive body hair. Both genders run the risk of cranial hair loss, increased incidence of acne, and aggression.[46] In addition, the abuse of AAS can stunt bone growth in adolescents and result in potentially permanent damage to the heart, liver, and kidneys.[120,163] Individuals who inject anabolic steroids with nonsterile needles also risk developing HIV, hepatitis, and other bloodborne infections.

Among male adolescents, steroid abuse is associated with worse self-esteem and higher rates of depressed mood and attempted suicide, worse knowledge, worse attitudes about health, greater participation in sports that emphasize weight and shape, greater parental concern about weight, and higher rates of disordered eating and substance use.[146] Among females, a similar but less consistent pattern of results also emerged.[146] Work by Goldberg and Elliot has substantiated the benefits of a gender-specific, sports team–centered approach to adolescent health risks and behaviors. For males, refer to the program entitled Adolescents Training and Learning to Avoid Steroids (ATLAS), and for females, Athletes Targeting Healthy Exercise and Nutrition Alternatives (ATHENA).[119]

Marijuana and Hashish. In addition to alcohol, marijuana has been the most widely used illicit drug for the 33 years of the MTF study.[154] Currently, 4 in 10 (42.6%) high school seniors, 29.9% of tenth graders, and 14.6% of eighth graders have tried marijuana. It continues to be easily accessible to students, with almost 39.3% of eighth graders, 67.4% of tenth graders, and 83.9% of high school seniors stating that they could easily obtain marijuana if they so desired. Over 80% of teens disapprove of "regular use" of marijuana, and most (60%) perceive it as carrying a risk of leading to other negative drug behaviors.[154]

Alcohol. Alcohol abuse and alcohol dependence are not only adult problems. They affect a significant number of adolescents between the ages of 12 and 20, even though the legal drinking age is 21 years. According to the AAP, almost 90% of 16- to 19-year-olds recall having their first alcoholic beverage after their eleventh birthday, and teens nationwide now average 5.5 days of drinking each month, with 16% reporting black-out spells because of heavy drinking.[165] Over 7 of 10 (71.9%) twelfth graders have consumed alcohol by the end of high school, with over half (58.3%) drinking by tenth grade, and almost 4 of 10 (38.9%) getting started by eighth grade. In 2008, over half (54.7%) of twelfth graders, 37.2% of tenth graders, and almost one fifth (18%) of eighth graders reported having been drunk at least once in their life.[154]

Adolescents who begin drinking before age 15 are 4 times more likely to develop alcohol dependence than those who begin drinking at age 21. More than 3 million teenagers are outright alcoholics, and several million others have serious drinking problems that will require professional help.[195] Dependence on alcohol (and other drugs) also has been associated with psychiatric problems such as depression, anxiety, oppositional defiant disorder, and antisocial personality disorder. Alcohol is a leading contributor to death in those 15 to 24 years old and is linked to the vast majority of young adult automobile crashes, homicides, suicides, and bicycle crashes.[40,140,195] As with any addictive behavior at any age, self-help groups, with advice and support from a health care professional, are the best way to address the addiction. Treatment also should involve family members (and peers) because family history may play a role in the origins of the problem, and treatment cannot succeed in isolation.[195]

Smoking and Smokeless Tobacco. Tobacco, in chewed or smoked form, has pervasive multisystem effects (e.g., addiction, back pain, cancer risks [bladder, cervical, esophageal, kidney, lung, oral, pharyngeal, and leukemia], CVD, delayed healing, diabetes, drug interactions, ear infections, emphysema, infertility, low birth weight, nutrition, osteoporosis, premature aging, respiratory ailments, stroke, tooth discoloration and decay).[21]

Smokeless Tobacco. Smokeless tobacco (e.g., snuff and chew) has been associated with halitosis, tooth loss, gum disease, and

oral and esophageal cancers. Thankfully, the use of smokeless tobacco by teens has fallen substantially from its all-time high of 32.4% of twelfth graders in 1992. The current lifetime rate of smokeless tobacco use is approximately 9.8% for eighth graders, 12.2% for tenth graders, and 15.6% for twelfth graders. With only about 2% of girls chewing tobacco, it is almost exclusively a male behavior. An estimated 34% to 48% of teens perceive smokeless tobacco as dangerous, and 82.1% of teens disapprove of persons who chew tobacco regularly.[154]

Cigarettes. Despite modest declines in the last decade, teenage smoking rates remain high.[154] Per MTF, the lifetime prevalence of cigarette use is 20.5% of eighth graders, 31.7% of tenth graders, and 44.7% of twelfth graders, down from a high level of 49.2% (eighth graders, 1996), 61.2% (tenth graders, 1996) and 65.4% (twelfth graders, 1997). Every day, 3600 American adolescents between 12 and 17 years of age begin smoking, with an estimated 1100 (30.6%) becoming regular smokers.[249] Half of adults who smoke were regular smokers by their 18th birthday, and 90% had started by the age of 21.[250]

Tobacco is a gateway to poor health, illicit drugs, and a host of unhealthy behaviors. Teenagers who smoke are less likely to engage in sports or other after-school activities, have less dynamic relationships with parents, and are more likely to get poor grades. Teens who smoke are 5.5 times more likely to have tried marijuana, 6 times more likely to get drunk at least once a month, and 3 times more likely to try an illegal drug in the future than teens who do not smoke.[250] Tobacco use in adolescence is also associated with a range of other unhealthy behaviors, including being involved in fights, carrying weapons, and engaging in high-risk sexual behavior.[250]

MENTAL HEALTH. Current global epidemiologic data consistently reports that up to 20% of children and adolescents suffer from a disabling mental illness, that suicide is the third leading cause of death among adolescents, and that up to 50% of all adult mental disorders have their onset in adolescence.[37] Worldwide, the conditions of poverty, physical and sexual abuse, war and dislocation, forced prostitution, child soldiering, and HIV and other diseases contribute to the ubiquitous and burdensome nature of pediatric mental illness.[37] Other societal factors that contribute to childhood suffering include teen pregnancy, divorce and single-parent homes, racial, ethnic or gender discrimination, substance abuse, and caregiver neglect. Costs of child and adolescent mental disorders are a long-standing problem for society and include lost economic productivity; crime and potential destabilization of communities; high rates of health care use; and burdens to the educational, criminal justice, and social welfare systems.[37]

A conservative estimate from the National Institute of Mental Health suggests that one in five American (15 million) children between the ages of 9 and 17 have a diagnosable mental or addictive disorder [196]. Chief mental health problems affecting children and adolescents include depressive disorders, anxiety disorders, attention-deficit/hyperactivity disorder (ADHD), EDs, autism, other pervasive developmental disorders (PDDs), and schizophrenia.[112] Noteworthy is the fact that some believe that the current International Statistical Classification of Diseases and Related Health Problems, 10th Revision (ICD-10) and *Diagnostic and Statistical Manual of Mental Disorders,*

4th Edition (DSM-IV) [112] diagnostic classifications for children and adolescents are woefully inadequate and of limited applicability in global epidemiologic studies. Aside from classification, there are also notable gaps in mental health resources for children, adolescents (and adults) that can be categorized into five broad categories: (1) economic, (2) manpower, (3) training, (4) services, and (5) policy.[37]

Depressive Disorders. Depressive disorders (e.g., major depressive disorder, dysthymic disorder, bipolar disorder) adversely affect mood, energy, interest, sleep, appetite, and overall functioning. Primary clues for depression include low self-esteem, anhedonia (failure to find pleasure in daily activities), sleep disorders, and difficulty concentrating or making decisions. Depressive disorders are associated with an increased risk of suicidal behavior. Among teenagers, suicide is the fourth leading cause of death among those 10 to 14 years old (6.3%) and the third leading cause of death in those 15 to 19 years old (12%). Evidence suggests that depressive disorders emerging early in life often continue into adulthood, and that early-onset depressive disorders may predict more severe illnesses in adult life.[234]

Screening for depressive disorders in the adolescent (and all patients) is recommended as a component of routine health maintenance assessment.[120,391] The Beck Depression Inventory (BDI-II) is an invaluable tool for depression screening and diagnosis.[35] This 21-item tool assesses the intensity of depression in clinical and normal individuals in an age range of 13 to 80 years. The BDI-II takes just 5 minutes to complete and also is used extensively to monitor therapeutic progress. Early diagnosis and treatment of depressive disorders in children and adolescents are critical in enabling young people to live up to their full potential.[196]

ANXIETY DISORDERS. Environmental, social, cultural, and psychosocial stresses can lead to anxiety for children and adolescents.[39,234] Anxiety disorders, including generalized anxiety disorder, obsessive-compulsive disorder (OCD), panic disorder,

post-traumatic stress disorder (PTSD), phobias, separation anxiety, and selective autism, are the most common mental, emotional, and behavioral problems to occur during childhood and adolescence. [249] The basic temperament of young people 6 to 8 years of age (i.e., being shy and restrained in unfamiliar places) and having a parent with an anxiety disorder may predispose children to the development of an anxiety disorder.[249] Researchers estimate that 13 of 100 U.S. children and adolescents ages 9 to 17 (girls more than boys) will have an anxiety-related disorder.[249] About half of children and adolescents with anxiety disorders have a second anxiety disorder or other mental or behavioral disorder, such as depression.[196] In addition, anxiety disorders may coexist with physical health conditions requiring treatment.

Children and adolescents with anxiety disorders typically experience intense fear, worry, or uneasiness that can last for long periods of time and significantly affect their lives. If not treated early, anxiety disorders can lead to repeated school absences or an inability to finish school, impaired relationships with peers, low self-esteem, alcohol or other drug use, problems adjusting to work situations, and anxiety disorders in adulthood.[249] Symptoms of anxiety, stress, and depression can be expressed in three primary modes, somatic, psychological, and behavioral (Table 16-14). These expressions of stress differ slightly across the life span and also depend somewhat on the individual and his or her level of psychosocial development.

Conversely, relaxation is a positively perceived state of mind and body in which a person feels relief from tension and strain. The three aims of relaxation training are following: (1) to protect the organs of the body from unnecessary wear; (2) to help relieve stress in conditions such as anxiety, essential HTN, tension headache, insomnia, asthma, HIV-AIDS, and panic; and (3) to create coping skills to calm the mind and allow thinking to be more clear and effective.[210] Various forms of psychotherapy, including cognitive-behavioral therapy, family therapy, and

---

TABLE 16-14

Modes of Anxiety Expressed by Body System and Recommended Treatment

Body System	Modes of Anxiety Expression	Treatment Methods
Somatic—physiologic changes	Increased HR (palpitations), BP, RR Increased sweating Reduced blood flow to the periphery (cold hands and feet) Raised blood coagulation rate Raised blood glucose level Muscle tension (headaches, neck, shoulder, low back pain) GI—indigestion, constipation, and diarrhea	Progressive relaxation techniques (Jacobson) Diaphragmatic breathing Physical interventions including stretching, aerobic exercise, yoga, tai chi, Feldenkrais, Alexander technique Biofeedback
Cognitive (mental)—symptoms reported by the patient	Tiredness or difficulty in sleeping Headache Difficulty concentrating, worry Impatience, feeling irritable, easily angered (patient also may report any of the above somatic changes)	Cognitive restructuring via self-statements and self-awareness activities Imagery Meditation
Behavioral—observable actions	Increased consumption of alcohol, tobacco, food Loss of appetite or excessive eating Restlessness Loss of sexual interest Tendency to experience accidents Acting-out behaviors (e.g., hitting, yelling)	Behavioral relaxation training Social and coping skills Autogenics—teaching the body and mind to relax (combines with cognitive)

Adapted from Payne RA: *Relaxation techniques: a practical handbook for the health care professional*, New York, 1995, Churchill Livingstone.

relaxation training, as well as certain medications, particularly selective serotonin reuptake inhibitors (SSRIs), are used to treat anxiety disorders in children and adolescents. Research on the safety and efficacy of these treatments is ongoing.[194]

Attention-Deficit/Hyperactivity Disorder and Learning Disabilities.

ADHD and learning disabilities (LDs) are among the most prevalent and widely researched diagnoses of American children. In 2008, the National Center for Health Statistics (NCHS) estimated that 5 million (8%) of children 3 to 17 years of age had ADHD with LD, 5 million (8%) had LD without ADHD,[45] and 5.9 million (3.7%) had both conditions.[209] Age, gender, race or ethnicity, family structure, and socioeconomic status all have diagnostic and treatment implications for these conditions. Boys were more likely than girls to have each diagnosis: ADHD without LD (boys, 10%; girls, 4.3%), LD without ADHD (boys, 10%; girls, 5%), and both conditions (boys, 5.1%; girls, 2.3%).[73,209] Older children (12 to 17 years of age) are more likely than younger children (6 to 11 years of age) to have each of the diagnoses.[209] Hispanic children were less likely to have ADHD or LD (4%, 6%) than non-Hispanic white children (10%, 9%) or non-Hispanic African American children (9%, 9%).[73] Children in single-mother families were more likely to have ADHD or LD (10%, 11%) compared with children in two-parent families (7%, 7%).[73] Children in low income families (less than $35,000/year) were twice as likely (12% to 6%) to have a LD as compared with children in high-income families ($100,000 or more).[73] When compared with children with an excellent or very good health status, children with a fair or poor health status were almost 5 times as likely to have an LD (27%, 7%) and more than twice as likely to have ADHD (19%, 7%).[73] Children with ADHD and LD are more likely than children with neither ADHD nor LD to have other chronic health conditions.[209]

The neurobiologic condition of ADHD is thought to be inherited, and symptoms persist into adulthood in as many as 60% of cases (approximately 4% of adults).[81] Up to 30% of children and 25% to 40% of adults with ADHD also have an associated anxiety disorder.[81,196] Diagnostically, there is no single medical, physical, or genetic test for ADHD[81] and its three core symptoms include inattention (lack of concentration and distractibility), hyperactivity, and impulsivity. Untreated children with ADHD often face long-standing problems with academic achievement, social relationships, life skills, vocational success, risk of injury, and functional independence.[18,81]

Treatment of this chronic condition includes behavioral therapy, parental training and guidance, collaboration with school personnel, and medications. Psychostimulant medications, including methylphenidate (Ritalin) and amphetamine (Dexedrine and Adderall), are the most widely researched and most prescribed first-line treatments for ADHD. Antidepressant medications (e.g., tricyclics, bupropion) represent a second-line pharmacologic treatment for ADHD. Over half of children with ADHD (56%) take medication for their disorder.[18] The economic effect of these conditions on families, schools, and the health care system is substantial, from $12,005 to $17,458 per individual or $36 to $52 billion dollars annually.[209] These costs in adolescence may still be warranted, because research suggests that treating ADHD in children and adolescents may reduce the likelihood of future drug and alcohol abuse.[18]

Eating Disorders During Puberty.

EDs entail serious disturbances in eating behavior, such as extreme and unhealthy reduction of food intake or severe overeating, as well as feelings of distress or extreme concern about body shape or weight. Risk factors that precede an ED diagnosis include gender (female), ethnicity, early childhood eating and gastrointestinal problems, elevated weight and shape concerns, negative self-evaluation (depression or anxiety), sexual abuse and other adverse experiences (substance abuse), and general psychiatric morbidity.[147] EDs are associated with a wide range of other health complications, including neuropathies, serious heart arrhythmias, and kidney failure, which may lead to death. Because of their complexity, EDs require a comprehensive treatment plan involving medical care and monitoring, psychotherapy, nutritional counseling and, when appropriate, medication management.[134,196]

Health care professionals working with adolescents should scrutinize for proper nutritional habits, behaviors, or personality changes that could indicate distorted eating habits or abuse of nutritional supplements or illicit drugs.[26] Box 16-4 discusses EDs, excessively low BMI, and clinical features of anorexia nervosa and bulimia nervosa. Females influenced by the cultural drive to be thin or psychosocial issues (e.g., history or depression, anxiety, rape, abuse) tend to result in more serious and devastating forms of EDs. For males, participation in sports can stimulate seasonal and transient distorted eating, but few seem to develop actual EDs.[230] Elite athletes, both male and female, competing in aesthetic sports (diving, figure skating, gymnastics, ballet) and weight-dependent sports (judo, karate, wrestling, lightweight rowing, distance running) have a significantly higher prevalence of EDs and ED symptoms (25%) than other athletes (12%) and nonathletes (5%).[54]

Anorexia nervosa (AN), bulimia nervosa (BN), binge-eating disorder (BED), compulsive overeating (CE), and emotional eating (EE) are classified as mental health disorders in the DSM-IV. Health professionals evaluate for EDs using a variety of testing tools (e.g., Eating Disorder Examination [EDE], Eating Disorder Examination Questionnaire [EDE-Q], Eating Disorder Inventory [EDI]).[26]

Tool selection is dependent on the disorder of interest (AN, BN, BED, or partial syndrome BN) and the likelihood of a concurrent personality disorder (PD). Personality traits (e.g., perfectionism, obsessive-compulsiveness, neuroticism, negative emotionality, harm avoidance, low self-directedness, low cooperativeness, high impulsivity, sensation seeking, novelty seeking) have been implicated in the onset, symptomatic expression, and maintenance of EDs.[59] The EDE-Q[107] is a valid paper and pencil screening tool that can be reliably administered by the PT to screen for disordered eating habits.[42,188,208] The PT should evaluate the entire context of the therapeutic situation, and referral to a nutritionist or qualified mental health professional who has experience in treating EDs is warranted.

Autism and Pervasive Developmental Disorders.

Autism and other PDDs, including Asperger's disorder, Rett's disorder, childhood disintegrative disorder, and pervasive developmental disorder, not otherwise specified (PDD-NOS), are brain disorders that occur in an estimated 2 to 6/1000 U.S. children. PDDs usually develop by 3 years of age and typically affect the ability to

BOX 16-4
Eating Disorders and Excessively Low Body Mass Index

In the United States, an estimated 5 to 10 million women and 1 million men suffer from eating disorders. These severe disturbances of eating behavior are often difficult to detect, especially in teens wearing baggy clothes or in individuals who binge and then induce vomiting or evacuation. Be familiar with the two principal eating disorders, anorexia nervosa and bulimia nervosa. Both conditions are characterized by distorted perceptions of body image and weight. Early detection is important, because prognosis improves when treatment occurs in the early stages of these disorders.

CLINICAL FEATURES

Anorexia Nervosa	Bulimia Nervosa
Refusal to maintain minimally normal body weight (or BMI above 17.5 kg/m^2)	Repeated binge eating followed by self-induced vomiting, misuse of laxatives, diuretics or other medications, fasting, or excessive exercise
Afraid of appearing fat	Often with normal weight
Frequently starving but in denial; lacking insight	Overeating at least twice a week during 3-mo period; large amounts of food consumed in short period (approximately 2 hr)
Often brought in by family members	Preoccupation with eating, craving and compulsion to eat, lack of control over eating, alternating with period of starvation
May present as failure to make expected weight gains in childhood or adolescence, amenorrhea in women, loss of libido or potency in men	Dread of fatness but may be obese
Associated with depressive symptoms such as depressed mood, irritability, social withdrawal, insomnia, decreased libido	Subtypes of
Additional features supporting diagnosis—self-induced vomiting or purging, excessive exercise, use of appetite suppressants and/or diuretics	• Purging—bulimic episodes accompanied by self-induced vomiting or use of laxatives, diuretics, or enemas
Biologic complications	• Nonpurging—bulimic episodes accompanied by compensatory behavior such as fasting, exercise, but without purging
• Neuroendocrine changes—amenorrhea, increased corticotropin-releasing factor, cortisol, growth hormone, serotonin; decreased diurnal cortisol fluctuation, luteinizing hormone, follicle-stimulating hormone, thyroid-stimulating hormone	Biologic complications
• Cardiovascular disorders—bradycardia, hypotension, arrhythmias, cardiomyopathy	See changes listed for anorexia nervosa, especially weakness, fatigue, mild cognitive disorders; also erosion of dental enamel, parotitis, pancreatic inflammation with elevated amylase levels, mild neuropathies, seizures, hypokalemia, hypochloremic metabolic acidosis, hypomagnesemia
• Metabolic disorders—hypokalemia, hypochloremic metabolic alkalosis, increased blood urea nitrogen level, edema	
• Other—dry skin, dental caries, delayed gastric emptying, constipation, anemia, osteoporosis	

Sources: World Health Organization: The ICD-10 classification of mental and behavioral disorders: diagnotisc criteria for research. Geneva, 1993, World Health Organization. American Psychiatric Association: *DSM-IV-TR: Diagnostic and statistical manual of mental disorders,* 4th ed. Washington, DC, 1994, American Psychiatric Association. Halmi KA: *Eating disorders:* In: Kalpan HI, Sadock BJ, eds. *Comprehensive textbook of psychiatry,* 7th ed. Philadelphia, 2000, Lippincott, Williams & Wilikins, 1663-1676. Melher PS. Bulimia nervosa. N Engl J Med 2003; 349(9):875-880.

communicate, form relationships with others, and respond appropriately to the outside world.[196]

Recent research has made it possible to identify earlier those children who show signs of developing a PDD and thus to initiate early intervention. Although no single treatment program is best for all children with PDDs, psychosocial and pharmacologic interventions can help improve their behavioral and cognitive functioning. The National Institutes of Mental Health (NIMH) is funding studies of behavioral treatments and medications to determine the best time to start treatment, optimum intensity and duration of treatment, and most effective methods to reach high- and low-functioning children.[196]

Schizophrenia. Schizophrenia is a chronic, severe, and disabling brain disorder that affects about 1% of the population during their lifetime. Symptoms include hallucinations, false beliefs, disordered thinking, and social withdrawal. Schizophrenia typically emerges in late adolescence or early adulthood. Researchers are just beginning to make headway into understanding its origins—genetic factors combined with developmental disturbances and environmental stressors.[196]

Treatments that help manage schizophrenia have improved significantly in recent years. Antipsychotic medications are especially helpful for reducing hallucinations and delusions in children and adolescents. The newer generation atypical antipsychotics, such as olanzapine and clozapine, also may help improve motivation and emotional expressiveness in some patients. Children with schizophrenia and their families also can benefit from supportive counseling, psychotherapies, and social skills training aimed at helping them cope with the illness. Special education or other accommodations may be necessary to help children with schizophrenia to succeed in the classroom.[196]

Musculoskeletal Disorders of Adolescence

Disorders and injuries of the MS system are many and of paramount concern to the orthopedic practitioner.[228] There are six major categories of MS disease: (1) congenital (see Table 16-3), (2) inflammatory, (3) metabolic, (4) vascular, (5) neoplastic, and (6) traumatic.[185] Age, gender, and race of the patient are important predictive variables in the differential diagnosis of MS disease.[56,120,228] Other variables include behavior of the lesion (osteoblastic or osteolytic), locus of the lesion (epiphysis, apophysis, metaphysis, diaphysis, or articular surface), shape and margins of the lesion, and a history of trauma.[185]

Radiologic evaluation, which requires a systematic approach, is absolutely essential to the management of these six categories of pediatric orthopedic conditions.[175,185] Radiographic diagnosis of orthopedic trauma and disease in the maturing skeleton can be a complicated process. First, only the ossified portions of bone have sufficient radiographic density to be imaged. Second, differentiation of fractures is complicated by the presence of epiphyseal plates, dense growth plates, dense growth lines, secondary centers of ossification, and large nutrient foramina, all of which may be confused with fracture lines. Comparison films of the uninvolved side often are obtained to assist in differential diagnosis.[175,185,228] Advanced diagnostic imaging techniques, including contrast-enhanced radiography, conventional tomography, CT, nuclear imaging (i.e., bone scan), and MRI, often are required for distinguishing osteocartilaginous and soft tissue structures located about a joint (see Chapter 14).[185]

Neoplastic and non-neoplastic (e.g., inflammatory, metabolic, and vascular) diseases characteristically manifest at specific bones or specific sites within bones and joints across the life span.[120,185,228] During the growth years, almost all bone neoplasms, benign and malignant, avoid the epiphysis. Epiphyseal growth plates are vulnerable to idiopathic necrosis (osteochondrosis), local growth disorders (dysplasias and osteochondritis dissecans), and a variety of traumatic conditions (e.g., apophysitis, epiphyseal fractures).[185,228] By contrast, the epiphyses tend to resist other afflictions. Hematogenous osteomyelitis, for example, never begins at the epiphysis and rarely spreads into it through the epiphyseal plate.[228]

Osteochondrosis (Avascular Necrosis of the Epiphyses)

The osteochondroses are idiopathic disorders seen in the immature skeleton, usually involving a secondary epiphyseal center or pressure epiphysis at the end of the long bone. They occasionally involve the primary epiphyseal center of a small bone, as in Kohler's disease (tarsal navicular), Kienböck's disease (lunate), and Calve's disease (vertebral body). Knowledge of the blood supply of epiphyses and their epiphyseal plates (physes) is pivotal to understanding these growth plate disorders. The epiphyses covered by the most articular cartilage (AC) (i.e., have the most precarious blood supply) are the most vulnerable (e.g., femoral head, capitellum).

Osteochondroses are most common in the middle years of growth, ages 3 to 10 years. They affect boys more than girls (4:1 ratio), affect lower limbs more than upper limbs, and have a bilateral presentation at any given epiphysis about 10% to 15% of the time.[228] Increased intracapsular joint pressure resulting from repetitive trauma, transient synovitis, infection, or granulation tissue is thought to disrupt blood flow and lead to the various conditions known as avascular necrosis, aseptic necrosis, and ischemic necrosis. In some of the osteochondroses particularly Legg-Calvé-Perthes (LCP) disease, there is a likely association with parental smoking during pregnancy, exposure to second-hand smoke in childhood, and hypofibrinolysis and thrombophilia (a deficiency in antithrombotic factor C or S, with an increased tendency toward thrombosis).[171,228]

These disorders are self-limiting (i.e., heal spontaneously) and follow four distinct stages:

- *Avascularity phase*: Involves obliteration of the blood vessels to the epiphysis (variety of causes) and kills the osteocytes and the bone-marrow cells within the epiphysis.
- *Revascularization phase*: Represents the vascular reaction of the surrounding tissues to dead bone and is characterized by revascularization of the dead epiphysis.
- *Bone healing phase*: Bone resorption ceases and bone deposition continues so that the fibrous and granulation tissue is slowly replaced by new bone.
- *Residual deformity phase*: When bony healing of the epiphysis is complete, its contours remain relatively unchanged.

LEGG-CALVÉ-PERTHES DISEASE. LCP disease is the most significant, most common, and most serious of the lower extremity osteochondroses. LCP disease involves the pressure epiphysis of the proximal femur, affects boys more than girls (a 5:1 ratio) and whites more than African Americans (10:1 ratio), and is bilateral 10% to 15% of the time.[56,228] The treatment goal is containment of the femoral head in the acetabulum via abduction casting. Prognosis is inversely related to age of onset and to gender (boys worse than girls). Of all patients, 50% have disabling osteoarthritis by the age of 50 years, and total hip arthroplasty is a typical long-term outcome.

FREIBERG'S DISEASE. Forefoot pain on weight bearing caused by osteochondrosis of the pressure epiphysis of the metatarsal heads (second more than third metatarsal) occurs most often in adolescent females. A congenitally long second metatarsal or short first metatarsal is a contributing factor. Shoe modifications (e.g., avoidance of heels, stiff rocker bottom sole) will redistribute weight, but occasionally surgical excision of the distorted portion of the metatarsal head is required.[228]

UPPER EXTREMITY OSTEOCHONDOSES. The upper extremity (UE) osteochondroses include Panner's disease (capitellum of the humerus) and Kienböck's disease (lunate). Panner's disease should be ruled out in children aged 3 to 11 years who present with pain, swelling, and limited range of motion (ROM) in the elbow joint. Conservative treatment via immobilization (sling during symptomatic period) usually leads to a good prognosis given the non–weight-bearing nature of the elbow joint.

Kienböck's disease has an inferior prognosis, and progression to degeneration of the wrist is common. Aching in the wrist, tenderness over the lunate, and swelling secondary to repetitive microtrauma (e.g., from occupations with vibration and wrist impact) in late adolescence and young adulthood characterize Kienböck's disease. The healing process is slower and often incomplete in adults compared with children and adolescents. Treatment is excision of the lunate before degenerative changes develop in the perilunar carpals.

SCHEUERMANN'S DISEASE. The most significant of the adolescent spinal osteochondroses is Scheuermann's disease (adolescent kyphosis or vertebral epiphysitis). It involves the ring epiphysis of the thoracic vertebra. It is more common in males aged 12 to 16 (and up to 19) years. Clinical manifestations include exaggerated kyphosis, with possible compensatory lumbar lordosis, prominent vertebral spinous process with or without pain, local MS pain, tenderness, and fatigue, stiffness on joint play assessment (JPA) of the spine, and possible Schmorl's nodes (vertically displaced nuclear material secondary to endplate degradation).[120,174,177] The treatment goal of this self-limiting disease is prevention of progressive deformity. Treatment includes therapeutic exercise (e.g., postural exercises, stretching, thoracic hyperextension), soft tissue and joint mobilization, traction and, occasionally, thoracic extension orthoses if the deformity advances rapidly (more than 60 degrees).[56,120]

Epiphyseal Dysplasia: Disorders of Epiphyseal Growth

Epiphyseal dysplasias begin during the growing years and tend to progress as long as the child is still growing. These disorders include: slipped capital femoral epiphysis (SCFE, or adolescent

TABLE 16-15

Disorders of Epiphyseal Growth

Epiphyseal Disorder	Incidence	Clinical Features and Diagnosis	Treatment and Outcome
Slipped capital femoral epiphysis (SCFE; adolescent coxa vara); most significant of lower limb epiphyseal plate disorders; most common hip disorder seen in adolescents	Males (13-16 yr) 2 to 5 times more likely to be affected than females (11-14 yr); 25%-33% bilateral, especially boys < 12 yr; more common in African Americans	Obesity (75% of cases); mild hip pain referred to medial aspect of knee; slight limp that increases with fatigue; positive Trendelenburg sign Posture —lower extremity unloaded into flexion, ER, and abduction to avoid impingement of metaphysis on anterior lip of acetabulum; reduced hip flexion, IR, abduction; diagnosis confirmed with x-ray (AP and lateral views helpful, but frog view with positive Kline's line is definitive)	Prescription—prevent further slip, maintain ROM, prevent OA, immobilize via a hip spica and non–weight-bearing (WB) status; if slip is <1 cm, screw or pin in situ, cast and WB after surgery
Blount's disease (tibia vara) — growth suppression with premature closure of the medial portion of the upper tibial epiphyseal plate	Girls > boys; infant type, <2-3 yr is most common; juvenile type, 4-10 yr; adolescent, >11 yr; Finland and Jamaica have highest incidence	Often seen in obese children who are early ambulators; lateral thrust during stance; tibial varum; early x-ray essential (displays defective ossification on medial side of tibia, beaked appearance of underlying metaphysis, obvious longitudinal growth disturbance)	Prescription — prevent progression of varus deformity; if unilateral infantile form (<3 yr),use hip, knee, ankle, foot, orthosis (HKAFO) 23 hr/day or night splints to correct varus deformity; if >4 yr, splinting usually fails, osteotomy of tibia is required (often must be repeated); African Americans girls have worst prognosis
Madelung's deformity— localized epiphyseal dysplasia on medial (ulnar) side of distal radial epiphysis	Adolescent onset; girls > boys; usually bilateral	Insidious onset of wrist pain; loss of forearm, wrist ROM (wrist flexion and supination); prominence of distal end of the ulna on dorsum of wrist and forward displacement of hand in relation to forearm	Correction of deformity via surgical excision of distal portion of ulna and osteotomy of deformed end of radius

ER, external rotation; *IR*, internal rotation.

coxa vara), Blount's disease (tibia vara), Madelung's deformity (epiphyseal dysplasia at the elbow), and idiopathic scoliosis. SCFE is the most significant epiphyseal plate disorder of the lower extremity, and the most common hip disorder seen in adolescents.[228] The incidence, clinical features, treatment, and prognosis of the extremity epiphyseal disorders are discussed in Table 16-15.

SCOLIOSIS: LATERAL DEVIATION OF THE SPINE. The pediatric spine is susceptible to growth plate interruption and external stresses that can cause abnormal skeletal modeling (structural scoliosis). MS injury or compensation can also cause nonstructural scoliosis. Structural scoliosis has three primary causes—neuromuscular, osteopathic, or idiopathic. Adolescent idiopathic scoliosis (AIS) is an epiphyseal disorder, and a diagnosis of exclusion, meaning that all other sources of lateral curvature of the spine have been ruled out.[174,228] AIS, which develops during the pediatric years, typically at the onset of puberty, is the most common form of scoliosis (75% to 80% of cases).

Neuromuscular causes of scoliosis (15% to 20% of cases) include cerebral palsy, myelomeningocele (spina bifida), neurofibromatosis, spinal cord injury, neuromuscular disorders (e.g., muscular dystrophy and spinal muscle atrophy), and myopathic diseases (e.g., amyotonia congenita or arthrogryposis).[56,174,228] Congenital osteopathic scoliosis (5% of cases) is caused by in-utero vertebral maldevelopment (e.g., wedge vertebrae, hemivertebrae, congenital bar, or block vertebrae). Persons with neuromuscular or congenital osteopathic scoliosis generally enter the medical system early in childhood and are typically managed by pediatric or neurologic physical therapy specialists. Cases of AIS or acquired osteopathic scoliosis can be caused by Scheuermann's disease, osteomalacia, nutritional deficits, rickets, traumatic sports-related conditions (e.g., compression fractures, spondylolysis, spondylolisthesis, endplate fractures, or Schmorl's nodes), or infection (e.g., diskitis, spondylitis, spondyloarthropathy) are more commonly managed by orthopedic physical therapy specialists.[56,120,177]

Scoliosis is named according to the shape (C or S), location, and convexity of the curve. Severity of curve is determined through radiographs (lateral and AP views of the spine) and the Cobb method (see Figure 16-7B) of measurement. Management is based on cause, gender, shape, location, and degree of curve. Structural scoliosis (regardless of type) is always accompanied by specific osseous changes in the vertebral column.[177]

Convex Side	Concave Side
Vertebral body rotation	Spinous process deviation
Posterior rib cage hump	Posterior rib cage hollow
Thoracic cage AP narrowing	Thoracic cage AP widening

Idiopathic scoliosis is broken down into four categories based on age: (1) infantile, children ages 3 and younger, (2) juvenile, 3 to 9 years old (mean age, 6 years), (3) adolescent, 10 to 18 years old; and (4) adult, after skeletal maturity.[56] Infantile idiopathic scoliosis typically creates a left thoracic curve and is more common in boys. Juvenile idiopathic scoliosis typically creates a right thoracic curve and displays an equal distribution among males and females (1.3% overall prevalence).[56] Idiopathic adolescent scoliosis has an overall prevalence of 2% to 4% in children 8 to 16 years of age.[56,112,120] The overall female-to-male ratio for adolescent idiopathic scoliosis is 3.6:1. It is significantly more common in females, especially as the magnitude of the curve increases. In curves of about 10 degrees, the female-to-male ratio is 1.4:1, whereas curves of 20 degrees or greater have a female-to-male ratio of 6.4:1.[56]

The Adam's forward bending test (specificity, 0.64; sensitivity, 0.56) is used as a screening tool to identify those with idiopathic scoliosis.[278] Its lack of reliability makes its general use in elementary school screenings controversial.[125,278] Children and adolescents suspected of having idiopathic scoliosis should be referred for medical examination. Monitoring of the curves via radiographs through growth spurts is crucial. The Risser sign (Figure 16-7B), or degree of iliac crest ossification (stages 1 to 5), is customarily used to determine chronologic bone age.[125]

A patient's skeletal maturity can determine the risk of progression of more severe scoliosis curves (lower numbers imply higher risk). In girls, Risser 4 generally corresponds with completion of spinal growth and the mean period between onset of iliac ossification and Risser 4 is 1 year. The Risser sign is considered a less reliable indicator in boys, with iliac ossification starting relatively early with respect to further growth potential.

The prognosis for idiopathic adolescent scoliosis is based on age of onset, gender, shape, location, and degree of curve. Younger patients, especially females before menarche, will have more growth potential and thus a greater risk of curve progression. Curves will progress in 19.3% of females compared with 1.2% of males. Double-curve patterns (S curve) carry a greater risk for progression than single-curve patterns (C curve). Curves with greater initial magnitude are always at risk to progress.

A progressive curve is defined by a continued increase of 5 degrees or more on two or more consecutive examinations occurring at 4- to 6-month intervals.[56,131] MRI is recommended for patients who display early onset of scoliosis (before age 8 years), rapid curve progression, unusual curve pattern, neurologic deficit, or pain.[125]

Mild deformities (curves of 10 to 20 degrees) are generally asymptomatic and respond well to conservative treatment.[131] Conservative therapy must address flexibility, strength, and muscle imbalance of the trunk, shoulder girdle, and pelvic girdle. Pelvic derotation (posterior pelvic tilt), proprioceptive exercises (pelvic clock), postural stabilization, and selective stretching are considered standard protocol.[56,120,131,159] Respiratory exercises should be added as necessary for thoracic mobility. Global movement programs such as yoga, Pilates, tai chi, and Feldenkrais all may prove useful, but more research is needed in this area.

Moderate deformities (curves of 25 to 40 degrees) typically create MS pain as well as cosmetic issues for the adolescent. Biomechanical bracing with end point control and redundant three-point pressure systems should be implemented when the apex of the curve is between 25 and 40 degrees, or when the curve appears progressive.[131] Goals of orthotic management include halting curve progression, gaining some permanent correction, and allowing for continued spinal growth.[56] Custom-molded total contact thoracolumbosacral orthoses (TLSO) are the current industry standard. Bracing requires strict compliance on the part of the patient (23 hours/day) and should be used in conjunction with a customized exercise program.[131]

Surgical correction of scoliosis is reserved for progressive curves of more than 45 to 50 degrees that compromise cardiovascular-pulmonary function, impair MS function, or result in intractable pain.[56,113,131] Spinal fusion, or arthrodesis, is achieved via internal fixation with Luque rods (L rods) or Harrington rods. The need for postoperative TLSO depends on the

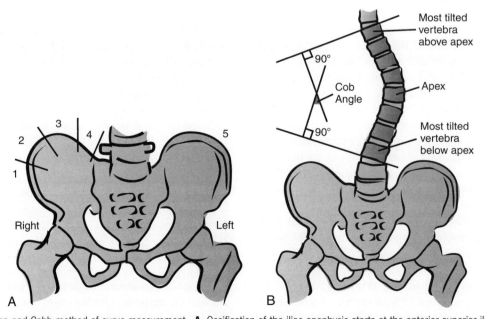

FIGURE 16-7 Risser sign and Cobb method of curve measurement . **A,** Ossification of the iliac apophysis starts at the anterior superior iliac spine and progresses posteromedially. The iliac crest is divided into quadrants, and the stage of maturity is designated as the number of ossified quadrants. For example, 50% ossified is a Risser grade 2. On the anatomic left (*right side of the figure*), all quadrants are ossified and the apophysis is fused to the iliac crest, for a Risser grade 5. **B,** Cobb method of curve measurement. (From Greiner KA. Adolescent idiopathic scoliosis: radiologic decision-making, *Am Fam Physician* 65:1817-1822, 2002.)

type of curve that was fused, type of instrumentation, postoperative alignment of the trunk, and surgeon's discretion.[56,113,115] A less invasive surgery, video-assisted thoracoscopic anterior spine fusion, is now available at several centers in the United States.[113,191]

Nonstructural scoliosis (no inherent osseous change in the vertebral column) can be caused by habitual posturing, pain or muscle hypertonicity (i.e., sciatic scoliosis often seen with low back pain [LBP]), leg length discrepancy (LLD; e.g., bony anomaly, slipped capital femoral epiphysis, Blount's disease, or growth retardation secondary to a prior epiphyseal injury), lower quarter biomechanical or pathoanatomic deformity (e.g., hyperpronation, internal-rotation deformity [IRD], external-rotation deformity [ERD]), or pelvic girdle lesion (e.g., anterior or posterior innominate lesion or innominate up slip).[159,174,232] Treatment for nonstructural scoliosis is always directed at the precipitating cause. Pelvic girdle lesions can be addressed via muscle energy techniques (METs) and direct mobilization or manipulation.[232,269] Other interventions include postural re-education, treatment of back pain and tone issues, treatment of muscular imbalances and orthopedic conditions in the lower kinetic chain, and compensation for a true bony LLD. Depending on the amount of LLD and the age and growth potential of the patient, treatment could range from a simple shoe lift or corrective foot orthosis to surgical osteotomy or a long-bone lengthening procedure (Ilizarov external fixator).

Osteochondritis Dissecans: Tangential Avascular Necrosis of a Pressure Epiphysis

The convex surfaces of certain pressure epiphyses are susceptible to avascular necrosis of a small tangential segment of subchondral bone that may become separated, or dissected, from the remaining portion of the epiphysis by reactive fibrous and granulation tissue—thus the name, osteochondritis dissecans (OCD).[228] Although a relatively uncommon disorder, OCD is seen most often in older children, adolescents, and young adults, and in boys more than girls. It is seen most often in the medial femoral condyle, undersurface of the patella, femoral head, dome of the talus, and capitulum of the humerus (Panner's disease).[228] In most cases, the cause of the initial avascular necrosis is unknown. Rotational or shearing trauma to a joint often is an aggravating variable in adolescents and adults.

The tangential area of avascular necrosis on the convex surface of the joint usually is no larger than 2 cm in diameter and is often smaller. The overlying AC, which is nourished by movement of synovial fluid, remains alive over the necrotic subchondral bone defect. The necrotic segment is eventually revascularized by a combination of bone resorption (osteoclasts) and bone deposition (osteoblasts). This can take up to 2 to 3 years. Juvenile-onset forms (i.e., with epiphyseal plates still open) have the best prognosis.[228]

The patient usually presents with little restriction in ROM, pain (particularly during the revascularization phase), moderate effusion, and disuse atrophy or reflex inhibition of the muscles crossing the joint of interest. Because these symptoms mirror other joint symptoms, tangential view radiographic imaging is imperative. MRI is a more powerful imaging tool to determine continuity of the overlying AC, whereas arthroscopy of

the joint is considered the most definitive diagnostic tool for OCD.[139,171,228]

The success of healing and the subsequent congruency of the joint surfaces depend on the size of the lesion, joint compressive forces, and the presence of concomitant joint-destabilizing forces (e.g., obesity, ligamentous laxity, muscle imbalances, muscle tightness, or poor proprioceptive control).[228] Gross rotational ligamentous laxity or meniscal lesions should be addressed surgically. Physical impairment (e.g., loss of ROM, muscle weakness, poor proprioceptive awareness) and functional limitations (e.g., gait disturbances, transfers, running, jumping) should be remediated with physical therapy.

Activity modification may be necessary to prevent fragment separation ("joint mouse") and subsequent abrasive wear inside the synovial joint. The knee and elbow joints are very susceptible to fragment separation. Detached loose bodies causing intermittent locking or catching should be surgically removed. Loose fragments larger than 2 cm in diameter, particularly in weight-bearing surfaces, should be fixated internally if feasible. If this is not possible, chondral resurfacing techniques (e.g., autologous cartilage implantation [ACI] or autogenous periosteal grafting) followed by continuous passive motion may be required to preserve the articular surface. Although the use of ACI and other chondral resurfacing techniques is becoming increasingly widespread, evidence regarding its superiority to other modalities (e.g., drilling, microfracture, abrasion arthroplasty) remains controversial.[85,118,139,178,270]

Neoplastic Disorders: Bone Tumors and Soft Tissue Tumors

Primary tumors of the MS system are rare, but this does not negate their importance. The childhood, adolescent, and young adult years show a predilection for malignant as well as benign bone tumors.[185] During the pediatric years, bone tumors tend to predominate in the ends of long bones that undergo the greatest growth and remodeling and have the greatest amount of cell activity.[120] Prevalence of bony tumor is as follows: distal end of the femur (53%), proximal tibia (26%), humerus (12%), fibula (5%), scapula (1%), ileum (1%), and other (2%; Figure 16-8).[120,228]

Benign tumors usually do not cause the constant severe pain that is associated with progressive malignant disease. Indeed, pain is the hallmark of malignant tumor development and progression.[120] Local signs such as soft tissue swelling, tenderness, joint pain, or the presence of a mass without a history of trauma should raise a red flag for the health care practitioner. Systemic warning signs of occult disease (e.g., night pain, pain unrelated to position, fever, weight loss, night sweats, fatigue) require referral for medical evaluation for potential bone tumor (infection or inflammatory condition).[50,120,185,228] Bony tumors sometimes manifest via a pathologic fracture during childhood or adolescent sporting events. If the lytic process affects a significant portion of the bone cortex (more than 50%) or occupies 60% of the bone diameter, the risk for fracture increases.[120]

Because sarcomas can readily metastasize to lung, liver, and other bone sites by hematogenous routes, early detection and treatment are warranted. Medical management of bony tumors and neoplasms includes several goals: (1) complete and permanent control of the primary tumor (amputation and limb-sparing

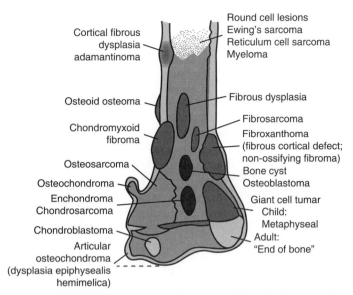

Round cell lesions
Ewing's sarcoma
Reticulum cell sarcoma
Myeloma

Cortical fibrous
dysplasia
adamantinoma

Osteoid osteoma

Fibrous dysplasia

Chondromyxoid
fibroma

Fibrosarcoma

Fibroxanthoma
(fibrous cortical defect;
non-ossifying fibroma)

Osteosarcoma

Bone cyst
Osteoblastoma

Osteochondroma
Enchondroma
Chondrosarcoma

Giant cell tumor
Child:
Metaphyseal
Adult:
"End of bone"

Chondroblastoma

Articular
osteochondroma
(dysplasia epiphysealis
hemimelica)

FIGURE 16-8 Bone cancer—composite diagram illustrating frequent sites of bone tumors. (From Goodman CC, Fuller KS: *Pathology: implications for the physical therapist*, 3rd ed, Philadelphia, 2009, Saunders-Elsevier.)

procedures), (2) control and prevention of microstatic (radiation therapy) and metastatic (chemotherapy) disease, and (3) preservation of function.[56] Amputation is decreasing as a result of early detection, reconstructive surgery, and improved cancer treatments.[56]

Persons caring for those undergoing radiation or chemotherapy treatments for malignant MS tumors must use a comprehensive treatment approach to address the physical and psychosocial needs of the young patient.[120] Chemotherapy drugs, radiation therapy, and amputation will compromise the physical endurance of the patient, necessitating pacing strategies and/or assistive technology to aid with functional activities. Young men should be told that most chemotherapy drugs will have no long-term effect on fertility, but some may reduce the number of spermatozoa. Young women should be taught that menses may become irregular or stop during chemotherapy, but that most often menses will return to normal after the treatment finishes. Long-term follow-up of women treated for bone cancer during childhood and adolescence indicates that the risk of permanent ovarian damage is very low (unless radiation was done in the immediate vicinity of the uterus or pituitary gland in the head).[19]

Children and adolescents who have received chemotherapy have a 10-fold greater chance of developing a second malignancy compared with a child who has never had cancer.[120,223] Patient and family education and support are crucial to the long-term physical and emotional recovery from childhood and adolescent cancer. The exact consequences of the late effects of cancer treatment on social, emotional, and economic (health care costs, return to work, societal dependency as an adult) variables are under ongoing investigation. The Cancer Information Service (http://cis.nih.gov) is the National Cancer Institute's link to the public, offering current scientific information in understandable language for health care professionals, the general public, patients, and their families.[74,223]

Traumatic Musculoskeletal Disorders

Traumatic injuries in childhood and adolescence are common. These injuries are intrinsic or extrinsic in origin. Intrinsic injuries arise from the patient's own physical activity (e.g., violent muscle contraction, awkward movement, fall, deceleration or pivot, inadequate physical conditioning or skill to tolerate the activity). Falls or blows from external forces or objects result in extrinsic injuries in which the adolescent "gets hurt" by something or someone else. Many accidents, as well as sports-related injuries, are preventable with primary prevention guidelines: use of seat belts and properly fitted helmets and protective equipment; common sense principles (don't drink and drive); adequate sport-specific training and conditioning; and abiding by sport-specific injury prevention guidelines ("heads up" tackling to avoid head or neck injury).

Elementary and middle school students participating in sports are less likely to suffer from severe injury because they are smaller and slower than older athletes (less inertia and momentum at impact). High school athletes are bigger, faster, stronger, and capable of delivering tremendous forces in contact sports, especially to younger smaller athletes who are skilled enough to play at the same competitive level. Traumatic injuries tend to be most common in organized and unorganized contact sports (e.g., football, basketball, soccer), bicycling, and roller sports (Box 16-5), whereas overuse injuries (e.g., tendinitis, apophysitis, stress fractures) are seen in repetitive impact loading sports (e.g., running, basketball, gymnastics) and throwing or racquet sports.[58]

Patterns of Adolescent Musculoskeletal Injury

Patterns of new injuries[254] ($N = 3,860,091$) and recurrent injuries ($N = 464,749$) by body site (ankle, knee, head and face, shoulder, low back, upper leg, other) and diagnoses (incomplete and complete sprain, strain, concussion, dislocation, contusion, other) among U.S. high school athletes (2005 to 2008) is shown in Figures 16-9 and 16-10. In a nationwide sample of 100 high schools, certified athletic trainers reported 24.4 injuries/10,000 athlete exposures. Recurrent injuries account for 10.5% of all injuries, and were 3.4 times more likely to cause end of participation (2.4%) versus first-time injuries (0.7%). Recurrent injuries most often involved the ankle (28.3%), knee (16.8%), head or face (12.1%), and shoulder (12.0%), and were most often incomplete ligament sprains (34.9%), incomplete muscle strains (13.3%), and concussion (11.6%). Recurrent injury rates and patterns of injury differ by sport (Table 16-16). To avoid deleterious consequences of injury, sports injury prevention must be a priority for all parents, coaches, teachers, and health care providers (Box 16-6).[254]

Connective Tissue Injuries

Integumentary (lacerations, abrasions) and soft tissue injuries (contusions) typically represent minor traumatic injuries that occur more often in physical education classes and free play sports than in organized team sports. For the most part, little time is lost from sports or general activities as a result of these injuries.[4] Injuries to other connective tissues (e.g., ligaments, tendons, menisci, articular cartilage) or the maturing skeleton

BOX 16-5

Bicycling and Roller Sports: Childhood Injuries and Safety Recommendations

Bicycle accidents have long been a source of unintentional injury and fatality for U.S. youth. Annually, approximately 140 children 0 to 14 years are killed, and another 250,000 to 275,000 children (~690/day) suffer nonfatal injuries as bicyclists. Roller sports including skateboarding (16%), roller skates (10%), and roller blades (4%) represent the remaining wheeled sports that kill and/or injure youth. Skateboarding accounts for approximately 61,000 injuries, including 18,743 head injuries (30.7%); roller skating injures another 38,155 youth/year. The foot-powered scooter, the new toy of the 21st millennium, represents another small-wheeled source of unintentional injury. In 2000, 5 million scooters were sold, and related emergency room injuries increased by 700%.

Those younger than 15 years account for 90% of injuries from roller sports, with the most injured age group being young adolescent males 10 to 14 years of age. One third of injuries occur in first-time participants. Head injuries occur almost exclusively to those participants not wearing a helmet. Almost 50% of all injuries occur in the after-school hours of 4 to 7 pm in residential and public areas. One of every two injurious falls results in a fracture (49% fracture; 51% soft tissue injuries), creating an increased risk for growth plate injury. The vast majority (85%) of fractures include wrist or elbow fractures from a fall on an outstretched hand (FOOSH injury). Seventy percent of soft tissue injuries also occur in the upper extremity. Only 5% of children wear protective limb or joint protective gear while involved in small-wheeled sports activities.

PREVENTION

National estimates report that bicycle helmet use among child bicyclists ranges from 15% to 25%. If just 85% of all cyclists ages 4 to 15 years wore helmets every time they rode bikes for 1 year, between 135 and 155 deaths, between 39,000 and 45,000 head injuries, and between 18,000 and 55,000 scalp and face injuries could be prevented annually. The lifetime medical cost savings could total between $134 million and $174 million —that is, every $11 spent on a bicycle helmet generates $570 in benefits to society.

Tips For Preventing Wheeled-Sport Injuries

- Learn to fall safely.
- Wear properly fit protective equipment – helmets, wrist guards, elbow guards, and kneepads, regardless of age, experience, or skating site.
- Minimize skating in the road, the most common setting of skating fall injuries. Avoid skating on streets with traffic, never skate against traffic, and be very careful at intersections. Pay attention to traffic lights, enter intersections cautiously, and watch out for vehicles, pedestrians, other skaters, and bicyclists.
- Keep speed consistent with experience, with the condition of the skating surface, and with the speed of other travelers.
- Do not skate at night because it is difficult to see and be seen.
- Check equipment often to make sure that it is in good working condition.
- Children younger than 8 years should be supervised.

Adapted from references 132, 133, and 226 and from Sheehan E, Mulhall KJ, Kearns S, McManus F, et al: Impact of dedicated skate parks on the severity and incidence of skateboard- and rollerblade-related pediatric fractures, *J Pediatr Orthop* 23:440-442, 2003.

(e.g., fractures, avulsion injuries), however, can constitute a more serious injury, with potential long-term consequences if improperly managed.

INTEGUMENTARY INJURIES: LACERATIONS AND ABRASIONS. When tissue injury has occurred, basic goals of wound management include the following: (1) protecting the wound and surrounding tissue from additional trauma, (2) reducing strain on the tissues near the wound, (3) protecting the tissue in the area of the wound from mechanical stress or movement, (4) reducing the number of pathogenic microorganisms in and around the wound, (5) expediting the healing process, and (6) reducing the formation of scar tissue.[213,253]

All open wounds run the risk of contamination from the environment. Similarly, the presence of blood necessitates the use of universal precautions to protect the health care provider and other persons in the vicinity of the injury from exposure to blood.[158,213] Universal precautions are the use of barriers such as gloves, gowns, masks, and eyewear when working with blood and other potentially infectious material (any and all body fluids, secretions, and excretions, except sweat) that pose the risk of bloodborne pathogens (e.g., HIV, HBV, HCV).[213] Young athletes and parents should be reassured that to date there have been no reported cases of HIV transmission in any sports, even football, basketball, and wrestling, in which abrasions are common.[158]

CONTUSIONS. Contusions (bruises) are the most common sports injury and rarely cause a student athlete to be sidelined. Contusions also are a common consequence of non–sports-related accidents (e.g., vehicular accidents, falls). A contusion occurs when blunt trauma causes bleeding in the underlying muscle or other soft tissues. No break occurs in the skin, and ecchymosis develops in the area.[130] Contusions may be graded as mild, moderate, or severe. If the ROM in the adjacent joint is two thirds that of normal, the contusion is considered mild. One third to two thirds of normal ROM constitutes a moderate contusion, and less than one third is classified as severe.[168] Prompt treatment for contusion, and for all connective tissue injuries, incorporates the PRICE principle[4,29,50,55,130,168]:

P Protection of the injured part (may include protective orthoses or assistive devices)

R Resting the injured part

I Ice application during the inflammation phase of injury

C Compression with elastic bandages to minimize soft tissue bleeding and edema

E Elevation of the injured part

Myositis Ossificans. Myositis ossificans (MO), or the formation of heterotopic bone within muscle, can be a complication of severe or poorly managed contusion.[29,130,168] In adolescent athletes, common sites for contusion and MO are the quadriceps and biceps brachii muscle bellies. Warning signs of severe contusion include a marked decrease in ROM, significant pain, a sympathetic associated joint effusion, and decreased function (loss of weight-bearing or antigravity muscle force production). If after several days of PRICE treatment a palpable mass develops at the site of injury, one should suspect MO. Initial radiographs will be negative. Bone scintigraphy and ultrasonography have been reported to reveal MO before it is visible on conventional plain radiographs, but MRI is the imaging test of choice for evaluating sports-related muscle injuries.[49] After 3 to 6 weeks, radiographs will reveal any heterotopic ossification, typically deep within the muscle and adjacent to the bone.[168]

Larson and colleagues[168] have described three phases for the treatment of muscle contusions and MO. Phase I consists of pain control via the following: (1) rest, compression, cooling, and elevation algorithm for 24 to 48 hours, regardless of injury severity; (2) positioning of the extremity so that the injured muscle is held out to length without additional pain; (3) 2 to 6 weeks of naproxen (750 mg daily) or indomethacin (50 mg twice daily) for moderate and severe contusions; and (4) analgesics such as acetaminophen (or hospitalization as needed) for pain control. Corticosteroids

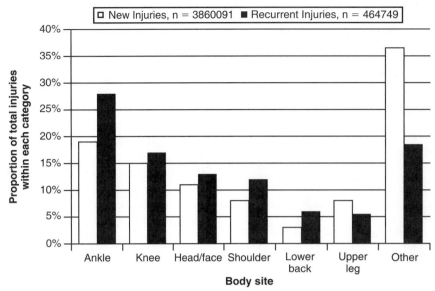

FIGURE 16-9 Most frequent body site injury for new and recurrent injuries. (From Swenson DM, Yard EE, Fields SK, Comstock RD: Patterns of recurrent injuries among U.S. high school athletes, 2005-2008, *Am J Sports Med* 37:1586-1593, 2009.)

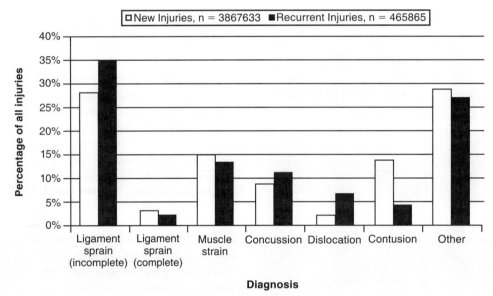

FIGURE 16-10 Most frequent diagnoses for injury for new and recurrent injuries. (From Swenson DM, Yard EE, Fields SK, Comstock RD: Patterns of recurrent injuries among U.S. high school athletes, 2005-2008, *Am J Sports Med* 37:1586-1593, 2009.)

should be avoided, but nonsteroidal anti-inflammatory drugs (NSAIDs) may reduce edema and the risk of heterotopic bone formation.[79,168] Phase II encompasses restoration of mobility via gentle active and passive ROM exercises and low-intensity aerobic exercise in functional patterns (e.g., walking, biking, upper body ergometer, aquatic activities). Phase III consists of functional rehabilitation (i.e., sports-specific activity). Protective padding is recommend for the injured muscle for 3 to 6 months after the injury.[168] Excision of the heterotopic bone is advocated if the mass is symptomatic, with continued muscle atrophy, limited joint motion, and pain after conservative treatment.

SPRAINS. Ligaments and joint capsules connect bone to bone, stabilize joints, restrict and guide joint movement, and allow for conscious kinesthesia.[201] Ligaments and tendons exhibit viscoelastic, or rate-dependent (time-dependent), behavior under loading. A slow rate of loading or sustained load over time is more likely to elongate collagen fibrils (creep tissue to a new length). At higher strain rates, ligaments and tendons can store more energy, require more force to rupture (increased stiffness), and undergo greater elongation.[202] If rate or intensity of load is too high, microfailure without laxity changes (grade I), microfailure with laxity changes (grade II), and complete rupture (grade III) can occur (Figure 16-11).

Signs and symptoms of sprain include the sound or feeling of a pop when the injury occurs, the feeling that a joint is loose or unstable, an inability to bear weight because of pain, loss of motion, and joint swelling with possible reflex muscle inhibition and loss of function.[4,130,177,202] The American Academy of

TABLE 16-16

Proportions of New and Recurrent Injuries by Diagnosis, Sport, and Gender, United States, 2005-2008 (%)*

Sport	Injury Type	Ligament Strain†	Muscle Strain†	Concussion	Contusion	Dislocation	Other‡	Total
Football	New	25.6	13.7	10.4	16.3	3.0	31.0	100
	Reinjury	29.8	12.3	12.4	6.6	9.4	29.5	100
Soccer								
Boys	New	23.8	18.5	9.2	17.3	1.5	29.8	100
	Reinjury	34.8	15.7	13.8	4.2	5.9	25.6	100
Girls	New	29.8	16.3	10.6	11.9	1.0	30.3	100
	Reinjury	37.2	14.0	19.1	2.8	1.9	25.0	100
Volleyball	New	48.5	13.8	4.4	4.8	1.5	27.0	100
	Reinjury	42.7	14.8	2.6	0.0	5.5	34.4	100
Basketball								
Boys	New	39.4	9.5	4.7	11.1	2.4	32.8	100
	Reinjury	58.4	8.0	2.2	1.0	5.8	24.4	100
Girls	New	35.6	11.8	9.1	7.1	1.7	34.6	100
	Reinjury	43.6	6.3	13.7	5.5	3.5	27.4	100
Wrestling	New	23.4	17.5	5.1	8.1	4.3	41.5	100
	Reinjury	20.1	18.4	9.6	5.9	14.8	31.2	100
Baseball	New	20.7	19.4	2.5	16.3	1.1	40.0	100
	Reinjury	24.9	31.9	4.4	4.8	5.2	28.8	100
Softball	New	20.7	15.4	5.3	18.7	2.3	37.6	100
	Reinjury	26.3	11.8	8.3	1.0	9.3	43.3	100

*These proportions reflect national estimates of new and recurrent injuries.

†Incomplete tears; complete tears represent a small minority of ligament sprains and muscle strains.

‡These diagnoses include, but are not limited to, tendon strains, fractures, tendinitis, infections, inflammation, and torn cartilage.

From Swenson DM, Yard EE, Fields SK, et al: Patterns of recurrent injuries among U.S. high school athletes, 2005-2008, *Am J Sports Med* 37:1586-1593, 2009.

Orthopaedic Surgeons (AAOS) classifies sprains on a three-point scale[130]:

- Grade I (mild) sprains occur when fibers are stretched without loss of continuity (i.e., damaged microscopically via intrasubstance rupture of cross links).
- Grade II (moderate) sprains result when some fibers are stretched and some are torn (i.e., plastic deformation has occurred on the stress-strain curve). These tears produce some joint laxity and often are very painful, given the fact that the remaining fibers and related soft tissues experience more stress because of the resultant joint instability.
- Grade III (severe) sprains are a complete or almost complete ligament rupture with resultant joint laxity, associated joint effusion, reflex inhibition, and loss of function.[130,202] After the initial injury, grade III sprains may not produce pain, because the ligaments and their stretch-sensitive receptors can no longer transmit noxious mechanical signals to the sensory cortex.

Older adolescents (closed epiphyseal plates) are more likely to have ligamentous sprain (rupture) whereas younger children and young teens (immature skeleton) are more likely to suffer an avulsion injury at the ligamentous-osseous junction. On physical examination and joint inspection, these avulsion fractures behave similarly to a midsubstance ligament rupture. In particular, a tibial eminence avulsion fracture in an 8- to 11- year old will have a history suspicious of anterior cruciate ligament rupture, and referral for diagnostic imaging is crucial to avoid mismanagement of the injury.

STRAINS. Contractile tissue (i.e., the musculotendinous unit) is composed of four elements: muscle, musculotendinous junction (MTJ), tendon, and tendon's interface with the bone.[177] A strain is an injury (a partial or complete tear) to any portion of the musculotendinous unit from an abrupt, excessive, or repeated muscle contraction that exceeds the tissue's tensile capability. The transition zones, tendon insertion (traction epiphysis or apophysis) and MTJ, are most susceptible to injury.[202] Strains, like ligamentous sprains, are classified as mild (grade I), moderate (grade II), or severe (grade III).[50,130] Clinical findings include pain, edema, loss of motion, tenderness on palpation, protective muscle spasm or cramping, and possible weakness.[130]

MTJ injuries are diagnosed by active or resistive contraction of the muscle (e.g., Cyriax's resisted motions in neutral [RMIN] classification system), passive elongation (stretching of the muscle), and palpation.[54,171,177] Radiographic imaging of muscle strain in adolescents is essential to rule out avulsion fractures (traumatic apophysis).[185]

Contact or ballistic sports such as soccer, football, hockey, boxing, wrestling, and track put people at risk for strains. Gymnastics, tennis, rowing, golf, and other sports that require extensive gripping can increase the risk of hand, forearm, and elbow strains. Strains of the upper and lower extremities sometimes occur in children and adolescents who lack proximal stability and kinesthetic control to participate in repetitive overhead activity

Pediatric and Adolescent Considerations in Sports Medicine

Approximately 35 million children age 5 to 18 years participate in organized sports in the United States.[243] Beyond organized sports, millions compete and participate in physical education classes, community intramural programs, church programs, and other recreational sporting activities.[4,29] Since the advent of Title IX in 1972, women's participation in physical activity and sports has increased dramatically (700%).[194] The American Academy of Pediatrics supports participation in sport for overall health benefits despite the fact that here has been an increase in acute and overuse injuries in young athletes over the past 20 to 30 years.[243] About 10% of youth (3.5 million) will be injured in sports each year, with about 95% being soft tissue injuries (contusions, muscle strain, ligament sprain, cuts and abrasions).[4]

There are an estimated 6 million emergency department (ED) visits annually in the United States for sports-related (SR) injuries in patients aged 5 to 24 (mean age, 13 years), with the highest percentage in 5- to 14-year-old boys.[52] Contact sports (basketball, football, and soccer) have the highest incidence of ED visits with sprains, contusions, and fractures each accounting for 20% to 30% of injuries.[243]

Studies show that 30% to 50% of all juvenile sports injuries are considered overuse (repetitive microtrauma) injuries. The American College of Sports Medicine estimates that 50% of overuse injuries in children and adolescents are avoidable.[228]

COMMON SENSE PRINCIPLES OF SPORTS INJURY PREVENTION[15,32]

- Obtain medical clearance for participation (including subjective history and a pre-participation physical examination [PPE]).[137]
- Immediately stop participation of any athlete with a sudden change in weight-bearing status or persistent pain, numbness, tingling, weakness, or altered function.
- Use and maintain proper protective equipment (covered head to toe).
- Evaluate field or court conditions before practice and competition.
- Study and apply the appropriate biomechanics of the sport (requires adequate coaching of technique).
- Enforce specific rules of safety (e.g., no spearing or clipping in football).
- Avoid the "no pain, no gain" mentality (many injuries are the result of fatigue).
- Promote psychological preparation in the athlete (visual practice, mental preparation, and training in stress management and relaxation).
- Foster high-quality communication on and off the field (recognize risks).
- Practice sound total conditioning principles (e.g., proper warm-up and cool-down, proper nutrition and fluid intake).[22]
- Prevent athlete burnout and susceptibility to overuse injuries via total conditioning principles (periodization).[32]
- Periodization—year-round training principles for the adolescent athlete. The off season is a key time to work on the fundamental skills of the sport.

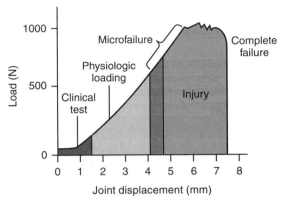

FIGURE 16-11 Stress-strain curve of a ligament. (From Nordin M, Frankel VH. *Basic biomechanics of the musculoskeletal system*, ed 3, 2001, Lippincott Williams & Wilkins.)

labrum), and positive orthopedic special tests can implicate FC injury.[177] MRI is the diagnostic imaging tool of choice for all FC injuries.[184] Plain radiographs may expose joint effusion, but they will not expose muscle, fat pads, fat lines, joint capsules and ligaments, periosteum, and menisci in the same fashion as MRI, especially given the confusion of the epiphyseal growth plates in the immature skeleton.[120,177,185]

Menisci. Knee meniscal injuries in children younger than 10 years are rare, and children younger than 15 years account for a small percentage (5% to 10%) of all meniscal injuries.[53,180,185] In late adolescence (15 to 19 years), decreased vascularity and resiliency of the knee menisci, coupled with increased sports participation, make meniscal injuries a common occurrence.[53,180,224]

In the 13- to 18-year-old group, almost 50% of all knee injuries involve the menisci.[53] Medial meniscus injuries are more common (88%) because of the medial meniscocapsular junction and the stress of closed kinetic chain pronation during pivoting and cutting activities. About one third (30% to 36%) of patients also display a concomitant anterior cruciate ligament (ACL) injury. In children, longitudinal tears parallel to the periphery account for 50% to 90% of meniscus tears.[53,180] The lateral meniscus is more prone to injury if the developmental abnormality, often called a discoid meniscus, is present. An abnormally wide lateral radiographic joint space is evident on the anteroposterior (AP) knee projection if discoid meniscus is present.[185]

Preservation of injured menisci should be the overarching goal of any surgical intervention. The patient's age, type of tear (radial, longitudinal, flap, or bucket handle tear), site of injury and blood supply (e.g., white zone [inner third], red-white zone [middle third], and red zone [outer third]) dictate whether selective débridement or meniscal repair is performed.[123,180,241] Concomitant ligamentous instability and/or osteochondral lesions should be surgically addressed, along with supervised physical therapy postoperatively to improve outcomes of any meniscus repair.

Glenoid Labrum. The glenoid labrum serves to deeper the socket and contributes to the intra-articular vacuum effect, thereby improving glenohumeral (GH) stability.[94] Glenoid labrum injury can result from traumatic GH dislocation (Bankart tear), recurrent subluxation or multidirectional instability (MDI), or

(e.g., racquet sports, volleyball, baseball) or repetitive lower quarter impact-loading sports (e.g., basketball, soccer, track).[4]

FIBROCARTILAGE DISORDERS. Three types of fibrocartilage (FC) are found in the body: (1) white (menisci, intervertebral disks [IVD], glenoid labrum, acetabular labrum, and pubic symphysis); (2) yellow (ears and epiglottis); and (3) hyaline AC.[201] FC structures are essential to the health of joints because they increase joint congruency, contact area and stability, and aid in shock absorption. For example, during activities, the menisci and AC attenuate up to 70% of the load across the knee.[180] The healing potential of FC depends on age, extent of injury, potential blood supply and, for AC, nutrition via low compressive load joint movement.[53,118,202]

The most pertinent FC structures include the knee menisci, shoulder glenoid labrum, and hyaline cartilage of all synovial joints. A report of locking or clicking with movement, joint effusion, loss of active and passive ROM, joint line pain, springy block end feel or excessive laxity (Bankart tear of the glenoid deceleration trauma at the insertion of the long head of biceps (LHB) from overhead, throwing, or racquet sports (SLAP lesion, or superior labral tear from anterior to posterior). Examination of the GH joint reveals pain and/or complaint of instability with overhead activities, joint clicking or catching, apprehension at end ROM, and positive glenoid labral special tests.[177] Bankart lesions are best handled via surgical repair to restore functional stability, whereas MDI is best managed with aggressive rehabilitation (90% to 95% success rate).[94] SLAP tears may require surgery if the LHB is rendered nonfunctional, associated rotator cuff injury is present, and the patient has failed conservative rehabilitation.[100]

Articular Hyaline Cartilage. AC is a highly specialized tissue (low cellular density, aneural, avascular, alymphatic) precisely suited for withstanding the highly loaded environment of a synovial joint.[202] AC can fail (osteochondral defect) under impact (compressive loads) or torsional loads, or via disease processes (inflammatory, metabolic, infectious disease). Stressing of the collagen-proteoglycan matrix (loss of water retention capabilities) is the underlying wear process in this highly specialized tissue. Joint pain, dysfunction and effusions and, in some cases, progressive joint degeneration, necessitate creating a healing environment for acutely damaged AC.

Cartilage has a poor reparative capacity, although it is unclear to what extent this may be dependent on age or maturation.[257] In general, AC heals best with low-load cyclic movement to foster joint lubrication and nutrition.[51,202] Use of continuous passive motion devices, unweighting systems, and aquatic therapy is advocated for the treatment of AC, meniscus, and other lower kinetic chain injuries that require selective weight-bearing progression.

A variety of treatments has the potential to improve healing of articular surfaces, including perforation of subchondral bone, altered joint loading, periosteal and perichondrial grafts, cell transplantation, growth factors, and artificial matrices. Selection of treatment for a patient with an AC injury should be guided by an understanding of the type of injury, the potential for healing, and the effects of treatment on joint surface restoration.[51] Gross ligamentous or directional instability or weak lower extremity musculature must be addressed before, or in conjunction with, fibrocartilaginous repair or transplantation.[118,130,201,202]

Fractures: Discontinuity of Osseous and Cartilaginous Structures

A fracture, whether of a bone, an epiphyseal plate, or a cartilaginous joint surface, is simply a structural break in continuity.[185] A fracture will always produce some degree of concomitant soft tissue injury (e.g., pain, tenderness, deformity, edema, ecchymosis) and loss of mobility and function.[120,202] The extent of injury depends on several factors, including the following: (1) type of bone fractured (cortical or cancellous), (2) location within the skeleton (intra-articular, extra-articular, or at a growth zone), (3) type of load (tension, compression, bending, shear, torsion, or combined loading), (4) amount and frequency of load (stress-strain or fatigue curve of the structure), (5) metabolic and disease status of the bone, and (6) overall fitness level and age of the individual.[120,185,202,228]

A bending force on a long bone causes a compressive failure on the concave side of the bone and an explosive tension failure (e.g., transverse or oblique fracture) on the convex side. In children and young adolescents, cortical bone is much more pliable, like green wood in a living young tree, and bending moments tend to create one of three incomplete fractures—greenstick, plastic bowing, or torus (buckling) fracture (see Chapter 14).

A twisting (torsional, rotational) force creates a spiraling tension fracture in long bones. Shear loads in children can create severe epiphyseal growth plate injuries, avulsion fractures, or ligamentous injuries, depending on skeletal maturity. A fracture that involves the AC of a joint is called an intra-articular fracture. The radiographic method used most often for the classification of pediatric epiphyseal fractures is the modified Salter-Harris classification system (see Chapter 14). Physeal fractures and apophyseal avulsions (15% to 20% of pediatric fractures) are unique to children and adolescents and warrant special attention given the risk for interrupted growth.[185,243]

Epidemiologic studies have demonstrated the incidence of fractures in adolescence to be 21.8/1000 (male, 31/1000; female, 13.1/1000).[186] Fractures account for about 20% to 30% of sports-related injuries.[243] The mean age of fracture is 12 years and there is a male predominance (2:1).[243] Two thirds of adolescent fractures occur in the UE (distal radius and ulna [43%] and fingers [23%]).[243] Rarely are the skull and spine fractured, and forceful hyperextension represents the most common mechanism of adolescent spinal fracture (e.g., spondylolysis, with or without spondylolisthesis).

Social deprivation appears to be predictive of the incidence of fracture in adolescent males and females,[88,186,247] especially upper limb and distal radius fractures in females and hand and carpus fractures in males.[186] There appears to be an association between low bone density and fractures in children and adolescents. A number of factors may be associated, including demographic variables (social deprivation, educational factors, ethnicity), skeletal fragility from disease (endocrine illness), diet and sun exposure (vitamin D),[89] and vigorous athletic activity.[86]

FRACTURE MANAGEMENT. The medical management of fracture depends on the following: (1) location of the fracture, (2) type of fracture, (3) need for reduction, (4) presence of instability after reduction, (5) extent of concomitant connective or neurovascular injury, and (6) functional requirements of the injured patient.[50,103,120,241] Fracture reduction is achieved through closed reduction (e.g., traction, reduction, immobilization) or open reduction methods. Surgical intervention (open reduction) includes bone grafts or bone substitutes (e.g., ceramic materials), internal fixation (e.g., metal plating, wiring, screws), or external fixation (e.g., Ilizarov external fixator). With or without surgical intervention, a period of immobilization is generally used after bone fracture to prevent longitudinal or shear stresses. Failure to stabilize the fracture site can result in pain, nonunion, or malunion.

Fractures in children usually heal in 4 to 6 weeks, in adolescents in 6 to 8 weeks, and in adults in 10 to 18 weeks.[120] Many factors, local and systemic, affect healing. Local factors include type, size, and location of fracture; postinjury infection or retained foreign body; movement or excessive pressure that compromises local blood supply; and electromagnetic energy

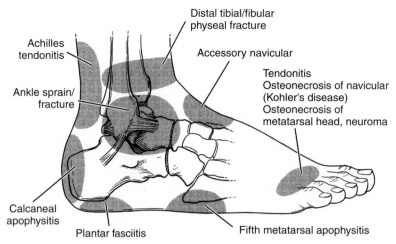

FIGURE 16-12 Common musculoskeletal conditions of the ankle. (From Lyon RM, Street CC: Pediatric sports injuries, *Pediatr Clin North Am* 45:221-244, 1998.)

or ultrasound (used when physicians anticipate healing problems).[55,103,120] Systemic factors affecting healing include age, metabolic status, general health (e.g., presence of comorbid conditions, medications that impede healing), nutrition, and avoidance of substances that inhibit bone formation (e.g., nicotine, corticosteroids, alcohol).[55,103,120]

Overuse Injuries

STRESS FRACTURES. Stress fractures (osseous overuse) are common injuries in adolescents and the prognosis mainly depends on early diagnosis and early initiated therapy (modification of weight-bearing loads).[138,229] Jumping and impact loading athletes (runners) in their late teens are most susceptible. Load-dependent pain is the main symptom of a stress fracture, and localized swelling and periosteal thickening may occur.[229] Differential diagnosis includes compartment syndrome, medial tibial stress syndrome (muscular shin splints), and/or nerve or artery entrapment syndromes. Data indicate that MRI is best suited to detect stress fractures of the juvenile skeletal system in early stages.[138]

Almost all stress fractures (95%) are in the lower extremity. The incidence of stress fracture is tibia (50%), metatarsals (25%), fibula (10% overall; 20% of children), proximal femur (5%), and other (10%; pelvis, navicular, medial epicondyle, humerus).[229] Recurrence is common; 60% of persons with a stress fracture have had a previous stress fracture.[229] Normally, 6 to 8 weeks (range, 2 to 24 weeks) of relative rest (rest from impact but not training) is required to heal stress fractures adequately. Anti-inflammatory strategies (e.g., ice, NSAIDs) are used symptomatically. During this time, contributing factors (inflexibility, proximal weakness [gluteus medius, quadriceps], and lack of shock absorption or overpronation [footwear and/or foot orthoses]) should be addressed before the patient begins a graduated return to activity, at a rate of less than 10% increase/week.[229]

SOFT TISSUE INJURIES. Because of their biomechanical makeup and relationship to external loads, the developing peripheral joints are particularly susceptible to overuse injury.[4,175] The most susceptible pediatric joints and potential differential diagnoses are illustrated in Figures 16-12 (ankle), 16-13 (knee), and 16-14 (elbow).[175] The increase in physeal injuries during adolescence is believed to be caused by biomechanical and structural weakness of the physeal cartilage during this stage of rapid MS growth. Long bone growth surges, muscle inflexibility, and increases in muscle mass and torque-generating capacity of muscle, because of the surge in testosterone, may explain why there are so many growth plate injuries. Young boys incur more physeal injuries as a result of four developmental factors: (1) males have a greater propensity for impact sports, (2) males have a higher overall rate of traumatic injury, (3) males have a greater percentage of increase in muscle mass, and (4) male growth plates remain open longer than those of girls.[185]

Apophysitis, or post-traumatic avulsion of the traction epiphysis, is typically a benign but annoying malady affecting the growing skeletons of active youngsters.[4] The symptoms of these growth plate conditions usually begin at 8 to 15 years of age. Clinical features of apophysitis include activity-related pain and swelling at the insertion site, associated loss of flexibility resulting from pain or secondary to growth spurts, reflex inhibition of the muscle secondary to pain and swelling, and functional limitations specific to the joint. The pain usually does not awaken the adolescent at night. The tenderness is well localized, and there are no other significant abnormalities of the joint.[171,175]

LOWER EXTREMITY INJURIES. Osgood-Schlatter disease is a partial avulsion of the patellar ligament at the tibial tubercle. It is most common in boys 10 to 15 years of age and girls 10 to 11 years of age, with a boy-to-girl ratio of 3:1. Like all osteochondroses, activity-related anterior knee pain is the presenting problem (e.g., kneeling, direct blow, forceful quadriceps contraction). Radiographs (AP and lateral) show irregular tibial tuberosity (fragmentation) and are necessary to rule out tumor.[185] Treatment consists of activity modification (rest), stretching, quadriceps strengthening, ice, iontophoresis, knee orthoses, and taping for comfort. Although usually self-limiting (heals in less than 2 years), débridement of avulsion bone fragments is sometimes required.[171, 228]

Sinding-Larsen-Johannson disease is a partial avulsion of the inferior pole of the patella and is most common in boys aged 10 to 15 years. No long-term disability is expected, and treatment is for symptoms only (see earlier, treatment of Osgood-Schlatter disease).[171]

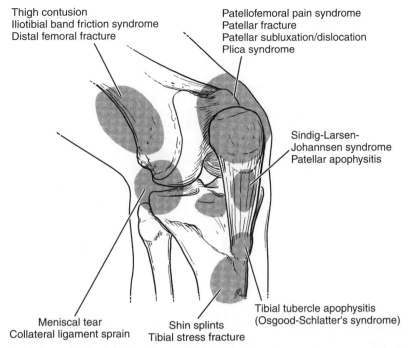

Thigh contusion
Iliotibial band friction syndrome
Distal femoral fracture

Patellofemoral pain syndrome
Patellar fracture
Patellar subluxation/dislocation
Plica syndrome

Sindig-Larsen-
Johannsen syndrome
Patellar apophysitis

Tibial tubercle apophysitis
(Osgood-Schlatter's syndrome)

Meniscal tear
Collateral ligament sprain

Shin splints
Tibial stress fracture

FIGURE 16-13 Common musculoskeletal conditions of the knee. (From Lyon RM, Street CC: Pediatric sports injuries, *Pediatr Clin North Am* 45:221-244, 1998.)

Sever's disease is a partial avulsion of the calcaneal apophysis. It is characterized by posterior heel pain (possibly bilateral), tenderness and swelling at the insertion of the Achilles, and calcaneal gait deviation (poor control of tibial advancement in midstance). It is most common in girls 5 to 10 years of age and often seen in boys aged 10 to 12 years. Radiographs are not diagnostic. Usually self-limiting (heals in less than 1 year), Sever's disease responds to rest, ice, stretching of one- and two-joint plantar flexors, iontophoresis, and a 1-cm heel lift to reduce stress on the tendon insertion.[171]

The sudden onset of anterior or posterior hip pain is more common in older adolescents and males than in females. Ballistic trauma (usually from sprinting) can cause avulsion of the rectus femoris at the anterior inferior iliac spine (AIIS) or a traction injury of the hamstring origin at the ischial tuberosity. For acute treatment, these injuries respond best to rest, ice, and gentle stretching of the involved one- and two-joint hip muscles. Postinjury strengthening (specifically eccentric exercise) is crucial after the initial healing phase. An elastic hip orthosis or neoprene sleeve to warm tissues and bias (protect) the muscle of interest also can offer the athlete postinjury protection.[171]

Long-term care of all lower extremity injuries should include proximal stabilization exercises (abdominals, gluteal musculature, and quadriceps) to create muscular balance to control lower kinetic chain forces.[57,236] Foot orthoses also may be indicated to control ground reaction forces.[4,241] Neural mobilization techniques may be indicated for chronic hamstring conditions.[141]

UPPER EXTREMITY INJURIES. Pain and inability to extend the elbow fully after a trivial injury or repetitive microtrauma in boys 5 to 10 years old (boys more than girls) could be Little Leaguer's elbow (medial epicondyle apophysis).[90,171,175] Radiographs are diagnostic, and rest via a sling and restriction of strenuous activity for the elbow are critical. If repetitive elbow trauma leads to lateral elbow pain, an osteochondritis dissecans of the capitellum

(Panner's disease) of the elbow can develop (11 to 15 years; boys more than girls).[90] If a fragment of bone from the capitellum loses its blood supply, loosens, and becomes a loose body in the joint, surgery often is required to correct the problem. Radiographs are diagnostic, and strict rest via a sling and avoidance of all strenuous activity for the elbow are essential to prevent long-term dysfunction and loss of elbow extension.[58]

Overhand-throwing athletes (boys more than girls) occasionally develop a stress fracture of the proximal humeral epiphysis (Little Leaguer's shoulder).[58] This condition must be differentiated from the many impingement-related conditions that can occur about the shoulder (rotator cuff tendinitis, biceps tendinitis, multidirectional instability, bursitis). Radiographs are diagnostic. Rest is essential for the healing of stress fractures and to prevent further damage.

Most adolescent shoulder and elbow overuse injuries are self-limiting and respond well to relative rest (avoidance of the precipitating mechanism), ice, and analgesics (acetaminophen or NSAIDs), followed by a comprehensive rehabilitation program.[34] The best way to prevent UE overuse injuries is to strengthen proximal musculature (scapular stabilizers) and core body muscles (abdominals, hip extensors, abductors).[94,271,272] Learning proper pitching technique, avoiding specialty pitches at a young age, and limiting the number of pitches allowed in Little League baseball (less than 350/week) is crucial.[34,94,271,272]

Lower Quarter Musculoskeletal Injuries

A comprehensive list of common lower quarter MS injuries is presented in Table 16-17, and Figure 16-12 (ankle) and Figure 16-13 (knee). Lower quarter MS injuries can be the result of macrotrauma or microtrauma. Knowledge of the mechanism of injury (MOI) can be useful in the differential diagnosis. Proximal injuries (i.e., pelvic ring, hip, and femur) typically are the

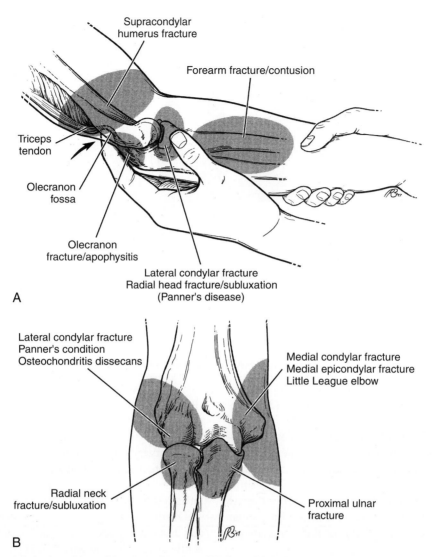

FIGURE 16-14 Common musculoskeletal conditions of the elbow. (From Lyon RM, Street CC: Pediatric sports injuries, *Pediatr Clin North Am* 45:221-244, 1998.)

result of high-energy trauma (e.g., motor vehicle or bicycle accidents, sports-related collisions, falls from a height). Rotational or pivoting forces in the lower limb are a significant contributor to injuries at both the knee and ankle.

ANKLE INJURIES. Across the life span, the most common foot and ankle conditions are ankle sprains, Achilles' tendinitis (strain), and plantar fasciitis.[220] Plantar flexion-inversion sprain of the anterior talofibular and calcaneofibular ligaments is the most common MOI (75% to 85%). Eversion (deltoid ligament, 15%) and high ankle (syndesmosis, 10%) sprains tend to be more serious and take twice as long to rehabilitate.[241] In the skeletally immature individual, physeal injuries should be considered after torsional ankle trauma; the distal tibial physis is the second most commonly injured physis in long bones.[225] Premature physeal closure has been reported at high rates (39.6%) in distal Salter-Harris types I and II fractures (see Chapter 14) of the tibia in both supination-external-rotation-type injuries (35%) and pronation-abduction-type injuries (54%).[225] Failure to fully rehabilitate an ankle sprain (loss of proprioceptive lower extremity control) in a young female has been linked to an increased risk of anterior cruciate ligament injury.[45]

KNEE INJURIES. The long contributing levers (femur and tibia) predispose the knee joint to injury from direct extrinsic blows as well as intrinsic pivoting, cutting, and deceleration injuries. Indeed, the knee is the second most commonly injured joint as a consequence of collisions, falls, and overuse occurring from childhood and adolescent sports (see Figure 16-9).[240,254] Figure 16-15 denotes major knee instabilities and Box 16-7 shows ligamentous tests often performed on the knee.[177] The skeletally mature teen will manifest injuries analogous to those of an adult, whereas physeal injuries (see Chapter 14) should be considered in the skeletally immature child or young teen.

Medial Collateral Ligament. In isolation, the medial collateral ligament (MCL) is the knee ligament most often sprained.[4,50,220,241] Most MCL sprains, including complete tears (grade III), can be treated conservatively. A bundle of the MCL is intimate with the medial joint capsule, posterior oblique ligament, and meniscotibial fibers, making the medial meniscus (along with the ACL) susceptible to forceful valgus rotation loads. The resultant injury—the terrible triad (MCL, ACL, and medial meniscus)—is best handled surgically to prevent long-term mechanical degradation of the knee (osteoarthrosis).

TABLE 16-17

Common Lower Extremity Injuries in the Adolescent*

| General Category | Specific Entity | | |
	Proximal Lower Extremity	Knee	Lower Leg, Ankle, and Foot
Instability	Sacroiliac joint (SIJ) instability	Patellar subluxation, dislocation	Ankle mortise dislocation and/or dislocation of any foot or toe joints
Ligamentous and/or capsular injury at joint of interest	Pubic symphysis instability Hip dislocation	Femoral-tibial subluxation, dislocation (with associated ligamentous damage) Ligamentous sprain (key ligaments of the knee—ACL, MCL, PCL, LCL) Tendon rupture (hamstrings, patellar tendon, ligament rupture)	Ligamentous sprain (key ligaments of the ankle—anterior talofibular [ATF], posterior talofibular [PTF], calcaneofibular [CF], deltoid) Tendon rupture (e.g., Achilles, tibialis posterior)
Impingement and/or nerve injuries	Hip labrum impingement (rare) Lumbosacral plexus injuries from trauma Lumbar radiculopathy from HNP (rare in adolescents) Piriformis syndrome	Peroneal nerve entrapment (complication of short leg casting) Fat pad impingement Plica syndrome	Tarsal tunnel syndrome (tibial nerve) Nerve entrapment at ankle retinaculum status post (s/p) trauma (peroneal, sural, or tibial branches)
Fractures	Pelvis (ischium, ilium, and pubis, and acetabular fractures) Sacrum Intracapsular (e.g., femoral head, subcapital, femoral neck fractures) Extracapsular (e.g., intertrochanteric, subtrochanteric, femoral shaft fractures) Apophyseal avulsion fractures Iliac crest—abdominals Anterior superior iliac spine—sartorius Anterior inferior iliac spine—rectus femoris Ischial tuberosity hamstrings	Distal femoral-shaft fractures Supracondylar fractures (e.g., displaced, nondisplaced, impacted, comminuted, condylar, intercondylar) Tibial avulsion fracture (mimics ACL instability) Patellar fractures (e.g., vertical, transverse, comminuted, or avulsion; all can be displaced and nondisplaced) Tibial plateau fractures (described on the Hohl classification system as type I-VI) Fractures of proximal fibula Osteochondritis dissecans (OCD)	Bimalleolar and trimalleolar fractures, including Tillaux fracture (juvenile triplane fracture with intra-articular anterolateral ankle mortise fracture) Calcaneus fractures (Rowe classification system types I-V) Talus fractures (described by location—body, dome, neck, head) Navicular fracture Tarsometatarsal fracture (Lisfranc) Metatarsal and phalangeal fractures
Soft tissue injuries (including overuse)	Muscle strain, tendinitis (any muscle about the hip) Contusion with potential complication of myositis ossificans (quads) Delayed-onset muscle soreness (DOMS) of proximal thigh musculature	Muscle strain, tendinitis (any muscle about the hip) Patellar tendon, ligament "tendinitis" Meniscus tears (e.g., vertical, horizontal, cleavage, bucket handle) Iliotibial band tendinitis (runner's knee) Osgood-Schlatter disease (jumper's knee) Sindig-Larsen-Johanssen disease Patellofemoral pain syndrome (PFPS)	Tibialis anterior and posterior tendinitis (shin splints) Achilles tendinitis Sever's disease Plantar fasciitis Contusions of foot, toes Nail bed injuries Compartment syndrome
Referred pain	Lumbar spine and knee referral (one joint above and below joint of interest) GI system referral Reproductive system referral Urinary system referral	Lumbar spine, pelvis, hip referral to knee	Lumbar spine, pelvis, hip, and knee referral to lower, leg, ankle, foot (LLAF)
Other	Degenerative joint disease (hip) Rheumatoid arthritis (hip) Avascular necrosis of hip Slipped femoral capital epiphysis Congenital dislocation of hip	Degenerative joint disease (knee) Rheumatoid arthritis (knee)	Degenerative joint disease (ankle) Rheumatoid arthritis (ankle) Gout (rare in children)

Lower extremity rehabilitation note: The PRICE principle is the focus of acute injury management. During the inflammatory phase of healing (days 0-6), connective tissue injuries should be treated with edema control, icing, and protection (i.e., motion control). Weight-bearing with an orthosis (brace or taping) is allowed as tolerated (as long as the athlete does not have a limp). Athletes should use assistive devices when and if a normal gait pattern cannot be tolerated. Protected motion with progressive strengthening and closed kinetic chain balance training are advanced individually, with return to sports allowed as early as a few days to 4 weeks for lesser sprains. Protection of ruptured ligaments during the first 3 weeks (proliferation phase) to 6 weeks (maturation phase) is crucial for optimal stabilization.[241] Strengthening and balance programs (i.e., closed kinetic chain training), impact loading, and sport-specific training are recommended for optimal return to sport function.[17] Prophylactic use of braces for ankle injuries is useful but controversial for the knee joint.[50,174,180,241]

*Hip, thigh, knee, lower leg, ankle, and foot.

Adapted from references 4, 175, 185, and 220.

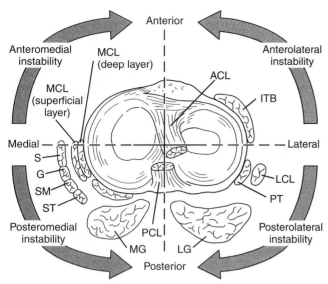

FIGURE 16-15 Knee instabilities. (From Magee DJ: *Orthopedic physical assessment*, 5th ed, Philadelphia, 2008, Saunders Elsevier.)

BOX 16-7

Ligamentous Tests Commonly Performed on the Knee

Test	Findings
One-plane medial instability	Valgus stress at 0 and 30 degrees
	Hughston valgus stress at 0 and 30 degrees
One-plane lateral instability	Varus stress at 0 and 30 degrees
	Hughston valgus stress at 0 and 30 degrees
One-plane anterior instability	Lachman test or its modifications
	Drawer test
	Active drawer test
One-plane posterior instability	Posterior sag
	Drawer test
	Active drawer test
	Godfrey test
Anteromedial rotary instability	Slocum test
Anterolateral rotary instability	Pivot shift test
	Losee test
	Hughston jerk test
	Slocum anterolateral rotatory instability test
	Crossover test
	Noyes flexion-rotation drawer test
Posteromedial rotary instability	Hughston posteromedial drawer test
	Posteromedial pivot shift test
Posterolateral rotary instability	Hughston posterolateral drawer test
	Jakob test
	External rotation recurvatum
	Loomer posterolateral rotary instability test
	Tibial external rotation test

From Magee DJ: *Orthopedic physical assessment*, 5th ed, Philadelphia, 2008, Saunders Elsevier.

Lateral Collateral Ligament. Isolated lateral collateral ligament (LCL) injuries (varus force) are the rarest form of athletic knee injuries. The ability to ambulate despite localized pain, stiffness, and swelling, without concomitant injury of the lateral meniscus, is typical. Instability or mechanical symptoms (e.g., locking or popping sensation) are uncommon. Isolated tenderness at the proximal LCL insertion or distal insertion sites may indicate an avulsion-type injury (biceps femoris or LCL), especially in the pediatric population.

It is noteworthy to discuss that the LCL is part of a complex of ligaments collectively named the posterolateral corner (PL-C). The structures in the PL-C include the LCL, popliteofibular ligament, popliteus ligament, arcuate ligament, short lateral ligament, and posterolateral joint capsule.[177] The patient with PL-C instability has sustained significant damage to the knee (cruciates, capsule, and LCL), and a Segund sign (avulsion fracture of the lateral tibia plateau) will likely be visible on an AP radiograph of the knee.[177,185]

Anterior Cruciate Ligament. The ACL is the primary restraint (85%)[180] of anterior translation of the tibia. It is supplemented by the MCL, LCL, middle third of the mediolateral capsule, popliteus corner, semimembranous corner, iliotibial band,[177] and dynamic synergistic muscle activity from the quadriceps, hamstrings, and hip external rotators and abductors (chiefly the gluteus medius). Across the life span, tear of the ACL is the most problematic of the ligamentous knee injuries. Most ACL injuries (78%)[204] are the result of a sudden cut (pivot) or deceleration injury (i.e., noncontact, intrinsic injury). The ACL also is susceptible to extrinsic blows to the posterolateral portion of the tibiofemoral joint and forced hyperextension.

The PT should take care to assess the stability of the medial and lateral knee structures if valgus or varus mechanisms were part of the mechanism of injury. Valgus stress can result in MCL injury, Salter I separation, distal femoral physeal injury, or meniscal injury.[241] Distal femoral physeal fractures are about 10 times as common as proximal tibial fractures. They can occur at any age but are seen most often in boys aged 10 to 14 years.

This age range is a time of significant growth, when the physis is weakest.[246] Joint line tenderness may be indicative of a meniscal injury.[177,241]

The PT should also assess stability of the patella to rule out a patellofemoral dislocation or subluxation. Standard knee radiographs include anteroposterior, lateral, tunnel, and sunrise (skyline) views. Varus and valgus stress views can differentiate between collateral ligament tears and physeal separations. MRI is considered the gold standard for the differential diagnosis of ACL and other associated knee injuries.[185,228,241]

In children and younger adolescents (8 to 11 years), anterior drawer laxity with the aforementioned signs and symptoms is most likely a tibial avulsion fracture.[246] Referral for imaging is paramount. Treatment (closed reduction or open reduction internal fixation) of tibial eminence avulsion fractures is dependent on the stability of the fracture. The long-term function of these patients is variable, with 74% having persistent anterior laxity, but only a small portion of these persons complain of clinical instability.[241,246]

If the physeal plates are near closure (Tanner stage IV or V), treatment of midsubstance ACL tears is similar to that of an adult, with intra-articular reconstruction using a graft of the surgeon's preference (e.g., middle third of the patellar tendon, hamstrings, allograft [cadaver]). In the child who is obviously skeletally immature, extra-articular reconstruction (iliotibial band tenodesis) may be attempted. This procedure may reduce the pivot shifting phenomenon but does not normalize the anterior translation, and long-term results are poor. Most observers advocate protective bracing and strict modification of activity (no pivoting, cutting, or impact sports) to prevent secondary instability, meniscus, or AC injury until the child is physically mature enough to have a more definitive intra-articular reconstruction. Nonsurgical treatment of ACL tears in the young population is unsuccessful.[241] The failure rate of rehabilitation and bracing is almost 100% if the patient returns to pivoting sports. The incidence of meniscal tears increases with chronic instability.[187,204]

Posterior Cruciate Ligament. The posterior cruciate ligament (PCL) functions as the knee's central axis of rotation, assists in the screw home mechanism of the knee, and acts as a secondary restraint of valgus and varus rotation (rotary stabilizer).[177] The reported incidence of PCL damage is between 3% and 44% of acute knee injuries, depending on the clinical setting.[122] Common mechanisms of PCL injury include a direct blow on the tibial tuberosity (i.e., a motor vehicle dashboard injury [45% of injuries]), direct blow because of sports trauma or a fall onto a flexed knee with the ankle plantar-flexed (40% of injuries),[122] hyperextension, and a combination of rotation and lateral force directed at the medial side of the knee.[180]

PCL injuries have attracted far less attention than ACL injuries because they occur less often and create much less functional disability. Persons with PCL instability report vague symptoms such as unsteadiness or insecurity of the knee and usually do not have incapacitating pain. Isolated grades I and II sprains are best managed conservatively, whereas surgical reconstruction is recommended when grade III PCL tears are combined with other ligamentous or soft tissue injury.[122] Once athletes have regained full ROM and 90% of the strength of the contralateral limb, they generally return to sport and suffer little or no functional loss.[122] Undiagnosed and untreated isolated PCL injuries may result in disability years later. Up to 80% to 90% report patellofemoral pain, and 67% of all subjects had grades II to IV cartilage lesions, with most found at the medial femoral condyle (49.7%) or patella (33.1%).[122]

Upper Quarter Musculoskeletal Injuries

A comprehensive list of common upper quarter MS injuries is presented in Table 16-18 and Figure 16-14 (elbow). A fall onto an outstretched hand (FOOSH) is the most common mechanism of upper quarter traumatic injury. Depending on the angle and speed of impact (compression load), a variety of upper quarter injuries are possible (e.g., fractures, dislocations, sprains, strains, contusions). Forceful traction (tensile) or rotational (shear) loads to the extremities typically will result in soft tissue damage (e.g., brachial plexus stretch, muscle strain, ligament sprain, GH subluxation or dislocation, radial head dislocation [nursemaid's elbow]).

STERNOCLAVICULAR JOINT SPRAIN. Traumatic posterior dislocation of the sternoclavicular (SC) joint is rare but constitutes a medical emergency. Complications include respiratory distress, venous congestion or arterial insufficiency, brachial plexus injury, and myocardial conduction abnormalities.

ACROMIOCLAVICULAR SEPARATION (SPRAIN). Acromioclavicular (AC) separation involves damage to the AC ligament and the two divisions of the coracoclavicular (CC) ligament—the trapezoid ligament (lateral portion of the CC ligament) and the more medial conoid ligament. AC sprains (separation) are graded via

bilateral AP radiographic views of the AC joint, with and without weights in the upper extremities[185]:
- Grade I (mild sprain): Minimal widening of the AC joint space with CC distance within normal limits
- Grade II (moderate sprain): Widening of the AC joint space to 1.0 to 1.5 cm with a 25% to 50% increase in the CC distance
- Grade III (severe sprain): Widening of the AC joint space 1.5 cm or more, with a 50% or more increase in the CC distance

With a grade III sprain, the AC joint is dislocated, and the clavicle is displaced superiorly.

Acute management of AC sprains consists of protection from further injury with a sling, ice, and pain medication. In the milder cases (grades I and II), the shoulder becomes relatively pain- free within 3 weeks, or by the end of the proliferation phase of healing.[29,34,55] If there is little danger of making the condition worse, activity can be determined by the symptoms. Grade III AC separation usually is treated conservatively, except in those patients who are unwilling to accept cosmetic deformity or who continue to have pain and dysfunction despite adequate conservative rehabilitation.

GLENOHUMERAL INJURIES. GH or shoulder joint problems are common in the adolescent population (see Figure 16-9). The GH joint is an inherently unstable joint and exhibits the greatest amount of motion of any joint in the body. From 90% to 97% of all shoulder dislocations are anterior. The primary mechanism of anterior dislocation is forceful shoulder external rotation and abduction via traumatic collision or a FOOSH mechanism. Posterior dislocations of the GH joint are rare (3% to 10%) and usually are the result of a posteriorly directed force through a flexed humerus.

Relocation can be spontaneous or can require emergency department care. The PT should rule out axillary nerve damage, which fortunately is rare, by sensory testing of the lateral shoulder (dermatome) and resisted testing (myotome) of the shoulder abductors (deltoid). Routine radiographs (AP with internal rotation; AP with lateral rotation) should be taken to rule out glenoid chip fractures, Hill-Sachs lesion, damage to the acromioclavicular arch, or acute supraspinatus rupture (may require contrast to be visualized). Specialty views, including the axillary and oblique views, are useful for shoulder dislocations, and the tangential view visualizes the bicipital groove.[185] An MRI will rule out associated injuries to the glenoid labrum. Surgical stabilization (e.g., Bankart repair, with or without capsular shift) often is indicated for the management of recurrent dislocation.[34]

Treatment of acute anterior dislocation consists of 1 to 2 weeks of GH immobilization with shoulder girdle and distal joint mobility exercises. Surgical repair of Bankart lesions is often required. Treatment of posterior GH dislocation is controversial, with surgical and nonoperative methods being reported. Recurrence of GH dislocation among young athletes is high and necessitates aggressive physical therapy. [34,94,271]

ELBOW, WRIST, AND HAND INJURIES. Figure 16-14 and Table 16-18 present the differential diagnoses that should be considered when the patient has areas of pain, swelling, tenderness, deformity, or loss of function in the distal UE. Persistent symptoms or a history of trauma make radiographic evaluation imperative. Referral to an orthopedic specialist (physician), occupational

TABLE 16-18

Common Upper Extremity Injuries in the Adolescent[*]

| General Category | Specific Entity | | |
	Shoulder	Elbow	Wrist and Hand
Instability	SC joint instability AC joint instability GH dislocation, subluxation GH unidirectional, bidirectional, and multidirectional instability (MDI) Labral tears	Radial head subluxation, dislocation Ulnar collateral ligament tear	Triangular fibrocartilage complex (TFCC) Collateral ligaments of the proximal interphalangeal (PIP) and distal interphalangeal (DIP) joints Ulnar collateral ligaments of thumb Dislocations of fingers and thumb
Impingement and/or nerve injuries	Rotator cuff tendinitis Biceps tendinitis Subacromial bursitis Impingement, primary or secondary, caused by MDI Brachial plexus injury (BPI)	Cubital tunnel syndrome (ulnar nerve) Pronator teres syndrome (median nerve) Ligament of Struthers (median nerve) Radial tunnel syndrome—arcade of Frohse in supinator (posterior interosseous branch of radial nerve)	Carpal tunnel syndrome (median nerve) De Quervain's tenosynovitis Guyon tunnel syndrome (ulnar nerve) Gymnast wrist
Fractures	Clavicle (described by location; including physeal fracture) Humerus—proximal shaft, neck, or avulsion fracture of tuberosity Scapula—rare; glenoid labrum rim fracture associated with traumatic GH dislocation	Distal fractures of humerus (supracondylar, transcondylar, intercondylar, condylar, articular, epicondylar classifications) Olecranon fractures (extra-articular and intra-articular groups) Radial head (Mason classification types I-IV) Radial and ulnar shaft (Monteggia's, Galeazzi's, and Colles' fractures) Osteochondritis dissecans (OCD) of elbow Panner's disease	Distal radius, ulna (Colles' fracture) Scaphoid (vulnerable blood supply) Hook of the hamate Metacarpal fractures (head, neck, shaft, base) Bennett's fracture—intra-articular avulsion fracture and subluxation of base of first metacarpal Rolando's fracture—comminuted fracture of base of first metacarpal Phalangeal fractures (stable, unstable, intra-articular) Mallet finger (avulsion of extensor tendon of distal phalanx) Jersey finger (rupture of flexor digitorum profundus; ring finger most often)
Soft tissue injuries (overuse)	Contusion (watch for complication of myositis ossificans in biceps brachii) Muscle strain Brachial plexus injuries Peripheral nerve injuries Delayed-onset muscle soreness (DOMS)	Tennis elbow (lateral epicondylitis) Golfer's elbow (medial epicondylitis) Olecranon bursitis (and/or infection)	Nail bed injuries Subungual hematoma Contusion
Referred pain	Cervical spine, elbow referral (one joint above and below joint of interest) Cardiac and pulmonary referral GI referral Gallbladder to right shoulder Spleen to left shoulder	Cervical spine, shoulder, wrist, hand referral to elbow	Cervical spine, shoulder, elbow referral to wrist, hand
Other	Thoracic outlet syndrome	Arterial injuries (Volkmann's ischemia as complication of perielbow fracture)	Swan neck deformity (PIP joint hyperextension with metacarpophalangeal [MCP] and DIP flexion caused by rupture of volar plate) Boutonnière deformity (extension of MCP and DIP and flexion of PIP caused by rupture of central tendinous slip of extensor hood) Rheumatoid arthritis

Upper extremity rehabilitation note: Proximal stability is a prerequisite for distal mobility and UE function. Full active and passive ROM and joint mobility are imperative. Joint mobilization can be useful in gating pain (grades I and II) or in stretching (grades III, IV, and V [thrust]) contributory joint hypomobility dysfunction.[272] Scapulohumeral rhythm must be restored. Suggested scapulothoracic muscles to target include serratus anterior, all fibers of the trapezius, levator scapulae, rhomboids, latissimus dorsi, and pectoralis major and minor. Rotator cuff and arm and forearm exercises also are advocated. [271,272] Closed kinetic chain (proprioceptive) exercises should be incorporated (pushups with emphasis on protracting scapula). The objective of a kinesthetic rehabilitation program is to facilitate the shoulder's performance of a complicated skill without conscious guidance.[94] Gradual return to functional activity via a variety of interval training programs is warranted for any of these UE injuries. Finally, improper technique, insufficient conditioning, and/or unsafe biomechanical practices must be addressed. Weakness, inflexibility, and poor proprioceptive control (lack of skill) in the lower quarter and/or trunk also can be contributory in sports that require repetitive overhead activity (e.g., throwing and racquet sports).

[*]Shoulder, elbow, wrist, and hand.

Adapted from references 4, 34, 177, and 185.

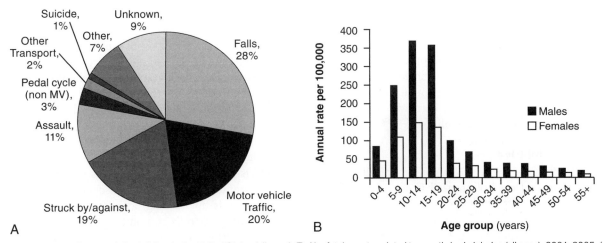

FIGURE 16-16 **A,** Causes of traumatic brain injury in the United States (all ages). **B,** Nonfatal, sports-related traumatic brain injuries (all ages), 2001-2005. (**A** from Centers for Disease Control and Prevention, National Center for Injury Prevention and Control: Traumatic brain injury in the United States [website]. http://www.cdc.gov/ncipc/tbi/TBI.htm. Accessed September 18, 2009; **B** from Centers for Disease Control and Prevention, Nonfatal Traumatic Brain Injuries [TBIs]: Injuries from Sports and Recreation Activities --- United States, 2001—2005 [website] http://www.cdc.gov/DataStatistics/2008/brainInjuries/116775_brain _injury_rev.gif. Accessed April 8, 2010.)

therapist, or certified hand therapist may be necessary to optimize the young patient's long-term UE function.

Traumatic Brain Injury

Traumatic brain injury (TBI) is a significant public health problem in the United States. An estimated 5.3 million survivors of TBI (about 2.5% of the U.S. population) currently live with neuropsychological impairments that result in disabilities affecting school, work, or social activities.[76] Of the 1.4 million in the United States who sustain a TBI each year, 1.1 million are treated and released from hospital emergency rooms, an average of 50,000 die, and 235,000 are hospitalized.[167] African Americans have the highest death rate from TBI, and African Americans and Native Americans and Alaskan Natives have the highest hospitalization rate.[167] At the turn of the century, the direct and indirect medical costs of TBI were an estimated $60 billion dollars.[110]

TBI in children and adolescents can result from multiple causes, including CNS infections, noninfectious disorders (epilepsy, hypoxia-ischemia, genetic or metabolic disorders), tumors, vascular abnormalities, and trauma (Figure 16-16A).[152] During 2001 to 2005, an estimated 207,830 patients with sports-related TBIs (concussions) were treated in the United States (see Figure 16-16B). Adolescent males 10 to 19 years of age are at greatest risk (1.5 times as likely as females) to sustain a sports-related TBI. The number of people, especially children and adolescents, with concussion who are not seen in an emergency department or who receive no care is unknown.[76]

The signs and symptoms of TBI vary and depend on the area of the brain injured: (1) cerebrum—cognitive aspects of motor control, memory, sensory awareness, speech, special senses (e.g., taste, vision, hearing); (2) cerebellum—coordinates and integrates motor behavior, balance problems, incoordination; (3) diencephalon (thalamus)—regulation of body temperature, control of emotions, information processing of the cerebrum; and (4) brainstem—control of respiratory and heart rates, peripheral blood flow control.[177] Prediction of outcomes is important to target interventions, allocate resources, provide education to family or caregivers, and begin appropriate planning for the future.[152]

Signs and symptoms of concussion, a summary of concussion classification systems, return to play guidelines, and behavioral therapies are discussed in greater detail in Chapter 7.

TBI not only affects the adolescent with the injury, but also greatly affects the family (higher rates of caregiver and sibling psychological distress). Behavioral problems such as disinhibition, irritability, restlessness, distractibility, and aggression are common after a TBI, and the persistence and severity of these problems can impair the brain-injured individual's reintegration into family, school, and community life.[242] PTs can assist families of those with a TBI by following these clinical guidelines: (1) select developmentally appropriate interventions; (2) match the intervention to the family; (3) provide advocacy; (4) provide injury education; (5) focus on family realignment; (6) appropriately adjust the child's environment; and (7) provide skills training to the family and child.[87]

Spinal Cord Injuries

Spinal cord injuries (SCIs) can be classified into traumatic (more than 80% of cases) and nontraumatic (e.g., tumor, infection) injuries. An SCI is a catastrophic event of low incidence (11,000/year) and high cost; the average lifetime expense for paraplegia is $428,000 and for quadriplegia is $1.35 million.[244] SCI predominantly (56%) occurs in young people between the ages of 16 and 30 years (most frequent age of injury, 19 years).[244] Young men (15 to 24 years) sustain 82% of all SCIs. The leading causes of SCI are motor vehicle accidents (37%), acts of violence (28%), falls (21%), sports (6% with two thirds from diving), and other (8%). Currently, about 250,000 persons in the United States are living with SCIs.[244] Patients suspected of having an SCI should be hospitalized in an intensive care unit and receive neurosurgical consultation. High-dose methylprednisolone given 1 to 2 days after injury will decrease the severity of injury (more likely to have incomplete SCI). The average length of stay for acute care is 15 days ($140,000) and 44 days for inpatient rehabilitation ($198,000).[244] Most persons with SCI (89%) are discharged home and 4.3% remain in nursing homes. Only 52% of SCI individuals are covered by private health insurance at the time of injury.[244] Physical therapy intervention is critical to the overall management of the patient with SCI and is typically performed by neurologic PTs. Rehabilitation includes psychosocial adjustment, physical skills training appropriate to the level of injury (e.g., survival skills, bed mobility, transfers, locomotion), health maintenance, and vocational adjustments. Given the fact that most SCIs involve young people, caregiver and external long-term support will need to be established.[120,264]

Peripheral Nerve Injuries

The peripheral nervous system (PNS) consists of all parts of the nervous system that are not encased in the vertebral column or skull (31 pairs of spinal nerve roots and the 12 cranial nerves).[264] Injury in the PNS will result in a lower motor neuron lesion (decreased tone, hyporeflexia, weakness), positive Tinel's (tapping) sign, and abnormal electromyographic findings. The more central the injury (closer to the cell body in the spinal cord), the worse the prognosis. The PNS can be damaged by the following: (1) disease (e.g., anterior horn cell degradation in poliomyelitis or amyotrophic lateral sclerosis [ALS], a demyelinating disease); (2) repetitive entrapment or compression syndromes (e.g., carpal tunnel syndrome, sciatica, thoracic outlet syndrome, double-crush syndromes); (3) tensile or traction injuries; and (4) trauma (e.g., lacerations, burns, or adolescent sports-related injury).

Brachial Plexus Injuries

Whereas neonatal brachial plexus injuries (BPIs) occur at a rate of 0.5 to 2/1000 live births,[120] approximately 30% to 65% of high school, college, or professional football players suffer a traumatic BPI (burner or stinger) during their careers.[156,245] Participants in other contact sports such as wrestling, rugby, and hockey also are susceptible to this neurovascular injury.[4] BPIs also can be caused by repetitive trauma (carrying a backpack that is too heavy), macrotrauma (car accidents), or incidental injuries (cradling a telephone under the neck while reaching for something). These all apply to the adolescent population.

The signs and symptoms of an acute BPI are immediate, sharp, burning or stinging pain that radiates from the clavicular region down the involved UE, associated numbness, and tingling or weakness of the arm ("flail arm") that may last for a few seconds to several minutes to months.[4,262] The musculature of the proximal upper trunk of the brachial plexus (C5 and C6) is most often involved (e.g., the deltoid, rotator cuff, biceps) and, rarely, the brachioradialis, supinator, and pronator teres (C5, C6, and C7) are involved. True neck pain should not appear with this injury; if it is present, one should suspect a cervical spine injury. Bilateral UE burning should be considered a major red flag for a significant cervical spine injury, and the victim should be treated with spinal precautions—cervical spine immobilization via a spine board.[261,262]

BPIs are classified by the degree or length of motor weakness and type of neurologic injury (neuropraxia, axonotmesis, or neurotmesis). The most common level or nerve root avulsion is C7, characterized by frank elbow extension weakness.[4] In severe cases, a concomitant Horner's syndrome, caused by disruption of the sympathetic nerve fibers, can be seen on the affected side. The classic signs are a drooping eyelid (ptosis), constricted pupil (miosis), and lack of sweat (anhidrosis) on the affected side. This situation is a medical emergency.[29]

Many professionals in sports medicine believe that a physician should examine all athletes after their first stinger, and that a complete cervical radiographic series should be taken.[4,29,261,262] The greatest concern is the presence of a Torg ratio (size of the vertebral canal relative to the vertebral body) of less than 0.80. Those with a Torg score less than 0.80 are 3 times more likely to suffer recurrent BPIs, especially if the mechanism of injury is extension or compression of the cervical spine.[261,262]

Sports-specific treatment for BPIs includes strengthening of the neck and shoulder girdle musculature, proper sports techniques (heads-up tackling, avoidance of spearing), protective equipment (neck rolls and built-up or elevated shoulder pads), and prohibition of contact if there is persistent strength loss. Return to normal sports is allowed when the athlete demonstrates normal strength and endurance in the affected shoulder.[262]

Environmental and Socioeconomic Factors of Adolescence

Dealing with adolescents has historically been a challenge for parents, caregivers, teachers, and community leaders, and the experience of health care providers can be no different. Although data suggest that 75% of adolescents and their families have a transitional experience that is trouble-free, many have described this period as one of "storm and stress."[126] The hormonal changes of puberty influence physical and sexual maturation, and emotional, mental, and social development. Beyond biologic influences, children, including teenagers, learn what they live.[126] The prevailing culture surrounding the young child and adolescent can lead to a wide range of attitudes, beliefs, and behaviors. Relevant environmental, social, and cultural factors must be considered by the health care professional (see Figure 16-3A).[251]

Environmental quality (e.g., exposure to ozone pollution and tobacco smoke, unsafe living conditions), geographic location, socioeconomic variables (e.g., race, ethnicity, family composition, income, access to education and health care), and contextual factors (i.e., family, school, peer group influences) are key determinants of adolescent behavior.[216,248] Relevant psychological variables include the adolescent's self-esteem, gender-role orientation, sense of mastery and control, and level of anxiety versus happiness and life satisfaction.[104,116,248,251,255] In early adolescence, the trend toward separation from family with increasing involvement in peer activities accelerates.[163] All these factors have the potential to affect overall health and have been found to correlate to physical dysfunction, disease, and illness.[251]

In today's society, adolescence is a prolonged developmental stage that lasts approximately 10 years, nominally between the ages of 11 and 22 years.[126] The prolonged duration of adolescence in the last century is twofold. First, there is an earlier onset of menarche and oigarche, which appears to be best explained by exposure to endocrine-disrupting chemicals, particularly the estrogen mimics and antiandrogens, and increased body fat.[105] Second, there is the notion that the legal age of 18 years equating to adulthood is somewhat arbitrary and not supported by new scientific evidence regarding brain development. These changes in the timing of puberty markers have potential adverse implications from a public health perspective.[105]

Adolescence is a period when many aspects of decision making appear adult-like, yet adolescents' decisions are inconsistent, which often leads to suboptimal or even dangerous behavior.[173] These inconsistencies manifest as risk-taking behaviors that can have long-term deleterious effects on health (e.g., poor nutrition leading to obesity, unprotected sex with risk of STDs or pregnancy, drug experimentation with risk of injury or death).

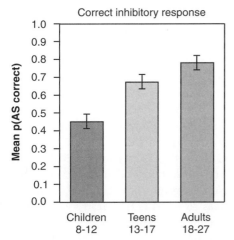

FIGURE 16-17 Development of the cognitive function of response inhibition (ages 8 to 27 years). Illustrated are the mean percentages of correct inhibitory responses (±1 SEM) for children (8-12 years), adolescents (13-17 years) and adults (18-27 years) generated while performing an antisaccade task inside an fMRI scanner. (Data from Velanova K, Wheeler ME, Luna B: Maturational changes in anterior cingulate and frontoparietal recruitment support the development of error processing and inhibitory control, *Cerebral Cortex* 18:2505-2522, 2008.)

Cognitive control is a function of the prefrontal cortex (PFC), and has two fundamental components, response inhibition and working memory. Response inhibition refers to the ability to voluntarily select a task-appropriate, goal-directed response while suppressing a more compelling but task-inappropriate response.[173] Working memory refers to the mental sketch pad that allows us to retain relevant information on-line to make a planned, goal-directed response.[173] Recent advances in functional MRI (fMRI) of the brain demonstrates that the skill of response inhibition, which is central to voluntary control of behavior, is not fully developed until early adulthood (Figure 16-17).[173]

Poverty in America: Our Children at Risk

The U.S. Census Bureau uses poverty data (income below $22,050 for a family of two adults and two children in 2009)[97] to evaluate the nation's economic status and national challenges, such as health care needs, educational needs, and employment opportunities. Children growing up in poverty are at double jeopardy because they face increased biologic risk factors such as prematurity, lead poisoning, and malnutrition, as well as increased social risk factors such as overcrowding, lower maternal education, exposure to violence, and lack of access to health care.[96,190] Key indicators of child well-being by race and ethnicity are shown in Table 16-19.

Because poor people in the United States are too diverse to be categorized along any one dimension, poverty rates are stratified by race and ethnicity, nativity, age, family composition, work experience, and geographic distribution. In 2007, the overall U.S. poverty rate was 12.5% (37.3 million). Poverty rate is stratified by race and ethnicity: Native American and Alaskan Native (25%); African American (24.5%); Hispanic-Latino (21.5%), Asian and Pacific Islanders (10.2%), and non-Hispanic white (8.2%).

TABLE 16-19

Ten Key Indicators of Child Well-Being*

Key Indicators	Total	Race or Ethnicity				
		White, Non-Hispanic	African American	Asian and Pacific Islander	Native American	Hispanic
Percentage of low birth rate (LBW) babies	8.3	7.3	13.6	8.1	7.5	7.0
Infant mortality rate (deaths per 1,000 live births)	6.7	5.6	13.3	3.6	8.2	5.5
Mortality rate (per 100,000)						
Children (1-14 years)	19	17	28	13	26	18
Teenagers (15-19 years)	64	59	85	37	95	65
Teen birth rate ((births per 1,000 females ages 15-19)	42	26	65	17	55	83
Percentage of teens who are high school dropouts (ages 16-19)	7	5	8	3	12	12
Percentage of teens not attending school and not working (ages 16-19)	8	6	13	4	15	12
Percentage of children living in families where no parent has full-time year-round employment	33	27	49	29	52	37
Percentage of children in poverty (income < $21,027 for family of two adults and two children)	18	11	35	12	33	27
Percentage of children in single-parent families	32	23	65	17	49	37

*By race and ethnicity profile, United States, 2006-2007.
Modified from Annie E. Casey Foundation: *2009 KIDS COUNT Data Book: state profiles of child well-being* (website). http://datacenter.kidscount.org/databook/2009/Default.aspx. Accessed February 25, 2010.

Ironically, foreign-born naturalized citizens have the second lowest poverty rate (9.5%), whereas noncitizens (21.3%) fare better than persons of color in this country. Poverty is most prevalent in the South (14.2%), followed by the West (12%), Northeast (11.4%), and Midwest (11.1%).[96]

The number of children living in poverty (13.3 million) continues on an upward trend, dating back to 2000. Persons younger than 18 years have the highest poverty rate (18%) of any age group in America.[96,189] Poverty rates for children by race and ethnicity are shown in Table 16-19.[189] The Children's Defense Fund (CDF) has noted that every day in America, 2483 babies are born into poverty, 2145 are born without health insurance, 1154 babies are born to teen mothers, and 928 babies are born at a low birth weight.[83]

Children (22.3 million) living in single-parent households have an overall poverty rate of 32%, which is 5.3 times the rate of their counterparts in married couple families (6%). Poverty rates for children living in single-parent households are shown in Table 16-19.[189] For children younger than 18 years living in a female-headed household and no male present, the rate of poverty is an astonishing 43%. Only one third of female-headed households reported receiving child support or alimony payments in 2006.[30]

Homelessness in America: Lost Educational Opportunities

Homeless families compromise roughly 34% of the total homeless population. Among industrialized nations, the United States has the largest number of homeless woman and children.[259] One in 50 children (over 1.5 million) experience homelessness in America each year. Homeless children face a barrage of stressful and traumatic experiences that have profound effects on their development and ability to learn.[260]

Homeless children have poor educational role models and insufficient access to educational, technologic, and health care opportunities.[149] Learning disabilities are twice as prevalent and, overall, these children are 4 times more likely to show delayed development.[260] Homeless children transfer among schools at 16 times the rate of the typical U.S. child. They are more likely than nonhomeless children to repeat a grade and to be placed in special education classes.[149]

Homeless children are sick 4 times more often than other children. They are 5 times more likely to have gastrointestinal problems, 4 times more likely to have respiratory infections or asthma, twice as likely to have ear infections, and 3 times more likely to experience emotional and behavior problems.[260] Despite going hungry at a rate twice that of their peers, they also have high rates of obesity because of poor nutrition.[260]

Furthermore, observers estimate that 20% to 25% of the single-adult homeless population suffers from some form of severe and persistent mental illness,[149] and that 50% of these have a co-occurring substance abuse disorder.[260] This means that homeless children in the United States not only confront a lack of food, shelter, clothing, and educational opportunities, but up to one in four persons that they meet on the streets has a mental disorder. Violence also plays a role in their lives, with almost 25% having witnessed acts of violence in their families. By age 12, 83% have been exposed to at least one serious violent event.[260]

Child Maltreatment and Neglect

The Children's Defense Fund has estimated that each day in the United States, 2421 children are confirmed as abused or neglected.[83] In 2007, state and local child protective services (CPS) investigated 3.2 million reports of children being abused or neglected (about 12 cases/1,000 children). These troubling numbers do not include potentially thousands of unreported cases. Types of child abuse included neglect (59%), physical abuse (11%), sexual abuse (8%), emotional abuse (4%), and other child maltreatment (18%). Victimization rates vary by race, with children of color being most significantly affected (per 1,000 children): African Americans (16.7), Native American and Alaskan Natives (14.2), and multiracial children (14.0). Overall, girls (52%) are at slightly higher risk than boys (48%).[266]

CPS reported that rates of maltreatment also vary by age (per 1000 children): 0 to 1year (21.9); 1 year (13.0); 2 years (12.6); 3 years (11.9), 4 to 7 years (11.5); 8 to 11 years (9.4), 12 to 15 years (8.7) and 16- to 17 years (5.4). In 2007, 1760 children (2.35/100,000) died from abuse of neglect. Adolescents represented 7% of all deaths (12 to 15 years [5%] and 16 to 17 years [2%]), while children younger than 4 years accounted for 76% of all deaths. Non-Hispanic white children accounted for 41% of deaths, whereas 26% and 17% of deaths were African American and Hispanic children, respectively.[62]

Observers estimate that one in every four children younger than 18 years in the United States is exposed to alcohol abuse or alcohol dependence in the family.[121] Substance abuse by the parent or caregiver is a factor in at least 70% of all reported cases of child maltreatment.[266] Adults with substance abuse disorders are 2.7 times more likely to report abusive behavior and 4.2 times more likely to report neglectful behavior toward their children. Maltreated children are more likely to suffer in all domains of wellness (physical, intellectual, social, emotional) and are at greater risk of developing substance abuse problems themselves.[266]

Given these facts, the health care provider working with adolescents must be vigilant for signs of injury resulting from neglect or physical, sexual, or emotional abuse. The PT should suspect physical abuse in the following situations:

- The patient has unexplained injuries that seem inconsistent with his or her story.
- The patient conceals injuries and appears embarrassed by them.
- The patient has delayed seeking medical care.
- The patient has a history of repeated injuries or accidents.
- A caregiver or person close to the patient has a history of substance abuse.[255]

The intimate physical signs that may indicate sexual abuse in children and adolescents (e.g., torn, stained, or bloody underclothing; pain or itching in the genital area; bruises or bleeding in external genitalia, vaginal, or anal regions; STD or pregnancy) are not typically within the domain of the physical examination by the PT. Any child with a concerning history or physical signs should be referred to a sexual abuse expert for a complete history and sexual abuse examination.[255]

FOSTER CARE. As of 2005, there were about 12 million alumni of foster care in the United States. Annually, about 500,000 children will spend all or part of the year in government-run foster care. Children are placed temporarily (average length of stay, 28.6 months) because of parental history of child abuse and neglect, domestic violence, substance abuse, or criminal offenses. The average age is 10 years and almost half (46%) are adolescents, with 28% aged 11 to 15 years and 18% aged 16 to 18 years. The male-to-female distribution into foster care is almost equal (52:48). Although child abuse and neglect occur at about the same rate in all racial and ethnic groups, there are more children of color in foster care than in the general U.S. population. By race and ethnicity, the foster care population versus general population statistics are as follows: African American (32% versus 15%); non-Hispanic white (41% versus 61%); Hispanic (18% versus 17%); Native American and Alaskan Native (2% versus 1%); and Asian–Pacific Islander (1% versus 3%). Of the young people leaving the system, 54% were reunited with their birth parents or primary caregivers.[111]

Each year, about 20,000 teens "age out" of the U.S. foster system. Without a lifelong connection to a caring adult, these older youth are often left vulnerable to a host of adverse situations. Just over half (54%) earn a high school diploma compared with the national average of 86.5%, and only 2% obtain a bachelor's degree or higher. Of these teens and young adults, 84% become a parent, over half (51%) are unemployed, and 30% are homeless, have no health insurance, or are receiving public assistance.[111]

LATCHKEY KIDS. The 2002 U.S. Census Bureau report noted that 5.8 million (15%) of all children between the ages of 5 and 14 years living with a mother care for themselves an average of 6.3 hours/week and 65% of those children spend between 2 and 9 hours home alone.[153] Comparatively, teenagers older than14 years spend increasingly more time alone or with peers (i.e. without adult supervision).

The effects of being a latchkey child differ with age. Although youngsters who are allowed to leave the house without an adult are more active and enjoy a richer social life than those who are constantly supervised, children who are unsupervised are also at risk of injury if the environments in which they wander alone are unsafe. Unsupervised youngsters are most at risk after school hours (3 to 8 PM).[153] Children younger than 10 years frequently report loneliness, boredom, and fear. In the early teens, there is a greater susceptibility to peer pressure, potentially resulting in alcohol abuse, smoking, and inappropriate sexual activity.[169]

Some communities offer services (e.g., after school programs, community, or police programs) to check in on latchkey kids. In the new millennium, cellular phones have provided a way for parents and caregivers to maintain contact with their children. For the past several decades, the *Children and Youth Services Review* has provided a forum for the critical analysis and assessment of social service programs designed to serve young people. The *Review* publishes full-length articles, current research and policy notes, and book reviews, and provides in-depth coverage on a variety of topics (child welfare, foster care, adoptions, child abuse and neglect, income support, mental health services, and social policy). It is available to health care providers at http://www.childwelfare.com/Kids/cysr.htm.

Crime: Adolescents as Victim, Perpetrator, or Both?

Vulnerability to violent crime (e.g., homicide, rape, sexual assault, robbery, aggravated assault) varies across the age spectrum. The victimization rate increases throughout the teenage years, crests at around age 20, and then steadily decreases. This pattern, with some exceptions, holds across all race, gender, and ethnic groups (Figure 16-18A).[211] U.S. adolescents and young adults (12 to 24 years) make up 35% of all murder victims and almost 50% of all victims of violent crime.[211] Adolescents are most often victimized by people they know, whether at home, in the community, or at school.[99]

TEENS AS VICTIMS. Adolescent victimization has distinct differences in gender and race. Late-adolescence males (18 to 21 years) of color are more likely than females to be victims of violent crime. Males are much more likely to be victims of violence inflicted by strangers, whereas females are more likely to be hurt by someone they know (93%), with 34.2% being family members, 58.7% acquaintances, and 7% strangers.[211]

One of six U.S. women (17.6%) has been the victim of an attempted or completed rape in their lifetime (14.8% completed rape; 2.8% attempted rape). Prevalence of rape by race was Asian and Pacific Islanders (6.8%), white women (17.7%), African American women (18.8%), Native American and Alaskan Native (34.1%). About 3% of U.S. men (1 in 33) have experienced an attempted or completed rape in their lifetime. Compared with their peers, victims of sexual assault are more likely to suffer depression (3 times more likely) and PTSD (6 times), and are more likely to abuse alcohol (13 times) or drugs (26 times) and/or to contemplate suicide (4 times).[219]

Young people living in the presence of substance abuse, alcoholism, homelessness, or poverty are at greatest risk.[96,121,221] Teens struggling with chronic illness or disability,[56] intellectual handicap,[233] or sexual orientation[116] are often victimized at higher rates than other children. This victimization ranges in severity from peer and public alienation to physical isolation and culminates in violent crimes such as robbery, physical abuse and neglect, sexual abuse, and even death.[266] Sadly, teenagers are the age group least likely to report a crime.[211]

TEENS AS PERPETRATORS. Many in the United States believe that today's youth are uniquely criminal, violent, and out of control. Juveniles, along with men 40 to 44 years of age, are the key perpetrators of crime, but adolescents (10 to 19 years) are doing far better today than the supposedly cerebrally developed midlifers (35 to 54 years) who are complaining about them. The behavior of middle-aged adults has deteriorated, even amid rising wealth, as adolescent behavior generally has improved, even amid rising poverty.[179]

A generational comparison between teenagers and adults from 1970 to 2005 demonstrates the following[179]:

Behavior and Condition	Teens, 10-19 yr	Adults, 35-54 yr
Drug overdose deaths	↑8%	↑279%
Suicidal deaths	↓12%	↑29%
Serious crime	↓29%	↑106%
Imprisonment	↓58%	↑467%
Income	↓15%	↑15%
Poverty	↑21%	↓5%

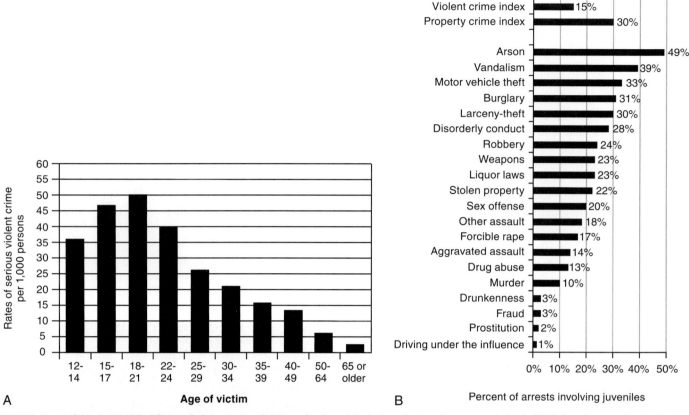

FIGURE 16-18 Crime in the United States. **A,** Age patterns of victims of serious violent crime. **B,** Juveniles as perpetrator. In 2001, juveniles were involved in about one in ten arrests for murder, one in eight arrests for a drug abuse violation, and one in three arrests for larceny-theft, burglary, or motor vehicle theft. **(A** from Perkins CA: *Age patterns of victims of serious violent crime* (website). http://www.ncjrs. gov/app/publications/abstract.aspx?ID=162031. Accessed February 26, 2010; **B** from Office of Juvenile Justice and Delinquency Prevention: *Crime in the United States 2001* (website). http://www.ncjrs.gov/html/ojjdp/201370/page2.html. Accessed March 9, 2010.)

Youth crime appears to be strongly related to socioeconomic status and not race. In U.S. regions where poverty is high, the crime rate is higher regardless of race. Nonwhites are statistically more likely to be burdened by poverty.[96] The high homicide rate among nonwhite youth is a direct result of industrial abandonment and joblessness, which forces young people into more dangerous alternatives, such as gangs.[206] Where youths, regardless of race, have the same socioeconomic status as adults, youths display murder and other crime rates lower than those of adults.[206] A health care provider is statistically more likely to care for a youth who has been a victim of a violent crime than to be a victim of a violent crime himself or herself.[211,266]

Indicators of School Crime and Safety

Schools are supposed to be safe havens for teaching and learning, free of crime and violence. Nonetheless, as of 2008, the vast majority (86%) of all schools reported at least one violent crime, theft, or other crime yearly. Any crime at school not only affects the individuals involved, but may also disrupt the educational process and affect innocent bystanders, the school itself, and/or the surrounding community.[99] The Bureau of Justice Statistics and the Institute of Educational Sciences regularly publish reports on school crime and school safety. Monitoring the indicators of crime (e.g., victimization, fights, bullying, alcohol) provides school administrators, police authorities, and legislators

with data to formulate policies for change that hopefully enhance the safety of students and staff and promote educational efforts.

Twenty-one indicators of school crime and safety have been indentified, encompassing six major categories: (1) violent deaths; (2) nonfatal student and teacher victimization; (3) school environment; (4) fights, weapons, and illegal substances; (5) fear and avoidance; and (6) discipline, safety, and security measures. In 2006 to 2007, 55.5 million students were enrolled in prekindergarten through grade 12 with 35 violent deaths (28 homicides and 8 suicides) being reported on school grounds. Among 12- to 18-year-olds, there were 1.7 million victims of nonfatal crimes at school, including 909,500 thefts and 767,000 serious crimes (rape, sexual assault, robbery, aggravated assault). The rate for serious violent crime was lower at school than away from school, but theft rates were higher. There was no measurable difference between the victimization rates for violent crime at or away from school.[99]

Twenty-three percent of students reported that gangs were present at their schools. Eight percent of students in grades 9 to 12 reported being threatened or injured by a weapon. Approximately 5% of those 12 to 18 years of age reported fear of attack or harm at school, compared with 3% away from school. Seven percent of students avoid school activities or places (cafeteria, restrooms) because of fear of attack or harm. On school grounds, 9% to 12% of students fight and 6% of students carry a weapon, whereas 3 times as many adolescents had been in a fight (36%) or carried a weapon (18%) anywhere.[99]

Ten percent of students reported hate-related words being directed at them, and 35% saw hate-related graffiti on school property. Bullying is prevalent; 32% to 38% reported verbal bullying and 4% indicated cyberbullying. Almost one quarter (22%) were offered, given, or sold drugs at school. Four percent of those in grades 9 to 12 drank or used marijuana on school property; 45% used alcohol and 20% used marijuana anywhere in the past 30 days.[99]

Disciplinary action is common, with 48% of schools reporting that they took serious disciplinary action against students, including suspension of 5 days (74%), expulsion (5%), and transfer to schools for special needs (20%). The CDF has estimated that each day in the United States, 2467 high school students drop out (lost educational potential), 18,221 public school students are suspended, and 1511 public school students are corporally punished.[83] The percentage of schools using security cameras has increased from 19% to 43% in recent years, and 66% of students were aware that cameras were being used.[99] Sadly, 7.2% of high school students self-rate their overall health as fair to poor. Having been in a physical fight, been injured in a physical fight, attempted suicide, and not gone to school because of safety concerns were significantly associated with fair or poor self-rated health after controlling for demographic characteristics and other potential confounders.[48]

Sexuality and Gender Identity

Gay, lesbian, bisexual, transgender, and questioning (GLBTQ) youth often face rejection from their families after coming out.[164] Schools (faculty and administration) often unwittingly or complicity reinforce that it is not healthy or safe to be gay, lesbian, or bisexual. Although some observers believe that peers tend to be more accepting of sexual ambiguity, research conducted in the last 20 years reports that the risk factors for suicide, self-harm, and substance abuse among GLBTQ youth have not decreased over time, not even in the most liberal parts of the nation.[192]

One in four (26%) of GLBTQ adolescents are thrown out of their homes. Forty-one percent suffer mistreatment from family, peers, or strangers, with almost half (46%) noting that family members were the perpetrators of violence. Up to 50% of gay males who leave home early turn to prostitution as a means of financial support placing them at greater higher risk for rape, assault, or infection (HIV or other STDs).[192] In 2005, the Youth Risk Behavior Survey reported that GLBTQ youth were more likely to have hurt themselves on purpose (44% versus 17%), to have seriously considered suicide (34% versus 11%) and to have made a suicide attempt in the past year (21% versus 5%).[192]

GLBTQ adolescents, like many teens, often cope with the problems that they encounter at home, school, or on the streets by using and often abusing alcohol and other drugs.[164] Sixty-eight percent of gay male adolescents reported alcohol use, with 26% using one or more times weekly. Forty-four percent reported drug use in addition to alcohol, and 8% considered themselves drug dependent. Lesbian adolescents reported high alcohol use (83%) and drug use (56%) and 11% specifically reported crack or cocaine use.[192]

Health care practitioners have an obligation to meet the health care needs of adolescents by practicing nonjudgmental acceptance and encouragement of individual social and sexual identity.[255] In conjunction with the federal government's *Healthy People 2010* project, the Gay and Lesbian Medical Association (GLMA) has published the first comprehensive document on the state of GLBTQ health. The *Healthy People 2010* Companion Document for GLBT Health is a comprehensive look at the multicultural GLBTQ community. It is written by and for health care consumers, providers, researchers, educators, government agencies, schools, clinics, advocates, and health professionals in all settings.[116]

Health Promotion and Counseling for Adolescents

An ounce of prevention is worth a pound of cure.
Benjamin Franklin (1706-1790)

Nowhere in health care is this sentiment more applicable than in the developing young person. Current medical literature is strewn with accounts of unhealthy children growing up to be unhealthy adults with multisystem health care problems.[44,205,268] Therefore, prevention strategies at a young age can improve health for many decades.

Health promotion has three fundamental components—primary, secondary, and tertiary prevention. Primary health prevention means preventing disease in a susceptible or potentially susceptible population via general health promotion and education. Secondary health prevention means reducing the duration of illness, severity of disease, and sequelae of disease via early diagnosis and prompt intervention. Tertiary health prevention means limiting the degree of disability and promoting rehabilitation and restoration of function in patients with chronic or irreversible conditions.[25] Health promotion for adolescents is not only the detection and prevention of disease, but also the promotion of well-being, which spans physical, cognitive, emotional, social, and spiritual domains.[255]

Health Promotion Topics Specific to Adolescents*

BACKPACK SAFETY GUIDELINES. A backpack and its contents should not exceed 10% to 15% of a child's body weight. Individual levels of fitness may affect this recommendation.[214] Extra weight can result in MS strain or pain in the back, shoulders, and neck. Parents and teens should look for the following features in a backpack:

- Wide, padded, and contoured shoulder straps. Avoid single-strap bags and slinging the backpack over one shoulder only.
- A padded back (contoured back a plus) to protect the vertebral spinous processes.
- A suspension bar in the backpack to distribute load more evenly.
- A padded waist belt to distribute some load to the pelvis.
- Compression straps that when tightened, compress the pack's contents to stabilize them.
- A size appropriate for the size of the child.[214]

---

*Disclaimer: This alphabetized list of adolescent health care topics is not meant to be all-inclusive or hierarchical in terms of health issues important to this age group.

Look for signs of MS strain: struggling to put on or take off the backpack, pain, red marks from straps, poor posture, and numbness and tingling in the upper extremities. These are signs that a backpack fits poorly or is overloaded.[214]

CELLULAR PHONE. Twenty-two percent of children 6 to 9 years of age, 60% of "tweens" (10 to 14 years) and 84% of teens (15 to 18 years) have a cell phone.[61] Although cell phones offer safety and convenience, the negatives can be significant (health risks, financial expense). Health risks of cell phones include cyber-bullying (psychological harassment), lack of sleep, eye strain, "digital thumb," bacteria and risk of illness, the possibility of brain tumors and low sperm count caused by electromagnetic radiation, increased risk (23x) of a motor vehicle accident[268a], and dependency; 37% of teens thought they wouldn't be able to live without a cell phone. The addictive, problematic use of cell phones has also been associated with dishonesty, low self-esteem, anxiety, and depression.[61]

Parents, caregivers, and teachers can promote the positive aspects of cell phone use by doing the following:
- Discuss the child's motivations for having a cell phone (should not be a status symbol).
- Develop a set of rules and responsibilities for a cell phone use, including rules about night use and driving abstinence.
- Consider a child-friendly cell phone for the young child ("mom-" and "dad-" only buttons).
- Teach children to only answer calls or view text messages from people they know.
- Help children save money and learn fiscal responsibility.[61]

SCREEN TIME GUIDELINES. Computers and television are an integral part of U.S. culture. Most teenagers (60%) spend on average of 20 hours/week in front of television and computer screens, a third spend almost 40 hours/week, and about 7% are exposed to more than 50 hours of screen time/week.[24] Television, computers, and the Internet can certainly have a profound effect on children's learning and development worldwide, but they similarly bring the consequences of repetitive strain. The six most common factors associated with the development of upper quadrant MS pain among children and adolescents are static postures, depression, stress, psychosomatic symptoms, gender, and age.[215]

The risk of long-term MS overuse injuries in young bodies is greater than ever. The primary care PT has an opportunity to make a difference in the general health of society, starting with its youngest television and computer-using members. The "Top 10 Ways to Monitor Kids' Computer Health" is available on the American Physical Therapy Association website (www.apta.org).[273]

SPORTS INJURY PREVENTION GUIDELINES. The AAP policy statement on "Intensive Training and Sports Specialization in Young Athletes" is a recommended reference for anyone working with highly competitive youngsters. Although intense sports competition among children raises many concerns, little scientific information is available to support or refute these risks.[16]

Health care providers must assist young athletes in avoiding the risks of early, excessive training and competition. Young athletes must obtain preparticipation physicals annually before the start of practice and competition.[95,137] Coaches should strive

for prevention, early recognition, and treatment of overuse injuries. Children should be encouraged to participate in sports at a level consistent with their abilities and interests. Pushing children beyond their limits is discouraged, as is specialization in a single sport before adolescence. Parents and health care providers should ensure that coaches know proper training techniques; signs of heat stress (see Table 16-6); biomechanics of the sport; safety equipment; and the unique physical, physiologic, and emotional characteristics of young competitors (see Box 16-6).

Given the underlying demands of adolescence for growth and development, young athletes should be monitored for adequate nutritional intake and growth. The intensely trained, specialized young athlete needs ongoing assessment of nutritional intake, with particular attention to total calories, a balanced diet, and intake of iron and calcium. Pediatric visits should focus on serial measurements of body composition, weight, and stature; cardiovascular findings (blood pressure, heart rate, and rhythm); sexual maturation; and evidence of emotional stress (psychosocial development). The pediatrician should watch for signs and symptoms of overtraining, including decline in performance, weight loss, anorexia in females and males, amenorrhea (in females), and sleep disturbances.

In 1997, the Red Cross and the U.S. Olympic Committee joined forces to develop a *Sport Safety Training Course* to teach coaches the basic first-aid skills and knowledge needed to care for athletic injuries.[27] The Red Cross also offers a full line of texts and courses on babysitting safety, water and swim safety, cardiopulmonary resuscitation (CPR), and first aid. Health care providers should be proficient and certified (depending on state practice act guidelines and employer specifications) in infant, child, and adult CPR. Competence in the use of the automated external defibrillator (AED) for cardiac arrest is now standard protocol for all health care providers.

Developing Healthy People 2020: The Road Ahead

Healthy People 2010 (see Box 16-1) recognizes the need to benefit from advances in quality of life and health, regardless of race, ethnicity, gender, geographic location, disability status, income, sexual or spiritual orientation, or educational level. Recognizing variations in patient populations is important to helping all health care professionals provide health-promoting and prevention programs.[120]

Health care professionals should view every interaction with an adolescent as an opportunity to advocate wellness (Box 16-8). The adolescent's intelligence mandates that the health care provider form a direct therapeutic alliance with the patient.[255] Caregivers, schoolteachers, coaches, and community leaders who interact with adolescents should be considered agents of change and appropriately educated by the health care team.

PHYSICAL ACTIVITY, OVERWEIGHT, AND OBESITY. Age-specific and gender-specific charts are available to assess the BMI of children and adolescents. BMI has three important categories: (1) youth below the fifth percentile, who are considered underweight; (2) children above the 95th percentile, who are considered overweight; and (3) children above the 85th percentile, who are considered at risk for being overweight.[267]

More than half of adults in the United States are estimated to be overweight or obese.[205] Between 16% and 33% of children

---

BOX 16-8

Components of a Health Supervision Visit for Adolescents 11-18 Years

DISCUSSION WITH PARENTS
- Address parent concerns
- Provide advice
- School, activities, social interactions
- Youth's behavior and habits, mental health

DISCUSSION WITH ADOLESCENT
- Social and emotional development—mental health, friends, family
- Physical development—puberty, self-concept
- Behavior and habits—nutrition, exercise, TV or computer screen time, drug, alcohol use
- Relationships and sexuality—dating, sexual activity, forced sex
- Family functioning—relations with parents and siblings
- School performance—activities, strengths

PHYSICAL EXAMINATION
- Perform a careful examination; note growth parameters, sexual maturity ratings

SCREENING TESTS
- Vision and hearing, blood pressure; consider hematocrit; assess emotional health and risk factors

IMMUNIZATIONS
- Recommended Immunization Schedule for Persons Aged 0 Through 6 Years—United States • 2010 http://www.cdc.gov/vaccines/recs/schedules/downloads/child/2010/10_0-6yrs-schedule-pr.pdf Accessed April 8, 2010[70]
- Recommended Immunization Schedule for Persons Aged 7 Through 18 Years—United States • 2010 http://www.cdc.gov/vaccines/recs/schedules/downloads/child/2010/10_7-18yrs-schedule-pr.pdf Accessed April 8, 2010[70]
- Catch-up Immunization Schedule for Persons Aged 4 Months Through 18 Years Who Start Late or Who Are More Than 1 Month Behind—United States • 2010 http://www.cdc.gov/vaccines/recs/schedules/downloads/child/2010/10_catchup-schedule-pr.pdf Accessed April 8, 2010[70]

ANTICIPATORY GUIDANCE—TEEN
Promote Healthy Habits and Behaviors
- Injury and illness prevention
- Seat belts, drunk driving, helmets, sun, weapons
- Nutrition
- Healthy meal and snacks, obesity prevention
- Oral health—dentist, brushing

Sexuality
- Confidentiality, sexual behaviors, safer sex, contraception if needed

Substance Abuse
- Prevention strategies, treatment if appropriate
- Parent-teen interaction
- Communication, rules

Social Achievement
- Activities, school, future
- Community interaction—resources, involvement

ANTICIPATORY GUIDANCE——PARENT
- Positive interactions, support, safety, limit setting, family values, modeling behaviors

From Bickley LS, Szilagyi PG: *Bates' guide to physical examination and history taking,* 10th ed, Philadelphia, 2008, Lippincott, Williams & Wilkins, p 839.

---

aged 6 to 19 years are overweight and/or obese. The proportion of adolescents from poor households who are overweight or obese is twice that of adolescents from middle-income and high-income households.[205] In modern society, declines in work-related physical activity and increases in sedentary behavior have tended to drive down the daily expenditure of energy. Conversely, energy intake is up. High-fat, energy-dense foods and large portion sizes in the fast foods industry have increased caloric intake. These changes are having widespread ill effects on health, including our children and adolescents.

Obesity in adolescence, as at any age, is difficult and discouraging to treat and is one of the most common presenting conditions in adolescent clinics.[36] Primary endocrine or metabolic disorders are uncommon; most cases are caused by the habit of eating more than is needed to meet the normal demands of the basal metabolic rate and activity. Secondary medical problems (e.g., low back pain, knee pain, HTN, diabetes) seen in overweight and obese adults also are found in pediatric patients. The obese adolescent often has a poor self-image and becomes more sedentary and socially withdrawn.[36]

Treatment should include the following: (1) education in proper nutrition (for the adolescent, caregivers, and food providers); (2) behavior modification, including reduction and control of caloric intake (i.e., permanent changes in eating habits); and (3) increased physical activity (aerobic activities coupled with strength training to burn calories and increase lean body mass).[7,32,36,183] Physical activity counseling by primary care providers is a key objective of the *Healthy People 2010* project. PTs have the requisite knowledge and expertise to address issues related to physical inactivity (Box 16-9). Activities that improve muscular strength, endurance, flexibility, and fitness (e.g., workplace, community, and school physical education programs) all have the potential to reduce the prevalence of obesity, coronary heart disease, and other chronic conditions.

TOBACCO USE. The greatest preventable cause of disease and mortality in the United States is cigarette smoking.[21,154,274] It is the strongest modifiable risk factor for coronary artery disease and numerous cancers, and significantly complicates the ramifications of other diseases (e.g., diabetes, low back pain, osteoporosis).[120] Preventing a teen from smoking today will pay off in the long run. According to research, if teens have not started smoking by the age of 20, chances are that they never will.[98] Prevention of tobacco use in adolescents is paramount, considering the serious health consequences of addiction, not to mention its monumental financial burden on the health care system.

SUBSTANCE ABUSE. Substance abuse is common among people of every age, social, economic, professional, and educational status. In recent years, health and human services organizations have emphasized the importance of developing adult-to-child mentoring programs to help children make better choices about drugs, alcohol, and tobacco. "Talk to your Kids" television advertisements[82] and Drug Abuse Resistance Education (DARE)[93] programs are two of these beacons of public information for children. Given the sheer scope of the substance abuse problems, health care workers should take advantage of any opportunity to deter a child from harmful addictions.

According to the National Institute on Drug Abuse (NIDA), successful drug abuse prevention programs embrace the

---

BOX 16-9

Health Promotion and Physical Activity: Strategies to Create Successful Exercise Programs and Biopsychosocial Benefits of Regular Activity and Exercise

STRATEGIES TO CREATE SUCCESSFUL EXERCISE PROGRAMS

- Ask the patient if he or she is currently exercising regularly (or was before illness or injury). Briefly describe the benefits that the person could achieve from such a program.
- Emphasize exercise benefits of improving health rather than achieving weight loss.
- Allow the person to respond to the recommendation for an exercise program. Encourage the person to verbalize any thoughts or reactions to your suggestions.
- Determine whether the person believes that an exercise program will benefit him or her personally. Help the individual set personal goals for exercise.
- Elicit from the patient a statement accepting an exercise program.
- Be aware of any cultural or philosophical beliefs the person may have about exercise.
- If resistance to the idea of an exercise program is encountered, give the person an opportunity to list potential barriers to exercise. Ask the person to suggest ways to overcome potential barriers.
- Whenever possible, provide a written description (preferably just pictures because of the potential of undisclosed illiteracy) of the proposed exercise program. Review progress and reward attempts, successes, and progression of the exercise program.
- Make it fun to foster a lifestyle approach characterized by long-term adherence.

BIOPSYCHOSOCIAL BENEFITS OF REGULAR ACTIVITY AND EXERCISE

- Reduces or prevents functional declines associated with aging.
- Maintains or improves cardiovascular function; improves submaximal exercise performance; reduces risk for high blood pressure; decreases myocardial oxygen demand.
- Aids in weight loss and weight control.
- Improves function of hormonal, metabolic, neurologic, respiratory, and hemodynamic systems.
- Alters carbohydrate-lipid metabolism, resulting in favorable increase in high-density lipoproteins.
- Strength training helps maintain muscle mass and strength, especially in the aging group.
- Reduces age-related bone loss; reduction in risk for osteoporosis.
- Improves flexibility, postural stability, and balance; reduces risk of falling and associated injuries.
- Psychological benefits (e.g., preserves cognitive function, alleviates symptoms/behavior of depression, improves self-awareness, promotes sense of well-being).
- Reduces disease risk factors.
- Improves functional capacity.
- Improves immune function (excessive exercise can inhibit immune function).
- Reduces age-related insulin resistance.
- Reduces incidence of some cancers (e.g., colon, breast).
- Contributes to social integration.
- Improves sleep pattern.

From Goodman CC, Fuller KS: *Pathology: implications for the physical therapist*, 3rd ed, Philadelphia, 2009, WB Saunders, pp 29-30.

BOX 16-10

The Hard Facts About Sexual Activity and Teen Pregnancy

- Sex is rare among very young teens, but becomes more common in the later teenage years.
- Six in10 teens who had sex say they wish they had waited.

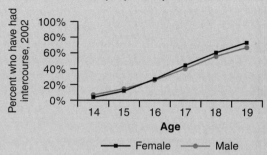

- A sexually active teen who does not use contraceptives has a 90% chance of becoming pregnant within a year.
- Each year, almost 750,000 teens aged 15 to 19 years of age become pregnant, with 82% of these pregnancies being unplanned.
- One third of girls in the United States becomes pregnant at least once by the age of 20.
- Almost two thirds (57%) of pregnancies are carried to term (birth), whereas 29% end in abortion and 14% end in miscarriage.
- Each year about 175 young women (15 to 19 years) die because of complications of childbirth.
- Teen childbearing in the United States costs taxpayers (federal, state, and local) at least $9.1 billion. Most of the costs of teen childbearing are associated with negative consequences for the children of teen mothers, including increased costs for health care, foster care, and incarceration (deadbeat dads and mothers convicted of child abuse).

Data from Guttmacher Institute: *Facts on U.S. teens' sexual and reproductive health, 2006* (website). http://www.guttmacher.org/pubs/fb_ATSRH.html. Accessed August 14, 2009.

---

first year and another 10 to 15 booster sessions), and (9) retain core elements of the effective intervention design (implementation fidelity), training, and monitoring, and undergo periodic evaluation.[195]

RESPONSIBLE SEXUAL BEHAVIOR. Responsible sexual behavior education for adolescents spans a wide continuum of topics: (1) abstinence as an option, (2) education in safe sex practices (condom use), (3) contraceptive education and use, (4) education on STDs, (5) prevention of unwanted pregnancy, and (6) identification and prevention of sexual abuse.[72,75] The disease ramifications of teenage promiscuity were previously discussed (see earlier). The hard facts about teen pregnancy (Box 16-10) are another weighty discussion for the health care provider to have with the adolescent. U.S. health care professionals reluctant to address sexual health issues with adolescents may be considered negligent in providing comprehensive health care. However, these professionals are caught between the adolescent's individual patient rights for confidentiality and the rights of caregivers and parents to know about the health of the minors in their care.

The 15- to 19-year-old teen pregnancy rate (72.2/1000) has declined in recent decades, but the United States still holds the dubious honor of the highest teen birth rate (42 births/1000 females) among industrialized nations.[256] Teen birth rates vary by race and ethnicity (per 1000): Hispanic (81.7), non-Hispanic

---

following nine criteria: (1) target the most critical age groups, (2) provide multiple years of intervention, (3) include a well-tested, standardized intervention with detailed lesson plans and student materials, (4) teach drug-resistance skills through interactive methods, (5) foster positive social bonding to the school and community, (6) contain appropriate content (e.g., teach social competence and drug resistance skills that are culturally and developmentally appropriate), (7) promote positive peer influence and antidrug social norms, (8) emphasize skills training teaching methods and include enough sessions (10 to 15 in the

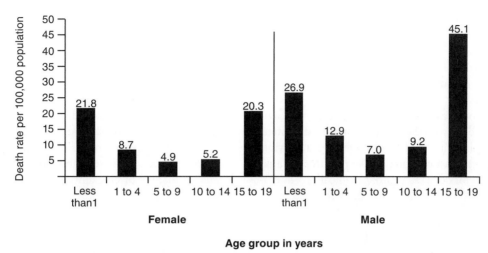

FIGURE 16-19 Unintentional injury death rates among children 0 to 19 years, by gender and age group, United States, 2000-2005. (Data from Centers for Disease Control and Prevention: *Unintentional injury deaths among children 0 to 19 Years, United States, 2000-2005* (website). http://www.amptoons.com/blog/ wp-content/ uploads/2009/01/accidental_deaths_age_sex1.png. Accessed March 9, 2010)

African American (64.3), Native Americans (59), non-Hispanic white (27.3), and Asian and Pacific Islanders (17.3). The decline in teen pregnancy rate is to the result of more consistent contraceptive use and a higher proportion of teens choosing to delay sexual activity.[231]

The American Medical Association believes that reducing the nation's rate of teen pregnancy is one of the best strategic means of improving overall child well-being in America. Teen pregnancy is closely linked to a host of other critical social issues—poverty and income, overall child well-being, out-of-wedlock births, responsible fatherhood, health issues, education, child welfare, and other risky behaviors.[258] Adolescent mothers frequently lack access to prenatal and postpartum care, increasing the risk for LBW and high infant mortality rates. Children born from unplanned pregnancies also face a range of developmental risks, such as poorer physical and mental health, lower cognitive scores, poverty, poorer school attendance records, high school dropout rate, lower college aspirations and, as adults, higher divorce rates. Simply put, if more children in this country were born to parents who were ready and able to care for them, we would see a significant reduction in a host of social problems afflicting children in the United States, from school failure and crime to child abuse and neglect.[258]

Homophobia, religious restrictions, and cultural attitudes about gender roles and condoms continue to hamper efforts to improve education about contraceptives and encourage consistent condom use in this country.[150] Health care providers and researchers agree that youth must be educated about drug use behaviors and safe sex practices for both same-gender and opposite-gender relationships.[6] In a review of 35 programs worldwide, the WHO has found that programs that teach only abstinence are less effective than programs that promote the delay of first sexual intercourse and teach about safer sex practices (contraception and condom use).[2] Peer-based interventions can reduce risk-associated behavior, increase condom acquisition and use, and reduce unprotected sexual intercourse, frequency of sexual intercourse, and the number of sexual partners.[150] Family factors, including a teens' perception of receiving warmth, love, and caring from

parents and parental disapproval of teen sexual activity, are protective in delaying initiation of sexual intercourse.[221]

MENTAL HEALTH. The future of our country, indeed of the world, depends on the mental health and strength of its youth. Research shows that half of all lifetime cases of mental illness begin by age 14.[160] Scientists are discovering that changes in the body leading to mental illness may start much earlier, before any symptoms appear.[196] What is most worrisome is that WHO predicts that by the year 2020, childhood neuropsychiatric disorders will rise by more than 50% internationally, to become one of the five most common causes of morbidity, mortality, and disability among the world's youth.[196]

The inclusion of mental health in the *Healthy People 2010* represents a shift in the federal government's concern for mental health as compared with previous decades. The Child and Adolescent Mental Health division of the National Institutes of Mental Health (NIMH) has made research on diagnosis, early intervention, and treatment of children an absolute priority.[196] Unfortunately, our society has insufficient resources to address this issue adequately, and fewer than one in five children who are mentally ill receive treatment. There is politically heated debate about the expense and proper roles of medications and psychotherapies for children at risk and children already suffering from mental illness. However, one thing is clear. Children who go untreated suffer, cannot learn, cannot form healthy relationships with peers and family, and are at increased risk of unemployment, homelessness, trouble with the law, and imprisonment.[234,266]

INJURY AND VIOLENCE.

Unintentional Injury. Unintentional injury accounts for about 45.1% of male and 20.3% of female adolescent deaths in those 15 to 19 years of age (Figure 16-19). Males are 2.2 times more likely to die of an unintentional injury and 5 times more likely to die of homicide or suicide. The gender difference is most pronounced in drowning; males are 10.6 times more likely to die than females of the same age. Alcohol abuse and risk-taking behaviors play a significant role in adolescent deaths and injuries. Adolescents are far less likely to use seat belts than any other age group.[75]

The Youth Risk Behavior Surveillance System (YRBSS) monitors the top six health risk behaviors among youth and young adults: unintentional injury and violence; tobacco use; alcohol and other drug use; sexual behaviors that contribute to unintended pregnancies and STDs, including HIV infection; unhealthy dietary behaviors and physical inactivity The YRBSS includes a national school-based survey conducted by the CDC and state, territorial, tribal, and local surveys conducted by state, territorial, and local education and health agencies and tribal governments. This is the most comprehensive resource for analyzing health risk behaviors of U.S. youth (the most recent edition is from 2008; the 2009 YRBSS results will be released in the summer 2010).[75]

ENVIRONMENTAL QUALITY. Allergic diseases affect more than 50 million people in the United States[3] and result in more than 20 million visits to physicians' offices annually.[120] The number of pediatric patients (those younger than 18 years of age) visiting physician offices for respiratory problems is dramatically rising.[205] Environmental quality is a key determinant of airway disease.[193]

Environmental quality encompasses six major areas in the *Healthy People 2010* project: (1) outdoor air quality (including exposure to ozone pollution); (2) water quality; (3) toxins and wastes; (4) healthy homes and healthy communities, including indoor air quality (i.e., exposure to second-hand smoke and allergens); (5) infrastructure and surveillance; and (6) global environmental health. Recommendations of the National Asthma Education and Prevention Program for addressing environmental allergens and irritants include the following:

- *Air pollution*: Consider limiting outdoor activities when levels of air pollution are high.
- *Animal dander*: Permanently remove pets from the house or at least keep pets away from the bedroom, carpeted areas, and upholstered furniture.
- *Cockroaches*: Use chemical measures and remove sources of food and water.
- *Dust mites*: Encase mattresses and pillows in vinyl or semipermeable covers; wash all bedding every 1 to 2 weeks in hot water of at least 54.4° C (130° F); other desirable measures include reducing indoor humidity to less than 50%, removing carpet from the bedroom and carpet over concrete, and avoid lying or sleeping on upholstered furniture.
- *Indoor mold*: Eliminate water leaks and damp areas associated with mold growth; consider reducing indoor humidity to less than 50%.
- *Pollens and outdoor molds*: Avoid outdoor activities when pollen and spore counts are high.
- *Tobacco*: Avoid exposure to active and passive tobacco smoke.[193]

IMMUNIZATION. The AAP has numerous policy statements regarding immunization on their website. [5,9-14,70] The recommended schedule for immunization of children and adolescents was revised and published in 2009.[14,70] There are three schedules: (1) children 0 to 6 years; (2) children 7 to 18 years; and (3) a catch-up immunization schedule for children and adolescents who start late or fall behind.[70] These schedules reflect current recommendations for the use of vaccines licensed by the FDA and include the following: (1) influenza vaccine for children 6 months through 18 years of age[11]; (2) oral rotavirus

vaccine; and (3) immunization against childhood diseases (e.g., diphtheria, tetanus, pertussis,[12] poliomyelitis, measles, mumps, rubella) and hepatitis B. These diseases are associated with birth defects, paralysis, brain damage, hearing loss, and liver cancer.

If a second dose of measles, mumps, and rubella (MMR) has not been given, it should be administered during adolescence. Adolescent females should be advised to avoid becoming pregnant within 3 months of vaccination. Varicella vaccine is recommended for susceptible adolescents—those who lack a reliable history of chickenpox or who have not been previously immunized.[13] Booster doses of tetanus and diphtheria (Td) are recommended at 10-year intervals. All adolescents should be immunized against hepatitis B virus. Adolescents (and adults) who plan to travel or work in a country with a high or intermediate rate of endemic hepatitis A or who live in a community with a high rate of hepatitis A are among those for whom vaccine should be considered. All adolescents should be immunized against HBV. Those at high risk of influenza and anyone who requests an immunization should receive an annual flu shot.[11] H1N1 ("swine flu") vaccinations are also recommended for all persons, especially children 6 months to 24 years, although the long-term success of these new vaccinations is still unknown.[5]

The Advisory Committee on Immunization Practices (ACIP) and AAP recommend informing parents of college students about meningococcal disease and its vaccine, and administering the vaccine if requested.[10] The American College Health Association (ACHA) recommends *Neisseria* meningitidis vaccine for all college students.[64] Most insurers currently will reimburse for routine meningococcal immunization for college freshmen. Some college health services offer meningococcal immunization at no cost or reduced cost for entering freshman. Healthy adolescents do not require pneumococcal immunization until age 65.

ACCESS TO HEALTH CARE. Access to health care is the last of the ten leading health care indicators of the *Healthy People 2010* project. Education, poverty, race, ethnicity, unemployment, and rising health care insurance premiums all adversely affect access to health care.[96] In the new millennium, the tragedy of September 11, 2001, international war, the dip in the economy, unemployment, and crises in federal and state budgets have reduced health care coverage for all age groups. While health care reform is on the horizon, presently, some 47 million people (15.5%) are without health insurance coverage in the United States. Among children, the likelihood of health care coverage varies by poverty status, age, and race. In 2006, 13.8% of adolescents 13 through 18 years of age and 28.4% of older adolescents aged 19 through 21 were uninsured. Adolescents at greatest risk of being uninsured are older, are Hispanic, and have low household income.[7]

Given these facts, the *Healthy People 2010* project has identified four key objectives in the delivery of health care to improve access to comprehensive, high-quality health care services:

- *Primary care objective*: Increase the proportion of people who have a specific source of ongoing care.
- *Clinical preventive care objective*: Increase the proportion of people with health insurance.

- *Emergency services objective*: Reduce the proportion of people who delay or have difficulty in getting emergency medical care (because delayed care typically incurs increased costs in the long run).
- *Long-term care and rehabilitative services objective*: Increase the access to the continuum of long-term care services for a greater proportion of people with these needs.[205]

Strong predictors of access to quality health care include having health insurance, a higher income level, and a regular primary care provider or other source of ongoing health care. Adults with health insurance are twice as likely to receive routine health checkups as adults without health insurance.

Adults can serve as important role models for children, demonstrating the importance of having a primary care provider, receiving appropriate preventive care (e.g., cancer screening, blood pressure, immunization, early prenatal care), and advocating wellness concepts. With health costs skyrocketing, PTs have an opportunity and a responsibility to play a vital role in providing primary and preventive care services to those of all ages.

The AAP 2009 recommendations for addressing the needs of underinsured adolescents should be read by every child health care provider and advocate for children and adolescents. These include guidelines for the improvement of preventive, reproductive, and behavioral health services, which are crucial for advancing adolescents' access to health care and improving their overall quality of life.[7]

Summary

When I look upon a child I am filled with admiration—not so much for what that child is today as for what it may become.

Louis Pasteur

All the topics addressed in this chapter affect not only the overall health and welfare of adolescents but also the future health of the United States. When talking to teens about health care issues, create an open, nonjudgmental environment that fosters safe, honest, and continuing dialogue. Juveniles are at a pivotal point in their physical, psychological, and psychosocial development, and health habits that start in adolescence can have long-lasting effects.

The successful treatment of adolescent conditions depends on early and accurate differential diagnoses and implementation of an appropriate rehabilitation program. Safe and efficacious exercise prescription integrates the three elements of evidenced-based medicine. The PT's clinical expertise ensures that the goals of therapy are directed at specific pathology, impairments, functional limitations, or disabilities. The PT also screens for specific contraindications and precautions (e.g., growth variables, injury and disease limitations, soft tissue healing constraints). The scientific merit for the intervention in the face of the presenting condition or medical history must be considered. Finally, patient values and motivation for physical therapy intervention, as well as caregiver or parental and peer support, must be incorporated into treatment planning. Cost, convenience, and availability of resources, and the safety of the exercise environment, always must be a priority.

Adolescents face many potential barriers to participating in health promotion activities and a healthy lifestyle. Cultural, family, and peer influences and self-esteem issues are the primary deterrents for adolescents.[255] Adolescents may cite variables such as cost, access, time, family opposition, or job or school constraints. Studies have shown that socioeconomic factors such as low income (no health insurance), low education, a difficult living environment, and lack of exposure to proper health promotion are key factors in failure to participate in health promotion activities. [7,205]

The adolescent or child with a chronic disease or disability faces increased environmental barriers, increased costs, and access constraints. [101, 268] PTs should readily refer at-risk or uninsured children and their families to state and federal agencies to see whether they qualify for federal or state aid for health care. Many national and international organizations offer research, educational materials, and health promotion guidelines for children and adolescents (see Appendix 16-1). The AAP has a plethora of policy statements for advancing the quality of life for children and adolescents with a disability (http://aappolicy.aappublications.org).

This chapter is intended to be the PT's first step in developing the communication, technical, and clinical decision making skills needed to provide safe, effective, and efficacious health care to adolescents. It is the first step in meeting the challenge of autonomous practice set forth by the Primary Care Special Interest Group of the Orthopedic Section of the American Physical Therapy Association. It is only the first step, however. Our ever-changing health care environment demands that all health care providers make a commitment to lifelong learning. Just as the youth of America grow and change, so must we as health care professionals.

REFERENCES

1. Adams RC. Spina bifida: life span management. In: Home Study Course 10.2.2: orthopaedic interventions for pediatric patients. La Crosse, WI: American Physical Therapy Association; 2002.
2. AIDS. Global public health goals thwarted by human rights violations, gender inequality, and stigma. Mexico City: XVII International AIDS Conference; 2008 (website). http://www.aids2008.org/admin/images/upload/825.pdf. Accessed February 23, 2010.
3. American Academy of Allergy, Asthma, and Immunology (AAAAI): The allergy report: science-based findings on the diagnosis and treatment of allergic disorders, 1996-2001 (website). http://www.aaaai.org/patients/gallery/prevention.asp?item=1a. Accessed February 23, 2010.
4. American Academy of Orthopedic Surgeons: Your orthopaedic connection (website). http://orthoinfo.aaos.org/. Accessed January 31, 2010.
5. American Academy of Pediatrics: H1N1 flu (swine flu) information (website). http://www.aap.org/advocacy/releases/swineflu.htm. Accessed September 29, 2009.
6. American Academy of Pediatrics. Committee on Adolescence: Emergency contraception. Pediatrics 2005;116:1026–35.
7. American Academy of Pediatrics. Committee on Adolescence: American Academy of Pediatrics Committee on Child Health Financing: Underinsurance of adolescents: recommendations for improved coverage of preventive, reproductive, and behavioral health care services. Pediatrics 2009;123:191–6.
8. American Academy of Pediatrics. Committee on Genetics: Health supervision for children with Down syndrome. Pediatrics 2001;107:442–9.
9. American Academy of Pediatrics. Committee on Infectious Diseases: Hepatitis A vaccine recommendations. Pediatrics 2007;120:189–99.
10. American Academy of Pediatrics. Committee on Infectious Diseases: Prevention and control of meningococcal disease: recommendations for use of meningococcal vaccines in pediatric patients. Pediatrics 2005;116:496–505.

11. American Academy of Pediatrics. Committee on Infectious Diseases: Prevention of influenza: recommendations for influenza immunization of children, 2007–2008. Pediatrics 2008;121; e1016-31.

12. American Academy of Pediatrics. Committee on Infectious Diseases: Prevention of pertussis among adolescents: recommendations for use of tetanus toxoid, reduced diphtheria toxoid, and acellular pertussis (Tdap) vaccine. Pediatrics 2006;117:965–78.

13. American Academy of Pediatrics. Committee on Infectious Diseases: Prevention of varicella: recommendations for use of varicella vaccines in children, including a recommendation for a routine 2-dose varicella immunization schedule. Pediatrics 2007;120:221–31.

14. American Academy of Pediatrics. Committee on Infectious Diseases: Recommended childhood immunization schedules—United States, 2009. Pediatrics 2009;123:189–90.

15. American Academy of Pediatrics. Committee on Sports Medicine and Fitness: Climatic heat stress and the exercising child and adolescent. Pediatrics 2000;106:158–9.

16. American Academy of Pediatrics. Committee on Sports Medicine and Fitness: Intensive training and sports specialization in young athletes. Pediatrics 2000;106:154–7 (reaffirmed February 1, 2010).

17. American Academy of Pediatrics. Council on Sports Medicine and Fitness; McCambridge TM, Stricker PR: Strength training by children and adolescents. Pediatrics 2008;121:835–40.

18. American Academy of Pediatrics. Subcommittee on Attention-Deficit/Hyperactivity Disorder and Committee on Quality Improvement: clinical practice guideline: treatment of the school-aged child with attention-deficit/hyperactivity disorder. Pediatrics 2001;108:1033–44.

19. American Cancer Association: Childhood cancer: late effects of cancer treatment (website). http://www.cancer.org/docroot/CRI/content/CRI_2_6x_Late_Effects_of_Childhood_Cancer.asp. Accessed September 9, 2009.

20. American Cancer Society: Cancer projected to become leading cause of death worldwide in 2010 (website). http://www.sciencedaily.com/releases/2008/12/081209111516.htm. Accessed February 23, 2010.

21. American Cancer Society. The dangers of tobacco. Patient Medical Assistant August 23, 1999. p 1.

22. American College of Sports Medicine: Sawka MN, Burke LM, Eichner ER, et al. Position stand: exercise and fluid replacement. Med Sci Sports Exerc 2007;39:377–90.

23. American Dental Association: Oral health topics A-Z: cleaning your teeth and gums (oral hygiene) (website). http://www.ada.org/public/topics/cleaning.asp. Accessed February 23, 2010.

24. American Heart Association: Many teens spend 30 hours a week on 'screen time' during high school (website). http://www.sciencedaily.com/releases/2008/03/080312172614.htm. Accessed September 9, 2009.

25. American Physical Therapy Association: Guide to Physical Therapist Practice. Second Edition. American Physical Therapy Association, Phys Ther 2001;81:9-746.

26. American Psychiatric Association. Eating disorders measures. In: Handbook of psychiatric measures. Washington DC: American Psychiatric Association; 2000. pp 647-73.

27. American Red Cross: American Red Cross sport safety training handbook, 2005 (website). http://www.redcrossstore.org/Shopper/Product.aspx?UniqueItemId=84. Accessed February 25, 2010.

28. American Social Health Association: Frequently asked questions about genital herpes (website). http://www.ashastd.org/pdfs/FAQ-HSV.pdf. Accessed February 25, 2010.

29. Anderson MK, Hall SJ, Parr GA. Foundations of athletic training: prevention, assessment, and management. 4th ed. Baltimore: Lippincott, Williams & Wilkins; 2009.

30. Annie E. Casey Foundation: 2009 KIDS COUNT Data Book: state profiles of child well-being (website). http://datacenter.kidscount.org/databook/2009/Default.aspx. Accessed February 25, 2010.

31. AVERT: HIV and AIDS in America (website). http://www.avert.org/america.htm. Accessed February 25, 2010.

32. Baechle TR, Earle RW, editors. Essentials of strength training and conditioning. 3rd ed. Champaign, IL: Human Kinetics; 2008.

33. Bar-Or O. Training considerations for children and adolescents with chronic disease. In: Hasson SM, editor. Clinical exercise physiology St. Louis: Mosby; 1994. pp 266–80.

34. Barrett J, Anderson MA, Palmer P, et al: Upper extremity injuries and rehabilitation of the pediatric athlete. In: Home Study Course 2000-2: Sports section, LaCrosse, WI: American Physical Therapy Association.

35. Beck AT, Steer RA, Garbin MG. Psychometric properties of the Beck Depression Inventory: twenty-five years of evaluation. Clin Psychol Rev 1988;8:77–100.

36. Beers MH, Porter RS, Jones TV, editors. Obesity: Merck manual of diagnosis and therapy. 18th ed. Rathway, NJ: Merck; 2006.

37. Belfer ML. Child and adolescent mental disorders: the magnitude of the problem across the globe. Child Psychol Psychiatry 2008;49:226–36.

38. Bernstein RM, Cozen H. Evaluation of back pain in children and adolescents. Am Fam Physician 2007;76:1669–76.

39. Bickley LS. Bates' guide to physical examination and history taking. 10th ed. Philadelphia: Lippincott, Williams & Wilkins; 2008.

40. Bicycle Helmet Safety Institute: Helmet-related statistics from many sources(website). http://www.bhsi.org/stats.htm. Accessed February 25, 2010.

41. Bienz D, Cori H, Hornig D. Adequate dosing of micronutrients for different groups in the life cycle. Food Nutr Bull 2003;24:S7–15.

42. Binford RB, Le Grange D, Jellar CC. Eating Disorders Examination versus Eating Disorders Examination-Questionnaire in adolescents with full and partial-syndrome bulimia nervosa and anorexia nervosa. Int J Eat Disord 2005;37:44–9.

43. Blythe MT. Committee on Adolescence, American Academy of Pediatrics: Underinsurance of adolescents: recommendations for improved coverage of preventive, reproductive, and behavioral health care services. Pediatrics 2009;123:191–6.

44. Booth FW, Chakravarthy MV, Gordon SE, et al. Waging war on physical inactivity: using modern molecular ammunition against an ancient enemy. J Appl Physiol 2002;93:3–30.

45. Borotikar BS, Newcomer R, Koppes R, et al. Combined effects of fatigue and decision making on female lower limb landing postures: central and peripheral contributions to ACL injury risk. Clin Biomech 2008;23:81–92.

46. Borowsky IW, Hogan M, Ireland M. Adolescent sexual aggression: risk and protective factors. Pediatrics 1997;100:E7.

47. Borse NN, Gilchrist J, Dellinger AM, et al. Unintentional childhood injuries in the United States: key findings for the CDC childhood injury report. J Safety Res 2009;40:71–4.

48. Bossarte RM, Swahn MH, Breiding M. Racial, ethnic, and sex differences in the associations between violence and self-reported health among U.S. high school students. J School Health 2009;79:74–81.

49. Boutin RD, Fritz RC, Steinbach LS. Imaging of sports-related muscle injuries. Radiol Clin North Am 2002;40:333–62.

50. Brotzman SB, Wilk KE. Clinical orthopaedic rehabilitation. 2nd ed. St. Louis: Mosby; 2003.

51. Buckwalter JA. Articular cartilage: injuries and potential for healing. J Orthop Sport Phys Ther 1998;28:192–202.

52. Burt CW, Overpeck MD. Emergency visits for sports-related injuries. Ann Emerg Med 2001;37:301–8.

53. Busch MT. Meniscal injuries in children and adolescents. Clin Sports Med 1990;9:661–80.

54. Byrne S, McLean N. Elite athletes: effects of the pressure to be thin. J Sci Med Sport 2002;5:80–94.

55. Cameron MH. Physical agents in rehabilitation: from research to practice. 3rd ed. Philadelphia: WB Saunders; 2009.

56. Campbell SK, Van der Linden DW, Palisano RJ, editors. Physical therapy for children. 3rd ed. Philadelphia: Saunders Elsevier; 2006.

57. Carlson C. The natural history and management of hamstring injuries. Curr Rev Musculoskelet Med 2008;1:120–3.

58. Cassas KJ, Cassettari-Wayhs A. Childhood and adolescent sports-related overuse injuries. Am Fam Physician 2006;73:1014–22.

59. Cassin SE, von Ranson KM. Personality and eating disorders: a decade in review. Clin Psychol Rev 2005;25:895–916.

60. Cech DJ, Martin S. Functional movement development across the life span. 2nd ed. Philadelphia: WB Saunders; 2002.

61. Center on Media and Child Health: Cell phones (website). http://www.cmch.tv/mentors/ hotTopic.asp?id=70. Accessed February 25, 2010.

62. Centers for Disease Control and Prevention (CDC): Child maltreatment: facts at a glance (website). http://www.cdc.gov/ViolencePrevention/pdf/CM-DataSheet-a.pdf. Accessed September 9, 2009.

63. Centers for Disease Control and Prevention (CDC): Clinical growth chart, May 30, 2000 (website). www.cdc.gov/ growthcharts. Accessed February 25, 2010.

64. Centers for Disease Control and Prevention (CDC): Fact sheet: meningococcal diseases and meningococcal vaccines as of April 25, 2006 (website). http://www.cdc.gov/vaccines/vpd-vac/mening/vac-mening-fs.htm#epi. Accessed August 28, 2009.

65. Centers for Disease Control and Prevention (CDC). Use of Supplements Containing Folic Acid Among Women of Childbearing Age — United States, 2007. MMWR Morb Mortal Wkly Rep 2008;57:5–8.

66. Centers for Disease Control and Prevention (CDC). Lyme disease—United States, 2003-2005. MMWR Morb Mortal Wkly Rep 2007;56:573–6.

67. Centers for Disease Control and Prevention (CDC): Oral health: preventing cavities, gum disease, and tooth loss, at a glance, April 2007 (website). http://www.cdc.gov/nccdphp/publications/aag/pdf/oh.pdf. Accessed May 11, 2009.

68. Centers for Disease Control and Prevention (CDC): Overweight and obesity (website). http://www.cdc.gov/nccdphp/dnpa/obesity/index.htm. Accessed February 26, 2010.

69. Centers for Disease Control and Prevention (CDC). Prevalence and most common causes of disability among adults—United States, 2005. MMWR Morb Mortal Wkly Rep 2009;58:421–6.

70. Centers for Disease Control and Prevention (CDC): Recommended immunization schedules for children and adolescents ages 0 through 18 years, United States, 2009 (website). http://www.cdc.gov/vaccines/recs/schedules/child-schedule.htm. Accessed February 25, 2010.

71. Centers for Disease Control and Prevention: Sexually transmitted diseases: STD health disparities—differences in STD rates by location, gender, age, and race (February 2009) (website). http://www.cdc.gov/std/health-disparities/default.htm. Accessed February 25, 2010.

72. Centers for Disease Control and Prevention (CDC): Sexually transmitted disease surveillance, 2007 (website). http://www.cdc.gov/std/pubs. Accessed August 11, 2009.

73. Centers for Disease Control and Prevention (CDC): Summary health statistics for U.S. children: National Health Interview Survey, 2008 (website). http://www.cdc.gov/nchs/ data/series/sr_10/sr10_244.pdf. Accessed February 25, 2010.

74. Centers for Disease Control and Prevention (CDC). Trends in childhood cancer mortality—United States, 1990-2004. MMWR Morb Mortal Wkly Rep 2007;56:1257–61.

75. Centers for Disease Control and Prevention: Youth risk behavior surveillance—United States, 2007(website). http://www.cdc.gov/healthyyouth/yrbs/pdf/yrbss07_mmwr.pdf. Accessed August 9, 2009.

76. Centers for Disease Control and Prevention, National Center for Injury Prevention and Control: Traumatic brain injury in the United States (website). http://www.cdc.gov/ncipc/tbi/TBI.htm. Accessed September 18, 2009.

77. Centers for Disease Control and Prevention, National Center for Injury Prevention and Control: WISQARS leading causes of death reports, 1999-2006 (website). http://webappa.cdc.gov/sasweb/ncipc/leadcaus10.html. Accessed August 1, 2009.

78. Cesario SK, Hughes LA. Precocious puberty: a comprehensive review of literature. J Obstet Gynecol Neonatal Nurs 2007;36:263–74.

79. Chao ST, Joyce MJ, Suh JH. Treatment of heterotopic ossification. Orthopedics 2007;30:457–64.

80. Chen MY, Wang EK, Jeng YK. Adequate sleep among adolescents is positively associated with health status and health-related behaviors. BMC Public Health 2006;6:59.

81. Children and Adults With Attention-Deficit/Hyperactivity Disorder (CHADD): Diagnosis of AD/HD in Adults (What We Know Series #9) (website). http://www.chadd.org. Accessed February 25, 2010.

82. Children Now: Talking with kids about drugs and alcohol (website). http://www.childrennow.org/index.php/learn/twk_drugs. Accessed February 26, 2010.

83. Children's Defense Fund: Each day in America (website). http://www.childrensdefense.org/child-research-data-publications/each-day-in-america.html. Accessed September 22, 2009.

84. Chugani HT. A critical period of brain development: studies of cerebral glucose utilization with PET. Prev Med 1998;7:184–8.

85. Clar C, Cummins E, McIntyre L, et al. Clinical and cost-effectiveness of autologous chondrocyte implantation for cartilage defects in knee joints: systematic review and economic evaluation. Health Technol Assess 2005;9:1–82.

86. Clark EM, Ness AR, Tobias JH. Vigorous physical activity increases fracture risk in children irrespective of bone mass: a prospective study of the independent risk factors for fractures in healthy children. J Bone Miner Res 2008;23:1012–22.

87. Cole WR, Paulos SK, Cole CA, et al. A review of family intervention guidelines for pediatric acquired brain injuries. Dev Disabil Res Rev 2009;15:159–66.

88. Cooper C, Dennison EM, Leufkens HG, et al. Epidemiology of childhood fractures in Britain: a study using the general practice research database. J Bone Miner Res 2004;19:1976–81.

89. Cranney A, Weiler HA, O'Donnell S, et al. Summary of evidence-based review on vitamin D efficacy and safety in relation to bone health. Am J Clin Nutr 2008;88:513S–9S.

90. Crowther M. Elbow pain in pediatrics. Curr Rev Musculoskelet Med 2009;2:83–7.

91. Cusick B. Lower extremity musculoskeletal development. In: Home Study Course 10.2.2: Orthopedic interventions for pediatric patients. La Crosse, WI: American Physical Therapy Association; 2002.

92. Daniels SR, Greer FR. Lipid screening and cardiovascular health in childhood. Pediatrics 2008;122:198–208.

93. DARE: Drug abuse resistance education (website). http://www.dare.com/home/default.asp. Accessed February 25, 2010.

94. Davies GJ, Wilk K, Ellenbecher T, et al. The shoulder: physical therapy patient management utilizing current evidence. In: Home Study Course 16.2.4: Orthopedic interventions for pediatric patients. La Crosse, WI: American Physical Therapy Association; 2002.

95. De La Torre DM, Snell BJ. Use of the preparticipation physical exam in screening for the female athlete triad among high school athletes. J Sch Nurs 2005;21:340–5.

96. DeNavas-Walt C, Proctor BD, Smith JC. U.S. Census Bureau, current population reports, income, poverty, and health insurance coverage in the United States: 2007. Washington DC: U.S. Government Printing Office; 2008. pp 60-235.

97. Department of Health and Human Services: The 2009 HHS federal poverty guidelines (website). http://aspe.hhs.gov/POVERTY/09poverty.shtml. Accessed September 22, 2009.

98. DiFranza JR, Savageau JA, Rigotti NA, et al. Development of symptoms of tobacco dependence in youths: 30-month follow-up data from the DANDY study. Tobacco Control 2002;11:228–35.

99. Dinkes R, Kemp J, Baum K: Indicators of school crime and safety 2008 (website). http://www.eric.ed.gov/ERICWebPortal/custom/portlets/record Details/detailmini.jsp?_nfpb=true&_&ERICExtSearch_SearchValue_0= ED504994&ERICExtSearch_SearchType_0=no&accno=ED504994 (NCES 2009-022/NCJ 226343). Accessed February 25, 2010.

100. Dodson CC, Altchek DW. SLAP lesions: an update on recognition and treatment. J Orthop Sports Phys Ther 2009;39:71–80.

101. Dougherty D. Children with chronic illness and disabilities. Rockville, MD: Agency for Healthcare Research Quality; 2002, Publication No 02–M025.

102. Dunger DB, Ahmed ML, Ong KK. Effects of obesity on growth and puberty. Best Pract Res Clin Endocrinol Metab 2005;19:375–90.

103. Eiff PM, Calmbach WL, Hatch RL. Fracture management for primary care. 2nd ed. Philadelphia: WB Saunders; 2002.

104. Erikson E. Childhood and society. 2nd ed. New York: Norton; 1963.

105. Euling SY, Selevan SG, Pescovitz OH, et al. Role of environmental factors in the timing of puberty. Pediatrics 2008; 121(Suppl. 3):S167–71.

106. Eyre H, Kahn R, Robertson RM, et al. Preventing cancer, cardiovascular disease, and diabetes: a common agenda for the American Cancer Society, the American Diabetes Association, and the American Heart Association, CA Cancer. J Clin 2004;54:190–207.

107. Fairburn CG, Cooper Z. Assessment of eating disorder psychopathology: interview of self-report questionnaire? Int J Eat Disord 1994;16:363–70.

108. Faure M. Management of acne in adolescents. Arch Pediatr 2007;14:1152.

109. Feudtner C, Feinstein JA, Satchell M, et al. Shifting place of death among children with complex chronic conditions in the United States, 1989-2003. JAMA 2007;294:2725–32.

110. Finkelstein E, Corso P, Miller T, et al. The incidence and economic burden of injuries in the United States. New York: Oxford University Press; 2006.

111. Foster Care Alumni of America: National facts about children in foster care (website). http://fostercarealumni.org/resources/foster_care_facts_and_statistics.htm. Accessed September 29, 2009.

112. Frances A, Pingus HA, First MB, editors. Diagnostic and statistical manual of mental disorders. 4th ed. Washington DC: American Psychiatric Association; 1994.

113. Franić M, Kovač V. Anterior instrumentation for correction of adolescent thoracic idiopathic scoliosis: historic prospective study. Croat Med J 2006;47:239–45.

114. Frisch RE. Body fat, menarche, fitness, and fertility. Hum Reprod 1987;6:521–33.

115. Gavin TM, Patwardhan AG, Ghanayem AJ, et al. Orthotics in the management of spinal dysfunction and instability. In: Lusardi MM, Nielson CC, editors. Orthotics and prosthetics in rehabilitation. 2nd ed. St. Louis: Saunders-Elsevier; 2007.

116. Gay and Lesbian Medical Association; LGBT health experts. Healthy People 2010 companion document for lesbian, gay, bisexual, and transgender (LGBT) health. San Francisco: Gay and Lesbian Medical Association; 2001.

117. Gidding SS, Dennison BA, Birch LL, et al. American Heart Association; American Academy of Pediatrics: Dietary recommendations for children and adolescents: a guide for practitioners. Pediatrics 2006;117:544–59.

118. Gillogly SD, Voight M, Blackburn T. Treatment of articular cartilage defects of the knee with autologous chondrocyte implantation. J Orthop Sport Phys Ther 1998;28:241–51.

119. Goldberg L, Elliot D. The adolescents training and learning to avoid steroids program: preventing drug use and promoting health behaviors. Arch Pediatr Adolesc Med 2000;154:332–8.

120. Goodman CC, Fuller KS. Pathology: implications for the physical therapist. 3rd ed. Philadelphia: Saunders-Elsevier; 2009.

121. Grant B. Estimates of U.S. children exposed to alcohol abuse and dependence in the family. Am J Publ Health 2000;90:112–5.

122. Grassmayr MJ, Parker DA, Coolican MR, et al. Posterior cruciate ligament deficiency: Biomechanical and biological consequences and the outcomes of conservative treatment: a systematic review. J Sci Med Sport 2008;11:433–43.

123. Gray JC. Neural and vascular anatomy of the menisci of the human knee. J Orthop Sport Phys Ther 1999;29:23–30.

124. Greer FA, Krebs NF. Committee on Nutrition: Optimizing bone health and calcium intakes in infants, children, and adolescents. Pediatrics 2006;117:578–85.

125. Greiner KA. Adolescent idiopathic scoliosis: radiologic decision-making. Am Fam Physician 2002;65:1817–22.

126. Gutgesell ME, Payne N. Issues of adolescent psychological development in the 21st century. Pediatr Rev 2004;25:79–85.

127. Guttmacher Institute: Facts on U.S. teens' sexual and reproductive health (website). http://www.guttmacher.org/pubs/fb_ATSRH.html. Accessed August 14, 2009.

128. Guttmacher Institute: U.S. teenage pregnancy statistics. National and state trends and trends by race and ethnicity, 1986–2006, January 2010 (website). http://www.guttmacher.org/pubs/USTPtrends.pdf. Accessed April 8, 2010.

129. Habif TP. Acne, rosacea, and related disorders. In: Habif TP, editor. Clinical dermatology. 5th ed. Philadelphia: Mosby Elsevier; 2009. pp 217–63.

130. Hall C, Thein-Brody L. Therapeutic exercise: moving towards function. 2nd ed. Philadelphia: Lippicott/Williams & Wilkins; 2005.

131. Harrigan TM. Orthotics and therapeutic interventions in the management of scoliosis. In: Lusardi MM, Nielson CC, editors. Orthotics and prosthetics in rehabilitation. 2nd ed. St. Louis: Saunders-Elsevier; 2007. pp 427–48.

132. Hassan I, Dorani BJ. Rollerblading and skateboarding injuries in children in northeast England. Emerg Med J 1999;16:348–50.

133. Heller DR, Routley V, Chambers S. Rollerblading injures in young children. J Pediatr Child Health 1996;32:35–8.

134. Henry BW, Ozier AD. Position of the American Dietetic Association: nutrition intervention in the treatment of anorexia nervosa, bulimia nervosa, and other eating disorders. J Am Diet Assoc 2006;106:2073–82.

135. Henry J, Kaiser Family Foundation: HIV/AIDS policy fact sheet: U.S. federal funding for HIV/AIDS: The President's FY 2010 budget request, May 2009 (website). http://www.kff. org/hivaids/upload/7029–05.pdf. Accessed August 14, 2009.

136. Henshaw SK. Disparities in rates of unintended pregnancy in the United States, 1994 and 2001. Perspect Sexl Reprod Health 2006;38:90–6.

137. Hergenroeder AC: The preparticipation sports examination in children and adolescents (website). http://www.uptodate.com/home/index.html. Accessed September 29, 2008.

138. Heyworth BE, Green DW. Lower extremity stress fractures in pediatric and adolescent athletes. Curr Opin Pediatr 2008;20:58–61.

139. Hixon Al, Gibbs LM. Osteochondritis dissecans: a diagnosis not to miss. Am Fam Physician 2000;61:151–6.

140. Holder HD, Gruenewald PJ, Ponicki WR, et al. Effect of community-based interventions on high-risk drinking and alcohol-related deaths. JAMA 2000;284:2341–7.

141. Hoskins W, Pollard H. Hamstring injury management—part 2: treatment. Man Ther 2005;10:180–90.

142. Humphrey LL, Fu R, Buckley DI, et al. Periodontal disease and coronary heart disease incidence: a systematic review and meta-analysis. J Gen Intern Med 2008;23:2079–86.

143. Ibáñez L, López-Bermejo A, Díaz M, et al. Metformin treatment for four years to reduce total and visceral fat in low birth weight girls with precocious pubarche. J Clin Endocrinol Metab 2008;93:1841–5.

144. Ibáñez L, Valls C, Marcos MV, et al. Insulin sensitization for girls with precocious pubarche and with risk for polycystic ovary syndrome: effects of prepubertal initiation and postpubertal discontinuation of metformin treatment. J Clin Endocrinol Metab 2004;89:4331–7.

145. Ibáñez L, Valls C, Ong K, et al. Metformin therapy during puberty delays menarche, prolongs pubertal growth, and augments adult height: a randomized study in low-birth-weight girls with early-normal onset of puberty. J Clin Endocrinol Metab 2006;91:2068–73.

146. Irving LM, Wall M, Neumark-Sztainer D, et al. Steroid use among adolescents: findings from Project EAT. J Adolesc Health 2002;30:243–52.

147. Jacobi C, Hayward C, deZwaan M, et al. Coming to terms with risk factors for eating disorders: application of risk terminology and suggestions for a general taxonomy. Psychol Bull 2004;130:19–65.

148. Janssen DF. First stirrings: cultural notes on orgasm, ejaculation, and wet dreams. J Sex Res 2007;44:122–34.

149. Jarvis C. Physical examination and health assessment. 5th ed. Philadelphia: WB Saunders; 2007.

150. Jemmott JB, Jemmott LS. Behavioral interventions with heterosexual adolescents. In: Reiss D, editor. NIH consensus development conference on interventions to prevent HIV risk behaviors. Bethesda, MD: National Institute of Health; 1997.

151. Jenny C. Committee on Child Abuse and Neglect: Evaluating infants and young children with multiple fractures. Pediatrics 2006;118:1299–303.

152. Johnson AR, DeMatt E, Salorio CF. Predictors of outcome following acquired brain injury in children. Dev Disabil Res Rev 2009;15:124–32.

153. Johnson JO. Who's minding the kids? Child care arrangements: Winter 2002 (website). http://www.census.gov/prod/2005pubs/p70-101.pdf. Accessed February 26, 2010.

154. Johnston LD, O'Malley PM, Bachman JG, et al. Monitoring the future: national results on adolescent drug use: overview of key findings, 2008. Bethesda, MD: National Institute on Drug Abuse; 2009, NIH Publication No. 09-7401.

155. Kaplowitz PB. Link between body fat and the timing of puberty. Pediatrics 2008;121(Suppl. 3):S208–17.

156. Kasow DB, Curl WW. "Stingers" in adolescent athletes. Instr Course Lect 2006;55:711–6.

157. Kavey R-EW, Daniels SR, Lauer RM, et al. American Heart Association guidelines for primary prevention of atherosclerotic cardiovascular disease beginning in childhood. Circulation 2003;107:1562–6.

158. Kell R, Jenkins AP. HIV transmission and sports: realities and recommendations. Strength Cond J 1998;20:58–61.

159. Kendall FP, McCreary EK, Provance PG, et al. Muscles—testing and function with posture and pain. 5th ed. Baltimore: Lippincott, Williams & Wilkins; 2005.

160. Kessler RC, Chiu WT, Demler O, et al. Prevalence, severity, and comorbidity of 12-month DSM-IV disorders in the National Comorbidity Survey Replication. Arch Gen Psychiatry 2005;62:617–27.

161. Kim WR. Epidemiology of hepatitis B in the United States. Hepatology 2009;49(Suppl.):S28–34.

162. Klein JD; Committee on Adolescence, American Academy of Pediatrics Policy Statement: Menstruation in girls and adolescents: using the menstrual cycle as a vital sign. Pediatrics 2006;118:2245–50.

163. Klingman RM, Behrman RE, Jenson HB, Stanton BF. Nelson textbook of pediatrics. 18th ed. Philadelphia: Saunders; 2007.

164. Kosciw JG, Diaz EM. The 2005 National School Climate Survey: the experiences of lesbian, gay, bisexual, and transgender youth in our nation's schools. New York: Gay, Lesbian and Straight Education Network (GLSEN); 2006.

165. Kulig JW. Committee on Substance Abuse: Tobacco, alcohol, and other drugs: the role of the pediatrician in prevention, identification, and management of substance abuse. Pediatrics 2005;115:816–21.

166. Kung HC, Hoyert DL, Xu JQ, et al. Deaths: Final data for 2005. Natl Vital Stat Rep 2008;56:1–20.

167. Langlois JA, Rutland-Brown W, Thomas KE. Traumatic brain injury in the United States: emergency department visits, hospitalizations, and deaths. Atlanta: Centers for Disease Control and Prevention, National Center for Injury Prevention and Control; 2006.

168. Larson CM, Almekinders LC, Karas SG, et al. Evaluating and managing muscle contusions and myositis ossificans. Phys Sports Med 2002;30:41–50.

169. Latchkey Kid: K12 academics (website). http://www.k12academics.com/pedagogy/latchkey-kid. Accessed September 29, 2009.

170. Lewis C: Physiological response to exercise in the child: considerations for the typically and atypically developing youngster, from Proceedings from the American Physical Therapy Association Combined Sections Meeting, San Antonio, TX, February 16, 2001.

171. Loth TS, Wadsworth CT. Orthopedic review for physical therapists. St. Louis: Mosby; 1998.

172. Luma GA, Spiotta RT. Hypertension in children and adolescents. Am Fam Physician 2006;73:1158–68.

173. Luna B, Padmanabhan A, O'Hearn K. What has fMRI told us about the development of cognitive control through adolescence? Brain Cogn 2010;72:101–13.

174. Lusardi MM, Nielsen CC. Orthotics and prosthetics in rehabilitation. 2nd ed. St Louis: Saunders-Elsevier; 2007.

175. Lyon RM, Street CC. Pediatric sports injuries. Pediatr Clin North Am 1998;45:221–44.

176. Ma NS, Geffner ME. Gynecomastia in prepubertal and pubertal men. Curr Opin Pediatr 2008;20:465–70.

177. Magee DJ. Orthopedic physical assessment. 5th ed. Philadelphia: Saunders Elsevier; 2008.

178. Magnussen RA, Dunn WR, Carey JL, et al. Treatment of focal articular cartilage defects in the knee: a systematic review. Clin Orthop Relat Res 2008;466:952–62.

179. Males M: The "teen brain" craze: new science or ancient politics? (website) http://youthfacts.org/brain.html. Accessed September 29, 2009.

180. Manal TJ, Strugill L. The knee: physical therapy patient management utilizing current evidence. In: Home Study Course 10.2.2: Orthopedic interventions for pediatric patients. LaCrosse, WI: American Physical Therapy Association; 2006.

181. Marshall WA, Tanner JM. Variations in the pattern of pubertal changes in boys. Arch Dis Child 1970;45:13–23.

182. Marshall WA, Tanner JM. Variations in the pattern of pubertal changes in girls. Arch Dis Child 1969;44:291–303.

183. McArdle WD, Katch FI, Katch VL. Exercise physiology: energy, nutrition, and human performance. 6th ed. Philadelphia: Lippincott, Williams & Wilkins; 2006.

184. McDevitt TM, Rowe PM: The United States in international context: 2000 (website). http://www.census.gov/prod/2002pubs/c2kbr01-11.pdf. Accessed February 25, 2010.

185. McKinnis LN. Fundamentals of musculoskeletal imaging. 2nd ed. Philadelphia: FA Davis; 2005.

187. Menon MR, Walker JL, Court-Brown CM. The epidemiology of fractures in adolescents with reference to social deprivation,. J Bone Joint Surg Br 2008;90:1482–6.

188. Mohtadi N, Grant J. Managing anterior cruciate ligament deficiency in the skeletally immature individual: a systematic review of the literature. Clin J Sports Med 2006;16:457–64.

189. Mond JM, Hay PJ, Rodgers B, et al. Validity of the Eating Disorder Examination Questionnaire (EDE-Q) in screening for eating disorders in community samples. Behav Res Ther 2004;42:551–67.

190. Moore KA, Redd Z, Burkhauser M, et al: Children in poverty: trends, consequences, and policy options (website). http://www.childtrends.org/files/child_trends-2009_04_07_rb_childreninpoverty.pdf. Accessed February 25, 2010.

191. More J. Children's bone health and meeting calcium needs. J Fam Health Care 2008;18:22–4.

191. Morgenstern WA. The results of selective anterior thoracic fusion for King II/Lenke type CL adolescent idiopathic scoliosis. J Bone Joint Surg Br 2002;125; 84-B SUPP IIabstract.

192. National Association of Social Workers: Suicide prevention current trends—risk factors and intervention strategies for gay, lesbian, bisexual, and transgender youth (website). http://www.helpstartshere.org/mind-and-spirit/suicide-prevention/lgbt-youth.html. Accessed February 26, 2010.

193. National Asthma Education and Prevention Program. National Asthma Education and Prevention Program. Expert Panel Report: Guidelines for the Diagnosis and Management of Asthma Update on Selected Topics—2002. J Allergy Clin Immunol 2002;110(Suppl):S141–219.

194. National Coalition for Women and Girls in Education: Title IX at 35: report card on gender equity (website). http://www.ncwge.org/pubs-reports.html. Accessed February 26, 2010.

195. National Institute on Alcohol Abuse and Alcoholism: Research findings on underage drinking and the minimum legal drinking age (website). http://www.niaaa.nih.gov/AboutNIAAA/NIAAASponsoredPrograms/drinkingage.htm. Accessed February 25, 2010.

196. National Institute of Mental Health: Brief notes on the mental health of children and adolescents (website). http://www.medhelp.org/nihlib/GF-233.html. Accessed February 25, 2010.

197. National Institute of Neurological Disorders and Stroke: Meningitis and encephalitis fact sheet (website). NIH Publication No. 04–4840. http://www.ninds.nih.gov/disorders/ encephalitis_meningitis/detail_encephalitis_meningitis.htm. Accessed February 25, 2010.

198. National Sleep Foundation: Children and sleep and Adolescent Sleep Needs and Patterns (website). http://www.sleepfoundation.org. Accessed April 8, 2010.

199. Nattiv A, Loucks AB, Manore MM, et al. American College of Sports Medicine: American American College of Sports Medicine Position stand: the female athlete triad. Med Sci Sports Exerc 2007;39:1867–82.

200. Nelson RM, Botkin JR, Kodish ED, et al. Ethical issues with genetic testing in pediatrics. Pediatrics 2001;107:1451–5.

201. Neumann DA. Kinesiology of the musculoskeletal system: foundations for physical rehabilitation. St. Louis: Mosby; 2002.

202. Norkin M, Frankel VH. Basic biomechanics of the musculoskeletal system. 3rd ed. Philadelphia: Lippincott, Williams & Wilkins; 2001.

203. Nordt CA, DiVasta AD. Gynecomastia in adolescents. Curr Opin Pediatr 2008;20:375–82.

204. Noyes FR, Mooar PA, Matthews DS, et al. The symptomatic anterior cruciate-deficient knee. Part I: the long-term functional disability in athletically active individuals. J Bone Joint Surg Am 1983;65:154–62.

205. Office of Disease Prevention and Health Promotion, U.S. Department of Health and Human Services: Healthy people 2010 (website). http://healthypeople.gov. Accessed February 25, 2010.

206. Office of Juvenile Justice and Delinquency Prevention: Juvenile arrests, 2001 (website). http://www.ncjrs.gov/html/ojjdp/201370/page2.html. Accessed August 22, 2009.

207. Ong KK, Emmett P, Northstone K, et al. Infancy weight gain predicts childhood body fat and age at menarche in girls. J Clin Endocrinol Metab 2009;94:1527–32.

208. Passi VA, Bryson SW, Lock J. Assessment of eating disorders in adolescents with anorexia nervosa: self-report questionnaire versus interview. Int J Eat Disord 2003;33:45–54.

209. Pastor PN, Reuben CA. Diagnosed attention deficit hyperactivity disorder and learning disability: United States, 2004-2006. Vital Health Stat 2008;10:1–4.

210. Payne RA. Relaxation techniques: a practical handbook for the health care professional. NewYork: Churchill Livingstone; 1995.

211. Perkins CA: Age patterns of victims of serious violent crime (website). http://www.ncjrs.gov/app/publications/abstract.aspx?ID=162031. Accessed February 26, 2010.

212. Perry M, Straker L, O'Sullivan P, et al. Fitness, motor competence, and body composition are weakly associated with adolescent back pain. J Orthop Sports Phys Ther 2009;39:439–49.

213. Pierson FM, Fairchild SL. Principles and techniques of patient care. 4th ed. Philadelphia: Saunders-Elsevier; 2008.

214. PT Magazine. For your health, backpack guidelines, September 17, 2001, p 13.

215. Prins Y, Crous L, Louw QA. A systematic review of posture and psychosocial factors as contributors to upper quadrant musculoskeletal pain in children and adolescents. Physiother Theory Pract 2008;24:221–42.

216. Pruitt D, editor. Your adolescent: emotional, behavioral, and cognitive development from early adolescence through the teen years. 2nd ed. New York: Harper Collins; 2000.

217. Rabinowicz T, de Courten-Myers GM, Petetot JM, et al. Human cortex development: estimates of neuronal numbers indicate major loss late in gestation. J Neuropathol Exp Neurol 1996;55:320–8.

218. Rao MS, Jacobson M, editors. Developmental neurobiology. 4th ed. New York: Kluwer Academic; 2007.

219. Rape, Abuse and Incest National Network: Who are the victims? Breakdown by gender and age (website). http://www.rainn.org/get-information/statistics/sexual-assault-victims. Accessed September 25, 2009.

220. Reischl SF, Noceti-DeWit LM. The foot and ankle: physical therapy patient management utilizing current evidence. Independent Study Course 16.2.11: Current Concepts of Orthopaedic Physical Therapy. 2nd ed. LaCrosse, WI: American Physical Therapy; 2006.

221. Resnick MD, Bearman PS, Blum RW, et al. Protecting adolescents from harm: findings from the national longitudinal study on adolescent health. JAMA 1997;278:823–32.

222. Rice SG. American Academy of Pediatrics Council on Sports Medicine and Fitness: Medical conditions affecting sports participation. Pediatrics 2008;121:841–8.

223. Ries LAG, Melbert D, Krapcho M, et al: SEER cancer statistics review, 1975-2006 (website). http://seer.cancer.gov/csr/1975_2006/index.html. Accessed February 26, 2010.

224. Roberts RA, Roberts SO. Exercise physiology: exercise, performance, and clinical applications. St. Louis: Mosby; 1997.

225. Rohmiller MT, Gaynor TP, Pawelek J, et al. Salter-Harris I and II fractures of the distal tibia: does mechanism of injury relate to premature physeal closure? J Pediatr Orthop 2006;26:322–8.

226. Ross M: CPSC reports as scooter sales skyrocket, injuries soar (website). http://www.kidsource.com/cpsc2/scooter.safety.html. Accessed February 26, 2010.

227. Sacks JJ, Helmick CG, Luo YH, et al. Prevalence of and annual ambulatory health care visits for pediatric arthritis and other rheumatologic conditions in the United States in 2001-2004. Arthritis Care Res 2007;57:1439–45.

228. Salter RB. Textbook of disorders and injuries of the musculoskeletal system. 3rd ed. Baltimore: Williams & Wilkins; 1999.

229. Sanderlin BW, Raspa RF. Common stress fractures. Am Fam Physician 2003;68:1527–32.

230. Sansone RA, Sawyer R. Male athletes and eating disorders [editorial]. Clin J Sports Med 2005;15:45–6.

231. Santelli JS, Lindberg LD, Finer LB, et al. Explaining recent declines in adolescent pregnancy in the United States: the contribution of abstinence and improved contraceptive use. Am J Public Health 2007;97:150–6.

232. Saunders HD, Saunders RS. Evaluation, treatment, and prevention of musculoskeletal disorders, vol. 1. 4th ed. Chaska, MN: The Saunders Group; 2004.

233. Senn CY: Vulnerable: Sexual abuse and people with an intellectual handicap (website). http://www.eric.ed.gov/ERICDocs/data/ericdocs2sql/content_storage_01/0000019b/80/1e/53/90.pdf. Accessed February 26, 2010.

234. Shaffer D, Fisher P, Dulcan MK, et al. The NIMH diagnostic interview schedule for children version 2.3 (DISC-2.3): description, acceptability, prevalence rates, and performance in the MECA study. Methods for the epidemiology of child and adolescent mental disorders study. J Am Acad Child Adolesc Psychiatry 1996;35:865–77.

235. Shalitin S, Phillip M. Role of obesity and leptin in the pubertal process and pubertal growth: a review. Int J Obes Relat Metab Disord 2003;27:869–74.

236. Sherry MA, Best TM. A comparison of two rehabilitation programs in the treatment of acute hamstring strains. J Orthop Sports Phys Ther 2004;34:116–25.

237. Shumway-Cook A, Woolacott MH. Motor control: translating research into clinical practice. 3rd ed. Baltimore: Lippincott, Williams & Wilkins; 2007.

238. Silk H, Romano-Clarke G: The seven tenets to teen oral health (website). http://contemporarypediatrics.modernmedicine.com/contpeds/Modern+Medicine+Now/The-seven-tenets-to-teen-oral-health/ArticleStandard/Article/detail/602066?context CategoryId=8648. Accessed August 15, 2009.

239. Silver EJ, Stein RE. Access to care, unmet health needs, and poverty status among children with and without chronic conditions. Ambul Pediatr 2001;1:314–20.

240. Siow HM, Cameron DB, Ganley TJ. Acute knee injuries in skeletally immature athletes. Phys Med Rehabil Clin North Am 2008;19:319–45.

241. Slawski DP, Seip R, Dahlgren G. Lower extremity injuries in the young athlete. In: Home Study Course 2000-2: Sports physical therapy section, pediatric. La Crosse, WI: American Physical Therapy Association; 2000.

242. Slifer KJ, Amari A. Behavior management for children and adolescents with acquired brain injury. Dev Disabil Res Rev 2009;15:144–51.

243. Soprano JV. Musculoskeletal injuries in the pediatric and adolescent athlete. Curr Sports Med Rep 2005;4:329–34.

244. Spinal Cord Injury Facts & Statistics: Who do spinal cord injuries affect in the United States (website)? http://www.sci-info-pages.com/facts.html. Accessed September 18, 2009.

245. Standaert C, Herring S. Expert opinion and controversies in musculoskeletal and sports medicine: stingers. Arch Phys Med Rehabil 2009;90:402–6.

246. Stanitski C, Sherman C. How I manage physeal fractures about the knee. Phys Sports Med 1996;4:59–70.

247. Stark AD, Bennet GC, Stone DH, et al. Association between childhood fractures and poverty: population based study. BMJ 2002;324:457.

248. Steinberg L. The ten basic principles of good parenting. New York: Simon and Shuster; 2004.

249. Substance Abuse and Mental Health Services Administration (SAMHSA), National Mental Health Information Center: Children and adolescents with anxiety disorders (website). http://mentalhealth.samhsa.gov/publications/allpubs/ca-0007/default.asp. Accessed September 6, 2009.

250. Substance Abuse and Mental Health Services Administration. Results from the 2007 national survey on drug use and health: national findings. Rockville, MD: U.S. Government Printing Office; 2008, DHHS Publication No. SMA 08-4343.

251. Sullivan PE, Markos PD. Clinical decision making in therapeutic exercise. Stamford, CT: Appleton & Lange; 1995.

252. Sun SS, Schubert CM, Chumlea WC, et al. National estimates of the timing of sexual maturation and racial differences among U.S. children. Pediatrics 2002;110:911–9.

253. Sussman C, Bates-Jensen B. Wound care: a collaborative manual for health care professionals. 3rd ed. Philadelphia: Lippincott, Wilkins & Williams; 2006.

254. Swenson DM, Yard EE, Fields SK, et al. Patterns of recurrent injuries among U.S. high school athletes, 2005-2008. Am J Sports Med 2009;37:1586–93.

255. Szilagyi PG. Assessing children: infancy through adolescence. In: Bickley LS, Szilagyi PG, editors. Bates' guide to physical examination and history taking. 10th ed. Philadelphia: Lippincott, Williams & Wilkins; 2009, p. 737–869.

256. Teen birth rates, 2006: How does the United States compare (website)? http://www.thenationalcampaign.org/resources/pdf/TBR_International Comparison2006.pdf. Accessed September 15, 2009.

257. Tew S, Redman S, Kwan A, et al. Differences in repair responses between immature and mature cartilage. Clin Orthop Relat Res 2001(391):S142–52.

258. The National Campaign to Prevent Teen Pregnancy: Teen pregnancy—why it matters (website). http://www.thenationalcampaign.org. Accessed September 15, 2009.

259. The National Center for Family Homelessness: The characteristics and needs of families experiencing homelessness (website). http://community.familyhomelessness.org/sites/default/files/NCFH%20Fact%20Sheet%204-08.pdf. Accessed September 22, 2009.

260. The National Center for Family Homelessness: What is family homelessness? (website). http://www.familyhomelessness.org/?q=node/5. Accessed September 22, 2009.

261. Torg JS. Cervical spinal stenosis with cord neurapraxia: evaluations and decisions regarding participation in athletics. Curr Sports Med Rep 2002;1:43–6.

262. Torg JS, Ramsey-Emrhein JA. Cervical spine and brachial plexus injuries: return-to-play recommendations. Phys Sports Med 1997;25:61–88.

263. Trotter TL, Hall JG. American Academy of Pediatrics Committee on Genetics: Health supervision for children with achondroplasia. Pediatrics 2005;116:771–83.

264. Umphred DA. Neurological rehabilitation. 5th ed. St. Louis: Mosby; 2007.

265. U.S. Census Bureau: U.S. and world population clocks (website). http://www.census.gov/main/www/popclock.html. Accessed February 27, 2009.

266. U.S. Department of Health and Human Services and Children's Bureau. Child maltreatment 2007: reports from the states to the National Child Abuse and Neglect Data System (NCANDS). Washington, DC: U.S. Government Printing Office; 2000.

267. U.S. Department of Health and Human Services. U.S. Department of Agriculture: Dietary guidelines for Americans. 6th ed. Washington, DC: U.S. Government Printing Office; 2005.

268. van der Lee JH, Mokkink LB, Grootenhuis MA, et al. Definitions and measurement of chronic health conditions in childhood: a systematic review. JAMA 2007;297:2741–51.

268a. Virginia Tech Transportation Institute: New data from VTTI provides insight into cell phone use and driving distraction (website). http://www.vtti.vt.edu/PDF/7-22-09-VTTIPress_Release_Cell_phones_and_Driver_Distraction.pdf. Accessed April 5, 2010.

269. Wainner RS, Flynn TW, Whitman J. Spinal and extremity manipulation: the basic skill set for physical therapists (CD-ROM). Minneapolis: Manipulations; 2001 (Available at OPTP.com.).

270. Wasiak J, Clar C, Villanueva E. Autologous cartilage implantation for full thickness articular cartilage defects of the knee. Cochrane Database Syst Rev 2006; (3):CD003323.

271. Wilk KE, Obma P, Simpson CD, et al. Shoulder injuries in the overhead athlete. J Orthop Sports Phys Ther 2009;39:38–54.

272. Wilk KE, Reinold MM, Andrews JR. Rehabilitation of the thrower's elbow. Clin Sports Med 2004;23:765–801.

273. Winter P: "Top 10" ways to monitor kids' computer health (website). http://www.pptjax.com/LinkClick.aspx?fileticket=6ymRVOmHpDQ%3D&tabid=189. Accessed February 26, 2010.

274. World Health Organization: Preventing cancer: promoting a healthy diet and physical activity in childhood (website). http://www.sho.int/cancer/prevention/children/en/pring/html. Accessed August 6, 2009.

275. Dabelea D, Bell RA, D'Agostino Jr RB, et al. Incidence of diabetes in youth in the United States. JAMA 2007;297:2716–24.

276. Wu T, Mendola P, Buck GM. Ethnic differences in the presence of secondary sex characteristics and menarche among U.S. girls: the Third National Health and Nutrition Examination Survey, 1988-1994. Pediatrics 2002;110:752–7.

277. Yan AC. Current concepts in acne management. Adolesc Med 2006;17:613–37.

278. Yawn BP, Yawn RA, Hodge D, et al. A population-based study of school scoliosis screening. JAMA 1999;282:1472–4.

Appendix **16-1** **Pediatric Health Care Organizations, References, and Resources**

- American Academy of Allergy Asthma & Immunology www.aaaai.org
- American Academy of Child & Adolescent Psychiatry www.aacap.org
- American Academy of Family Physicians www.aafp.org
- American Academy of Orthopaedic Surgeons www.aaos.org
- American Academy of Pediatrics www.aap.org
- American Cancer Society www.cancer.org
- American College of Allergy, Asthma & Immunology www.acaai.org
- American Dental Association www.ada.org
- American Red Cross www.redcross.org
- Bicycle Helmet Safety Institute www.bhsi.org
- Centers for Disease Control and Prevention (CDC) www.cdc.gov
- CDC Growth Charts www.cdc.gov/growthcharts
- Drug Abuse Resistance Education (DARE) www.dare.com
- Gay & Lesbian Medical Association www.glma.org
- Guttmacher Institute www.guttmacher.org
- Healthy People 2010 www.healthypeople.gov
- Immunization Schedules www.cdc.gov/vaccines/recs/schedules
- Monitoring the Future www.monitoringthefuture.org
- National Eating Disorders Association www.nationaleatingdisorders.org
- National Heart Lung and Blood Institute www.nhlbi.nih.gov
- National Institute of Arthritis and Musculoskeletal and Skin Diseases (NIAMS) www.niams.nih.gov
- National Institute of Drug Abuse www.drugabuse.gov
- National Institute of Mental Health www.nimh.nih.gov
- National Interscholastic Athletic Administrators Association www.niaaa.org
- National Organization for Rare Diseases www.rarediseases.org
- National Osteoporosis Foundation www.nof.org
- National Sleep Foundation www.sleepfoundation.org
- National Youth Sports Safety Foundation www.nyssf.org
- Prader-Willi Syndrome Association www.pwsausa.org
- Sickle Cell Disease Association of America, Inc. www.sicklecelldisease.org
- State Children's Health Insurance Program (CHIP) www.ncsl.org/programs/health/chiphome.htm
- Talking with Kids About Tough Issues www.talkingwithkids.org
- The Henry J. Kaiser Family Foundation www.kff.org
- U.S. Census Bureau www.census.gov
- U.S. Department of Agriculture www.usda.gov
- Youth Risk Behavior Surveillance System (YRBSS) www.cdc.gov/HealthyYouth/yrbs/index.htm

Jill Schiff Boissonnault, PT, PhD
Rebecca G. Stephenson, PT, DPT, MS, WCS

Objectives

After reading the chapter, the reader will be able to:

1. Describe the roles of the primary caregivers for the obstetric client.
2. Define terms unique to pregnancy and the postpartum period.
3. Describe the anatomic and physiologic changes in pregnancy and the postpartum period.
4. Describe the common medical conditions and symptoms of pregnancy and the postpartum period, including those that warrant referral.
5. Describe the common symptoms and diseases that occur in pregnancy that imitate musculoskeletal conditions.
6. Describe examination modifications necessary for this population.
7. Describe the special issues of pregnant women with disabilities or chronic illness.
8. Describe medial diagnostic and pharmacologic challenges in the childbearing years.

Prenatal and Postpartum Issues

Interest in obstetric physical therapy has expanded concomitantly with increased attention directed toward research and advocacy for a broad range of women's health issues. As movement specialists, physical therapists (PTs) are ideally suited to adapt and expand their knowledge base to include evaluation and treatment of the pregnant and postpartum patient. This chapter highlights the anatomic and physiologic changes in pregnancy and the postpartum period, common medical conditions, and screenings that warrant referral. Special conditions in pregnancy, examination modifications, medication concerns, and diagnostic challenges are also covered.

This chapter is designed to assist the outpatient PT in understanding the nomenclature necessary for interdisciplinary communication, the changes that occur during pregnancy and the postpartum period, the systems changes that affect the childbearing year, coverage of selected disease response to pregnancy, and information that might directly affect intervention or examination.

Armed with the information presented in this chapter, any PT should be able to examine confidently and refer an obstetric patient whose symptoms demand medical attention or specialty women's health physical therapy. In addition, this chapter was written to enable PTs to treat pregnant and postpartum women without worry of unsafe positioning or intervention modalities. This information should allow for more holistic care of this population and increased PT comfort in providing services for these women.

Defining Obstetric Terms

Many terms are used to describe number of pregnancies and deliveries and the stages of pregnancy, labor, and postpartum period (Table 17-1). These definitions are relevant to understanding the prenatal medical record and aid in communication with other health care practitioners.

Para, from the French word *parere*, meaning "to give birth," is the base word for the number of times a woman has given birth, regardless of the number of infants born (e.g., twins, triplets). *Gravida*, from the French word *gravis*, meaning "heavy," describes a woman who is or has been pregnant, regardless of the pregnancy outcome.

Past obstetric history can be documented in two different written forms. The gravida para method notes the number of pregnancies and births; for example, "gravida 3 para 2" means that a woman has been pregnant three times and has delivered two infants. The second, more complete method, indicates reproductive history and is indicated by a series of numbers separated by dashes. The first number refers to the number of term infants, the second the number of preterm infants, the third the number of abortions, and the fourth the number of children currently alive. For example, an obstetric history in a chart with a number sequence of 3-1-2-3 indicates that the woman had three term deliveries, one preterm delivery, two abortions, and three children currently living.[43]

The Caregivers: Who They Are and Their Differences in Philosophy and Practice

Many health care professions are involved in the care of the pregnant woman. Overlap occurs in some of the roles.

Registered nurses can train to work in obstetrics by becoming additionally trained as a family, gynecologic, or women's health nurse practitioner. These programs consist of a formal curriculum leading to a certificate or master's degree in nursing. Nurse practitioners typically work under the supervision of a physician and can order diagnostic procedures.

A direct-entry midwife has a certificate of midwifery studies without any other prerequisite. They have a limited scope of practice that is particular to home births, but they may also practice in birth centers. Direct-entry midwives learn by apprenticeship. Their birth philosophy is generally holistic and noninterventionist.

A nurse-midwife is trained in both nursing and midwifery and attends to births in the hospital, the birthing center, and the home. Most of these births (94%) are in the hospital.[76] Nurse-midwives practice in collaboration with physicians and are skilled at risk screening to make referrals to a physician when

TABLE 17-1

Classification of Maternal Circumstance by Number of Pregnancies, Live Births, and Period During the Childbearing Year

Term	Definition
Nullipara	A woman who has not completed a pregnancy beyond 20 wk of gestation. She may or may not have been pregnant or have had an abortion or spontaneous miscarriage.
Primipara	A woman who has had one delivery beyond 20 wk of gestation.
Multipara	A woman who has delivered two or more pregnancies beyond 20 wk of gestation, regardless of whether the fetuses were born live or stillborn (not the number of fetuses delivered).
Grand multipara	A woman who has carried six or more pregnancies to a viable stage.
Nulligravida	A woman who is not now or who never has been pregnant.
Primigravida	A woman who has been pregnant once, regardless of outcome.
Multigravida	A woman who has had more than one pregnancy, regardless of the outcome. The number represents the number of pregnancies.
Postpartum	The period after childbirth, usually noted as the first 3-6 mo after birth.
Puerpera	Puerpera refers to a woman who has just delivered. The puerperal period is from the end of labor until the uterus returns to prepregnancy size, generally from 3-6 wk postpartum.
Gestation	Duration of the pregnancy, usually 280 days, or 40 wk, marked from the first day of the last menstrual period.
Trimester	Division of weeks of pregnancy: first trimester, 1-13; second, 14-27; third, 28-40.
EDC, EDD	"Expected date of confinement" (EDC) is an old-fashioned term indicating the date that a woman was expected to deliver and be confined. A more modern term, estimated date of delivery (EDD), is now commonly used.
Parturient	A woman in labor.
Preterm labor	Labor that starts after the twentieth but before the thirty-seventh week.
Term labor	Labor initiated after the thirty-seventh week of pregnancy but before the forty-second week.
Post-term, postdates	Post-term or postdate is defined as a pregnancy that extends to 42 wk and beyond.

needed. They provide prenatal care, labor and delivery assistance, postpartum care, well-woman gynecology, normal newborn care, and family planning. They practice within the medical model but are less interventionist and more aligned with conservative care models than allopathic physicians.

An obstetrician is a physician who has specialized in the management of pregnancy, labor, and postpartum care. He or she can manage all types of pregnancies; some may have subspecialty training in high-risk pregnancies. Perinatologists are obstetricians specializing in high-risk care.

Family practice physicians also attend deliveries and provide prenatal care but do not manage high-risk pregnancies.

REFERRALS TO THE PHYSICIAN OR MIDWIFE. Table 17-2 lists some common prenatal and postnatal conditions and their corresponding symptoms and signs. The signs may not be available to the PT, as in the case of medically ordered diagnostic test results. The table lists some of the more likely conditions that a PT working in an outpatient setting might encounter in the prenatal and postnatal population that necessitate communication with the obstetric caregiver.

Referral to a Women's Health Specialist

Specialist certification has recently been developed by the American Physical Therapy Association (APTA) Section on Women's Health. The specialist certification program was established to provide formal recognition for PTs with advanced clinical knowledge, experience, and skills as a women's health certified specialist (WCS) to assist consumers and the health care community in identifying these PTs. Coordination of this program is provided by the American Board of Physical Therapy Specialties (ABPTS).

Common referrals to women's health PTs are listed in Table 17-3. See Appendix 17-2 for an additional list of clinician resources.

Precautionary Notes for Examination and Treatment

Restrictions guide the PT when planning and administering an examination of obstetric patients. These constraints may impede standard physical therapy procedures, and accommodations must be made accordingly. Pregnant women should avoid the following:

- Positions that involve abdominal compression in mid to late pregnancy (e.g., flat prone lying); largely related to maternal comfort and requirement of a level examination surface[167]
- Positions that maintain the supine position for longer than a few minutes after the fourth month of pregnancy; concerns about supine hypotension syndrome[43,157]
- Activities that strain the pelvic floor and abdominal muscles; risk of prolapse, incontinence, and diastasis recti abdominis
- Positions that involve rapid uncontrolled bouncing or swinging movements; balance concerns
- Positions that encourage vigorous stretching of hip adductors; concern for pubic symphysis integrity[167]
- Overheating; fetal concerns related to increased maternal core temperature[67]
- Deep heat modalities or electrical stimulation over the trunk[25,166,167]

These restrictions are lifted once the mother has delivered. Consequently, most exercise positions and physical agents can be used for treatment in the postpartum period. Lactation may result in breast tenderness, especially early in the postpartum period, and this may interfere with comfortable prone lying.

TABLE 17-2

Screening for Common Conditions of Pregnancy and Postpartum Period that Warrant Communication with Midwife or Physician

Condition	Symptoms	Sign or Positive Test Result
Preeclampsia	Headache, blurred vision	Edema (sudden onset, may be global), high blood pressure, proteinuria
Pregnancy-induced hypertension	Headache, blurred vision*	High blood pressure
Ectopic pregnancy	Severe lower abdominal pain,* dizziness or lightheadedness, nausea	Blood tests for progesterone and human chorionic gonadotropin levels; ultrasonography
Abruptio placentae	Severe lower abdominal pain,* vaginal bleeding	Positive ultrasonography
Fetal distress or demise	Decreased fetal movement*	Positive nonstress test or ultrasonography
Osteoporosis of pregnancy	Pain in hip or low back, pain with weight bearing	Empty or spasm end-feel in hip flexion; loss of height
Placenta previa	Vaginal bleeding*	Positive ultrasonography (US)
Retained placenta	Increased postpartum bleeding*	Uterine tenderness to palpation uterine cramping, pelvic pain
Mastitis	Localized breast tenderness	Localized breast redness, edema; fever may be present
Urinary tract infection		
Cystitis	Pain or burning, frequency or urgency of urine, suprapubic pain	Positive urine culture or urinalysis
Acute pyelonephritis	Flank pain, fever, chills, malaise; may have frequency or urgency	Positive urine culture or urinalysis; serum leukocytosis
Deep venous thrombosis	Localized calf, popliteal; or anterior thigh or groin pain; calf or lower extremity swelling; pitting edema*	Well's clinical decision rule for DVT score; D-dimer blood test; Doppler duplex US

*An urgent referral back to the care provider is warranted.
Wells P, Anderson DR, Bormanis J, et al. Value of assessment of pretest probability of deep-vein thrombosis in clinical management. *Lancet* 350:1795-1798, 1997.

TABLE 17-3

Common Referrals to a Women's Health Physical Therapist

Condition	Symptom	Sign or Positive Test Result
Anal and urinary incontinence; urinary urgency	Urinary, fecal leakage, staining, uncontrolled gas	Unable to stop urine flow or hold urine for 2 hr
Pubic symphysis pain	Pain in pubic symphysis pre- or postpartum	Exquisitely tender pubic symphysis; separation on radiograph >10 mm
Sacroiliac pain	Pain in sacroiliac joint (SIJ) pre- or postpartum	Positive pelvic pain provocation (4P), Faber test, active straight leg test
Rib pain	Pain in rib cage with trunk movement on inspiration, expiration	Reproduction of pain at costotransverse or costovertebral joint
Low back pain in pregnancy or postpartum	Pain in low back	Positive long dorsal ligament pain, pain on palpation
Diastasis recti abdominis (DR)	Bulging or separation of recti muscles	Positive DR test >2 cm (or two fingertips)
Pelvic floor muscle tenderness or pain	Pelvic pain, painful intercourse, pain with gynecologic examination	Tenderness on internal examination, palpation of pelvic floor muscles
Pelvic floor muscle weakness	Urinary frequency, urgency, incontinence, prolapsed pelvic organs	Positive leakage with cough, sneeze, laugh, lifting; inability to hold pelvic floor muscles for 5 sec during digital vaginal muscle test
Postpartum neuromusculoskeletal injury	Neurologic loss; SIJ, pubic symphysis injury (e.g., separation); coccyx fracture or dislocation	Muscle weakness in lower extremities; pain on palpation of coccyx, SIJ, pubic symphysis; positive radiographic findings; positive provocation tests

Adapted from Vleeming A, Albert HB, Ostgaard HC, et al: European guidelines for the diagnosis and treatment of pelvic girdle pain, *Eur Spine J* 17:794-819, 2008.

Modifications to the History and Physical Examination

HISTORY. A few additions to a standard subjective examination for musculoskeletal symptoms will ensure patient and fetal safety and assist the PT in making a physical therapy diagnosis. Special questions for the pregnant patient are listed in Table 17-4. Special questions for the postpartum patient are listed in Table 17-5.

PHYSICAL EXAMINATION. In addition to an awareness of the normal anatomic and physiologic changes occurring in the pregnant and postpartum woman, PTs must also consider alterations in

TABLE 17-4

History Taking of the Pregnant Patient

Special Questions	Ramifications
Any complications with this pregnancy (e.g., uterine bleeding, premature contractions, incompetent cervix, pregnancy-induced hypertension, preeclampsia, or other need for special tests or bed rest)?	A positive response may alter the rigor of the physical examination and any exercise prescription given by the PT and may necessitate monitoring of vital signs and other signs and symptoms with each visit.
Any complications with a previous pregnancy or delivery that is placing you at high risk now? Were you considered high risk in a previous pregnancy?	For example, preterm labor in one pregnancy places a woman at risk for a similar outcome in subsequent pregnancies. Monitoring a woman for signs of preterm labor should occur with each visit.
Did you have any of your current musculoskeletal symptoms during a previous pregnancy and, if so, what was done for them? Was the treatment successful?	This information can aid the PT in treatment planning.
What medications are currently being taken and what medications did you stop because of your pregnancy?	Medications such as nonsteroidal anti-inflammatory drugs, antidepressants, and migraine prescriptions that are contraindicated in pregnancy can affect symptoms of the musculoskeletal system and a patient's pain perception and affect.
Are you currently having any urinary or anal incontinence?	Recognition of this condition will aid the PT and patient in treatment before and after delivery.

From Boissonnault JS, Bookhout MM: Course notes for physical therapy management of musculoskeletal dysfunction in the pregnant client, 2008; and Bookhout MM, Boissonnault WG: Physical therapy management of musculoskeletal disorders during pregnancy. In Wilder E, ed: *Obstetric and gynecological physical therapy: clinics in physical therapy*, New York, 1988, Churchill Livingstone, pp. 17-62.

TABLE 17-5

History Taking of the Postpartum Patient

Special Questions	Ramifications
Were you on bed rest during pregnancy? If so, for how long?	Debilitation may have resulted from prolonged bed rest and may necessitate treatment or modifications.
Did any of the following occur during delivery: regional anesthetic injection; forceps or vacuum extraction; episiotomy or tears of the perineum; cesarean?	Specific tissues may be affected by these procedures or occurrences and may necessitate treatment by or referral to a PT with training in women's health.
Do you now have symptoms of urinary or anal incontinence or organ prolapse?	Referral to a PT with training in rehabilitation of the pelvic floor would be appropriate.
Did you have your current symptoms during your pregnancy or after a previous pregnancy and, if so, was there any treatment that was successful in ameliorating these symptoms?	A positive response may assist in determining cause, interventions, and prognosis.

From Boissonnault JS, Bookhout MM: Course notes for physical therapy management of musculoskeletal dysfunction in the pregnant client, 2008; and Bookhout MM, Boissonnault WG: Physical therapy management of musculoskeletal disorders during pregnancy. In Wilder E, ed: *Obstetric and gynecological physical therapy: clinics in physical therapy*, New York, 1988, Churchill Livingstone, pp. 17-62.

positioning for examination and treatment of this population. Supine hypotension syndrome, which occurs in approximately 10% of the pregnant population, can occur when women in the second half of pregnancy lie supine, compressing returning blood flow by the inferior vena cava,[43,157] which can also affect the aorta.[136] These women do not have adequate collateral circulation to the brain to avoid symptoms of shock,[105] resulting in nausea, bradycardia, and syncope.[43]

It is important for PTs to follow accepted medical guidelines regarding the positioning of pregnant women during the second half of pregnancy. Although only a small percentage of women have overt signs of distress during supine lying, some research has shown that pregnant women have decreased cardiac output as a result of caval and aortic occlusion, with a subsequent decrease in uterine blood flow.[3,136] The American College of Obstetricians and Gynecologists discourages exercise in the supine position in the second and third trimesters of pregnancy.[3] Extrapolation of these guidelines to PT practice infers avoidance of prolonged supine lying during examination and treatment, as well as in exercise classes and home exercise sessions. Use of the supine position for brief palpation and treatment is sometimes necessary, but practices that require longer supine positioning should be performed with the women turned 30 degrees to the left, supported with pillows or cushions under the right side.[105,157] This positioning is sufficient to shift the uterus to the left and relieve caval occlusion.

Modifications to examination and treatment in prone lying become necessary once the gravid uterus rises above the brim of the pelvis (12 to 16 weeks of gestation). Placing a pillow above or below the baby to create a nest for the belly or using an adaptive cushion system both work well for some women until late pregnancy. Women may become nauseated in prone lying, even with these modifications. Mobilization tables with a cutout for the gravid uterus are available in some locations. If prone lying is not possible, almost all examination and treatment techniques can be adapted to a sitting, side-lying, or four-point position.

Medications: Pregnancy and Lactation

Many prescription and some over-the-counter (OTC) medications are contraindicated in pregnancy because of the risk to the fetus or the mother. Many texts are available to assist health professionals' decision making related to prescription drugs. Patients often take OTC medications or herbal remedies without their physician's knowledge. If the PT discovers such use, an awareness of any safety issues regarding these substances helps determine whether communication to the obstetric caregiver is warranted. Table 17-6 presents a list of the most common OTC medications used during pregnancy and by the lactating woman after birth. In general, a nursing mother who needs medication should be encouraged to take any OTC medication 30 to 60 minutes after nursing and 3 to 4 hours before the next feeding.[48] In general, herbal remedies are not proven to be safe during pregnancy, so their use is discouraged.[43] PTs are also encouraged to visit the U.S. Food and Drug Administration (FDA) website (www.fda.gov) and to be cognizant of the FDA categories for medications and drugs in pregnancy. A brief explanation of the FDA categories follows:

- Category A: Controlled studies in human beings have demonstrated no fetal risks.
- Category B: Animal studies indicate no fetal risks (no human studies are available). It also can mean that adverse effects have occurred in some animal studies but not in well-controlled human studies.
- Category C: No adequate human or animal studies, or there are no human studies to substantiate negative animal studies. Risks cannot be ruled out in humans.
- Category D: Evidence to indicate fetal risk, but benefits are thought to outweigh these risks.
- Category X: Drugs contraindicated in human pregnancy. Fetal risks outweigh any potential benefits.

Medical Diagnostic Challenges

Diagnostic Imaging

RADIOGRAPHY. Plain films should be avoided during the first trimester, and overall fetal x-ray exposure should be limited because of the risk of malformation with fetal exposure to more than 0.015 Gy (1.5 rad).[56] The total risk of fetal malformation is increased 1% with exposure to more than 0.1 Gy (10 rad). Abdominal lead shields will reduce the fetal radiation exposure to right-angle scatter by approximately 0.01 mGy (1 mrad), except in filming the lumbar spines and myelography, which should be especially avoided during the first trimester.[56] Standard x-ray films of the thoracic and lumbar spines will expose the fetus to 5 mGy (500 mrad) and 10 mGy (1000 mrad), respectively. Plain films are not an absolute contraindication after the first trimester and may be needed for diagnosis. A trauma series of an extremity, skull, or rib series delivers low doses to the fetus because of the distance from the screened area. A single-view pyelogram can locate a urolithiasis or other urinary obstruction that cannot be proved by ultrasound.[43]

COMPUTED TOMOGRAPHY SCAN. Computed tomography (CT) scans taken of the head and neck expose the fetus to the same minimal dose of radiation as a plain radiograph of the skull and cervical spine.[55] CT is commonly used when rapid diagnosis is needed to differentiate medical and surgical management. Chen and colleagues,[30] in a recently published evidenced-based guideline for CT and magnetic resonance imaging (MRI) in pregnancy and lactation, have suggested that CT studies are not recommended in any trimester of pregnancy, mostly because of the risk of carcinogenesis in the fetus.[30]

MAGNETIC RESONANCE IMAGING. MRI is believed to be safe in pregnancy and is considered low risk. However, MRI is not recommended for elective studies or for use in the first trimester.[30] MRI can be used in pregnancy to diagnose arteriovenous malformations, nervous system abnormalities, spinal cord diseases, spine pathology, and demyelinating diseases. MRI is the preferred method of imaging the thoracic and lumbar regions when considering maternal spinal pathology because there is believed to be little or no effect on the fetus.[56]

DIAGNOSTIC ULTRASOUND. Diagnostic ultrasound has been in existence since the late 1950s and is considered safe.[121] The sound waves are delivered at a high frequency, 3.5 to 5 MHz for transabdominal and 5 to 7.5 MHz for transvaginal transducers. Increased frequency will give a better resolution but less tissue penetration.[132] Diagnostic ultrasound is frequently used to determine fetal age and well-being, position, fetal cardiac activity, placenta placement, and amount of amniotic fluid. It is not currently recommended by the American College of Obstetricians and Gynecologists in routine low-risk pregnancies.[43]

In 1992, obstetric ultrasonography devices were outfitted with video displays that provided the diagnostician with indications of any ultrasound-induced bioeffects. The two effects of potential concern are (1) the thermal index, which indicates ultrasound-induced tissue heating, and (2) the mechanical index, which indicates inertial cavitation in body fluids and tissues. The concern with ultrasonography is in the third trimester, when the fetus becomes somewhat warmer than the mother's core temperature. If the mother is febrile, her core temperature will rise, and diagnostic ultrasound may be contraindicated.[121]

Laboratory Tests

In pregnancy, the intravascular volume in the blood results in dilutional anemia. Although there is an elevated erythropoietin level, which will lead to a compensatory increase in total red cell mass, some anemia is never fully corrected. There is a modest increase in white blood cell count during pregnancy and a marked elevation during labor and immediately after delivery. Pregnancy is a hypercoagulable state, and this increase protects the mother from too much blood loss at delivery but also enhances the risk of thromboembolism fivefold.[23,132]

A variety of blood tests are routinely performed in pregnancy. The most common are listed in Table 17-7.

CHORIONIC VILLUS SAMPLING. Chorionic villus sampling (CVS) is an early detection test of genetic disorders that can be performed at 10 to 13 weeks of gestation and quickly provide results. This ultrasound-guided procedure removes some of the placental villi through the cervix, abdominal wall, or vagina. The chance of miscarriage is 1% to 2%.[132]

TABLE 17-6

Over-the-Counter Medications and Herbal Remedies for Pregnant and Lactating Women

Name of Drug	FDA Category	Recommendation in Pregnancy	Recommendation for Lactating Women	Negative Side Effects
Aspirin	D	Generally not recommended in pregnancy, especially in third trimester	Not recommended but may be taken in normal doses if breast-feeding delayed for a few hours after ingestion; ibuprofen preferred to aspirin use in lactating women	In third trimester, >100 mg can lead to maternal and fetal platelet disorders, additional fetal and maternal complications; postpartum concerns are similar
Acetaminophen	B	Recommended pain reliever in pregnancy	Recommended pain reliever during lactation	None
NSAID	B in first and second trimesters, D in third trimester	Not recommended during pregnancy	Ibuprofen is recommended NSAID during lactation; naproxen to be avoided (long acting)	Concerns about fetal complications in pregnancy as seen with aspirin, but not well studied; naproxen may cause bleeding problems, gastrointestinal upset in neonate from breast milk
Antacids	B	General usage approved; prolonged use should be checked with physician or midwife	Safe to use in lactating women	Potential toxicity if used long term in pregnancy
Antihistamines	Chlorpheniramine, B	Some OTC versions found in cold medications acceptable for use during pregnancy; chlorpheniramine is antihistamine of choice in pregnancy	Less sedating agents preferred; recommended to avoid breast-feeding for a few hours after ingestion	No large studies have shown ill effects on fetus or mother in pregnancy; in postpartum period, sedating effects on infants with older, sedating antihistamines; some concern about inhibition of lactation
Decongestants	Pseudoephedrine hydrochloride, B	Discouraged in pregnancy, but based on little research; pseudoephedrine hydrochloride is oral decongestant of choice	Nasal spray recommended over oral route	In pregnancy, may cause fetal tachycardia, increased fetal activity; in postpartum period, may cause infant irritability and suppress lactation
Laxatives	Lactulose, magnesium sulfate, B; docusate, docusate sodium, mineral oil, C	Mineral oil may interfere with absorption of fat-soluble vitamins; castor oil's irritant effects may induce premature labor	Avoid products containing aloe, cascara, anthraquinone, or phenolphthalein in lactating women; bulking agents safe, as are stool softeners such as docusate	Laxative effect on breast-fed infant
Antidiarrheals	Kaolin-pectin, loperamide, B	Kaolin-pectin products are preferred to other antidiarrheals; loperamide not well studied	Kaolin-pectin products safe, preferred to other antidiarrheals	Those with salicylates contraindicated because of aspirin-like effects

FDA, U.S. Food and Drug Administration; *NSAID*, nonsteroidal anti-inflammatory drug.
Adapted from Anderson PO, Knoben JE, Troutman WG: *Handbook of clinical drug data*, 10th ed, New York, 2002, McGraw-Hill; Cunningham FG, Leveno KJ, Bloom SL, et al: *Williams obstetrics*, 22nd ed, New York, 2005, McGraw-Hill; Lawrence RM: *The breast and the physiology of lactation*. In Creasy RK, Resnick RR, eds: *Creasy and Resnik's maternal fetal medicine, principles and practice*, 6th ed, Philadelphia, 2009, WB Saunders; *Drug facts and comparisons: pocket version 2009*, St. Louis, 2010, Mosby; and Das BP, Joshi M, Pant CR: An overview of over the counter drugs in pregnancy and lactation. *Kathmandu U Med J (KUMJ)* 4;545-551, 2006.

AMNIOCENTESIS. Amniocentesis tests for genetic disorders and abnormalities in growth patterns and is usually performed after 15 weeks of gestation. A physician inserts a hollow needle into the amniotic sac and withdraws fluid while being guided simultaneously by abdominal ultrasound. There is a 1 in 270 chance of a spontaneous miscarriage caused by the procedure. Consequently, amniocentesis is used for women older than 35 years and those with high-risk pregnancies.[43,132]

GLUCOSE TESTING. Screening and diagnosis of diabetes in pregnancy are done by using a glucose tolerance test. A 100-g dose of oral glucose is ingested and blood levels are measured every hour for 3 hours. A diagnosis of gestational diabetes is made when any two values in Table 17-8 are met or exceeded.

Common Medical Conditions and Symptoms of Pregnant and Postpartum Women

Table 17-9 presents an overview of common medical conditions and symptoms of pregnancy.

Differentiating Between High-Risk and Low-Risk Pregnancy

A high-risk pregnancy is distinguished by any fetal or maternal condition that can adversely affect the successful outcome of the pregnancy, often resulting in premature infants. In 2004, in the United States, more than 500,000 infants were born prematurely at a rate of 12.5%.[74] By identifying pregnancies that are

TABLE 17-7

Common Tests and Procedures in Pregnancy

Gestational Stage (wk)	Test	Indication/Reason for Test
4-8	Transvaginal ultrasound	High-risk pregnancy, early diagnosis of multiple pregnancies
4; first prenatal visit	Blood screening	Hematocrit, blood group, Rh, antibody, rubella status, syphilis, hepatitis B surface antigen, human immunodeficiency virus
Every prenatal visit	Urinalysis, urine culture	Protein and glucose levels
10-12	Chorionic villus sampling	Placental tissue tested for chromosomal and genetic information
16-18	Amniocentesis	Amniotic fluid tested for chromosomal and genetic disorders
16-18	Alpha-fetoprotein	Determine risk for neural tube disorder, Down syndrome
16-18	Triple screening	Alpha-fetoprotein, human chorionic gonadotropin, unconjugated estriol levels to screen for Down syndrome
16-18	Quadruple screening	Same as triple screening for Down syndrome with addition of inhibin A, protein produced by placenta and ovaries; false-positive rate lower than triple screening
18-20	Abdominal ultrasound	Measure fetal growth, check for placental position, congenital anomalies
24-28	Glucose screening	Blood test for gestational diabetes
Only when medically indicated	Radiography	Determining fractures
35-37	Group B streptococcus bacteria screening	To prevent passing it from mother to baby during delivery

Data from Cunningham FG, Leveno KJ, Bloom SL, et al: *Williams obstetrics*, 22nd ed, New York, 2001, McGraw-Hill; and Hayman B: *A miracle in the making,* Chicago, 2000, Budlong Press.

TABLE 17-8

Gestational Diabetes: Diagnostic Values

Diagnostic 100-g Oral Glucose Tolerance Test	Plasma Glucose Level (mg/dL)*
Fasting	105
1 hr	190
2 hr	165
3 hr	145

*National Diabetes Data Group conversion.
Adapted from Lucas MJ: Diabetes complicating pregnancy, *Obstet Gynecol Clin North Am* 28:513-536, 2001.

high risk, extra attention is given to those mothers who need the most medical care. Preexisting maternal conditions such as heart and lung disease, diabetes, chronic illness, and disability can be identified before conception or within the first trimester and managed so that mortality and morbidity rates for the mother and child are decreased. Other women may start with a low-risk pregnancy but have complications develop (e.g., preeclampsia, premature labor, or multiple gestation) that can threaten the outcome of the pregnancy.[113]

Bed rest is prescribed for 18.2% of high-risk pregnant women in the United States,[113] which is more than 1 million U.S. women who are experiencing pregnancy complications.[110,111] Bed rest may be prescribed for preterm labor, premature rupture of membranes, amniotic fluid volume disorders, placental abnormalities, pregnancy-induced hypertension,[110-112] pulmonary edema, hyperemesis gravidarum, cardiomyopathy, and a multifetal pregnancy.[166]

Examinations of the high-risk pregnant woman must assess the patient within the physical restrictions set by her primary practitioner, and examination positions should be adapted to these restrictions. Her home setup and support available should be part of the overall PT assessment.

The physiologic effects of bed rest have been studied by aerospace scientists who have used it as a model for weightlessness in space. Bed rest results in a shift in body fluids toward the head, and reduced weight bearing rapidly induces changes in every physiologic system.[112] In addition, psychological changes result from isolation and reduced kinesthetic and sensory stimuli.[111]

Classifications of bed rest activity limitations are listed in Table 17-10.[64]

Overview of Physiologic and Anatomic Changes Associated with Pregnancy

The dynamic process of pregnancy changes the woman's anatomy and physiology, with changes occurring in every system. The pregnant woman's body changes internally and externally as she adjusts to fetal growth. Table 17-11 presents an overview of these anatomic and physiologic changes by gestational month. Table 17-12 presents an overview of changes during pregnancy categorized by body system. Most of the changes listed in these tables are covered in more detail throughout the chapter.

Psychosocial Issues in Pregnancy and the Postpartum Period

The periods before and after childbirth are ones of great transition and adjustment for the pregnant woman and her family. PTs who commonly work with women during this life event are

TABLE 17-9
Common Medical Conditions and Symptoms of Pregnancy*

Condition	Symptom and Cause
Backache	Reported by 50% to 90% of pregnant women; can be related to muscles, joints, or ligaments
Breast tenderness	Tingling and tenderness experienced in early pregnancy; breast size can increase by 500-800 g; veins become visible, nipples enlarge
Carpal tunnel syndrome	Increased fluid volume in wrist causes compression of median nerve, resulting in wrist and hand pain, sensation change
Constipation	Decreased elimination from decreased motility of small bowel, increased ingestion of iron; muscular relaxation of colon, with increased absorption of water
Edema	Increased weight, gravity, progesterone cause venous engorgement, swelling
Fainting	Vasodilation in early pregnancy, uterine pressure on inferior vena cava in late pregnancy
Fatigue	Increase in fatigue, excessive sleep in early pregnancy may be caused by progesterone; usually subsides by fourth month of pregnancy
Headache	Frequent symptom in early pregnancy that decreases by midpregnancy; cause usually not demonstrated; severe headaches in later pregnancy may be related to hypertensive disorders
Heartburn	Common symptom caused by gastric reflux into lower esophagus, relaxation of lower esophageal sphincter, upward displacement and compression of stomach by the uterus
Hemorrhoids	Varicosities of rectal veins related to increased pressure by obstruction of venous return of expanding uterus, with tendency toward constipation
Insomnia	Increase in physical discomfort with increasing pregnancy; anxiety, vivid dreams may decrease sleep
Muscle cramps	Increased pressure of the expanding uterus on lower extremity nerves may cause ischemia
Nausea, vomiting	Morning sickness often starts after the first 6 wk of pregnancy; many theories about cause
Urinary frequency	Pressure of uterus on bladder as pregnancy progresses
Varicosities of lower extremities, vulva, or rectum	Increased blood volume, pressure of uterus on pelvic veins, swelling of veins, causing regurgitation

*Adapted from references 43, 134, 137, 142, 145, and 149.

TABLE 17-10
Activity Restrictions for Pregnant Women on Bed Rest

Limitations of Activity	Toileting	Positions for Eating
Ad lib activity	No restrictions	No restrictions
Bed rest with bathroom privileges	May use toilet or bedside commode; shower in a shower chair	Limited sitting
Strict bed rest; no upright activity	Bedpan for all toileting; bed bath	Woman may prop herself up on elbow or elevate head of bed 30-45 degrees for eating
Strict bed rest in Trendelenburg position, head of bed 15 degrees lower than foot of bed; no upright activity	Bedpan for toileting; bed bath	May roll side to side; may prop herself on elbow for eating

From Frahm J, Welsh RA: Physical therapy management of the high-risk antepartum patient, *Clin Management* 9:4:15, 1989.

familiar with the signs of the emotional work that women do during this time in their lives. Coombes and Darken[41] have suggested that "Each trimester of pregnancy can generally be related to one of three psychological states: acknowledgment, consolidation and preparation" and that "A woman's mechanisms of coping throughout each stage are dependent upon such variables as her physical condition, social and family support networks, the reaction evoked in the woman by her pregnancy, and the significance she attaches to it." Anxiety, insecurity, joy and elation, stress, and irritability are all emotions or experiences likely to surface in pregnant and postpartum women. Any PT treating or examining women during the childbearing years needs to be aware of the tremendous emotional challenges these women face.

The emotional status and childbirth practices of women are also influenced by culture and ethnicity. Multiple resources exist in today's literature that introduce the health care provider to cultural beliefs and practices common during pregnancy, childbirth, and the postpartum period.*

Gaining perspective on a particular woman's emotional health necessitates an awareness of her cultural belief system. See Chapter 3 for additional information on diversity and multiculturalism.

*References 69, 97, 99, 103, 140, and 164.

TABLE 17-11

Overview of Anatomy and Physiology During Pregnancy

Month	Maternal and Physiologic Changes	Anatomic Changes
1	Rise in temperature, vomiting, fatigue, breast discomfort, end of menses	Ovulation, fertilization, implantation of ovum, thickening of uterine lining from increased estrogen and progesterone
2	Positive pregnancy test; nausea subsiding; profuse, thick vaginal discharge; breast enlargement	Mucus plug forming in cervix; pressure on bladder with frequency of urination
3	Colostrum leaking from breasts; nausea subsiding; bladder pressure less	Placenta completely formed and secreting estrogen; uterine cavity filled; uterus rising from pelvic cavity into abdomen
4	Abdominal appearance of pregnancy; backache	Blood volume increasing; fundus halfway between symphysis and umbilicus
5	Fetal movement, called quickening	Placenta covers half of uterine wall
6	Stretch marks; linea nigra appears; possible chloasma (around eyes); period of greatest weight gain starts	Height of fundus at umbilicus; period of lowest hemoglobin level
7	Braxton Hicks contractions palpable; intermittent uterine contractions	Blood volume highest
8	Braxton Hicks contractions stronger; stretch marks more pronounced; backache possible	Longitudinal stretching of uterus
9	Umbilicus protrudes; shortness of breath, varicosities, swelling; descent of fetal head; lightening (baby drops); easier breathing; urinary frequency	Fundus just under diaphragm (before lightening); lightening more common in primiparas but can occur in multiparas; may drop just before birth

From Stephenson RG, O'Connor LJ: *Obstetric and gynecologic care in physical therapy,* 2nd ed, Thorofare, NJ, 2000, Slack.

TABLE 17-12

Overview of Pregnancy Changes by Function

Function	Change
Gastrointestinal	Nausea and vomiting may occur in early pregnancy, intestinal motility slows, constipation can develop.
Urogenital	Glomerular filtration rate increases by 50%, renal function increases with increased urinary output, reproductive organs hypertrophy from edema and increased vascularity.
Cardiovascular	Blood volume increases 40%-50%; stroke volume increases 20%-40% in midpregnancy, then decreases after 28-32 wk until term; resting heart rate increases average of 20 beats/min throughout pregnancy; cardiac output increases at wk 12, peaks at 28-32 wk.
Endocrine	Adrenal, thyroid, parathyroid, and pituitary glands enlarge; hormones increase to support the pregnancy and placenta and to prepare mother's body for labor; hormones cause generalized increase in joint laxity and return to prepregnant values by 3-6 mo postpartum.
Respiratory	Oxygen consumption increases by 18%, carbon dioxide output increases, tidal volume increases 40%, vital capacity increases 5%, residual volume decreases 20%, ventilation increases up to 40%, diaphragm elevates, central part flattens; breathing is more costal than abdominal.
Metabolic	Increased demand for tissue growth; insulin level is elevated from plasma expansion and blood glucose level is reduced for a given insulin load; renal threshold for glucose drops because of increased glomerular filtration rate; fats and minerals are stored for maternal use; increase in sodium and water retention.
Musculoskeletal	Diaphragm rises approximately 4 cm, rib cage circumference increases 6 cm, increasing the subcostal angle appreciably, and the transverse diameter increases by 2 cm; rectus muscles may separate and form a diastasis; posture changes caused by change in center of gravity, weight gain, and decrease in spinal curves.
Neurologic	Swelling and increased fluid volume can cause nerve compression at the thoracic outlet, wrists, or groin (brachial plexus, median nerve, lateral femoral cutaneous nerves, respectively).
Integumentary	Pigmentation may increase around eyes, face, linea alba, areolas; spider nevi, telangiectasia, and palmar erythema appear because of increase in estrogen level and capillary dilations; striae gravidarum (stretch marks) appear; increases in sweating, hirsutism, and varices may appear but resolve postpartum.
Psychiatric	Pregnancy-related depression and postpartum depression may occur.

Data from Crapo RO: Normal cardiopulmonary physiology during pregnancy, *Clin Obstet Gynecol* 39:3-16, 1996; and Cunningham FG, Gant NF, Leveno KJ, et al: *Williams Obstetrics,* 22nd ed, New York, 2005, McGraw-Hill.

Although a certain amount of emotional uncertainty and stress is normal during pregnancy, some studies have demonstrated that undue stress and high job strain (high demand, low control) correlate with preterm delivery, pregnancy-induced hypertension, and preeclampsia.[98,114] The PT may choose to alert the medical care provider if patients admit to being under a great deal of stress or when their conversations indicate very high-stress lives; that is, this should signal a red flag for the PT involved in the care of such patients.

The following sections outline two additional issues facing pregnant and postpartum women in the psychosocial realm—domestic violence in pregnancy and prenatal and postnatal depression.

Domestic Violence in Pregnancy

Domestic violence, or battering, may be defined as "A pattern of physical, psychological, or sexual abuse between intimate partners."[31] The abuse is often episodic and chronic and can cause both physical and psychological injury.[31] The incidence of domestic violence in pregnancy is estimated to be approximately 10%, with a range of 4% to 20% reported in the literature, thus making it one of the most common complications of pregnancy.[31,73,116] Battering may begin during pregnancy, although the prevalence of battering is lower in pregnancy than before pregnancy[147]; estimates are that as many as 25% to 45% of women who are victims of domestic violence before pregnancy will continue to experience it during pregnancy.[31,120] Adolescents and unintended pregnancies carry an even greater risk of abuse than intended pregnancies or those begun in adulthood.[73]

Nannini and associates[129] have studied pregnant women hospitalized for assault in pregnancy and found that injury occurred most often to a woman's head, neck, then torso, and finally, her extremities.[129] Pregnant women often experience physical abuse directly to the abdomen.[31,120] Outcome studies on women who have suffered abuse during pregnancy have demonstrated negative outcomes, including preterm labor and birth, antepartum hemorrhage, intrauterine growth retardation, low-birth-weight babies, and perinatal death,[31,79,150] and can include a host of other maternal and fetal complications. Some of these complications (e.g., fetal injury or death, maternal fractures) are a direct result of violent encounters and some are from indirect effects of violence, such as emotional stress or decreased access to health care.[150] Table 17-13 lists potential adverse effects of domestic violence perpetrated during pregnancy.

The clinical presentation is likely to be extremely variable. Patients who are victims of domestic violence may have symptoms directly related to the injury that they have sustained from the violent encounter but will more likely have vague physical and psychological symptoms, such as headache, chronic pelvic pain, sleep disorders, and depression or anxiety.[31] Particularly telling for physical therapy patients is the common denominator of patients seeking care for relatively minor symptoms and those who do not comply with prescribed treatment regimens, although the latter is a scenario that PTs also encounter in the general physical therapy population.

A partner who does not allow a patient to speak for herself, refuses to let the PT interview the patient alone or leave the area during examination or treatment, or in some other way seems overly protective should raise the suspicion of domestic abuse. Every PT should have training in spotting domestic violence and should have a plan of how to question patients regarding abuse and how to offer assistance if such violence is disclosed. Because battering is so common during pregnancy, the primary care PT should consider it a possibility with every pregnant patient seen and should routinely screen for it. Suggestions for specific, direct questions related to abuse detection in pregnancy can be found in many hospital policies and in multiple texts and articles. Examples of such questions include the following:

- Since you have been pregnant, have you been hit, slapped, kicked, or otherwise physically hurt by someone?[31]
- Have you been afraid of a current or former intimate partner during your pregnancy?[79]

TABLE 17-13

Adverse Perinatal Effects Caused by Domestic Abuse of Mother

Direct	Indirect
Abruptio placentae	Elevated maternal stress
Fetal fracture	Isolation of mother
Uterine rupture	Inadequate health care
Rupture of maternal liver	Inadequate nutrition
Rupture of maternal spleen	Substance abuse
Pelvic fracture	Late entry into prenatal care
Antepartum hemorrhage	Unintended pregnancy
Preterm labor, delivery	Lack of breast-feeding
Preterm premature rupture of the membranes	Sexually transmitted disease

Data from Dattel BJ: Domestic violence. In Sanfilippo JS, Smith RP, eds: *Primary care in obstetrics and gynecology: a handbook for clinicians*, New York, 1998, Springer-Verlag, p 216.

Additional information on domestic violence as it applies to the primary care PT, as well as general questions related to abuse detection, are found in Chapter 8.

Perinatal Depression

Perinatal depression has been documented to occur in 5% to 20%[29,57,81,131] of all pregnant and postpartum women, with 3% to 5% of these cases representing major depression per the *Diagnostic and Statistical Manual IV*.[7a,53,57] Josefsson[81] and coworkers[46] have found the prevalence of depressive symptoms during late pregnancy (35 to 36 weeks of gestation) to be 17%, higher than their postpartum prevalence of 13%. Depressive postpartum disorders range from "postpartum blues," which occur in approximately 30% of women, are self-limiting, and typically resolve in 2 to 3 weeks postpartum,[57,62] to postpartum depression and postpartum psychosis. The latter two are more serious conditions and require medical or social intervention to avoid serious ramifications to the family unit. The baby blues appear within the first few postpartum days and are characterized by episodes of crying, mood swings, irritability, and sadness.[62] The cause of the more serious postpartum depression is still unclear, but studies have shown that depression during pregnancy or in a previous postpartum period is often predictive of postpartum depression.[29,57,81] Other factors such as maternal age, parity, prepregnancy history of affective disorders, low socioeconomic status, non-European race, social isolation, and thoughts of death and symptoms of insomnia in the first postpartum month have all been demonstrated in the literature to be predictive of prenatal and postpartum depression.[29,57,81,131]

New-onset abnormalities of autoimmune postpartum thyroid function are said to occur in up to 10% of the population[128] and may account for some postpartum depression. Postpartum thyroiditis is a condition marked by a transient swing between a thyrotoxic phase, with symptoms of fatigue, weight loss, palpitations, and dizziness, followed by a hypothyroid phase, with symptoms of fatigue and weight gain. The thyrotoxic phase is most common at 6 weeks to 6 months postpartum, with the hypothyroid phase following and lasting up to 1 year postpartum.[128] Depression is a common symptom associated with hypothyroidism and has been successfully treated with thyroid hormone therapy.[128] Nader[128] has stated that "Women who present with symptoms [of postpartum thyroiditis including depression] should have a TSH assay performed. High-risk women (i.e., women with a history of postpartum thyroiditis and women with type 1 diabetes) should be screened."[128] The most vulnerable time for development of postpartum depression seems to be within the first 3 months after delivery,[128] with an outside range of 6 to 12 months.[57] It has been shown that postpartum depression can affect the cognitive development of the infant[35] and is theorized to have an effect on a woman's marital relationship, mother-infant relationship, and even survival of the infant.[81] Prenatal depression has been shown to increase the risk of preterm birth, possibly from increased levels of cortisol.[57]

A commonly used validated screening tool for postpartum depression, the Edinburgh Postnatal Depression Scale,[42] is one tool the PT can use to assess for possible postpartum depression. The tool is easily administered in 5 minutes and has demonstrated good specificity and sensitivity.[42,81] A validation study has shown that mothers who score greater then threshold (92.3%) are likely to have a depressive illness of varying severity.[42] The authors warn that the score should not override clinical judgment. Once the screen has been used and a score of more than 10 has been achieved, a referral to medical care is warranted. The tool is simply a screen and does not diagnose depression. The scale indicates how the mother has felt during the previous week; in doubtful cases it may be repeated after 2 weeks. The scale does not detect mothers with anxiety, neuroses, phobias, or personality disorder.[42] The Edinburgh Postnatal Depression Scale is presented in Appendix 17-1.

Postpartum psychosis is a much more serious disorder, occurring in approximately 1 to 2/1000 women and should be treated as a medical emergency.[41] Signs of postpartum psychosis include symptoms of mania and depression. The woman may experience hallucinations and delusions, especially concerning her child, with the disorder placing the woman at risk for suicide and infanticide.[41] This condition usually occurs within the first 2 weeks postpartum and may be related to the hormonal changes mentioned in relation to the postpartum blues.[41] Early recognition and proper treatment are imperative for the safety of the mother and baby.

Additional information on depression related to the primary care PT can be found in Chapters 5 and 8.

Gastrointestinal System

Common gastrointestinal (GI) symptoms during pregnancy include nausea and vomiting, esophageal reflux, intestinal motility, and an increase in the incidence and symptoms of gallbladder disease. Of these, only the gallbladder problems present a diagnostic challenge to the primary care PT; gallbladder symptoms can mimic musculoskeletal dysfunction and pain, and accurate differential diagnosis is helpful in preserving the health of the mother. The other issues interfere with the woman's quality of life, but only in rare cases do they present significant morbidity concerns. Anal incontinence is a very troubling GI symptom but will be covered in the next section of this chapter.

NAUSEA, VOMITING, AND HYPEREMESIS. Nausea is reported to occur in approximately 50% to 80% of pregnancies,[12,43,61,86] with vomiting complicating approximately 40% of pregnancies.[86] In general, these symptoms are confined to the first 16 weeks of pregnancy but occasionally remain throughout the entire 10 lunar months. Women carrying multiple fetuses may have more intense or prolonged symptoms than women carrying one fetus. Vellacott and colleagues[172] have reported that 25% of the pregnant women reporting nausea and vomiting require time off from work because of these symptoms and that almost 50% of employed women cite job inefficiency as a result of this early complication.

Hyperemesis gravidarum, a condition resulting from continued and prolonged vomiting in pregnancy, occurs in 5% or fewer of pregnant women[12] but may require hospitalization and nutritional and fluid support, as well as electrolyte balancing. Hyperemesis gravidarum can result in weight loss, dehydration, acidosis from starvation, alkalosis from loss of hydrochloric acid in vomitus, and hypokalemia.[43] Patients reporting severe vomiting and weight loss should be encouraged to contact their obstetric caregiver or primary care provider if they have not yet seen a midwife, obstetrician, or obstetric family practitioner.

ESOPHAGEAL REFLUX AND HEARTBURN. Fifty percent to 80% of women report heartburn (pyrosis) during pregnancy, with its incidence peaking in the third trimester.[43,61,86] In general, pregnant women are not thought to be at risk for esophagitis or occult esophagitis and stricture and therefore are not candidates for invasive diagnostic studies or aggressive treatment. They are treated for the nuisance and discomfort, with advice on posture (assuming an upright posture and avoiding forward bending activities after meals), reduction in volume but increase in frequency of meals, diet modification (decrease fatty and spicy foods), smoking cessation, and medications such as antacids or acid-suppressing drugs when necessary.

MOTILITY ISSUES AND CONSTIPATION. Whether the GI system in pregnancy slows down or not is a matter of controversy. Minimal and conflicting scientific investigation exists on the matter. Of pregnant women, 10% to 40% experience constipation in pregnancy secondary to decreased intestinal motility and increased absorption of water and sodium.[43,86] When present, symptoms of constipation may be distressing for the pregnant woman and may include abdominal bloating and straining to pass stool, with potential pelvic floor dysfunction exacerbation (prolapse of organs) and hemorrhoids. To ensure that a woman with this problem obtains symptomatic relief, the PT should encourage the woman to report her symptoms to her obstetric caregiver.

GALLBLADDER DISORDERS. Pregnancy increases a woman's risk of cholelithiasis (gallstones),[43,61,141,161] most likely from the following: (1) increased bile production with a concomitant increase in the percentage of cholesterol in the bile and (2) decreased gallbladder emptying time or incomplete emptying.[43,161] Smith[161] has reported a symptomatic incidence of 3% to 4% in pregnant women, with increased parity a significant risk factor.

Symptoms of gallstones include intermittent right upper abdominal quadrant pain referred to the back and scapular areas.

In addition, fatty food intolerance and nausea and vomiting may be present. Because these latter symptoms are common in pregnancy, gallstones may be overlooked as the source of these symptoms. Differential diagnosis to rule out musculoskeletal dysfunction as a source of the upper quadrant symptoms may be necessary.

Ultrasonography is the preferred diagnostic tool for this condition. Confirmed diagnosis may require surgical intervention, especially when acute cholecystitis results.[43] Safe outcomes for mother and fetus have been reported, especially in the second trimester. Laparoscopic cholecystectomy is the procedure now commonly performed.[43]

Urogenital System and Anorectal Issues

Anatomic and hormonal changes during pregnancy place the pregnant woman at risk for both lower and upper urinary tract infections and for urinary incontinence. Events of labor and delivery (the puerperium) place a woman at risk for de novo development of urinary and anal incontinence (inadvertent loss of stool, gas, or rectal mucous) and pelvic organ prolapse. Although PTs are not responsible for the treatment of urogenital infection during pregnancy, they need to recognize the symptoms of such infections (see Chapter 9) and refer the patient to the primary physician or obstetric caregiver. Differentiating signs and symptoms of upper and lower urinary tract infections from symptoms of back or pelvic pain of musculoskeletal origin is a primary function of any PT treating pregnant women.

Pregnant and postpartum women with incontinence symptoms (anal and urinary) and urogenital supportive dysfunction, such as prolapsed uterus, prolapsed bladder (cystocele), or prolapsed rectum (rectocele), should be referred to PTs specializing in this area of practice. The Section on Women's Health, APTA, can assist in locating such specialized practitioners. The primary care PT is in a unique position to screen for these common disorders in postpartum women and should take advantage of the opportunity to improve the quality of life for the women they treat and perhaps prevent additional or continued urogenital dysfunction in later years.

URINARY TRACT INFECTIONS. The frequency of upper (kidney, acute pyelonephritis) and lower (bladder, acute cystitis) urinary tract infections is increased during pregnancy. The anatomic and physiologic changes of pregnancy place the pregnant woman at greater risk for these infections. These changes include dilation of ureters and kidneys, compression of the ureters at the pelvic rim by midpregnancy, and softening of the angle of insertion at the ureterovesical junction. All contribute to vesicoureteral reflux and increased risk of kidney infection.[43,186] Increased glomerular filtration rate, decreased bladder capacity and emptying, decreased drainage of blood and lymph of the bladder, and urinary stasis because of collagenous changes in the urinary tract contribute to increased risk of acute cystitis.[43,125,186]

Pyelonephritis is said to be the most common serious medical complication of pregnancy and remains the leading cause of septic shock during this period.[43] In perhaps as many as 40% of untreated cases of acute cystitis, the infection ascends to the kidneys and results in acute pyelonephritis.[43] Thus, identification and subsequent treatment of both of these entities are imperative for maternal-fetal well-being.

ACUTE CYSTITIS. Acute cystitis occurs in approximately 1% of pregnancies.[186] Symptoms of acute cystitis may include urinary frequency, urinary urgency, suprapubic discomfort or pain, and pain and burning with voiding.[43,186] Referred pain may be experienced over the sacral spine (see Chapter 6). Some of these symptoms are difficult to distinguish from the normal symptoms of pregnancy (frequency and urgency, abdominal discomfort) or from musculoskeletal dysfunction (sacroiliac [SI] joint problems), further complicating differential diagnosis. Medical treatment should be sought and most commonly includes 3-day antimicrobial treatment.[43]

ACUTE PYELONEPHRITIS. Acute pyelonephritis occurs in approximately 2% of pregnancies.[186] Symptoms include flank pain; fever; nausea and vomiting; and, although not in all cases, symptoms of lower urinary tract involvement such as urgency, frequency, and dysuria.[43,186] Percussion over the costovertebral angle usually elicits flank tenderness, but this may also be present with musculoskeletal dysfunction of the lower rib cage in pregnancy and therefore may be diagnostically less than helpful. Pyelonephritis during pregnancy usually requires hospitalization, and suspicions of this condition should be immediately reported to the patient's medical care provider. Women with acute pyelonephritis in pregnancy are at risk for relapse and recurrence,[61] thus warranting continued vigilance of those women who have had such an occurrence.

An interesting aside to urinary tract infections in pregnancy is the apparently rare incidence of sacroiliitis associated with pyelonephritis. Egerman and colleagues[60] have described such a case and review the literature on this infection and "unusual cause[s] of back pain." Recent history of peripartal infection with failure to reduce symptoms of SI dysfunction should lead the PT to consider referral to the primary care provider for further investigation of the pain symptoms.

URINARY INCONTINENCE. Current literature supports the long-held belief that women have an increased incidence of urinary incontinence during pregnancy.[156,182-185] Prevalence rates of self-reported stress urinary incontinence (incontinence resulting from increased intra-abdominal pressure, such as a cough or sneeze) range from 21% to 46%,[156,182-184] with most researchers noting rates between 25% and 46%.[156,182-184] Researchers report prevalence rates of stress incontinence in the general population before pregnancy in the range of 11%[107] to 15%[183] in women who had never been pregnant, which demonstrates an increased prevalence of urinary incontinence during pregnancy over pre-pregnancy rates in nulliparas. Estimates of the prevalence of urinary incontinence (urge and stress incontinence) after birth vary, but, in general, range from 17% to 31%[19,182,184] and include statistics of the numbers of women who have urinary incontinence develop de novo and those whose incontinence began during pregnancy and did not resolve in the postpartum period. Some studies report a decrease in incontinence symptoms in postpartum women whose incontinence began in pregnancy,[169,184] although Viktrup and Lose,[174] in a 12-year follow-up study, have found that symptoms of incontinence fluctuate after delivery and in many women do not resolve in ensuing years.

Clearly, urinary incontinence is an issue affecting many women during and after pregnancy and could easily be screened for by the primary care PT who sees these women incidentally.

ANAL INCONTINENCE. Urinary incontinence has gained more recognition over the past decades, with patients consulting medical practitioners about this problem more readily than in the past. This has not occurred to the same degree with anal incontinence. There has been a significant increase in research dollars spent on the investigation of anal incontinence resulting from labor and delivery, but this has not affected public awareness. Patients rarely volunteer information on involuntary loss of stool, mucous, or gas, even though they often demonstrate profound changes in quality of life. Screening and obtaining treatment for these issues can become part of a primary care PT's common practice with a little background knowledge and the right set of questions to ask the patient. These questions, like those that screen for urinary incontinence, can be incorporated into the health history questionnaire (see Chapters 8 and 9).

The incidence of anal incontinence is much lower than that of urinary incontinence. Postpartum estimates of fecal incontinence range from 4% to 15%.[11,133] Research on the cause of anal incontinence points to pudendal nerve damage or anal sphincter disruption and damage, both occurring during delivery.[49,149] Symptoms may include rectal urgency or urge incontinence of stool or passive or insensitive loss of rectal contents, including stool or gas.[149]

Organ Prolapse Related to Obstetrics

Compared with incontinence, there is very little written or researched in medical literature about postpartum urogenital prolapse. Sapsford and Markwell[149] have briefly discussed postpartum uterine, bladder (cystocele), rectal (rectocele), and intestinal prolapse (enterocele) and the need for pelvic floor rehabilitation to provide support for these entities. Surgical repair is commonly performed for cystocele or rectocele that compromise normal voiding or defecation functions, and hysterectomy is commonly performed for a uterine prolapse that protrudes beyond the introitus (opening of the vaginal vault). Theoretically, the combination of endocrine changes of pregnancy with resultant connective tissue laxity and trauma occurring within the maternal pelvis during fetal descent can result in any one or a combination of these supportive disorders. Mild prolapse of organs often spontaneously resolves by 3 to 6 months postpartum. Moderate prolapse may be given a trial of pelvic floor rehabilitation before surgical options are explored. The pessary, a supportive device, may be another nonsurgical option for women with cystocele or uterine prolapse.

Symptoms of prolapse may include a feeling of incomplete emptying of the bladder or rectum, depending on the organ involved,[149] and rubbing or irritation at the introitus. Patients with uterine prolapse sometimes report aching in the area of the sacrum, possibly because of increased torsion placed on the uterosacral ligament.

Endocrine System

Endocrine system changes during pregnancy occur as a result of physiologic alterations in the secretions of the endocrine glands. This system is extremely sensitive and is vital to the support of a thriving pregnancy. The endocrine system regulates how the body responds to thermal changes. As the pregnant woman's metabolism increases, surplus heat is dissipated by peripheral vasodilation and acceleration of sweating occurs. Consequently, she may frequently experience heat intolerance and exhaustion after minimal activity.[167] The functions of many hormones change during pregnancy, including the action of hormones on the musculoskeletal system. (See Table 17-12 for information on effects of the endocrine system and hormones on the musculoskeletal system.) Certain diseases of the endocrine system are common to pregnancy and, with close medical supervision, can coexist with a successful outcome.

GESTATIONAL DIABETES. Gestational diabetes mellitus (GDM) is defined as carbohydrate intolerance diagnosed during pregnancy, regardless of whether insulin is required for treatment. The development of this disease during pregnancy may be caused by exaggerated physiologic changes in carbohydrate metabolism, which affect 1% to 14% of the population.[4] GDM may also be a maturity onset of type 2 diabetes that is uncovered during pregnancy.[43] There is a 33% to 50% probability of gestational diabetes in subsequent pregnancies and a 50% increased lifetime risk of developing non–insulin-dependent diabetes mellitus.[6,122] Women with GDM and all types of diabetes are at an increased risk of developing hypertensive disorders and preeclampsia and require a cesarean delivery.[6,106] There is additional evidence for long-term obesity and diabetes in the offspring of diabetic mothers.[43]

GDM is associated with an increased risk of congenital malformations, macrosomia (infants large or heavy for gestational age), and perinatal morbidity and death.[122] Large infants can be difficult to deliver and have a greater chance of developing shoulder dystocia with resulting brachial plexus neuropathy from prolonged compression during delivery.

There is controversy regarding the optimal approach to screening for GDM because of the lack of data from well-designed studies.[6,43] Typical protocols call for all pregnant women to be screened for GDM with a 50-g oral glucose load between weeks 24 and 26 of pregnancy. If the blood glucose level is greater than 130 to 140 mg/dL, then a full 3-hour glucose tolerance test with a 100-g oral glucose load follows the initial screening.[106,122]

Women with GDM must strictly monitor and control their blood glucose level through dietary changes during pregnancy, monitor and decrease strenuous work and lifestyle, and have other medications checked with a primary care physician.[6] At the 6-week postpartum checkup, women should have their blood glucose level rechecked.

INSULIN-DEPENDENT DIABETES MELLITUS. Insulin-dependent diabetes mellitus (IDDM) was formerly known as type 1 diabetes mellitus. The risk of malformations in infants of mothers with type 1 diabetes mellitus is two to three times that of the general population.[106] An increased rate of stillborn and macrosomic newborns is also attributed to pregestational diabetes.[106] Management of pregnant women with type 1 diabetes includes treatment with insulin, frequent monitoring of blood glucose levels, diet control, and repeat sonograms to measure for infant size. There is usually a decrease in insulin needed in the third trimester, and hypoglycemia needs to be monitored because fetal loss is associated with a low blood sugar level.[106]

Cesarean sections are performed in 50% to 75% of insulin-treated diabetic mothers.[106] Prophylactic cesarean deliveries are sometimes performed if the fetal weight is estimated to exceed 4500 g. The PT working with this population may be involved with exercise regulation and abdominal rehabilitation after delivery.

NON–INSULIN-DEPENDENT DIABETES MELLITUS. Non-IDDM was previously known as type 2 diabetes mellitus. Type 2 diabetes occurs when there is abnormal insulin secretion and insulin resistance in the target tissues.[43] Type 2 diabetes is more common in women, especially in those with a history of gestational diabetes.[170] Most patients have inherited the disease and are obese. It is speculated that peripheral insulin resistance, which is induced by obesity, leads to beta cell exhaustion.[43] During the postpartum period, the newborn should be monitored for low glucose levels, low blood calcium and magnesium levels, excess of red blood cells, neonatal jaundice, and breathing problems. The mother will likely have a change in her insulin levels after delivery and should be routinely monitored.

EXERCISE FOR PREGNANT WOMEN WITH DIABETES. Control of all forms of diabetes during pregnancy requires home monitoring, diet change, exercise, insulin or other medications, and prenatal care. Pregnant women with diabetes should regularly exercise to enhance insulin sensitivity, decrease cardiovascular risk factors, and increase muscular strength and sense of well-being.[170] Because exercise reduces the amount of insulin necessary for normal blood glucose levels and the effect of exercise on metabolism is complex, the woman with diabetes and her health care practitioner should decide which type of exercise is best.[5,122]

For women with GDM, a program involving cardiovascular conditioning improves glycemic control better than diet control alone.[82] Women with type 1 diabetes should monitor their glucose levels closely, because they are vulnerable to exercise-related hypoglycemia.[43] Exercise levels can be safely increased without fear of fetal distress if, during exercise, the lower body is kept from an excessive weight-bearing load. Consequently, upper extremity exercise is a good choice for pregnant women because as it places little mechanical stress on the trunk region.[43] Jovanovic-Peterson and Peterson[83] have reported that, with upper body cardiovascular training, a decrease in glucose levels becomes apparent after 4 weeks of exercise. PTs working with diabetic pregnant women should provide counsel on adequate hydration and not becoming tachycardic or dyspneic.

Cardiovascular System

Cardiovascular problems can arise in pregnancy and in the postpartum period as a result of preexisting diseases, disorders, or physiologic changes in pregnancy. The cardiovascular system normally undergoes rapid and broad changes because the blood volume increases by 40%.[132] The combined effect of underlying cardiovascular disease and physiologic changes in pregnancy puts the mother and fetus at risk for serious complications.

Advances in cardiac surgery and medical therapy have increased the number of women with congenital heart disease living to reproductive age. Pulmonary hypertension and cyanotic disease present a 50% risk of maternal death, so antenatal counseling should be tailored to their specific condition.[108]

The PT involved in the care of pregnant women with cardiovascular disease needs to obtain guidelines from the cardiologist,

---

BOX 17-1

Clinical Indicators of Heart Disease During Pregnancy

SYMPTOMS
Progressive dyspnea or orthopnea
Nocturnal cough
Hemoptysis
Syncope
Chest pain

CLINICAL FINDINGS
Cyanosis
Clubbing of fingers
Persistent neck vein distention
Systolic murmur, grade 3/6 or higher
Diastolic murmur
Cardiomegaly
Persistent arrhythmia
Persistent split-second sound
Criteria for pulmonary hypertension

From Cunningham FG, Leveno KJ, Bloom SL, et al: *Williams obstetrics*, 22nd ed, New York, 2005, McGraw-Hill, p 1183.

TABLE 17-14

New York Heart Association Classification of Maternal Heart Disease

Class	Degree of Compromise	Features
I	Uncompromised	Patients are asymptomatic in all situations
II	Slightly compromised	Patients are symptomatic with greater than normal exertion
III	Markedly compromised	Patients are symptomatic with normal activities
IV	Severely compromised	Patients are symptomatic at rest

Adapted from Norwitz E, Schorge J: *Obstetrics and gynecology at a glance*, Oxford, England, 2001, Blackwell Science; Cunningham FG, Leveno KJ, Bloom SL, et al: *Williams obstetrics*, 22nd ed, New York, McGraw-Hill, 2005; Hauptman PJ, Rich MW, Heidenreich PA, et al; Heart Failure Society of America: The heart failure clinic: a consensus statement of the Heart Failure Society of America, *J Card Fail* 14:801-815, 2008.

---

obstetrician, or midwife who is managing the mother's overall care before planning a physical therapy program. PTs working with pregnant patients should be aware of the clinical indicators of heart disease during pregnancy (Box 17-1).

The prognosis for pregnant women with heart disease depends on functional cardiac capacity, clinical conditions, medications, and the specific nature of the condition. Cardiac function has been classified by the New York Heart Association (Table 17-14).

Sickle Cell Disease

Sickle cell anemia decreases the blood cells' ability to transport oxygen throughout the body and complicates 1 in every 500 African American pregnancies.[124,126] In this condition, blood cells clump together and can cause clogging in capillaries. The blockage causes a decrease in blood flow and can bring on a painful crisis in the pregnant woman.[124] Oxygen flow to the uterus can be compromised as blood is shunted to vital organs, resulting in decreased oxygenation to the fetus, which may become severely compromised.

More than 90% of patients with sickle cell disease now reach the age of 20 years, and the median life expectancy of these patients is at least 50 years in countries with advanced health care systems. Adults with homozygous sickle cell disease have increasingly frequent chronic osteoarticular, renal, cardiorespiratory, ocular, cutaneous, and cerebral complications.[43]

Pregnancy is a high risk for women with sickle cell disease, who are at increased risk for preterm labor, abruptio placentae, placenta previa, and toxemia of pregnancy.[43,89] All tissues and organs are at risk for an ischemic injury because of decreased blood flow. Symptoms of the hypoxic injury are often acute and are delineated by painful episodes. PTs working with this population should be aware of the patient's preexisting condition, because a painful crisis may mimic musculoskeletal conditions. The PT needs to quickly differentiate symptoms of a sickle cell crisis from musculoskeletal disorders so that the woman can obtain appropriate care (see Table 17-18).

Patients with sickle cell disease have increased likelihood of seizure activity, thrombosis, and hemorrhage. Headaches can often be the first sign of an acute central nervous system event.[89] Patients with sickle cell disease also have the potential for acute, pleuritic-type chest pain, urinary tract infections, and acute cholecystitis.

Supine Hypotension Syndrome

Supine hypotension syndrome is defined as a hypotensive state brought on by compression of the inferior vena cava (and sometimes the aorta) by the gravid uterus, resulting in decreased venous return, decreased cardiac output, and a drop in blood pressure[43] when the woman assumes a supine position or during prolonged standing or semirecumbent sitting.[3] Symptoms may include nausea, bradycardia, and syncope. Only 8% to 10% of women seem to demonstrate any signs or symptoms of hypotension; these women are said to have inadequate collateral paravertebral circulation.[105] It appears that all women in the latter half of pregnancy have decreased cardiac output in a fully supine position, but the effect on the fetus is not fully understood. There is disagreement concerning at which point in pregnancy the gravid uterus is large enough to cause the occlusion, but the American College of Obstetricians and Gynecologists has suggested that women in the second trimester of pregnancy and beyond follow the recommendation to avoid exercise in the supine position.[3] Consensus opinion considers right or left side-lying or turning 30 degrees to the left from supine to relieve the caval occlusion.

Hypertensive Disorders in Pregnancy

Hypertensive disorders complicate 5% to 10% of all pregnancies and are the most common medical risk factor. These disorders are responsible for 15% maternal morbidity.[43,45,104] Of pregnant women with chronic renal disease, essential hypertension, diabetes mellitus, or lupus erythematosus, 20% to 40% will have hypertensive complications.[45] Hypertensive disorders complicating pregnancy have been divided into five types—gestational hypertension (pregnancy-induced hypertension), preeclampsia, eclampsia, preeclampsia superimposed on chronic hypertension, and chronic hypertension. In total, 30% of hypertensive disorders in pregnancy are caused by chronic hypertension and 70% by gestational hypertension.[43]

Despite decades of research, the relationship between pregnancy and aggravation of hypertension remains unknown.[43] Hypertension is diagnosed when blood pressure is 140/90 mm Hg or higher, and these measurements must be present on at least two occasions, at least 6 hours apart but not more than 1 week apart.[43] Edema is no longer a diagnostic criterion for hypertension because too many normal pregnant women also have edema.[2] Table 17-15 summarizes the types of hypertension in pregnancy and defines the disorders, including preeclampsia and eclampsia. Edema occurs in approximately 50% of pregnant women and is seen in such nondependent regions as the face, hands, or lungs. Consequently, a sudden weight gain of 5 pounds or more in a week is another indication of fluid retention.[43]

A severe form of preeclampsia is the HELLP syndrome (**h**emolysis, **e**levated **l**iver enzymes, and **l**ow **p**latelet count) and is found in 10% of pregnancies complicated by severe preeclampsia. Laboratory findings are consistent with hemolysis and indicate elevated levels of thrombocytopenia and impaired liver function. Blood pressure may be only slightly elevated, but the patient would still be classified as having severe preeclampsia. The clinical picture is of multiparous white female patients diagnosed at less than 35 weeks of gestation. Symptoms consist of vague complaints of general malaise and/or epigastric or right upper quadrant pain (67%), vomiting (30%), and nonspecific viral-like complaints.[43]

PTs should check the pregnant woman's blood pressure if she has not had it taken within the last week and look for sudden onset of edema. Signs of hypertension such as visual changes, headaches, blood pressure change above baseline, and sudden onset of edema should be reported to the primary caregiver. Abruption of the placenta (when the placenta breaks away, or abrupts, from the wall of the uterus before the baby is born) is a possible sequela to hypertension, preeclampsia, or eclampsia in pregnancy (see Table 17-15). Abruptio placentae may mimic groin pain but will be long lasting and not mechanical in origin.

Venous Thromboembolism

Venous thromboembolism (VTE) is a complicating factor in 1 in 1000 to 2000 pregnancies, a rate five times higher than in nonpregnant women of similar age.[8,43,101] Pulmonary embolism, a complication of VTE, is the primary cause of maternal death in the United States[54,100] and the United Kingdom.[157] In untreated cases of deep venous thrombosis (DVT), pulmonary embolism will develop in 24% of pregnant women, resulting in a mortality rate of 15%.[8] However, patients who are managed will have less risk (4.5%) of pulmonary embolism and a less than 1% mortality rate.[8]

All the risk factors for VTE (all potentially present in pregnancy)—hypercoagulability, venous stasis, vascular damage, and changes in the coagulation system—contribute to increased risk for VTE.[8] Additional risk factors for pregnancy-associated DVT and pulmonary embolism are tobacco smoking, prior superficial vein thrombosis, and varicose veins. Women who smoke or have varicose veins also have a risk for overall primary pulmonary embolism during the postpartum period.[47]

Risk factors for VTE in the postpartum period include age older than 40 years, smoking, obesity, blood group other than type O, congenital or acquired thrombophilia, immobility, congestive heart failure, malignancy, hypertension, delivery by

TABLE 17-15

Types of Hypertension During Pregnancy

Disorder, Incidence	Definition	Diagnostic Criteria	Signs and Symptoms
Gestational hypertension: affects nulliparous women most often during second half of pregnancy or in the first 24 hr postpartum	Diagnosis made retrospectively when preeclampsia does not develop and blood pressure returns to normal by wk 12 postpartum	Blood pressure ≥140/99 mm Hg for first time during pregnancy; no proteinuria; blood pressure returns to normal by postpartum wk 12	Epigastric pain, thrombocytopenia, headache
Preeclampsia: 5% incidence influenced by parity, race, ethnicity, environmental factors; occurs after wk 20 of gestation; 6%-7% in primigravidas, 3%-4% in multiparous women	Pregnancy-specific syndrome defined by hypertension, proteinuria, symptoms; results in reduced organ perfusion from vasospasm and endothelial activation; can cause intracranial hemorrhage, renal failure, retinal detachment, pulmonary edema, liver rupture, abruptio placentae, death	Blood pressure ≥140/90 mm Hg after wk 20 of gestation; proteinuria— ≥300 mg of urinary protein in 24-hr period or persistent level of 30 mg/dL in random urine samples	The more severe the hypertension or proteinuria, the more certain is the severity of preeclampsia; symptoms of eclampsia, such as headache, cerebral or visual disturbance, epigastric or right upper quadrant pain
Eclampsia: 0.05% to 0.1% in United States, higher in developing countries; maternal mortality rate is 4.2%, perinatal mortality is 13%-30%; occurs antepartum (50%), intrapartum (25%), or postpartum (25%)	Seizures in pregnant woman with preeclampsia not assigned to other causes	Grand mal seizures appearing before, during, or after labor; in nulliparas, seizures may develop 48 hours to 10 days after delivery	Mother may develop abruptio placentae, neurologic deficits, aspiration pneumonia, pulmonary edema, cardiopulmonary arrest, acute renal failure; may result in maternal death
Superimposed preeclampsia on chronic hypertension	Chronic hypertensive disorders predispose to development of superimposed preeclampsia, eclampsia	New-onset proteinuria ≥300 mg in 24 hr in hypertensive women; no proteinuria before wk 20 of gestation	Risk of abruptio placentae; fetus at risk for growth restriction and death
Chronic hypertension: strong familial history of essential hypertension and/or multiparous women with hypertension complicated by previous pregnancy beyond the first one; occurs in 1%-5% of pregnancies	Hypertension that persists longer than 6 wk after delivery, or elevated blood pressure prior to wk 20 of gestation; women with chronic hypertension at risk of developing superimposed preeclampsia	Hypertension ≥140/90 mm Hg before pregnancy; hypertension ≥140/90 mm Hg detected before wk 20 of gestation; persistent hypertension long after delivery	Risk of abruptio placentae; fetus at risk for growth restriction and death; pulmonary edema; hypertensive encephalopathy; renal failure

Adapted from ACOG Committee on Practice Bulletins: ACOG Practice Bulletin. Chronic hypertension in pregnancy. ACOG Committee on Practice Bulletins, *Obstet Gynecol* 98:177-185, 2001; Cunningham FG, Gant NF, Leveno KJ, et al: *Williams obstetrics*, 22nd ed, New York, 2005, McGraw-Hill; and Livingston JC, Baha MS: Chronic hypertension in pregnancy, *Obstet Gynecol Clin North Am* 28:447-463, 2001.

cesarean section, preeclampsia, and eclampsia.[159] Simpson and associates[159] have estimated that 38% of puerperal DVT and 22% of puerperal pulmonary emboli manifest after discharge from the hospital. Consequently, twice as many postnatal as antenatal events are identified.[159]

PTs working with pregnant and postpartum women should be aware of the acute symptoms of DVT, because patients may report these symptoms occurring in the iliofemoral region or veins of the calf during classes or therapy. Symptoms include pain in the proximal thigh, inguinal region, or calf. Often, these symptoms are nonspecific, with the patient reporting diffuse tenderness and leg pain. Signs of DVT include skin discoloration, edema, prominent superficial veins, and a positive Homans' sign.[155] Homans' sign is positive if the ankle is passively dorsiflexed and the patient reports any sudden increase of pain in the calf or popliteal space.[144]

Pulmonary embolism is uncommon during pregnancy and the puerperium but is responsible for approximately 15% of maternal deaths.[43] This incidence averages approximately 1 in 7000 pregnancies, divided equally in the antepartum and postpartum periods.[43] The common symptoms of pulmonary embolism disease are dyspnea, chest pain, cough, tachycardia, syncope, and hemoptysis. Sometimes, there is an increased pulmonic closure sound, rales, or a friction rub on auscultation.

Respiratory System

Disorders of the respiratory system severe enough to cause respiratory distress are rare in pregnancy. Comfort and oxygen exchange issues influence physical therapy treatment of the pregnant patient.

Dyspnea, often one of the first signs of pregnancy, occurs as the level of progesterone increases. The mother initiates "overbreathing" in response to increased sensitivity of the respiratory center in the brain to carbon dioxide.[34] Sixty percent of pregnant women report dyspnea. The elevation of the diaphragm by approximately 4 cm and the flaring of the lower ribs during pregnancy improve the mother's capacity to breathe deeply, ensuring an oxygen supply to the fetus.[9,34] Implications for the PT include consideration of dyspnea during maternal exercise.

Asthma

Asthma in pregnancy occurs in 4% to 5% of the population, which is the same for the general population.[78] During the course of pregnancy, one third will get better, one third will get worse, and one third will have no change in their asthma.[78,181] Effects of asthma on pregnancy include increased incidence of preterm low-birth-weight infants, preeclampsia, and perinatal morbidity.[181] There is also an association of pregnancy-induced hypertension in women with asthma.[181] The fetus is susceptible to maternal respiratory changes; the placenta consequently functions as a concurrent oxygen exchange organ. The fetus may develop hypoxemia before maternal perception of any respiratory compromise.

Exercise-induced asthma is brought on by smooth muscle constriction in the walls of the airways that respond to changes in airway temperature and hydration. The constriction increases the resistance to air flow, making it difficult to breathe deeply fast enough to keep up with oxygen needs for exercise. Hormonal changes in pregnancy decrease smooth muscle constriction, thereby improving symptoms. Adequate hydration and use of respiratory inhalers before exercise can prevent exercise-induced asthma.[34]

Cystic Fibrosis

Cystic fibrosis (CF) is a genetic disease marked by exocrine gland dysfunction, with the production of thick, viscous secretions. The eccrine sweat gland is the foundation for the sweat test, characterized by elevated chloride, potassium, and sodium levels.

The frequency of CF is estimated to be 1 per 1500 white births and 1 per 17,000 African American births. The median survival rate has increased from 14 years in 1969 to 30 years in 1995,[117] and those born after 2000 are expected to live into their fifties.[158a] Because of improved diagnostics and treatment, 80% of women with CF will likely survive to adulthood, and the North American Cystic Fibrosis Foundation estimates that 4% of women with CF become pregnant each year.

The concern for a pregnant patient with CF relates to her ability to support her own pulmonary and nutritional needs, as well as those of a fetus. Chronic lung disease, hypoxia, and frequent lung infections can be dangerous to the fetus. Cor pulmonale and pancreatic dysfunction frequently develop. Pulmonary involvement, hypoxia, and repeated lung infections can be harmful to pregnancy. The patient with CF who chooses to become pregnant is best managed with serial pulmonary function testing for infection, development of diabetes, and heart failure. Heart failure is reported in 13% of pregnant women with CF, and pancreatic dysfunction can also contribute significantly to inferior maternal nutrition.[43]

Pregnant women with CF can have a successful pregnancy. The Shwachman-Kulczycki, or Taussig, score (0 to 100) is used to rate the severity of CF symptoms based on radiologic and clinical criteria. Women who have a Shwachman-Kulczycki score higher than 75, good nutrition, and a forced expiratory volume in 1 second of 70% usually tolerate pregnancy well.[43] Physical therapy may be indicated for postural drainage and respiratory therapy for bronchodilation.

The PT working with mothers with CF should know that preterm labor and delivery are a significant risk to fetal well-being. Perinatal death rates are higher in infants of women with CF because of preterm deliveries.[43] Patients with any signs of preterm labor such as increased vaginal discharge, vaginal bleeding, onset of regular contractions, and increased uterine pressure sensation should be referred to their primary obstetric caregiver as an emergency. For operative delivery, epidural anesthesia is recommended. Postpartum, breast-feeding is not contraindicated as long as the mother can provide adequate caloric intake for herself and for the production of breast milk.

Musculoskeletal System

Pregnancy and the postpartum period present a unique challenge to the musculoskeletal system of a woman. At no other time in a woman's life does she experience the need for such a relatively quick adjustment in posture, profound alteration in the distensibility and load requirements of the abdominal wall or pelvic floor, or increase in the amount of joint play available in and around the bony pelvis. A number of pathologic conditions of the musculoskeletal system are more prevalent during the childbearing year, such as transient osteoporosis of the hip, spine, and wrist and diastasis recti abdominis, a separation at the tendinous aponeurosis that lays between the two bellies of the rectus abdominis. Low back pain, said to occur in approximately 38% to 70% of pregnant women[21,165,179]; pelvic ring pain (pain in the joints of the SI or pubic symphysis), with a prevalence of 20%[176]; patellofemoral dysfunction and pain; rib and thoracic spine pain; coccydynia; and headaches are some of the commonly occurring musculoskeletal dysfunctions seen in the pregnant population.

The primary care PT needs to be aware of the relative ligamentous laxity, both capsular and extracapsular, exhibited by many pregnant women, especially at the SI joints and pubis. Increased extensibility of many of the soft tissues of the body occurs in most pregnant women[24,115,152] and, when combined with increased weight gain and fluid retention, may lead to conditions otherwise normally seen only as a result of trauma or repetitive stress. In pregnancy, it may take very little force or torque to result in significant dysfunction. Soft tissue injury or dysfunction may also occur without concomitant joint dysfunction, as in diastasis recti abdominis or urinary stress incontinence. However, it is also important to recognize that even though there is generalized increased soft tissue mobility, localized soft tissue or joint restriction may also occur. Joint or soft tissue mobilization is appropriate in these cases. PTs must respect soft tissue laxity by avoiding positioning that places joints in closed-packed, end-range positions and by using treatment techniques that impart the least amount of force needed to accomplish the treatment goal. Treatment-based classification schemes have become popular in recent years[51,66] and may provide assistance in classifying the musculoskeletal dysfunction seen in pregnancy. Some of the pregnancy-related musculoskeletal dysfunction would fall under the "Stabilization" category, some under the "Manipulation" category, and some under the "Specific Exercise" category in the treatment-based scheme proposed by Delitto and coworkers in 1995 and refined by Fritz and colleagues in 2007.[51,66] Each category has concomitant intervention procedures that can be applied, sometimes with modifications, to the obstetric population. Awareness of these issues and of the more common musculoskeletal conditions in pregnancy may assist the PT in appropriate treatment strategies and in developing the prognosis.

Any PT working with this population should recognize the potential for significant postural changes in the pregnant woman and the need for relatively quick adaptation to postural change in the postpartum period. In general, the curves of the cervical, thoracic, and lumbar spines all increase in the pregnant woman, as does the inclination of the sacrum.[157] Although the center of gravity shifts anteriorly in response to weight gain and the growing uterus, research has shown that the change in curvature is not correlated with the onset of low back pain.[20,65]

Low Back Pain in Pregnancy

As noted, the prevalence of low back pain in pregnancy is high. PTs usually get involved in management of low back pain in pregnancy when it affects a woman's ability to function at work (at home or outside the home) or during her leisure time.

The actual incidence of disk herniation first occurring in pregnancy is reported to be 1 in 10,000,[93] and exacerbation of existing disk disease has not been reported. Because the annulus is considered a ligamentous structure and ligaments soften during pregnancy, it could be speculated that disk herniation would be higher during this period than in the nonpregnant state. However, statistics do not bear this out. Disk herniation does occur in pregnancy and the presentation in pregnancy is unlikely to be significantly different than in the nonpregnant state, although changes in bowel and bladder habits may be harder to discern because of changes commonly seen in these functions during pregnancy. MRI can be safely used in pregnancy to make a definitive diagnosis but is generally reserved for surgical candidates.[68,93] A pregnant woman will occasionally have a very flattened lumbar spine unrelated to disk disease and a lumbar lateral trunk shift. One explanation for this may be that, in some women, tight dorsolumbar fascia exerts an overwhelming pull on the spine in the frontal plane, disallowing significant sagittal plane mobility. PTs should not be fooled into thinking that all flat backs represent signs of disk lesions.

Mechanical low back pain is much more common than disk herniation or disk degeneration in this population and can be assessed in pregnancy just as in the nonpregnant state.[16] The pregnant woman in the first trimester may have increased range of active trunk motion compared with her nonpregnant state. In later pregnancy, active movements of the spine may be limited because of the bulk of the fetus and the stretch on dorsolumbar fascia. PTs may note what would normally be considered increased mobility to posteroanterior pressures of the spine during this period. This hypermobility should be considered normal in the pregnant woman when it is generalized to the whole spine.

PTs should always consider the possibility of kidney infection as a source of back pain in pregnancy. As noted, pregnant women are at greater risk for kidney infections than the nonpregnant population, and therefore PTs should screen all patients with symptoms of thoracolumbar or posterior rib pain for this condition.

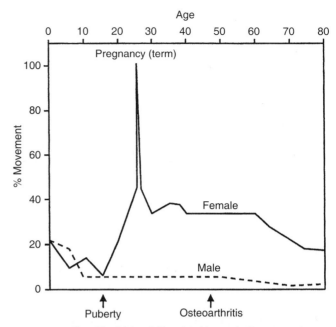

FIGURE 17-1 Sacroiliac joint mobility related to age in the man and woman. (From Bookhout MM, Boissonnault JS: Musculoskeletal dysfunction in the female pelvis, *Orthop Phys Ther Clin North Am* 5:23-45, 1996.)

Sacroiliac Joint Dysfunction

The point prevalence of pelvic ring dysfunction, also commonly called *pelvic girdle pain, pelvic insufficiency,* or *symptom-giving pelvic girdle relaxation,* in pregnancy has been estimated at 20%.[176] This syndrome includes posterior pelvic pain, which is discussed here as SI joint pain, and pain around the pubic symphysis. Aggravation of SI pain occurs during weight-shifting activities such as sitting to standing, rolling in bed, donning shoes or socks, getting up from a chair, and gait or stair climbing.[75,95] Women with SI joint pain commonly report sharp pain in and around the sacrum and buttocks, with referral around the entire pelvic region and often down one or both lower extremities to the knee. The literature notes that referral is possible down the lower extremities, occasionally to the foot.[13] This pain pattern may make differentiation between nerve root compression with radicular pain and SI dysfunction a challenge.

There is much debate in the literature concerning the role of the hormone relaxin in the cause of SI joint dysfunction in pregnancy,[115] but it is agreed that increased SI joint mobility, whatever the mechanism, allows the condition to occur. Figure 17-1 depicts the significant increase in SI joint mobility during pregnancy compared with men and nonpregnant women throughout the lifespan.

Albert and associates[1] have developed a scheme to determine the prognosis for pelvic ring dysfunction that begins in pregnancy. According to their classification, women who exhibit symptoms unilaterally or bilaterally at the sacrum or pubis are much more likely to have their symptoms resolve within 6 months after delivery. It took up to 2 years in women who had pain in all three joints for their symptoms to resolve. The women with three-joint involvement fare the worst regarding disablement.

In addition to joint and soft tissue mobility, examination of the pelvic ring should include assessment of intrinsic support about the pelvis, body mechanics and posture, environmental factors such as chairs and bed cushioning (softer is often better in this population), and job and family demands.

Observation of unusual presentation should suggest conditions that warrant referral back to the obstetric caregiver or primary care physician. Sacroiliitis, a condition of inflammation and erosion of the bone at the margins of the SI joints caused by infection, can present with signs and symptoms similar to the more typical SI joint dysfunction encountered in pregnancy. However, the condition will not respond to joint or soft tissue mobilization but may improve with external stabilization (e.g., a belt or support). Sacroiliitis has been reported as a complication of peripartal infection, including urinary tract infection or after surgery of the urogenital system.[60] Postpartum medical imaging or perinatal MRI will demonstrate changes indicative of this condition. Intensity of symptoms with difficulty in resolution should raise suspicion for this condition. Similarly, transient osteoporosis of the spine or hip may be confused with mechanical dysfunction at the lumbar spine or pelvic ring; PTs should consider it as a possible cause of pain around the hips and pelvis.

Pubic Symphysis Dysfunction

Groin or pubic pain, with possible referral to the medial thigh(s) or along the pubic rami, is also a relatively common musculoskeletal symptom during the childbearing year. There is potential for increased incidence of pubic symphysis dysfunction in pregnancy and the postpartum period because of increased joint mobility around the pelvis before and after delivery and because of significant force on the joint during parturition. Owens and coworkers[135] have reported a prevalence of 1 in 36 over a 2-year period in pregnant women seen in a physiotherapy clinic. Dysfunction may include a relatively simple shifting of the rami cephalad or caudad (pubic shears) or a more complex and painful condition called *pubic symphysis separation*. In later postpartum months, the condition of osteitis pubis may occur, perhaps as a result of periosteal trauma that has occurred during pregnancy or the puerperium. Lentz,[100] in a review article on osteitis pubis, has stated that "although the pathogenesis of osteitis pubis is not clear, periosteal trauma seems to be an important initiating event."

All three types of pubic dysfunction may share common symptoms of painful gait and weight-shifting activities, especially in bed mobility activities, as well as painful abduction of the lower extremities. In general, a separated symphysis results in greater intensity of symptoms. Pubic shears will yield positive palpatory findings of asymmetry at the pubic tubercles. Pubic symphysis separation and osteitis pubis can be confirmed with medical imaging techniques. Plain radiographic findings may lag behind the symptoms of osteitis pubis by as much as 4 weeks, but the results of bone scans will be positive much sooner.[100] Scriven and colleagues[153] have recommended ultrasound as the medical imaging modality of choice for separated symphyses because of its ability to detect trauma to organs and other soft tissues associated with the separation and because of its relatively low cost. However, plain radiographs provide an adequate picture of the bony separation (Figure 17-2).

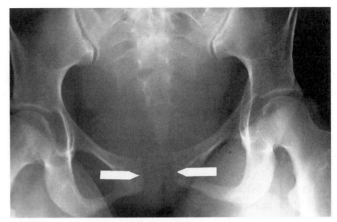

FIGURE 17-2 Plain radiograph, anteroposterior view, illustrating postpartum separated pubis.

There are few estimates of the incidence of pubic symphysis separation during pregnancy, but postpartum incidence ranges from 1 in 300 to 30,000 births, with a general consensus of 1 in 600 births.[18,26,162] Separation is generally defined as a widening at the pubis of greater than 10 mm.[52,102] The woman who has this separation is generally aware of her inability to get out of bed and walk immediately after birth and will require significant family support to get through the first 3 to 6 postpartum weeks. Physical therapy is appropriate for these patients and includes provision of external support (a trochanteric belt), education in appropriate body mechanics and bed mobility techniques, limited weight bearing, and eventually (6 to 12 weeks postpartum) joint mobilization and stabilization exercises.[10,176] The PT should consider the diagnosis of separated symphysis under the following conditions: significant pain at the pubis and surrounding tissues, with onset immediately postpartum or occasionally prenatally; inability to bear or shift weight fully on the lower extremities; lack of positive palpatory findings other than pain at the pubis; and occasional bladder dysfunction (inability to void or hematuria).

Osteitis pubis is more of a chronic condition and, as noted, is more likely to occur later in the postpartum period but has been reported as early as 3 weeks postpartum after a woman participates in a household move.[72] This condition is also seen after bladder repair[84,175] and in athletes. This latter population is often treated aggressively with joint injections and short-term immobilization with a strong trochanteric belt.[77] Postpartum women who demonstrate radiographic signs of loss of smooth cortical periphery at the pubic symphysis, superficial bone destruction and sclerosis, and occasional heterotopic ossification, coupled with symptoms of pain at the joint or in surrounding tissues, aggravated with weight shift or abduction, and in whom joint infection and separation have been ruled out, may be diagnosed similarly.[100] The treatment offered to athletes with osteitis pubis can be effective for the postpartum population. Because the condition is often more chronic in postpartum women, external support may be necessary for many months compared with the few weeks common with an acute athletic injury.

Thoracic Spine and Rib Dysfunction

The rib cage undergoes significant anatomic changes during pregnancy (Figure 17-3; see Table 17-11) and does not fully revert to the nonpregnant state once childbirth has occurred.

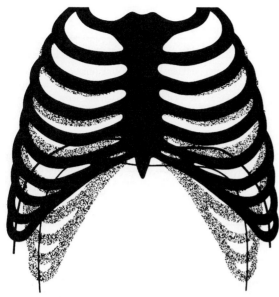

FIGURE 17-3 The rib cage in pregnancy *(black)* and in the nonpregnant state *(stippled)* showing the increased subcostal angle, increased transverse diameter, and raised diaphragm in pregnancy. (From deSwiet M: The respiratory system. In Hyten FE, Chamberlain G, eds: *Clinical physiology in obstetrics*, 2nd ed, Oxford, England, 1991, Blackwell Scientific, p 88.)

These profound changes likely account for the joint dysfunction that may occur at the sternocostal joints anteriorly or at the costotransverse joints and costovertebral joints posteriorly. Women who demonstrate this type of dysfunction often report pain, stiffness, or pressure in the vicinity of the mechanical problem but may also demonstrate referred pain, with or without concomitant soft tissue restrictions and trigger points. In the third trimester, when the fundus of the uterus is elevated nearly to the xiphoid process, decreased trunk mobility coupled with an elevated diaphragm and thoracocostal or sternocostal dysfunction can produce significant impediment to daily function. The woman may not be able to sit or work in a seated position (especially during keyboarding or desk tasks) or assume a recumbent position without disabling pain or discomfort. Understanding the anatomic changes and propensity for dysfunction in this body region may assist the primary care PT in recognizing these issues and result in prompt therapeutic intervention. As noted, screening for kidney infection is an important step in the examination of the pregnant woman with symptoms in the posterior thoracolumbar region.

Headaches and Cervical Spine Dysfunction

Headaches in pregnancy are usually migraines or tension headaches.[63] A certain proportion of prepregnancy headaches get better during pregnancy, supposedly because of the increase in estrogen during this period. A large prospective study using the International Headache Society's definition criteria showed that by the third trimester of pregnancy, 89% of women who had a history of prepregnancy migraines had either no attacks or fewer attacks.[71,118] Headache in pregnancy may be the result of endocrine system–mediated effects on the neurotransmitters or on the vascular system of the brain.[63] However, upper cervical mechanical dysfunction and stress and tension, with associated soft tissue changes, have also been implicated in headaches in the general population.[63]

Migraines are seldom said to begin in pregnancy.[118] A summary of symptoms and treatments for these types of headaches during pregnancy can be found in Table 17-16.[63] Headaches may also be caused by various pathologic processes, such as pregnancy-induced hypertension and preeclampsia. These conditions are discussed in the cardiovascular section of this chapter, and the differential diagnosis of these conditions should be part of the screening process for any pregnant patient with headaches.

Physical therapy of existing soft tissue and joint dysfunction, along with any positive neural tension signs, is one intervention used to reduce headaches in this population. In pregnancy, with the increase of curvature throughout the spine,[21] there exists a potential for aggravation of facet joint problems where the normal lordosis is increased, as in the lumbar and cervical regions. The same anatomic changes predispose women to adaptive shortening of the posterior musculature and soft tissues in the suboccipital area, which can lead to increased soft tissue tension and potentially to pressure on the suboccipital nerve. The soft tissue tension and nerve compression can result in headaches. Reducing forward head posture and addressing needed workstation adaptations may reduce the need for additional acute, hands-on intervention. Because stress plays such a large role in all headaches, screening for undue stress and assisting women in obtaining appropriate stress-reduction strategies or therapies should be part of an overall prenatal PT headache treatment plan.

Postpartum headache may be a result of postdural puncture after spinal anesthesia has been given during labor.[28] Resolution generally occurs, unless the dural puncture has resulted in a subdural hematoma, which is quite rare, but a blood patch may be required.[171] Early postpartum migraine headaches, during the first weeks, are said to be common in women with a history of prepregnancy headaches.[71]

Extremity Dysfunction

Lower leg, ankle, and foot problems are not as common as back or pelvic ring pain in pregnancy but have been found to be more common than in the general population.[177] Nerve entrapment syndromes and neuropathies of peripheral and cranial nerves are detailed in Table 17-17. Patellofemoral dysfunction in the form of chondromalacia patellae is said to occur with greater frequency in pregnancy because of ligamentous laxity,[166] increased load on the knees, and increased fluid retention.[9] Symptoms of pain at the patella during prolonged or end-range flexion of the joint and patellar tracking problems are likely with this diagnosis.[9] Treatment can be similar to that offered during nonpregnancy but, because of the transient mechanical changes, should not involve the purchase of expensive orthotics.

The same advice holds true for changes to the foot during pregnancy. Because the changes may not be permanent or may continue into the postpartum period and not stabilize for many months, expensive foot orthotics should be avoided during this period. Off-the-shelf or temporary orthotics that support the arch of the foot and provide some cushioning are preferred in pregnancy. The foot may undergo anatomic change during pregnancy because of ligamentous laxity, including softening

TABLE 17-16

Symptoms and Treatment for Tension-Type and Migraine Headache During Pregnancy

Type of Headache	Symptoms	Treatment
Tension-type	Bilateral, dull, steady pain that worsens throughout the day; pressure that feels like a tight rubber band around the head; lasts 4 to 24 hr; areas of tenderness on head and neck; onset gradual and sometimes slight; anxiety, nausea, or dizziness present	Identify stress- and tension-producing situations; develop new ways of coping; rest, use of ice packs; biofeedback, relaxation techniques, physical therapy; analgesics, sedatives, other medications that have no or few effects on fetus
Migraine	Severe, throbbing, one-sided pain; lasts 4 to 72 hr; may be accompanied by nausea, vomiting, dizziness, tremors, increased sensitivity to sound and light; classic migraine (with aura)—warning symptoms include visual disturbance, numbness in extremities, strange olfactory sensations, possible hallucinations	Avoid triggering factors such as foods high in tyramine, nitrites and nitrates, MSG, alcohol, weather changes, activity changes, stress, hunger, changes in sleep patterns; develop lifestyle changes; biofeedback; analgesics, beta blockers, sedatives, other medications that have no or few adverse effects on fetus

From Feller CM, Franko-Filipasis KJ: Headaches during pregnancy, *J Perinatal Neonatal Nurs* 7:1-10, 1993.

TABLE 17-17

Nerve Entrapments and Palsies Found in Pregnancy and Postpartum Period

Nerve Injury	Mechanism and Structure	Result
Bell's palsy (cranial nerve VII)	Compression on facial nerve five times more common in pregnant than in nonpregnant women	Facial paralysis, pain, numbness; poorer prognosis for spontaneous recovery in pregnancy
Thoracic outlet syndrome (C5-C8, T1)	Caused by pregnancy-related posture changes of head and neck forward, causing compression of brachial plexus nerve fibers, subclavian artery, vein at cervico-thoracic dorsal outlet	Pain and paresthesia in neck, shoulder, or hand; vascular and autonomic changes in the hand
Carpal tunnel syndrome (C6-C8, T1)	Compression of the median nerve by flexor retinaculum, increased fluid volumes of pregnancy	Numbness, tingling, and pain in thumb, index, middle fingers, lateral aspect of ring finger; positive Tinel's sign
Radial nerve palsy (C5-C8)	Squatting with forearms resting over birthing bar	Weakness of forearm and wrist extensors
Lumbosacral plexus injury (T12-L4)	Compression on lumbosacral plexus by fetal head and forceps or retractor against pelvic wall	Lumbosacral plexopathy; unilateral footdrop
Ilioinguinal neuropathy (L1)	Entrapment after low and wide abdominal incision (Pfannenstiel)	Paresthesia of mons pubis, labium, medial thigh
Iliohypogastric neuropathy (T12-L1)	Entrapment after low and wide abdominal incision	Paresthesia in hypogastric region
Genitofemoral neuropathy (L1-L2)	Injury under inguinal ligament	Paresthesia in lateral thigh and labium
Meralgia paresthetica or lateral femoral cutaneous neuropathy (L2-L3)	Painful dysesthesia in third trimester results from entrapment of sensory lateral femoral cutaneous nerve between inguinal ligament and enlarging abdomen and iliacus fascia; postpartum from prolonged pushing in thigh-flexed position or from Pfannenstiel incision during cesarean section	Unilateral or bilateral paresthesias, numbness and tingling over lateral aspect of thigh; spontaneously resolves after delivery when present before labor
Femoral neuropathy (L2-L4)	Compression on femoral nerve with retractor during cesarean section or prolonged dorsolithotomy or thigh-flexed positions	Paresthesia in anterior thigh, weak quadriceps and/or iliopsoas
Obturator neuropathy (L2-L4)	Compression through labor and lithotomy position or postpartum hematoma 2° pudendal nerve blocks or trauma	Paresthesia in medial thigh, weakness in thigh muscles
Pudendal neuropathy (S2-S4)	Pudendal block, forceps, prolonged labor, or fetal head pressure during delivery	Perineal neuralgia Levator ani weakness
Common peroneal, fibular neuropathy (L4, L5-S1, S2)	Pressure on the common peroneal nerve between leg-holders and fibular head during labor	Footdrop; dorsiflexors and evertors affected

Data from references 36, 43, 55, 88, 158, and 187.

of the supportive ligaments, with resultant loss of arches and increased size. These changes may or may not produce symptoms. Cognizance of the possibility of this type of anatomic change in the feet will improve holistic therapeutic management of many musculoskeletal symptoms during pregnancy.

Osteoporosis in Pregnancy

Osteoporosis in pregnancy is said to be transient and to affect the lumbar spine, hip, and wrist most commonly,[67,148] although reports have described cases with osteoporosis at the knee and ankle.[46,173] The condition is not always associated with any symptoms and rarely causes a hip or wrist fracture, although compression fractures of the spine and subcapital femoral fracture have been reported.[160,188] The decreased bone density can, and does, result in significant pain and disability in some women, probably because of joint effusion and irritation.[17] A suspected diagnosis is made by ruling out other mechanical causes of pain coupled with pain that does not change with physical therapy interventions, such as joint mobilization, soft tissue work, or physical agents, although some relief may be achieved by ameliorating secondary symptoms of edema and muscle spasm. Empty or spasm end-feels at the hip, spine, and wrist are also possible signs. In general, there will be no history of trauma as a precipitating factor of the patient's pain. Onset of pain in transient osteoporosis of the hip has been cited as most commonly occurring in the third trimester and with an antalgic gait or inability to bear weight on the affected side.[160] Pregnancy-related osteoporosis of the spine will also present most commonly in the third trimester and may be associated with back pain and change in height from compression fracture of the vertebral column.[160] A confirmed diagnosis is made postpartum, when medical imaging techniques can demonstrate the decreased bone density necessary for a diagnosis of osteoporosis.

Every PT who cares for pregnant women must keep the possibility of this diagnosis in mind when examining patients. The incidence of osteoporosis in pregnancy is unknown. There are numerous cases of transient osteoporosis of the hip in pregnancy found in the literature,[17,67,92,94,151] but there are no large epidemiologic studies that attempt to estimate the incidence, prevalence, or true longevity of this condition during the childbearing year. There are many theories regarding the cause of osteoporosis in pregnancy,[27,33,59] but none has been substantiated through clinical investigation. However, preexisting osteopenia has been shown to predispose a pregnant woman to this condition.[87] Prolonged use of corticosteroids, heparin, cigarettes, and alcohol are risk factors for osteopenia and should raise suspicion of this condition in women with this type of history. In addition, numerous other diseases place a woman at risk of osteopenia and osteoporosis. These include rheumatoid arthritis; hyperthyroidism and hyperparathyroidism; eating disorders; and cancers such as multiple myeloma, lymphoma, and leukemia.[96]

Treatment of osteoporosis in pregnancy, when symptomatic, is largely aimed at preserving joint integrity and minimizing disability. During pregnancy, for the spine and hip, minimizing weight bearing with lifestyle changes and gait aids, education in positioning for rest and sleep, and general body mechanics instruction are the main intervention strategies used. Osteoporosis at the wrist may benefit from adaptive activities of daily living strategies, with likely referral to occupational therapy. After a definitive diagnosis is made, the postpartum patient can gradually progress through a gentle mobility and strengthening program. Aquatic therapy is a safe way to begin.[17] Eventually, weight-bearing exercise should be implemented as pain resolves and the danger of joint collapse or damage diminishes. Schapira and colleagues[151] have discussed a successfully treated postpartum case via intravenous bisphosphonate therapy,[94] Laktasic-Zerjavic and associates[94] have described successful management via the use of postpartum calcitonin, and La Montagna and coworkers[92] have described a case managed with intramuscular injections of neridronate.

Abdominal Musculature and Diastasis Recti Abdominis

Diastasis recti abdominis (DR) is defined clinically as a separation of greater than two fingertip widths of the two bellies of the rectus abdominis muscle at the linea alba (or linea nigra, in pregnancy).[15] It has been studied in cadavers and categorized in women younger than 45 years as a separation or diastasis when the separation exceeds 10 mm above the umbilicus, 27 mm at the umbilical ring, and 9 mm below the umbilicus.[143] This painless condition occurs most frequently in relation to pregnancy but can be found in patients with chronic pulmonary conditions, in children younger than 2 years, and in men with "beer bellies."[14] Because the condition changes the integrity of the abdominal wall and trunk, it has theoretically been linked to low back pain and urinary incontinence; dysfunction may correlate with altered intra-abdominal pressure gradients or abdominal muscle function. However, the repercussions of DR are not well researched.

DR is commonly noted in primiparas in the third trimester and seems to resolve spontaneously in most women as they progress through the postpartum period.[15] However, DR will not resolve spontaneously in all women. Coldron and colleagues[38] have used ultrasound to measure recti muscles in a group of postpartum women and found that even at 12 months postpartum, the mean distance between recti bellies was still greater than the mean distance in a group of nulliparous women. Exercise aimed at strengthening the recti without increasing intra-abdominal pressure is commonly used to reduce the gap.[14,15,166] Some case design evidence suggests that strengthening the transversus abdominis may enhance resolution of the separation as well.[39] The separation may be noted anywhere along the linea alba (or nigra) and may or may not appear as a distinct bulge noted during movements that involve abdominal contraction with increased intra-abdominal pressure (e.g., a curl-up). The most common assessment technique for this condition is to have the woman perform a curl-up while the PT palpates horizontally between the two sides of the contracted recti. The PT notes the number of fingertips that he or she is able to place within the potential separation of the two bellies of the muscle. More than two fingertips is considered a diastasis[15,166] (Figure 17-4).

It is suggested that women work to eliminate DR after birth and before resuming more stressful abdominal muscle strengthening, such as curl-ups.[70] Transversus abdominis work or other exercises for the abdominals that do not result in increased intra-abdominal pressure should be safe, even in the presence of DR. During pregnancy, because of the changes in hormones and the advancing weight and size of the fetus, resolution of this condition is not possible, but abdominal exercise in pregnancy that focuses on the transversus abdominis muscle may decrease the likelihood of developing the condition.[32] The abdominal wall changes considerably during pregnancy as the fetus exerts force against it, and increased maternal hormones soften its structures. The rectus abdominis elongates during pregnancy and seems to curve around the gravid uterus rather than maintain its nonpregnant linear orientation.[70]

After delivery, the rectus suffers from stretch weakness. The linea alba, which has darkened and become the linea nigra, also stretches to accommodate fetal growth; in some women, it tears, but in most, it becomes elongated and flaccid (moved beyond its

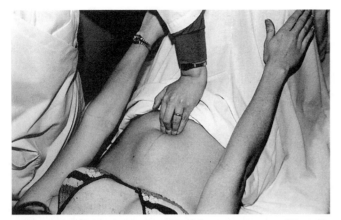

FIGURE 17-4 Diastasis recti abdominis assessment with patient supine. This patient had a diastasis recti of four finger widths. (From Boissonnault JS, Kotarinas RK: Diastasis recti. In Wilder E, editor: *Obstetric and gynecologic physical therapy*, New York, 1988, Churchill Livingstone, p 75.)

elastic limit).[90] Because the linea alba is a tendinous aponeurosis and not composed of contractile tissue, it cannot resume its prepregnancy condition and will therefore remain loose, even as the rectus regains its size and tensile force. As the two sides of the rectus regain their prepregnancy position, the linea alba will continue to lay between them as an overstretched, sagging structure. This makes the likelihood of DR in subsequent pregnancies high, although this has not been established in the literature.

The abdominal wall, with or without DR, exhibits diminished functional capacity as pregnancy progresses. Gilleard and Brown[70] have examined the ability of pregnant women to stabilize the pelvis against resistance. They found that pregnant women, when compared with nonpregnant control subjects, could not accomplish this task in the later stages of pregnancy. Pregnancy and the early postpartum period are times of great stress on the abdominal wall and times of relative weakness of these structures. Proper rehabilitation may have a significant effect on a woman's urogenital and musculoskeletal health throughout her life. Referral to a women's health PT specialist is appropriate to accomplish this rehabilitation when DR is noted by the primary care PT.

Coccydynia

Coccydynia is defined as pain in and around the region of the coccyx.[189] Perinatal coccydynia is most likely to result from parturition-related trauma such as sacrococcygeal subluxation or fracture or a stretch injury to the sacrococcygeal ligaments or sacrococcygeal or intercoccygeal disks.[85,138,146] Patients will have pain in the region of the coccyx or perineum, with sitting as the most common aggravating factor. In addition to the localized trauma to the joint and bone itself, there may be associated soft tissue dysfunction, often classified as levator ani syndrome, particularly in the coccygeal and levator ani musculature that make up part of the pelvic floor.[168,189]

Providing the patient with seating adaptation to lessen the weight on the coccyx, which can be done simply by placing toweling under each thigh or by purchasing an appropriate cushion, and to support the lumbar spine to maintain lordosis and disallow lumbar flexion with posterior pelvic tilt will aid in healing

of tissues and should provide some pain relief. If the patient is still symptomatic after following this postural adaptation for a few weeks postpartum, manual therapy to treat any joint subluxation or concomitant soft tissue dysfunction should be initiated.[16] Some PTs have advocated the use of iontophoresis with dexamethasone for this condition, especially if there is significant pain provoked on the dorsal surface of the sacrococcygeal surface. High-volt galvanic stimulation to the area via rectal probe has been suggested,[163] as has internal soft tissue mobilization.[168] Wray and associates[189] have reported on a series of patients with coccydynia (some were postpartum women) and found that combining joint manipulation with the patient under general anesthesia and injection around the coccyx provided the best results. A more recent randomized trial has found that mobilization and manipulation, sometimes combined with levator stretching, produces the best results.[109]

Primary coccydynia (i.e., pain in the coccyx region that emanates directly from these tissues) that begins during pregnancy is uncommon. Because coccydynia is such a difficult condition to overcome, some women will continue to have symptoms from this dysfunction into their subsequent pregnancies. Legitimate fear of delivery trauma may bring them to a PT during a subsequent pregnancy. Instruction in sitting and body mechanics, along with suggestions for positions in labor and delivery that allow for full mobility of the coccyx, are welcome therapeutic interventions for this population.

Symptoms that Can Mimic Musculoskeletal Conditions in Pregnancy

Table 17-18 contains a partial list of symptoms during pregnancy that may result from musculoskeletal dysfunction or from medical conditions. The table lists common presenting symptoms, the pregnancy-related condition, the musculoskeletal dysfunction that might be responsible, and differential tests.

Neurologic System

Chronic neurologic diseases are common in women of childbearing age[43] and do not preclude a successful pregnancy. Neurologic diseases can contribute to maternal mortality. Most women with neurologic disease have been diagnosed before pregnancy and may require individual treatment.

Neurodiagnostic procedures are not contraindicated during pregnancy. Electromyography and electroencephalography can be undertaken without risk. Pregnancy does not alter the cerebrospinal fluid or the indications for its examination.[55,56] It is wise to limit fetal x-ray exposure, although there is no absolute contraindication for any neuroradiologic study. During the first trimester, x-ray exposure should be limited because there is an increased risk of malformation with fetal exposure to more than 0.015 Gy (1.5 rad).

Neurologic disorders of the central nervous system are rare in pregnancy. Brain tumor incidence in pregnancy is 1 in 1000,[43] and epilepsy is said to complicate 1 in 200 pregnancies.[132] Peripheral nervous system disorders are more common. These are summarized in Table 17-17 by structure, mechanism of injury, and results of commonly found peripheral nerve entrapments and palsies in pregnancy and the postpartum period.

TABLE 17-18

Symptoms that Can Mimic Musculoskeletal Conditions in Pregnancy

Symptoms	Possible Medical Condition	Possible Musculoskeletal Dysfunction	Differentiating Tests or Measures
Calf, proximal thigh, or inguinal pain	Deep venous thrombosis	Gastrocnemius-soleus sprain; radicular symptoms from nerve root impingement; compartment syndrome; pubic symphysis dysfunction	Duplex ultrasonography; positive Homans' sign; assessment of response to treatment and provocation of pain by musculoskeletal examination of pelvis and lower quadrant
Urinary incontinence	Urinary tract infection	Pelvic floor muscle dysfunction; cauda equina syndrome	Urinalysis; assessment of onset (acute or gradual) and aggravating factors
Lower abdominal pain	Abruption of the placenta; ectopic pregnancy; sickle cell disease	Pubic symphysis dysfunction (shears or separation)	Assessment of nature of pain (constant or intermittent) and aggravating factors; provocation of pain by musculoskeletal assessment of the pelvis; diagnostic ultrasound; blood testing
Low back pain or hip pain	Osteoporosis of pregnancy with or without fracture	Mechanical dysfunction of low back or pelvic ring; disk disease; spondylolisthesis	Height assessment; pain pattern assessment; objective findings (e.g., provocation tests, palpatory findings, neurologic findings, end-feels)
Flank pain	Upper urinary tract infection (kidney)	Rib or thoracic spine dysfunction	Percussion over ribs; assessment of response to therapy and provocation of pain by musculoskeletal examination of thorax; fever assessment; urinalysis
Right upper quadrant, scapular pain	Gallstones	Shoulder girdle or thoracic spine or rib dysfunction	Diagnostic ultrasound; assessment of response to treatment and nature of symptoms (whether pain is constant or provoked by activity)
Headache	Pregnancy-induced hypertension or preeclampsia; sickle cell disease	Upper cervical dysfunction or tension-type headache	Blood pressure assessment for hypertension; signs of recent onset of edema; provocation of headache by musculoskeletal assessment of upper cervical spine; sickle cell disease assessment

Peripheral Nervous System Disorders

Peripheral nervous system disorders can result from compression injuries and surgical neuropathies. Increases in extracellular fluid and weight gain, along with hormonal changes, are largely responsible for the neuropathic conditions seen during pregnancy. Most postpartum peripheral nervous system damage is caused by trauma incurred during labor and delivery, such as radial nerve palsies from holding on to the squat bar incorrectly or femoral nerve damage from the lithotomy position. In addition, pelvic floor dysfunction may develop as a result of sacral plexus or pudendal nerve damage from vaginal delivery or the use of forceps and vacuum extractors (see Table 17-17).

Epilepsy

Epilepsy affects 1.1 million women of childbearing age and complicates 1 in 200 pregnancies.[43] Pregnancy can change the pattern of seizures and how a woman's body reacts to her antiepileptic drugs (AEDs), possibly by exacerbating the epilepsy by altering the metabolism of the anticonvulsant medications.[43] Seizures need to be avoided because of the risk of congenital malformation for the growing fetus. There is cause for concern because as many as one third of epileptic women will have an increase in the number of seizures during pregnancy, despite taking AEDs.[43] In addition, these women will have an increase in high blood pressure. Seizures can also increase the risk of falls, which can result in serious injury.

There is a 2% to 3% increase in fetal anomalies found in pregnant women who take anticonvulsant drugs. Children born to mothers with epilepsy have a fourfold increase of developing a seizure disorder.[132] During labor and delivery, women are monitored, and the experience is usually uneventful. AEDs will need to be readjusted after delivery, and these mothers will need counseling because all anticonvulsant medications will cross into breast milk to some degree, although this is not a contraindication to breast-feeding.[132,139] Studies of seizure frequency have shown that 35% of pregnant women will have an increase in seizures, 15% will report a decrease, and 50% will find no change in seizure activity.[43] In women with an increased rate of seizures, there is a return to prepregnancy seizure rates after delivery.[139]

Multiple Sclerosis

The prevalence of multiple sclerosis (MS) during pregnancy is 120/100,000 and affects women twice as much as men, usually occurring in the 20s and 30s during susceptible childbearing years.[43] During pregnancy, there is a trend toward lower relapse rates, followed by an increase in relapse during the 6-month postpartum period. Initial onset of MS during pregnancy is uncommon and occurs in fewer than 10% of patients with MS.[44] Women with MS who have a singleton infant are no more likely to have complications in pregnancy or during delivery than women without MS. However, they are more likely be hospitalized during the first 3 postpartum months.[127] Damek and Shuster[44] have also shown that women who have had children before or after their MS diagnosis may have positively altered the course of the disease over the long term.

Physical therapy management of pregnant women with MS is the same as for nonaffected women. Evaluation should include careful attention to the effects of potential balance and gait disturbances and spasticity on activities of daily living and functional activities. The enlarging uterus can affect the function of an already neurogenic bladder and increase the episodes of cystitis. Labor itself remains unchanged, but extensor or flexor spasms can be triggered by labor pain.[56]

In the postpartum period, the PT can assist the new mother by encouraging her to obtain adequate rest, arrange for adequate child care, and obtain community support if she has an exacerbation.

Spinal Cord Injury

In the United States, there are 11,000 spinal cord injuries (SCIs) each year; half of these affect people in their reproductive years, and 18% are women.[7] Patients with SCI with cervical or thoracic lesions caused by trauma or tumor are not a contraindication to conception, pregnancy, or delivery. Women with SCIs have lower-birth-weight infants and have more complications in pregnancy. These complications include bacteriuria, urinary tract infections, pyelonephritis, pressure sores of the insensate skin, bowel dysfunction, respiratory problems, preterm contractions, and autonomic dysreflexia.[43,180] The perinatal mortality rate is 3.9% and the preterm delivery rate is 20%.[43]

In lesions above T10, respiratory function and cough reflex will be compromised, which can affect pulmonary function in pregnancy. Women with lesions above T10 may need ventilatory support in late pregnancy or during labor. In lesions at or above T6, autonomic hyperreflexia can occur, which is a potentially life-threatening situation. The splanchnic nerves are excited and are not dampened because of the lack of central inhibition.

Concomitantly, sudden sympathetic stimulation of nerves below the cord lesion can cause throbbing headaches, facial flushing, sweating, bradycardia, and paroxysmal hypertension. Culpable stimuli could include examination of pelvic structures; uterine contractions; cervical dilation; and urethral bladder, rectal, or cervical distention and catheterization. This can precipitate dangerous hypertension and require immediate attention. Support during labor often includes spinal or epidural anesthesia; these measures can prevent dysreflexia and are initiated at the start of labor.

The level of the lesion does not affect uterine contractions for all spinal cord lesions. In lesions below T12, contractions are felt normally. Women with lesions above T12 are instructed in how to palpate uterine contractions or monitor with home tocodynamometry. The American College of Obstetricians and Gynecologists recommends continuous cardiac and intra-arterial pressure monitoring.[22]

During the postpartum period, the mother with an SCI may have poor episiotomy healing and DVT. Blood loss during delivery may complicate the anemia commonly seen in pregnancy. This can lead to decreased energy levels and difficulty in the extra demands that can accompany parenting.[180] PTs can teach safe transfer techniques to avoid injury when the mother is fatigued.

Spina Bifida

Spina bifida (SB) is diagnosed in 2000 infants every year in the United States.[180] Through corrective surgery and adaptive technology, many women with spina bifida have full lives, including pregnancy. The incidence of women with SB giving birth to infants with SB is 2% to 4% higher than the general population.[180] Folic acid intake needs to be increased if a woman has already had one child with SB.

Poorly developed pelvic floor structures of these women can influence labor. Complications can result from previous bladder and bowel surgeries, resulting in renal function deterioration, pain with intraperitoneal adhesions, increased incontinence, urinary tract infections, pyelonephritis, and obstruction with shifting of the intra-abdominal contents as the uterus expands.[180]

MRI pelvimetry may be necessary for pregnant women who have SB and a contracted pelvis. The deformity can result in an obstructed birth, with cephalopelvic disproportion. Labor and delivery can be protracted, resulting in permanent loss in perineal muscle strength. Women with SB are at higher risk for pelvic organ prolapse without any effect of vaginal delivery. Spinal anesthesia for these women can be complex because of the level of their spinal lesion.

Guillain-Barré Syndrome

Guillain-Barré syndrome is an acute demyelinating polyradiculoneuropathy. In more that 67% of patients, there is clinical evidence of viral infection, such as cytomegalovirus or Epstein-Barr virus. Approximately 10% of cases develop within weeks of a surgical procedure.[91] There is no increased incidence of Guillain-Barré syndrome in pregnancy, but there is a threefold increase in the first 30 days after delivery.[43]

Migraine

See the musculoskeletal section of this chapter for discussion of migraine headaches.

Integumentary System

Changes to the integumentary system during pregnancy usually occur for one of three reasons—physiologic skin changes, dermatologic conditions unique to pregnancy, or preexisting skin diseases that complicate pregnancy. These conditions are rarely harmful to the pregnant patient but can be inconvenient and bothersome. PTs have a responsibility and opportunity to report any unusual skin changes because they see large areas of the patient's skin when examining and treating. It is helpful for clinicians to know what these skin changes are so that they can act as a resource for the patient and refer the patient for further consultation (see Chapter 10).

Physiologic Changes

Hormonal changes during pregnancy have an extensive effect on the skin. These changes include hyperpigmentation, connective tissue and collagen changes, hair growth, vascular modifications, and glandular activity.

Increased skin darkening is observed in 90% of all pregnant women and is one of the most recognized changes of pregnancy.[80] This hyperpigmentation can occur in the nipples, areolae, linea alba, perineum, recent scars, moles, freckles, vulva, and perianal region. These areas of pigmentation usually increase in the first trimester, especially in dark-complected and dark-haired women, and fade in the postpartum period. However, the pigmentation seldom returns to the prepregnancy level.[80]

Chloasma, or melasma, also called the mask of pregnancy, consists of irregular brownish patches of pigmentation that occur in 50% of pregnant women.[43] The pattern of increased pigmentation can cover the forehead, cheeks, upper lip, nose, and chin. Other separated patterns are limited to the cheeks, nose, and mandible. Melasma also occurs in 30% of women taking oral contraceptives. All these pigmentation changes are thought to be mediated by hormonal responses. No medical treatment is needed for chloasma.[43]

Vascular changes can affect the skin, causing edema in the face and hands in approximately 50% of all pregnant women. Edema of the legs, not associated with preeclampsia, develops in 80% of all pregnancies.[80] The swelling is worse in the morning; is nonpitting; and is caused by increases in fluid retention, vascular permeability; and blood flow and decreased colloid osmotic plasma pressure. PTs can assist in management of the edema by patient education in the appropriate use of gradient pressure stockings and body positioning for optimal return of blood and lymph.

Spider nevi—dilated arterioles, or angioma, in the skin, with radiating capillary branches[58]—and palmar erythema (redness in the palms) are thought to appear because of an increase in estrogen production.[166] Spider nevi appear between the second and fifth months of pregnancy in approximately 57% of white and 10% of African American women.[80] They usually occur in the areas drained by the superior vena cava on the upper trunk and face and disappear by the seventh postpartum week. Palmar erythema develops in the first trimester in 70% of white and 35% of African American women, resolving quickly after delivery.[80]

Varices most often involve the saphenous veins in the legs, vulva, and hemorrhoidal tissue. These dilated vessels result from increased venous pressure from compression of the pelvic and femoral veins by the enlarging uterus, increased blood volume, increased collagen fragility, and hereditary tendency to varicose veins. As the vein swells, the valve inside the vein does not close completely, and retrograde flow forms varices. These subside after birth, but often not fully. Treatment includes rest with the legs elevated and support stockings to increase the pressure on the leg or vulva, decreasing the swelling within the vein, and might prevent varices.

There is a familial tendency for connective tissue changes affecting the skin that occur most often in the second half of pregnancy.[80] These striae gravidarum, or stretch marks, are most commonly clustered on the abdomen, breasts, and thighs. The collagen and elastic fibers rupture with the increased stretching of the abdominal wall. Estrogen and relaxin are thought to increase the separation of the collagen fibers.[80] During the second half of pregnancy, skin tags may develop on the pregnant woman's face, neck, and axillae and under the breasts. These usually recede postpartum.

Dermatoses

Five types of dermatoses are unique to pregnancy—herpes gestationis, polymorphic eruption of pregnancy, prurigo of pregnancy, pruritic folliculitis of pregnancy, and cholestasis-related pruritus of pregnancy. PTs need to be alert to skin changes because they may be seeing a woman during a skin eruption, necessitating a referral to a dermatologist.

Herpes gestationis, or pemphigoid gestationis, is a rare autoimmune condition characterized by intensely pruritic papules with blistering skin eruptions in the second or third trimester of pregnancy on the abdomen and extremities.[43] It occurs in 1 in 10,000 multiparous women.[43] In subsequent pregnancies, herpes

gestationis is likely to appear earlier and with increased severity. It can sometimes appear in early pregnancy and up to 1 week after birth. These lesions vary in form from erythematous and edematous papules to large, tense bullae and vesicles.[43] Babies born to mothers with herpes gestationis may have a tendency for premature delivery, which may put the infant at risk for increased morbidity.[80] Treatment includes antipruritics, topical corticosteroids, and oral corticosteroids if the symptoms are severe.

Pruritic urticarial papules and plaques of pregnancy (PUPPs), also referred to as polymorphic eruption of pregnancy, is the most common of the pruritic dermatoses of pregnancy, occurring in 0.25% to 1% of pregnancies.[43] These intensely pruritic cutaneous eruptions, which can be patchy or generalized, appear in late pregnancy, developing on the abdomen around the striae and spreading to the buttocks, thighs, and extremities. This disease is common in nulliparas and is not known to recur in later pregnancies. The pathogenetic pathology is unknown. Treatment with topical corticosteroid ointments and oral corticosteroids helps if itching is severe. The rash most usually disappears within several days of delivery, and there is no evidence of perinatal morbidity.

Prurigo of pregnancy, also known as prurigo gestationis or papular dermatitis, is uncommon, with an incidence of 1 in 300 to 2400 pregnancies. This type of dermatosis is characterized by small skin eruptions on the forearms and trunk. The lesions appear at 25 to 30 weeks of gestation with no adverse outcome to mother or fetus. The itching is controlled by antihistamines and topical corticosteroid creams.

Impetigo herpetiformis is a rare skin eruption seen in late pregnancy, consisting of pustules that form around the margin of erythematous patches. Itching is not severe but there are signs of nausea, vomiting, diarrhea, chills, and fever. The pustules may become infected after rupture, and sepsis can be a major concern. Treatment consists of systemic corticosteroids and antimicrobials to treat secondary infection. This disease can persist for several months after delivery, or may not fully resolve, and fetal morbidity and mortality rates can be affected by the severity of the maternal infection.[43]

Cholestasis (inflammation of the gallbladder) is common in 1% to 2% of pregnancies and involves intense pruritus without lesions, resolving after birth. This skin disease is a mild form of cholestatic jaundice with onset in the third trimester generalized throughout the body. There is an increase in the rate of perinatal morbidity.[43]

Preexisting Skin Diseases

The hormones of pregnancy can affect existing skin diseases. An improvement of psoriasis during pregnancy occurs in 65% of women, but 90% report a flare of the psoriasis in the postpartum period.[43] Psoriasis may remain unchanged, clear, worsen, or appear for the first time during pregnancy.[80] The effect of pregnancy on acne is unpredictable. Acne can improve or worsen in pregnancy. It can also appear for the first time, along with hirsutism. Retinoids and tetracyclines are highly teratogenic during pregnancy and are contraindicated. As a result, the withdrawal of these drugs may cause a flare of the acne. Candidiasis is 10 to 20 times more common in pregnancy because the lowered vaginal pH and increased sweating create a favorable environment. Treatment is topical, with nystatin or miconazole.[80]

Special Considerations During Pregnancy and the Postpartum Period

Systemic Lupus Erythematosus

Systemic lupus erythematosus (SLE) is an autoimmune disorder that can be affected by the hormonal changes of pregnancy. SLE in pregnancy has three main outcomes—it increases late pregnancy miscarriage from hypertension and renal failure, it can cause heart block and other cardiac defects in the newborn, and it can increase the risk of idiopathic abortion. The main risk factors for adverse pregnancy outcome are active disease; nephritis with proteinuria; hypertension; and maternal serum antibodies to SSA/Ro, SSB/La, cardiolipin, beta$_2$-glycoprotein 1, and lupus antiocoagulant.[123]

SLE is a fluctuating illness and pregnancy does not affect the long-term prognosis of the disease as long as the disease is stable,[123] but it may cause more flare-ups, particularly in the postpartum period. If the fetus survives to full gestation, there is an increased risk of fetal distress.[50] Women with SLE can have many complications of hypertension and renal failure or may have no medical complications.

Rheumatoid Arthritis

Pregnancy usually improves the inflammatory component of rheumatoid arthritis (RA) in 75% of women who have RA.[130] Symptoms and complications occurring during pregnancy are rare.[43,50] The pregnant woman with RA may feel a relief of her pain and stiffness in the first trimester. However, in the postpartum period, there is a sixfold likelihood of exacerbation within the first 3 to 4 months. Some medications can be used safely during pregnancy and lactation without injury to the baby.[130] There is a small risk of congenital heart block in the newborn. The PT working with these pregnant women can caution against potential problems resulting from abduction of the mother's legs during delivery and hyperextension of her neck for intubation during general anesthesia.[50]

Women who have juvenile RA report similar results of decreased disease activity during pregnancy, with flare-ups in the postpartum period. In addition, joint deformities are common, and cesarean deliveries are performed for contracted pelves or joint prostheses.

Teen Pregnancy

The rate of teen and adolescent pregnancies fluctuates with the success rate of pregnancy prevention programs. Adolescents are at increased risk for preterm labor and psychological problems.[43] By 1996, the teenage birth rate was 54.7 live births per 1000 population. Ninety percent of these teens described their pregnancies as unintended.[40] Milwaukee conducted a trend analysis for teen birth rates between 1991 and 2006 to forecast and set a birth rate goal for 2015. Their projection was 35.9 births per 1000 females aged 15 to 17 years. The leaders of the Milwaukee project set a goal of 30 births per 1000 females aged 15 to17 years, which would be an overall 46% reduction from the 2006 rate.[68a,124a]

Teen pregnancies are complicated by incomplete pelvic growth, lack of psychological maturity, lack of prenatal care, and inadequate weight gain. As the teen continues to grow herself, she must gain enough for her own nutritional needs, as well as for the growing fetus. Pregnant teens grow at a slower rate than their nonpregnant peers. Consequently, pregnant adolescents have more than twice the mortality rate of adult pregnant women.[178]

The PT involved with this population can support the teenager in understanding the nutritional, physical, emotional, and nurturing changes with which she will be confronted (see Chapter 16). The PT can serve as a resource outside the family unit.

Cesarean Deliveries

Cesarean, or abdominal birth, is the delivery of the infant through the abdominal wall. In 2004, a record high cesarean delivery rate was reported at 29.1% of all births in the United States, an increase of 8%.[43,119]

There are many reasons for cesarean deliveries. More than 89.4% are performed because of prior cesareans, labor dystocia, fetal distress, and breech presentation.[43,74] In subsequent pregnancies, women who have had a cesarean delivery may be given a chance to try a vaginal delivery as long as the risk factors are low. Vaginal birth after cesarean delivery can be associated with a small but significant risk of uterine rupture, with poor outcomes for the mother and infant.[43]

Most often, the surgical approach is made transversely through the lower uterine segment above the pubic bone. The classic cesarean incision vertically from umbilicus to pubis is now reserved for emergency situations. For a planned procedure, the patient may have options for anesthesia.

Early postpartum management by the PT is similar to any surgical patient—active movement of the extremities to prevent venous stasis and peripheral edema. Some women may have labored for an extensive period before requiring a cesarean section and may need assistance in recovery from major abdominal surgery, as well as from labor. In the later postpartum period, the PT can assist the patient in the full recovery of body mechanics, activities of daily living, abdominal wall strengthening, and return to an endurance and exercise program.

REFERENCES

1. Albert H, Godskesen M, Westergaard J. Prognosis in four syndromes of pregnancy-related pelvic pain. Acta Obstet Gynecol Scand 2001;80:505–10.
2. American College of Obstetricians and Gynecologists. ACOG Practice Bulletin. Chronic hypertension in pregnancy. Obstet Gynecol 2001;98:177–85.
3. American College of Obstetricians and Gynecologists: Committee Obstetric Practice: ACOG Committee opinion. Number 267, January 2002: Exercise during pregnancy and the postpartum period. Obstet Gynecol 2002;99:171–3.
4. American College of Obstetricians and Gynecologists: Diabetes during pregnancy, 2009 (website). http://www.acog.org/publications/patient_education/bp051.cfm. Accessed March 14, 2010.
5. American College of Obstetricians and Gynecologists. Exercise during pregnancy and the postpartum period. ACOG Technical Bulletin Number 189—February 1994. Int J Gynaecol Obstet 1994;45:65–70.
6. American College of Obstetricians and Gynecologists Committee on Practice Bulletins—Obstetrics: ACOG Practice Bulletin. Clinical management guidelines for obstetrician-gynecologists. Number 30, September 2001 (replaces Technical Bulletin Number 200, December 1994). Gestational diabetes. Obstet Gynecol 2001;98:525–38.
7. American College of Obstetricians and Gynecologists: ACOG Committee Opinion: Number 275, September 2002. Obstetric management of patients with spinal cord injuries. Obstet Gynecol 2002;100:625–7.
7a. American Psychiatric Association: Diagnostic and statistical manual of mental disorders. 4th ed. Washington DC: American Psychiatric Association; 2000.

8. Andres RL, Miles A. Venous thromboembolism and pregnancy. Obstet Gynecol Clin North Am 2001;28:613–30.

9. Artal Mittelmark R, Wiswell RA. Drinkwater BL: Exercise in pregnancy. Baltimore: Williams & Wilkins; 1991.

10. Association of Chartered Physiotherapists in Women's Health: Pregnancy-related pelvic girdle pain: guidance for professionals, 2007 (website). http://www.acpwh.org.uk/docs/ACPWH-PGP_HP.pdf. Accessed March 14, 2010.

11. Baydock SA, Flood C, Schulz JA, et al. Prevalence and risk factors for urinary and fecal incontinence four months after vaginal delivery. J Obstet Gynaecol Can 2009;31:36–41.

12. Belluomini J, Litt RC, Lee KA, Katz M. Acupressure for nausea and vomiting of pregnancy: a randomized, blinded study. Obstet Gynecol 1994;84:245–8.

13. Berg G, Hammar M, Moller-Nielsen J, et al. Low back pain during pregnancy. Obstet Gynecol 1988;71:71–5.

14. Boissonnault JS, Kotarinos RK. Diastasis recti. In: Wilder E, editor. Obstetric and gynecologic physical therapy: clinics in physical therapy. New York: Churchill Livingstone; 1988.

15. Boissonnault JS, Blaschak MJ. Incidence of diastasis recti abdominis during the childbearing years. Phys Ther 1988;68:1082–6.

16. Boissonnault JS. Physical therapy management of musculoskeletal dysfunction during pregnancy. In: Irion GL, editor. Women's health in physical therapy. Philadelphia: Lippincott, Williams & Wilkins; 2009.p. 226–51.

17. Boissonnault WG, Boissonnault JS. Transient osteoporosis of the hip associated with pregnancy. J Orthop Sports Phys Ther 2001;31:359–65.

18. Bolland BF. Spraration of symphysis pubis: report of ten cases occurring during delivery. N Engl J Med 1933;208:431–8.

19. Boyles SH, Li H, Mori T, et al. Effect of mode of delivery on the incidence of urinary incontinence in primiparous women. Obstet Gynecol 2009;113:134–41.

20. Bullock JE, Jull GA, Bullock MI. The relationship of low back pain to postural changes during pregnancy. Aust J Physiother 1987;33:10–7.

21. Bullock-Saxton J. Musculoskeletal changes associated with the perinatal period. In: Sapsford R, Bullock-Saxton J, Markwell S, editors. Women's health. A textbook for physiotherapists. Philadelphia: WB Saunders; 1998. pp. 134–61.

22. Burns AS, Jackson AB. Gynecologic and reproductive issues in women with spinal cord injury. Phys Med Rehabil Clin North Am 2001;12:183–99.

23. Burtis CA, Ashwood ER, Bruns DE. Tietz textbook of clinical chemistry and molecular diagnostics. St. Louis: Saunders Elsevier; 2006.

24. Calguneri M, Bird HA, Wright V. Changes in joint laxity occurring during pregnancy. Ann Rheum Dis 1982;41:126–8.

25. Cameron MH. Physical agents in rehabilitation: from research to practice. St. Louis: Saunders Elsevier; 2009.

26. Cappiello GA, Oliver BC. Rupture of symphysis pubis caused by forceful and excessive abduction of the thighs with labor epidural anesthesia. J Fla Med Assoc 1995;82:261–3.

27. Carbonne LD, Palmieri GMH, Graves SC, et al. Osteoporosis of pregnancy: long term follow-up of patients and their offspring. Obstet Gynecol 1995;86:664–6.

28. Chan TM, Ahmed E, Yentis SM, Holdcroft A. Obstetric Anaesthetists' Association, NOAD Steering Group: Postpartum headaches: summary report of the National Obstetric Anaesthetic Database (NOAD) 1999. Int J Obstet Anesth 2003;12:107–12.

29. Chaudron LH, Klein MH, Remington P, et al. Predictors, prodromes and incidence of postpartum depression. J Psychosom Obstet Gynaecol 2001;22:102–3.

30. Chen MM, Coakley FV, Kaimal A, Laro Jr RK. Guidelines for computed tomography and magnetic resonance imaging use during pregnancy and lactation. Obstet Gynecol 2008;112:333–40.

31. Chez RA. Women battering in pregnancy. In: Sapsford R, Bullock-Saxton J, Markwell S, editors. Women's health. A textbook for physiotherapists. Philadelphia: WB Saunders,; 1998.

32. Chiarello CM, Falzone LA, McCaslin KE, et al. The effects of an exercise program on diastasis recti abdominis in pregnant women. J Womens Health Phys Ther 2005;29:11–6.

33. Chigira M, Watanabe H, Udagawa E. Transient osteoporosis of the hip in the first trimester of pregnancy. A case report and review of Japanese literature. Arch Orthop Trauma Surg 1988;107:178–80.

34. Clapp III JF. Exercising through your pregnancy. Omaha, NE: Addicus Books; 2002.

35. Cogill SR, Caplan HL, Alexandra H, et al. Impact of maternal postnatal depression on cognitive development of young children. Br Med J (Clin Res Ed) 1986;292:1165–7.

36. Cohen Y, Lavie O, Granovsky-Grisaru S, et al. Bell palsy complicating pregnancy: a review. Obstet Gynecol Surv 2000;55:184–8.

37. Cokkinides VE, Coker AL, Sanderson M, et al. Physical violence during pregnancy: maternal complications and birth outcomes. Obstet Gynecol 1999;93:661–6.

38. Coldron Y, Stokes MJ, Newham DJ, Cook K. Postpartum characteristics of rectus abdominis on ultrasound imaging. Man Ther 2008;13:112–21.

39. Collie ME, Harris BA. Physical therapy treatment for diastasis recti: a case report. J Sect Womens Health 2004;28:11–5.

40. Committee on Adolescence. Adolescent pregnancy: current trends and issues. Pediatrics 1999;103:516–20.

41. Coombes K, Darken R. The psychological and emotional aspects of childbearing. In: Sapsford R, Bullock-Saxton J, Markwell S, editors. Women's health. A textbook for physiotherapists. Philadelphia: WB Saunders; 1998. p. 125–31.

42. Cox JL, Holden JM, Sagovsky R. Detection of postnatal depression. Development of the 10-item Edinburgh Postnatal Depression Scale. Br J Psychiatry 1987;150:782–6.

43. Cunningham FG, Leveno KJ, Bloom SL, et al. Williams obstetrics. 22nd ed. New York: McGraw-Hill; 2005.

44. Damek DE, Shuster EA. Pregnancy and multiple sclerosis. Mayo Clin Proc 1997;72:977–89.

45. Danforth DN, Scott JR. Obstetrics and gynecology. Philadelphia: JB Lippincott; 1986.

46. Daniel RS, Farrar EK, Norton HR, Nussbaum AI. Bilateral transient osteoporosis of the talus in pregnancy. Osteoporos Int 2009;20:1973–5.

47. Danilenko-Dixon DR, Heit JA, Silverstein MD, et al. Risk factors for deep vein thrombosis and pulmonary embolism during pregnancy or post partum: a population-based, case-control study. Am J Obstet Gynecol 2001;184:104–10.

48. Das BP, Joshi M, Pant CR. An overview of over the counter drugs in pregnancy and lactation. Kathmandu Univ Med J (KUMJ) 2006;4:545–51.

49. De Leeuw JW, Vierhout ME, Struijk PC, et al. Anal sphincter damage after vaginal delivery: functional outcome and risk factors for fecal incontinence. Acta Obstet Gynecol Scand 2001;80:830–4.

50. de Swiet M. Systemic lupus erythematosus and other connective tissue diseases. In: de Swiet M, editor. Medical disorders in obstetric practice. 4th ed. Malden, MA: Wiley-Blackwell; 2002 pp. 267–81.

51. Delitto A, Erhard RE, Bowling RW. A treatment-based classification approach to low back syndrome: identifying and staging patients for conservative treatment,. Phys Ther 1995;75:470–85.

52. Dhar S, Anderton JM. Rupture of the symphysis pubis during labor. Clin Orthop Relat Res 1992 Oct;(283):252–7.

53. Dietz PM, Williams SB, Callaghan WM, et al. Clinically identified maternal depression before, during, and after pregnancies ending in live births. Am J Psychiatry 2007;164:1515–20.

54. Dixon-Townson D. Pregnancy-related venous thromboembolism. Clin Obstet Gynecol 2002;45:363–8.

55. Donaldson JO. Neurologic complications. In: Burrow GN, Duffy TP, editors. Medical complications during pregnancy. 5th ed. Philadelphia: WB Saunders; 1999. p. 401–14.

56. Donaldson JO. Neurological disorders. In: de Swiet M, editor. Medical disorders in obstetric practice. 4th ed. Malden, MA: Wiley-Blackwell; 2002. p. 486–500.

57. Dossett EC. Perinatal depression. Obstet Gynecol Clin North Am 2008;35:419–34.

58. Dox IG, Melloni BJ, Eisner GM, Melloni JL. Melloni's illustrated medical dictionary. London: Parthenon; 2002.

59. Dunne F, Walters B, Marshall T, Heath DA. Pregnancy-associated osteoporosis. Clin Endocrinol (Oxf) 1993;39:487–90.

60. Egerman RS, Mabie WC, Eifrid M, et al. Sacroiliitis associated with pyelonephritis in pregnancy. Obstet Gynecol 1995;85:834–5.

61. Enkin E, Keirse MJNC, Neilson J. A guide to effective care in pregnancy and childbirth. New York: Oxford University Press; 2000.

62. Faisal-Cury A, Menezes PR, Tedesco JJ, et al. Maternity "blues": prevalence and risk factors. Span J Psychol 2008;11:593–9.

62a. Felice ME, Feinstein RA, Fisher MM, et al. Adolescent pregnancy: current trends and issues: 1998 American Academy of Pediatrics Committee on Adolescence, 1998-1999. Pediatrics 1999;103:516–20.

63. Feller CM, Franko-Filipasic KJ. Headaches during pregnancy: diagnosis and management. J Perinat Neonatal Nurs 1993;7:1–10.

64. Frahm J, Welsh RA. Physical therapy management of the high-risk antepartum patient. Clin Management 1989;9(4):15.

65. Franklin ME, Conner-Kerr T. An analysis of posture and back pain in the first and third trimesters of pregnancy. J Orthop Sports Phys Ther 1998;28:133–8.

66. Fritz JM, Cleland JA, Childs JD. Subgrouping patients with low back pain: evolution of a classification approach to physical therapy. J Orthop Sports Phys Ther 2007;37:290–302.

67. Funk JL, Shoback DM, Genant HK. Transient osteoporosis of the hip in pregnancy: natural history of changes in bone mineral density. Clin Endocrinol (Oxf) 1995;43:373–82.

68. Garmel SH, Guzelian GA, D'Alton JG, D'Alton ME. Lumbar disk disease in pregnancy. Obstet Gynecol 1997;89:821–2.

68a. Gavin L, MacKay AP, Brown K, et al. Centers for Disease Control and Prevention (CDC). Sexual and reproductive health of persons aged 10-24 years—United States, 2002-2007. MMWR Surveill Summ 2009;58(6):1–58; Jul 17.

69. Giger JN, Davidhizar RE. Transcultural nursing: assessment and intervention. St. Louis: Mosby Elsevier; 2008.

70. Gilleard WL, Brown JM. Structure and function of the abdominal muscles in primigravid subjects during pregnancy and the immediate postbirth period. Phys Ther 1996;76:750–62.

71. Goadsby PJ, Goldberg J, Silberstein SD. Migraine in pregnancy. BMJ 2008;336:1502–4.

72. Gonik B, Stringer CA. Postpartum osteitis pubis. South Med J 1985;78:213–4.

73. Goodwin MM, Gazmararian JA, Johnson CH, et al. Pregnancy intendedness and physical abuse around the time of pregnancy: findings from the pregnancy risk assessment monitoring system, 1996-1997. PRAMS Working Group. Pregnancy Risk Assessment Monitoring System. Matern Child Health J 2000;4:85–92.

74. Hamilton BE, Martin JA, Ventura SJ, et al. Births: preliminary data for 2004. Natl Vital Stat Rep 2005;54:1–7.

75. Hansen A, Jensen DV, Wormslev M, et al. Symptom-giving pelvic girdle relaxation in pregnancy. II: Symptoms and clinical signs. Acta Obstet Gynecol Scand 1999;78:111–5.

76. Hayman B. A miracle in the making. Chicago: Budlong Press; 2000.

77. Holt MA, Keene JS, Graf BK, Helwig DC. Treatment of osteitis pubis in athletes. Results of corticosteroid injections. Am J Sports Med 1995;23:601–6.

78. James AW. Asthma. Obstet Gynecol Clin North Am 2001;28:305–20.

79. Janssen PA, Holt VL, Sugg NK, et al. Intimate partner violence and adverse pregnancy outcomes: a population-based study. Am J Obstet Gynecol 2003; 188:1341–7.

80. Jones SV, Black MM. Skin diseases in pregnancy. In: de Swiet M, editor. Medical disorders in obstetric practice. 4th ed. Malden, MA: Wiley-Blackwell; 2002. p. 566.

81. Josefsson A, Berg G, Nordin C, Sydsjo G. Prevalence of depressive symptoms in late pregnancy and postpartum. Acta Obstet Gynecol Scand 2001;80:251–5.

82. Jovanovic-Peterson L, Durak EP, Peters CM. Randomized trial of diet versus diet plus cardiovascular conditioning on glucose levels in gestational diabetes. Am J Obstet Gynecol 1989;161:415.

83. Jovanovic-Peterson L, Peterson CM. Dietary manipulation as a primary treatment strategy for pregnancies complicated by diabetes. J Am Coll Nutr 1990;9:320.

84. Kammerer-Doak DN, Cornella JL, Magrina JF, et al. Osteitis pubis after Marshall-Marchetti-Krantz urethropexy: a pubic osteomyelitis. Am J Obstet Gynecol 1998;179:586–90.

85. Kaushal R, Bhanot A, Luthra S, et al. Intrapartum coccygeal fracture, a cause for postpartum coccydynia: a case report. J Surg Orthop Adv 2005;14:136–7.

86. Kelly TF, Savides TJ. Gastrointestinal disease in pregnancy. In: Creasy RK, Resnik R, Iams JD, editors. Creasy and Resnik's maternal-fetal medicine: principles and practice. 6th ed. Philadelphia: Saunders Elsevier; 2009. p. 1041–53.

87. Khastgir G, Studd JW, King H, et al. Changes in bone density and biochemical markers of bone turnover in pregnancy-associated osteoporosis. Br J Obstet Gynaecol 1996;103:716–8.

88. Kopell HP, Thompson WAL. Peripheral entrapment neuropathies. Huntington, NY: Robert E. Krieger; 1976.

89. Koshy M, Burd L. Management of pregnancy in sickle cell syndromes. Hematol Oncol Clin North Am 1991;5:585–96.

90. Kotarinos R. Diastasis recti: clinical assessment versus surgical observation. J Obstet Gynecol Phys Ther 1991;15:9–12.

91. Kuwabara S. Guillain-Barré syndrome: epidemiology, pathophysiology and management. Drugs 2004;64:597–610.

92. La Montagna G, Malesci D, Tirri R, Valentini G. Successful neridronate therapy in transient osteoporosis of the hip. Clin Rheumatol 2005;24:67–9.

93. LaBan MM, Viola S, Williams DA, Wang AM. Magnetic resonance imaging of the lumbar herniated disk in pregnancy. Am J Phys Med Rehabil 1995;74:59–61.

94. Laktasic-Zerjavic N, Curkovic B, Babic-Naglic D, et al. Transient osteoporosis of the hip in pregnancy. Successful treatment with calcitonin: a case report. Z Rheumatol 2007;66:510–3.

95. Larsen EC, Wilken-Jensen C, Hansen A, et al. Symptom-giving pelvic girdle relaxation in pregnancy. I: Prevalence and risk factors. Acta Obstet Gynecol Scand 1999;78:105–10.

96. Larson J. Osteoporosis and the physiotherapist. In: Sapsford R, Bullock-Saxton J, Markwell S, editors. Women's health: a textbook for physiotherapists. Philadelphia: WB Saunders; 1998. p. 412–53.

97. Leavitt R. Cross-cultural rehabilitation: an international perspective. Philadelphia: WB Saunders; 2001.

98. Leeners B, Neumaier-Wagner P, Kuse S, et al. Emotional stress and the risk to develop hypertensive diseases in pregnancy. Hypertens Pregnancy 2007;26:211–26.

99. Leininger M, McFarland M. Transcultural nursing: concepts, theories, research and practice. New York: McGraw Hill; 2002.

100. Lentz SS. Osteitis pubis: a review. Obstet Gynecol Surv 1995;50:310–5.

101. Lepercq J, Conard J, Borel-Derlon A, et al. Venous thromboembolism during pregnancy: a retrospective study of enoxaparin safety in 624 pregnancies. BJOG 2001;108:1134–40.

102. Lindsey RW, Leggon RE, Wright DG, Nolasco DR. Separation of the symphysis pubis in association with childbearing. A case report. J Bone Joint Surg Am 1988;70:289–92.

103. Lipson JG, Dibble SL. Culture and clinical care. San Francisco: UCSF Nursing Press; 2005.

104. Livingstone L. Postnatal management. In: Sapsford R, Bullock-Saxton J, Markwell S, editors. Women's health. A textbook for physiotherapists. Philadelphia: WB Saunders; 1998. p. 220–46.

105. Livingstone L. Physiology of labour. In: Sapsford R, Bullock-Saxton J, Markwell S, editors. Women's health. A textbook for physiotherapists. Philadelphia: WB Saunders; 1998. p. 192–219.

106. Lucas MJ. Diabetes complicating pregnancy. Obstet Gynecol Clin North Am 2001;28:513–36.

107. Lukacz ES, Lawrence JM, Contreras R, et al. Parity, mode of delivery, and pelvic floor disorders. Obstet Gynecol 2006;107:1253–60.

108. Lupton M, Oteng-Ntim E, Ayida G, Steer PJ. Cardiac disease in pregnancy. Curr Opin Obstet Gynecol 2002;14:137–43.

109. Maigne JY, Chatellier G, Faou ML, Archambeau M. The treatment of chronic coccydynia with intrarectal manipulation: a randomized controlled study. Spine 2006;31:E621–7.

110. Maloni JA, Park S, Anthony MK, Musil CM. Measurement of antepartum depressive symptoms during high-risk pregnancy. Res Nurs Health 2005;28:16–26.

111. Maloni JA, Park S. Postpartum symptoms after antepartum bed rest. J Obstet Gynecol Neonatal Nurs 2005;34:163–71.

112. Maloni JA, Schneider BS. Inactivity: symptoms associated with gastrocnemius muscle disuse during pregnancy. AACN Clin Issues 2002;13:248–62.

113. Maloni JA. Bed rest and high-risk pregnancy. Differentiating the effects of diagnosis, setting, and treatment. Nurs Clin North Am 1996;31:313–25.

114. Marcoux S, Berube S, Brisson C, Mondor M. Job strain and pregnancy-induced hypertension. Epidemiology 1999;10:376–82.

115. Marnach ML, Ramin KD, Ramsey PS, et al. Characterization of the relationship between joint laxity and maternal hormones in pregnancy. Obstet Gynecol 2003;101:331–5.

116. Martin SL, Mackie L, Kuppe LL, et al. Physical abuse of women before, during, and after pregnancy. JAMA 2001;285:1581–4.

117. McMullen AH, Pasta DJ, Frederick PD, et al. Impact of pregnancy on women with cystic fibrosis. Chest 2006;129:706–11.

118. Melhado EM, Maciel Jr JA, Guerreiro CA. Headache during gestation: evaluation of 1101 women. Can J Neurol Sci 2007;34:187–92.

119. Menacker F, Hamilton BE. Recent trends in cesarean delivery in the United States. NCHS data brief, no 35. Hyattsville, MD: National Center for Health Statistics; 2010.

120. Mezey GC, Bewley S. Domestic violence and pregnancy. Br J Obstet Gynaecol 1997;104:528–31.

121. Miller MW, Brayman AA, Abramowicz JS. Obstetric ultrasonography: a biophysical consideration of patient safety—the "rules" have changed. Am J Obstet Gynecol 1998;179:241–54.

122. Mokshagundam S, Broadstone V. Diabetes mellitus. In: Sanfilippo JS, Smith RP, editors. Primary care in obstetrics and gynecology: a handbook for clinicians. 2nd ed. New York: Springer-Verlag; 2007. p. 309–541.

123. Molad Y. Systemic lupus erythematosus and pregnancy. Curr Opin Obstet Gynecol 2006;18:613–7.

124. Montgomery KS. Caring for the pregnant woman with sickle cell disease. MCN Am J Matern Child Nurs 1996;21:224–8.

124a. Mori N, Blair KA, Ward TC, Bergstrorn J, Galvão L, Cisler RA. Setting a goal to reduce teen births in Milwaukee by 2015. Wisc Medical J (WMJ) 2009 Oct;108(7):365–9.

125. Morin KH. Urologic consequences of childbirth: a review of the literature. Urol Nurs 1994;14:41–7.

126. Mou Sun P, Wilburn W, Raynor BD, et al. Sickle cell disease in pregnancy: twenty years of experience at Grady Memorial Hospital, Atlanta, Georgia. Am J Obstet Gynecol 2001;184:1127–30.

127. Mueller BA, Zhang J, Critchlow CW. Birth outcomes and need for hospitalization after delivery among women with multiple sclerosis. Am J Obstet Gynecol 2002;186:446–52.

128. Nader S. Thyroid disease of pregnancy. In: Creasy RK, Resnik R, Iams JD, editors. Creasy and Resnik's maternal-fetal medicine: principles and practice. 6th ed. Philadelphia: Saunders Elsevier; 2009. p. 995–1014.

129. Nannini A, Lazar J, Berg C, et al. Physical injuries reported on hospital visits for assault during the pregnancy-associated period. Nurs Res 2008;57:144–9.

130. Nelson JL, Ostensen M. Pregnancy and rheumatoid arthritis. Rheum Dis Clin North Am 1997;23:195–212.

131. Nielsen Forman D, Videbech P, Hedegaard M, et al. Postpartum depression: identification of women at risk. BJOG 2000;107:1210–7.

132. Norwitz E, Schorge JO. Obstetrics and gynecology at a glance. Malden, MA: Blackwell Science; 2001.

133. O'Boyle AL, O'Boyle JD, Magann EF, et al. Anorectal symptoms in pregnancy and the postpartum period. J Reprod Med 2008;53:151–4.

134. Ostergaard GC, Rubin RJ, Salvati EP, et al. Electrogalvanic stimulation in the treatment of levator ani syndrome. Dis Colon Rectum 1998;28:662–3.

135. Owens K, Pearson A, Mason G. Symphysis pubis dysfunction—a cause of significant obstetric morbidity. Eur J Obstet Gynecol Reprod Biol 2002;105:143–6.

136. Paech MJ. Should we take a different angle in managing pregnant women at delivery? Attempting to avoid the 'supine hypotensive syndrome'. Anaesth Intensive Care 2008;36:775–7.

137. Perkins J, Hammer RL, Louber P. Identification and management of pregnancy-related low back pain. J Nurse Midwifery 1998;43:31–40.

138. Peyton FW. Coccygodynia in women. Indiana Med 1988;81:697–8.

139. Pschirrer ER, Monga M. Seizure disorders in pregnancy. Obstet Gynecol Clin North Am 2001;28:601–11.

140. Purnell LD, Paulanka BJ. Transcultural health care: a culturally competent approach. Philadelphia: FA Davis; 2008.

141. Ramin KD, Ramsey PS. Disease of the gallbladder and pancreas in pregnancy. Obstet Gynecol Clin North Am 2001;28:571–80.

142. Rath JD, Rath R, Mielcarski E, et al. Low back pain during pregnancy: helping patients take control. J Musculoskel Med 2000;17:223–32.

143. Rath AM, Attali P, Dumas JL, et al. The abdominal linea alba: an anatomo-radiologic and biomechanical study. Surg Radiol Anat 1996;18:281–8.

144. Rothstein JM, Roy SH, Wolf SL, Scalzitti D. The rehabilitation specialist's handbook. Philadelphia: FA Davis; 2005.

145. Rungee JL. Low back pain during pregnancy. Orthopedics 1993;16:1339–44.

146. Ryder I, Alexander J. Coccydynia: a woman's tail. Midwifery 2000;16:155–60.

147. Saltzman LE, Johnson CH, Gilbert BC, Goodwin MM. Physical abuse around the time of pregnancy: an examination of prevalence and risk factors in 16 states. Matern Child Health J 2003;7:31–43.

148. Samdani A, Lachmann E, Nagler W. Transient osteoporosis of the hip during pregnancy: a case report. Am J Phys Med Rehabil 1998;77:153–6.

149. Sapsford R, Markwell S. Pelvic floor dysfunction in the perinatal period. In: Sapsford R, Bullock-Saxton J, Markwell S, editors. Women's health. A textbook for physiotherapists. Philadelphia: WB Saunders; 1998. p. 529.

150. Sarkar NN. The impact of intimate partner violence on women's reproductive health and pregnancy outcome. J Obstet Gynaecol 2008;28:266–71.

151. Schapira D, Braun Moscovici Y, Gutierrez G, Nahir AM. Severe transient osteoporosis of the hip during pregnancy. Successful treatment with intravenous biphosphonates. Clin Exp Rheumatol 2003;21:107–10.

152. Schauberger CW, Rooney BL, Goldsmith L, et al. Peripheral joint laxity increases in pregnancy but does not correlate with serum relaxin levels. Am J Obstet Gynecol 1996;174:667–71.

153. Scriven MW, Jones DA, McKnight L. The importance of pubic pain following childbirth: a clinical and ultrasonographic study of diastasis of the pubic symphysis. J R Soc Med 1995;88:28–30.

154. Seely BL, Burrow GN. Thyroid disease and pregnancy. In: Creasy RK, Resnik R, Iams JD, editors. Creasy and Resnik's maternal-fetal medicine: principles and practice. 6th ed. Philadelphia: Saunders Elsevier; 2009.

155. Shankman G. Thromboembolic disease anticoagulation therapy. Orthop Pract 2001;13:14–5.

156. Sharma JB, Aggarwal S, Singhal S, et al. Prevalence of urinary incontinence and other urological problems during pregnancy: a questionnaire based study. Arch Gynecol Obstet 2009;279:845–51.

157. Sharpe R. Pregnancy and puerperism: physiological changes. In: Sapsford R, Bullock-Saxton J, Markwell S, editors. Women's health. A textbook for physiotherapists. Philadelphia: WB Saunders; 1998. p. 112–24.

158. Silva M, Mallinson C, Reynolds F. Sciatic nerve palsy following childbirth. Anaesthesia 1996;51:1144–8.

158a. Simcox AM, et al. Decision making about reproduction and pregnancy by women with cystic fibrosis. Br J Hosp Med (Lond) 2009 Nov;70(11):639–43.

159. Simpson EL, Lawrenson RA, Nightingale AL, Farmer RD. Venous thromboembolism in pregnancy and the puerperium: incidence and additional risk factors from a London perinatal database. BJOG 2001;108:56–60.

160. Smith R, Ostlere S, Athanasou N, Vipond S. Pregnancy-associated osteoporosis. Lancet 1996;348:402–3.

161. Smith RP. Gastrointestinal disorders. In: Sanfilippo JS, Smith RP, editors. Primary care in obstetrics and gynecology: a handbook for clinicians. 2nd ed. New York: Springer-Verlag; 2007. p. 327–38.

162. Snow RE, Neubert AG. Peripartum pubic symphysis separation: a case series and review of the literature. Obstet Gynecol Surv 1997;52:438–43.

163. Sohn N, Weinstein MA, Robbins RD. The levator syndrome and its treatment with high-voltage electrogalvanic stimulation. Am J Surg 1982; 144:580–2.

164. Spector RE. Cultural diversity in health and illness. 7th ed. Upper Saddle River, NJ: Pearson; 2008.

165. Stapleton DB, MacLennan AH, Kristiansson P. The prevalence of recalled low back pain during and after pregnancy: a South Australian population survey. Aust N Z J Obstet Gynaecol 2002;42:482–5.

166. Stephenson RG, O'Connor LJ. Obstetric and gynecologic care in physical therapy. Thorofare, NJ: Slack; 2000.

167. Strauhal MJ. Therapeutic exercise in obstetrics. In: Hall CM, Brody LT, editors. Therapeutic exercise: moving toward function. 2nd ed. Philadelphia: Lippincott, Williams & Wilkins; 2005. p. 213–32.

168. Thiele GH. Coccygeus and piriformis muscles: its relationship to coccygodynia and pain in the region of the hip and down the leg. Transcript Am Proct Soc 1936;37:145–55.

169. Thorp Jr JM, Norton PA, Wall LL, et al. Urinary incontinence in pregnancy and the puerperium: a prospective study. Am J Obstet Gynecol 1999;181:266–73.

170. Umpierrez GE, Kitabchi AE. Management of type 2 diabetes: evolving strategies for treatment. Obstet Gynecol Clin North Am 2001;28:401–19.

171. Vaughan DJ, Stirrup CA, Robinson PN. Cranial subdural haematoma associated with dural puncture in labour. Br J Anaesth 2000;84:518–20.

172. Vellacott ID, Cooke EJ, James CE. Nausea and vomiting in early pregnancy. Int J Gynaecol Obstet 1988;27:57–62.

173. Ververidis AN, Drosos GI, Kazakos KJ, et al. Bilateral transient bone marrow edema or transient osteoporosis of the knee in pregnancy. Knee Surg Sports Traumatol Arthrosc 2009;17:1061–4.

174. Viktrup L, Lose G. Incidence and remission of lower urinary tract symptoms during 12 years after the first delivery: a cohort study. J Urol 2008;180:992–7.

175. Vincent C. Osteitis pubis. J Am Board Fam Pract 1993;6:492–6.

176. Vleeming A, Albert HB, Ostgaard HC, et al. European guidelines for the diagnosis and treatment of pelvic girdle pain. Eur Spine J 2008;7:794–819.

177. Vullo VJ, Richardson JK, Hurvitz EA. Hip, knee, and foot pain during pregnancy and the postpartum period. J Fam Pract 1996;43:63–8.

178. Wahl R. Nutrition in the adolescent. Pediatr Ann 1999;28:107–11.

179. Wang SM, Dezinno P, Maranets I, et al. Low back pain during pregnancy: prevalence, risk factors, and outcomes. Obstet Gynecol 2004;104:65–70.

180. Welner S. Pregnancy in women with disabilities. In: Cohen WR, editor. Cherry and Merkatz's complications of pregnancy. 5th ed. Philadelphia: Lippincott, Williams & Wilkins; 2000. p. 829–38.

181. Wendel PJ. Asthma in pregnancy. Obstet Gynecol Clin North Am 2001;28:537–51.

182. Wesnes SL, Hunskaar S, Bo K, Rortveit G. The effect of urinary incontinence status during pregnancy and delivery mode on incontinence postpartum. A cohort study. BJOG 2009;116:700–7.

183. Wesnes SL, Rortveit G, Bo K, Hunskaar S. Urinary incontinence during pregnancy. Obstet Gynecol 2007;109:922–8.

184. Wijma J, Potters AE, de Wolf BT, et al. Anatomical and functional changes in the lower urinary tract following spontaneous vaginal delivery. BJOG 2003;110:658–63.

185. Wijma J, Weis Potters AE, de Wolf BT, et al. Anatomical and functional changes in the lower urinary tract during pregnancy. BJOG 2001;108: 726–32.

186. Williams DJ, Davison JM. Renal disorders. In: Creasy RK, Resnik R, Iams JD, editors. Creasy and Resnik's maternal-fetal medicine: principles and practice. 6th ed. Philadelphia: Saunders Elsevier; 2009. p. 905–26.

187. Wong CA, Scavone BM, Dugan S, et al. Incidence of postpartum lumbosacral spine and lower extremity nerve injuries. Obstet Gynecol 2003;101: 279–88.

188. Wood ML, Larson CM, Dahners LE. Late presentation of a displaced subcapital fracture of the hip in transient osteoporosis of pregnancy. J Orthop Trauma 2003;17:582–4.

189. Wray CC, Easom S, Hoskinson J. Coccydynia. Aetiology and treatment. J Bone Joint Surg Br 1991;73:335–8.

Appendix **17-1** Edinburgh Postnatal Depression Scale (EPDS)

INSTRUCTIONS FOR ADMINISTRATORS

The mother is asked to underline the response that comes closest to how she has been feeling in the previous 7 days. All 10 items must be completed.

Care should be taken to avoid the possibility of the mother discussing her answers with others. The mother should complete the scale herself unless she has limited English or difficulty with reading.

The EPDS may be used at 6 to 8 weeks after delivery to screen postnatal women. The child health clinic, postnatal checkup, or home visit may provide suitable opportunities for its completion.

A score of 10 or higher warrants referral to a primary care or mental health provider for further evaluation.

INSTRUCTIONS FOR USERS

Because you have recently had a baby, we would like to know how you are feeling. Please UNDERLINE the answer that comes closest to how you have felt IN THE PAST 7 DAYS, not just how you feel today.

1. **I have been able to laugh and see the funny side of things.**
   As much as I always could
   Not quite so much now
   Definitely not so much now
   Not at all

2. **I have looked forward with enjoyment to things.**
   As much as I ever did
   Rather less than I used to
   Definitely less than I used to
   Hardly at all

3. **I have blamed myself unnecessarily when things went wrong.***
   Yes, most of the time
   Yes, some of the time
   Not very often
   No, never

4. **I have been anxious or worried for no good reason.**
   No, not at all
   Hardly ever
   Yes, sometimes
   Yes, very often

5. **I have felt scared or panicky for no very good reason.***
   Yes, quite a lot
   Yes, sometimes
   No, not much
   No, not at all

6. **Things have been getting on top of me.***
   Yes, most of the time I haven't been able to cope at all.
   Yes, sometimes I haven't been coping as well as usual.
   No, most of the time I have coped quite well.
   No, I have been coping as well as ever.

7. **I have been so unhappy that I have had difficulty sleeping.***
   Yes, most of the time
   Yes, sometimes
   Not very often
   No, not at all

8. **I have felt sad or miserable.***
   Yes, most of the time
   Yes, quite often
   Not very often
   No, not at all

9. **I have been so unhappy that I have been crying.***
   Yes, most of the time
   Yes, quite often
   Only occasionally
   No, never

10. **The thought of harming myself has occurred to me.***
    Yes, quite often
    Sometimes
    Hardly ever
    Never

Response categories are scored 0, 1, 2, and 3, according to increased severity of the symptoms. Items marked with an asterisk are reverse-coded (3, 2, 1, and 0). The total score is calculated by adding together the scores for each of the 10 items.[42]

Appendix **17-2 Obstetric Resources**

Maternal-Child Health Organizations
American Academy of Husband-Coached Childbirth (AAHCC)
The Bradley Method
PO Box 5224
Sherman Oaks, CA 91413-5224
818-788-6662
800-422-4784
www.bradleybirth.com
American College of Nurse-Midwives (ACNM)
8403 Colesville Rd., Suite 1550
Silver Spring, MD 20910
240-485-1800
www.acnm.org
Gives listing of nurse-midwives and nurse-midwifery training programs.
American College of Obstetricians and Gynecologists (ACOG)
409 12th Street, SW
PO Box 96920
Washington, DC 20090-6920
202-638-5577
www.acog.org
Brochure: "Exercise and Fitness: A Guide for Women and Women and Exercise"
Technical Bulletins: *Women and Exercise, Exercise During Pregnancy and the Postpartum Period*
Birth Works, Inc.
PO Box 2045
Medford, NJ 08055
888-862-4784
www.birthworks.org
Offers a holistic approach to childbirth and provides information from a holistic standpoint.
Council of Childbirth Education Specialists, Inc.
PO Box 2000
Williamsburg, VA 23187-2000
757-258-5282
www.councilces.org
Childbirth organization offering certification to nurses and PTs; offers introductory and advanced seminars.
International Childbirth Education Association (ICEA)
1500 Sunday Drive, Suite 102
Raleigh, NC 27607
919-863-9487
800-624-4934
www.icea.org
Certifies childbirth educators, has mail order bookstore, and offers information about pregnancy and childbirth education.

International Organization of Physical Therapists in Women's Health (IOPTWH)
Subgroup of the World Confederation for Physical Therapy (WCPT)
335 Main Street
Medfield, MA 02052
508-359-2427
www.ioptwh.org
La Leche League International (LLLI)
PO Box 4079
Schaumburg, IL 60168-4079
847-519-7730
800-LALECHE (525-3243)
www.llli.org
Headquarters for the 3000 groups throughout the world offering support for breast-feeding through individual counseling and education.
Lamaze International (formerly known as the American Society for Psychoprophylaxis in Obstetrics)
2025 M Street NW, Suite 800
Washington, DC 20036-3309
800-368-4404
202-367-1128 (international calls)
www.lamaze.org
Offers certification in Lamaze method of childbirth preparation, publishes the *Lamaze Parents* magazine, and provides information about pregnancy and childbirth-related topics.
National Domestic Violence Hotline
800-799-SAFE
National Family Violence HelpLine
800-222-2000
National Institutes of Health (NIH)
U.S. Department of Health and Human Services
9000 Rockville Pike
Bethesda, MD 20892
301-496-4000
www.nih.gov
Offers all NIH publications and information on antenatal diagnosis, cesarean birth, toxoplasmosis, and ultrasound imaging.
Association of Women's Health, Obstetric and Neonatal Nurses (AWHONN)
2000 L Street, NW, Suite 740
Washington, DC 20036
800-673-8499
www.awhonn.org
Organization for nurses specializing in obstetric, gynecologic, and neonatal nursing, with many publications related to pregnancy and childbirth, continuing education programs, and current maternal and child health information.

Sidelines National High Risk Pregnancy Support Network
PO Box 1808
Laguna Beach, CA 92652
714-497-2265
602-941-0176
www.sidelines.org
Support for women with high-risk pregnancies.

U.S. Department of Agriculture
WIC Supplemental Food Section
1400 Independence Ave SW
Washington, DC 20250
www.usda.gov
Offers information on nutrition for pregnant and nursing women.

AUDIOVISUAL AIDS FOR PATIENT EDUCATION

American Physical Therapy Association
Section on Women's Health
1111 North Fairfax St.
Alexandria, VA 22314
703-684-2782
800-999-2782
www.womenshealthapta.org

Lamaze International
2025 M Street NW, Suite 800
Washington, DC 20036-3309
202-367-1128
800-368-4404
www.lamaze.org

Childbirth Graphics
5045 Franklin Ave
Waco, TX 76710
254-776-6461, ext 287
800-299-3366, ext 287
www.childbirthgraphics.com
Perinatal education materials company providing more than 1100 products, including models, posters, slides, and brochures.

International Childbirth Education Association (ICEA)
1500 Sunday Drive, Suite 102
Raleigh, NC 27607
919-863-9487
800-624-4934
www.icea.org
Materials include patient education booklets, community education programs in slide format, pelvic floor evaluation forms, courses, and PT referral forms.

Sue Wenker, PT, MS, GCS
Maureen Euhardy, PT, MS, GCS

The Geriatric Population | 18

Objectives

After reading this chapter, the reader will be able to:

1. Explain the distinctions between normal and pathologic aging.
2. Describe the working definitions of frailty and screening as they apply to the geriatric population.
3. Describe the medical diagnostic challenges associated with the geriatric population, including polypharmacy, falls, nutritional deficits, dehydration, and changes in cognition.
4. Explain the clinical diagnoses associated with diseases common to the geriatric population.

There are currently "80 million baby boomers born between 1946 and 1964 constituting a third of the U.S. population, raising the specter of more disease and more costs for the healthcare system."[12] From a rehabilitative, physical therapy perspective, observers predict that this new cohort of older adults, the aging boomers, will crave vigor, vitality, and extended life. The U.S. population aged 65 years and older is expected to double within the next 25 years. By 2030, almost 1 of every 5 Americans, some 72 million people, will be 65 years or older. In percentage terms, the portion of the U.S. population that is 65 or older is expected to rise from 12% to almost 20%.[26] The age group 85 years and older is now the fastest growing segment of the U.S. population.[12] The number of the "oldest old," those who are 80 and older, is also expected to almost double, from 11 to 20 million. The irony of past medical successes is that many long-living older adults now struggle with long-term disability that the American health care system is ill prepared to handle, such as heart disease, cancer, arthritis, osteoporosis, and Alzheimer's disease.[11] This results in many older adults needing rehabilitative services in primary care outpatient clinics.

The good news is that with proper preventive interventions, which can be incorporated into the primary care setting, there is potential to produce a healthier version of aging at a lower cost than the current health care delivery system. Physical therapy is poised to help meet the aging population's primary care needs. Through direct access, physical therapists (PTs) often will be the practitioner of choice for many of these patients. In addition to our traditional roles in rehabilitation, we will shift our clinical interventions toward prevention of disease, injury, and disability. PTs in the primary care venue should be an integral part of the interdisciplinary approach inherent in a family or general medicine practice or non–hospital-based outpatient physical therapy clinic.

PTs in primary care outpatient settings encounter geriatric patients each day, and in many clinics, older patients make up a significant proportion of the hospital and non–hospital-based ambulatory care patient population. Therefore, it is essential that PTs develop expertise in the management of geriatric patients in this environment. This chapter's overall goal is to provide clinicians working in primary care settings with an understanding of the principles and practices necessary to address the physical therapy needs of an aging patient population competently.

Primary Care in Geriatric Physical Therapy

The *Guide to Physical Therapist Practice* describes primary care as "the provision of integrated, accessible health care services by clinicians who are accountable for addressing a large majority of personal health care needs, developing a sustained partnership with patients, and practicing within the context of family and community."[3] These components are crucial to the holistic and comprehensive care of aged individuals.

Because physical therpay is the potential patient entry point into a primary care clinic, a sound educational background in differential diagnosis and acute management of musculoskeletal conditions and other pathologies specific to the older population, as well as a working knowledge of radiology, pharmacology, nutrition, laboratory technology, team building, and communication skills, are essential. Having a geriatric clinical specialist (GCS) on staff who is knowledgeable and capable of providing high-quality care for older patients with more complex health concerns is important. However, all PTs in general outpatient clinics should be competent in providing most aspects of primary care to an older adult.

The value of interdisciplinary teams for the care of older adults with complex care needs has been increasingly acknowledged in recent years.[26] Still, health care professionals are typically trained separately by discipline, which fosters ideas of hierarchy and responsibility for individual decision making.[26] As a subspecialty, geriatric physical therapy must go beyond traditional physical therapy models of care and work closely with those in other health care fields, such as social work, nursing, dietetics, medicine, occupational therapy, and pharmacy in providing clinical services and education in a primary care setting. Geriatrics should be seen as a *perspective* concerned with a stage of life that calls for an interdisciplinary approach, with collaboration among specialties. This is the core premise of primary care in the physical therapy management of the geriatric patient.

Geriatric Assessment and Managed Care

With the reorganization of the financing of health care and the creation of systems of care, it is possible to design and implement organizational interventions to improve the care of older adults. The Balanced Budget Act of 1997 brought several changes in

This chapter includes contributions by Jennifer Bottomley from the first edition of *Primary Care for the Physical Therapist, Examination and Triage.*

Medicare managed care. However, the need to serve the aging population better continues to be a dynamic progress, and identifying successful models of care is only the first challenge to improving the health care of older adults.[15] Older adults have diverse health care needs, and a variety of health care delivery models exists to meet those needs. Currently, multiple models of managed care are available for the older adult, including the Geriatric Resources for Assessment and Care of Elders (GRACE), Program of All-inclusive Care for the Elderly (PACE), and Family Care (Wisconsin).[18,56] Risk and value of services are central concepts that affect managed care of this population. Changing the structure of delivery to an interdisciplinary, primary care model is a potentially powerful method of influencing health care and maintaining the health of older persons. The result would be an efficient and effective model delivering appropriate screening and appraisal of health and functional risks identifying those older individuals who are at greatest risk of developing morbidity and disability.

Cohen and associates,[14] in a controlled trial, found that primary care in inpatient geriatric units and outpatient geriatric clinics have no significant effects on survival. However, there were significant reductions in functional decline with inpatient geriatric evaluations and management. Improvements were also noted in mental health and functional status with outpatient primary care evaluation and management, with no increase in costs.[1]

Effective new strategies that complement primary care are needed to reduce disability risks and to improve the self-management of chronic illness in frail older people living in the community. The models of health care noted earlier speak to new methods of delivering high-quality care. There continue to be barriers, such as limited geriatric education in the field of medicine, a ratio of aging adults that far outweighs the number of health care professionals able to provide care, and an increased burnout rate for health care workers in the field of geriatrics. However, the need to be trained as an effective interdisciplinary team member is of utmost importance in providing the best care possible for the older adult.

Ideally, in traditional fee-for-service primary care practices, comprehensive assessment of older patients is provided at the site of care by an interdisciplinary team. Targeting this complex, costly, and time-consuming process to individuals who have the potential to benefit the most from subsequent interventions (i.e., the highest-risk older population) is vital to the success of primary care within a managed care environment. An example is a one-time physical examination, in addition to education and counseling about preventive services, including certain screenings, shots, and referrals for other care if needed, when an adult enrolls in the Medicare Part B program. Starting January 1, 2009, Medicare covered this examination within the first 12 months for the patient who has Medicare Part B. The patient pays 20% of the Medicare-approved amount, and the Part B deductible no longer applies. A person becomes eligible for Medicare Part B or an advantage plan in the 7-month period that begins 3 months before a person turns 65, includes the month the person turns 65, and ends 3 months after the month he or she turns 65.[13,84]

It is often difficult for most Medicare providers to conduct all-inclusive examinations because of the time and personnel required for interdisciplinary geriatric care. However, the economic and clinical forces of managed care promote creativity and innovation in the development of targeted programs that provide the most efficient and effective interventions for geriatric patients. For example, disease management programs generally include the identification of high-risk members and the targeting of coordinated care to those individuals.[67]

A model in physical therapy would be screening for risk of falls; identifying those older adults most likely to experience a fall; and intervening by strengthening weak muscles, promoting erect posture, and facilitating sensory organization strategies to accommodate for instability around the center of gravity. Treating before a fall is intuitively much less costly than intervening after a fall. Targeting allows the available resources of the interdisciplinary geriatric team to be directed to individuals with the greatest potential to benefit. High-risk screening or health risk appraisals often are used to identify older adults requiring primary, secondary, or tertiary preventive health interventions. Ideally, it would be beneficial if high-risk individuals could then be triaged to interventions such as physical therapy.

Unique Clinical Characteristics of the Aging Population

One primary concept associated with the geriatric population is that of heterogeneity. More than any other age group, older adults vary in their level of functional capabilities. In the clinic, we often see 65-year-old individuals who are severely physically disabled sitting right next to individuals of the same age who are still working full time and who are extremely active. Even in the "old-old" category, variability in physical and cognitive functioning is remarkable.[46]

Another important concept in geriatric physical therapy is the concept of activity versus inactivity. "The most common reason for losses in functional capabilities in the aged is inactivity or immobility."[7] Older adults become immobilized for many reasons. Acute immobilization often is considered to be accidental and can be associated with acute catastrophic trauma or illnesses, including severe blood loss, trauma, head injury, cerebral vascular accident, burns, and hip fracture. "The patient's activity level often is severely curtailed until the acute illnesses become medically stable."[46]

Chronic immobilization may result from long-standing problems that are undertreated or left untreated; these include amputations, arthritis, cardiac disease, pulmonary disease, and low back pain. Environmental barriers are a major cause of accidental immobilization in the acute and chronic care settings. These include bed rails, the height of the bed, physical restraints, an inappropriate chair, lack of physical assistance, fall precautions imposed by medical staff, lack of orders in the chart for mobilization, social isolation, and physical obstacles (e.g., stairs or doorway thresholds). Cognitive impairments, central nervous system (CNS) disorders (e.g., stroke, Parkinson's disease, multiple sclerosis), peripheral neuropathies resulting from diabetes, and pain with movement also can severely reduce mobility. Affective disorders such as depression, anxiety, or fear of falling also may lead to accidental immobilization. In addition, sensory changes, terminal illnesses (e.g., cancer, cirrhosis of the liver), acute episodes of illness such as pneumonia or cellulitis, or an attitude of "I'm too sick to get up" can reduce mobility.[7]

A third key concept in geriatric rehabilitation is the principle of optimal health. The World Health Organization defines health as a state of complete physical, mental, and social well-being, not merely the absence of disease or infirmity.[58] The presence of complete physical health refers to the absence of disease, limitation in activities, or participation restrictions and is achievable. Mental and social well-being within the person's community are closely related and possibly less easy to obtain in this age cohort. The World Health Organization defines mental health as a state of well-being in which the individual realizes his or her own abilities, can cope with the normal stresses of life, can work productively and fruitfully, and is able to make a contribution to his or her community.[35] The social components of health include living situation, social roles (e.g., mother, daughter, vocation), and economic status.[35]

The clinician must consider these unique clinical characteristics of aging as part of a comprehensive screening and examination of an older individual entering the primary care environment. Many myths exist regarding aging. Box 18-1 provides the reader with facts to correct some of these inaccurate orphans perceptions.

Normal Version Pathologic Aging

Aging is considered a normal physiologic process because of its universality. As much as the aging process may affect the predisposition to disease, aging in and of itself is not considered to be pathologic. This distinction seems conceptually clear, but the fine line between aging and disease often is blurred, with some degree of decline in biologic, physiologic, anatomic, and functional capabilities occurring as one ages. Some degree of atrophy is evident in all tissues of the body.[46] A variety of degenerative processes are called normal aging until they proceed far enough to cause clinically significant disability.

Although aging may not be considered a disease process, the time-dependent loss of structure and function in all organ systems leads to pathologic end states. Age brings a general decline in structure, function, and number of many cell types. Consider the following examples. Cellular aging is accompanied by denaturation of extracellular proteins, and the elastin of the skin becomes irreversibly crystalline and broken. The hyaline cartilage on articular surfaces of joints becomes fibrillar and fragmented, and the beautifully ordered structure of the eye lens becomes brittle and chaotic as lens protein is gradually

---

BOX 18-1

General Facts about Aging

- Approximately 50% of decreased function is attributed to pathology rather than "normal" aging changes.
- Organ systems decline at a rate of approximately 0.75% to 1% per year starting at the age of 30 years.
- Hip surgery is the third-most-common surgery for those older than 65 years.
- The risk of hip surgery doubles every 5 years after the age of 60 years.
- The overall efficiency of body systems decreases.
- Many physiologic responses that are normal in younger individuals are blunted or slowed in the older adult population.
- The presence of chronic illnesses also may affect response to exercise.

---

denatured. However, the most important aging changes occur at the molecular level. Small injuries occurring within the molecule result in the loss of genetic memory and progressive cross-linking of collagen, the chief structural protein in the body.

Disease is defined as the reaction to injury.[40] If aging is a gradual accumulation of incompletely repaired injuries caused by microtrauma throughout life, aging may not be normal, despite its universality. Perhaps "aging" is a pathologic process resulting from tissue reactions to imperceptible injuries that could have been avoided.[49]

In the primary care model, PTs play a major role in preventing the disabilities that result from these insidious microtraumas. Screening and subsequent evaluation, and interventions for the limitations and disabilities identified, could preserve health and function. For example, preventive strengthening and conditioning exercises, positioning, joint and tissue mobilization, and many other treatments all affect functional capabilities, especially in an older population. Preventing disabilities that can result from pathologic processes greatly improves the level of function and quality of life. Certainly, some changes that occur with aging need not be inevitable.[46]

Anatomic and Physiologic Features of the Aging Process

Many changes are associated with aging throughout adulthood and into old age. Box 18-2 summarizes these system changes. Box 18-3 summarizes changes related to exercise in older adults. One must remember that individuals age at different rates. Therefore, although it is useful to summarize age-related changes, the PT must remember that any one individual may vary remarkably from her or his peers.

Defining Frailty

Defining the term *frailty* is difficult, but the image of frailty is well understood in geriatric rehabilitation. The concept of frailty invokes a clear mental image for most clinicians; the components of frailty may include compromises in cognition, reductions in sensorimotor input and integration, polypharmacy, dehydration, and malnutrition. The decline in muscle strength and mass, decreased respiratory reserve and cardiovascular functioning, kyphotic postural changes, compromised eyesight, poor hydration and marginal nutritional intake, and many other physiologic and physical changes associated with inactivity and aging lead to frailty. Concomitant diseases such as congestive heart failure, renal disease, osteoporosis, diabetes, chronic lung disease, and arthritis all add to the level of frailty. Lack of mobility can further manifest a sense of frailty. Extended periods of bed rest may also contribute to frailty. Box 18-4 is a summary of the effects of bed rest on a person's body. Any of these conditions, in isolation or in combination, can create frailty.

Screening the Geriatric Population

As the entry point into the primary care setting, PTs should be routinely triaging patients for need of referral. Many diseases can be prevented or forestalled by identifying and avoiding high-risk

BOX 18-2
Summary of Multisystem Changes in Older Adults

MUSCULOSKELETAL SYSTEM

- Muscle mass and strength decrease at a rate of about 30% between the ages of 60 and 90 years.
- Loss of muscle fiber type—type II fibers (white, fast twitch) decrease by about 50%.
- Change in clear differentiation of fiber type, with the red increasing in speed of contraction and the white fibers decreasing in the speed of contraction.
- Decrease in recruitment of motor units.
- Decrease in the speed of movement.
- Decreased tensile strength of bone (more than 30% of women older than 65 years have osteoporosis).
- Women lose about 30% of bone mass by the age of 70 years; men lose about 15% by the age of 70 years.
- Joint flexibility is reduced by 25% to 30% in those older than 70 years.
- Decrease in enzymatic activity, cell count, and metabolic substrates in cartilage (collagen fibers increase their cross-linking, resulting in increase in soft tissue density).

NEUROMUSCULAR SYSTEM

- Atrophy of neurons; nerve fibers decrease and change in structure.
- Myoneural junction decreases in transmission speed.
- Mitochondrial activity decreases.
- Dopamine level depletion.
- Decrease in nerve conduction velocity by about 0.4% per year after age 70 years.
- Slowing of motor neuron conduction, which contributes to alterations in the autonomic system.
- Decreases in reflexes result from a decrease in nerve conduction. In a population of those 70 to 80 years old, ankle jerk is absent in about 70%, and knee and biceps jerk are absent in about 15%.
- Overall, slowed and decreased responsiveness in reaction time.
- Linear increase in postural sway (less in women than in men).
- Changes in sleep patterns affect neuromuscular functioning.

NEUROSENSORY SYSTEM

- Decrease in sweating (implications for modalities and exercise).
- 10% to 20% decrease in brain weight by age 90 years.
- Decrease in mechanoreceptors.
- Decrease in efficiency of the neuroendocrine system (i.e., decrease in calcium control, affecting heart contraction and causing osteoporosis; thymus function decreases 90% between ages 20 and 80 years).
- Decrease in visual acuity and ability to accommodate to lighting changes resulting from increased density of lens.
- Decrease in hearing, especially high frequencies.
- Decrease in the senses of smell and taste; decreased number of taste buds.

CARDIOVASCULAR AND PULMONARY SYSTEMS

- Decrease in cardiac output by about 0.7% per year after 20 years of age (5 L/min CO at age 20 versus 3.5 L/min by age 75 years).
- Increased vascular resistance.

- Decreased arterial elasticity.
- Decreased cardiac reserve, decreased physical response to stress.
- Decrease in lipid catabolism, which may increase risk for heart disease. About 50% of adults between ages 65 and 74 years have evidence of heart disease, and about 30% in this age range have sustained myocardial infarction (MI), even in the absence of symptoms of ischemia (with congestive heart failure, MIs exceed 50%).
- Decrease in lung function (from age 25 to 85 years, as much as a 50% decrease in maximal voluntary ventilation caused by an increase in air resistance and approximately a 40% decrease in vital capacity).
- Respiratory gas exchange surface area decreases at a rate of about 0.27 m²/year.
- Decrease in elastin in the lungs (increased rigidity) and chest wall soft tissues results in decrease in chest wall compliance.
- Decreases in vital capacity and in pulmonary blood flow contribute to lower oxygen saturation levels.
- Residual volume doubles.
- Decreased cough reflex.
- Decreased ciliary response.
- Work capacity declines about 30% between the ages of 40 and 70 years.

UROGENITAL AND RENAL SYSTEMS

- Gradual overall structure change in all renal components.
- Decreased glomerular filtration rate and creatinine clearance.
- Muscle hypertrophy in the urethra and bladder.
- Decreased ability to concentrate urine.

GASTROINTESTINAL SYSTEM

- Decreased peristalsis.
- Diminished secretions of pepsin and acid in the stomach.
- Decrease in hepatic and pancreatic enzymes.

INTEGUMENTARY SYSTEM

- Slower healing time of damaged tissues.
- Increased vulnerability of tissue trauma from shear and frictional forces.
- Decreased oxidative and nutritive state of tissues.
- Increased risk of arterial, venous, and pressure ulcers.
- Increased rate of wound dehiscence.
- Decreased tensile strength.
- Skin feels thinner.

IMMUNE SYSTEM

- Decrease in overall function with increased susceptibility to infection.
- Decreased temperature regulation.
- Decrease in number of T cells.
- Decrease in neuroendocrine system efficiency, diminishing responsiveness.
- Training.

Adapted from Bottomley JM: Summary of system changes. Comparing and contrasting age-related changes. In Bottomley JM, Lewis CB: *Geriatric rehabilitation: a clinical approach*, 3rd ed, Upper Saddleback, NJ, 2008, Prentice Hall.

behaviors. As a result of initiatives implemented by the Surgeon General in the early 1980s, many agencies now offer preventive health programs, including screening for high-risk behaviors and the presence of disease.[46] Health screening and early detection of disease processes should substantially reduce health care costs.

Screening programs for older adults often address behavior patterns such as smoking, level of activity, dietary habits, living environment, health care needs such as dental and foot care, and immunization history. These programs should have a follow-up mechanism for patient education or referral sources for evaluating and treating physical or medical problems identified during

the screening. *The Guide to Physical Therapist Practice*[3] presents the various definitions of prevention, including the following:

1. Primary prevention programs include immunizations; screening for falls; posture and flexibility assessment; and assessment of health-risk behaviors such as smoking, poor nutrition, inactivity, isolation, and other psychosocial factors.
2. Secondary prevention focuses on early detection and treatment of disease and is particularly applicable in disorders such as hypertension, vision and hearing impairments, musculoskeletal problems, neuromuscular conditions, depression, and iatrogenic adverse drug effects.

BOX 18-3

Effects of Exercise on Aging

- 10 weeks of aerobic training results in a 10% to 15% increase in maximal oxygen consumption, stroke volume, and cardiac output.
- Maximal oxygen consumption in those older than 80 years increases by 0% to 38% with endurance training of as little as 6 weeks.
- 1 hour of exercise class (seated exercises) four times a week has shown a favorable effect on aerobic parameters.
- Exercise for 70-year-olds, three times a week for 12 weeks (45-minute sessions), increases static and dynamic strength at all velocities, increases type II muscle fibers, and improves enzymatic responses.
- Muscle activation (neural factors) increases with little muscle hypertrophy in older adults related to strength training.
- Less stretch is required to produce maximal twitch tension after resistance training in individuals 70 to 95 years of age.
- Balance exercises improve postural control, trunk strength, and speed of reaction time in adults older than 70 years.
- There are significant improvements in muscle strength and muscle cross-sectional area, improved mobility (including increased walking speed, improved stair-climbing ability, and higher functional capabilities), improved dietary intake, and increased spontaneous physical activity in frail older adults with high-intensity, progressive resistance exercise.

Adapted from Bottomley JM: Summary of system changes. Comparing and contrasting age-related changes. In Bottomley JM, Lewis CB: *Geriatric rehabilitation: a clinical approach*, 3rd ed, Upper Saddleback, NJ, 2008, Prentice Hall.

BOX 18-4

Effects of Bed Rest

- Maximal oxygen uptake decreases by 20% to 40% within 3 days.
- Ventilatory volume at rest and during functional activity declines by as much as 50% within the first week of bed rest.
- Stroke volume decreases by about 10% within the first week and decreases by about 10% each week thereafter.
- Work capacity declines as much as 25% after 3 weeks of bed rest, declining at a rate of about 1% per day.
- Blood volume decreases by 700 to 800 mL, resulting in hypovolemic manifestations of tachycardia and orthostatic hypotension, as well as increasing thromboembolic risk within the first 3 days.
- Nitrogen spilling into urine increases, indicative of protein wasting, within 3 days.
- Bone mass is lost at a rate of up to 1.4% per day without weight bearing (starting on day 1). About 40% of bone mass can be lost after 6 weeks of bed rest.
- Skeletal muscle mass and contractile strength and efficiency decrease by about 10% to 15% within the first week of bed rest.

---

3. Tertiary prevention focuses on functional assessment and maximizing physical potential and environmental efficiency to prevent the progression of functional decline.

The U.S. Preventive Services Task Force[92,93] has identified screening interventions that successfully alter the outcomes of various diseases. Its recommendations emphasize the importance of educating the older population about modifications of high-risk behaviors. For example, the Task Force advises that older adults be given educational material about the benefits of physical activity in disease prevention; recommendations for selecting appropriate exercise levels and modes of exercise should be provided individually to each person screened. Other components in the Task Force's recommendations include smoking cessation programs, dietary modification to prevent diseases associated with dietary excesses or imbalances (e.g., osteoporosis, heart disease, some cancers, cerebral vascular accident, dental diseases), alcohol cessation programs when abuse is identified, home modification screening to reduce the potential for accidental injuries, vaccination programs for *Pneumococcus* and influenza, tetanus immunization, and screening for preventive chemoprophylaxis programs such as low-dose aspirin therapy (e.g., 80 mg/day) for those at risk for cardiovascular disease and calcium supplements for women at increased risk for the development of osteoporosis.

Medical Complexity and Multisystem Involvement

The potential for an increased number of comorbidities and multisystem involvement increases with age. Any older person who is admitted for acute illness or injury faces significant short-term deterioration in mobility and other functional domains.[91] Decline in physical function, although a negative outcome in itself, also has been associated with many adverse consequences such as falls, disability, and mortality.[27,28,91]

Functional dependence develops in approximately 10% of nondisabled community-dwelling persons older than 75 years annually.[27] Increasing levels of disability are associated with substantial morbidity, leading to the adverse outcomes of hospitalization and nursing home placement and greater use of home care services.[28] Functional dependence leads to increasing levels of frailty, especially in the medically complex, multisystem-involved older adult. With each medical insult and hospitalization, the patient faces a decreasing level of physiologic capacity, which is associated with greater difficulty in recovering his or her premorbid functional abilities.[10,60] Therefore, the primary care PT needs to be cognizant of the patient's medical and social history, along with his or her current condition and future plans. The medically complex patient may require increased time spent on evaluation compared with younger patients. This initial increase in evaluation time may decrease future patient needs and cost.

Polypharmacy

The presence of multiple diagnoses in the older adult leads to multiple drug and nutrient interactions and complex medical management, with the resulting side effects of progressive loss of functional reserve and physiologic homeostasis.

Many medications are absorbed, distributed, metabolized, and excreted (pharmacokinetics) differently in older adults, and the action of drugs (pharmacodynamics) may be exaggerated or reduced[25] (see Chapter 4). Different drugs interact with each other by pharmacokinetic inhibition or induction of drug metabolism or by pharmacodynamic potentiation or antagonism. Knowledge of these pharmacologic pathways has a profound effect on the quality of care. There are multiple definitions of polypharmacy, ranging from the concurrent use of two to five prescription medications; however, a more useful definition is proposed focusing on whether medications are clinically indicated.

Many drugs have paradoxical or bizarre side effects when given to the older adult. One should be suspicious of every drug that the patient is taking, including over-the-counter medications, especially when CNS-related abnormalities are noted during the examination. The potential for drug interactions increases as the number of drugs increases, and older adults are often taking a number of medications[46] (see Chapter 4).

Medication mishaps in older adults occur for many reasons. Multiple providers often are unaware of one another's new prescriptions or medication changes, especially after hospitalization. This problem may diminish as electronic records become more mainstream. Older patients often have visual or cognitive impairments (or both) that lead to errors in self-administration. Patients may be unable to afford their medicines, so they may take only some of what is prescribed based on how they are feeling, or they cut doses to save money and extend the life of their prescription. Functional illiteracy can make adherence to a medical regimen difficult. Cultural beliefs also affect some older adults' perceptions about the value of taking a certain medication when some natural alternative has been used for centuries in their culture to treat the same condition.[46]

PTs in a primary care setting must understand the actions and interactions of drugs for several reasons[14]:

1. With direct access, and PTs being the entry point of care, screening for drug interactions and side effects of the multipharmacy regimen is critical.
2. Drugs often have side effects, or desired actions, that affect physical therapy interventions. For example, the use of a beta blocker will lower the heart rate and cardiac output. Therefore, the response to exercise may be blunted.
3. PTs design and monitor exercise programs that can affect the pharmacokinetics of drugs. Fat-soluble drugs, for example, may be affected by a person's decrease in fat after participation in an exercise program, so dosages will need to be adjusted accordingly.

If adequately educated in pharmacology, PTs can communicate with physicians, contributing to modifications of drug regimens. Appropriate medication management is an interdisciplinary concern. Other health care team members, not just the physician or nurse practitioner, must take responsibility for the supervision and coordination of drug interventions, especially in a primary care setting.

Falls

Falls are not a part of the normal aging process. Among older adults, falls are the leading cause of death from injury. The Centers for Disease Control and Prevention estimates that approximately one third of people 65 years and older fall each year. Falls are the most common cause of traumatic brain injuries (TBIs).[17,37] In 2000, TBIs accounted for 46% of fatal falls in older adults.[78] Most fractures that occur in older adults are caused by falls,[6] with the most common fracture sites being the spine, hip, forearm, leg, ankle, pelvis, upper arm, and hand.[72] Approximately 1 in 5 patients who have suffered a hip fracture die within 1 year of the injury.[14]

Many people who fall, even those who are not injured, develop a fear of falling. This fear may cause them to limit their activities, leading to reduced mobility and physical fitness, and increasing their actual risk of falling.[86] There are numerous steps that older adults can take to protect their independence

and reduce their risk of falling. Box 18-5 outlines several of these interventions.

Women tend to fall more often than men. In 2005, the rate for women was almost 49% higher than for men.[15] Figures 18-1 and 18-2 illustrate the higher incidence of falls with injuries for women versus men and the geographic distribution of women who are injured as a result of falls across the United States, respectively.[12]

Clinical Features of Malnutrition

There may be several factors contributing to an older adult's reduced nutritional reserve. Malnutrition is another example of the complexities when evaluating an older adult because of the diversity of symptoms. Poor nutritional status may contribute to postoperative confusion, delayed recovery times of homeostatic function, delayed wound healing, and increased susceptibility to infection.[31]

The clinical assessment, including the history and physical examination, may reveal findings associated with nutritional deficiencies.[21,87] This clinical assessment should include weight history (current and usual), assessment of changes in diet, symptoms affecting nutrition including nausea and vomiting, diarrhea, constipation, stomatitis, mucositis, dry mouth, taste or olfactory abnormalities, pain medications that may affect intake or metabolic requirements, and other medical conditions that may affect nutritional intake or nutrition intervention options. Physical examination entails a general assessment of physical

---

BOX 18-5

Interventions to Minimize Risk of Falls

- Exercise regularly; exercise programs such as tai chi that increase strength and improve balance are especially effective.
- Ask a physician or pharmacist to review medicines, prescription and over the counter, to reduce side effects and interactions.
- Have eyes checked by an optometrist or ophthalmologist at least once a year.
- Improve lighting in the home.
- Reduce hazards in the home that can lead to falls—for example, minimize clutter and keep walkways clear of obstacles.

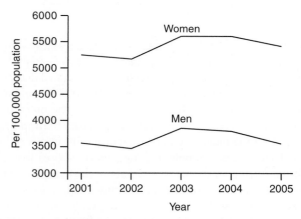

FIGURE 18-1 Age-adjusted nonfatal fall injury rates among men and women aged 65 years and older, United States, 2001-2005. (From Centers for Disease Control Prevention: *Injury prevention & control: data & statistics [WISQARS]*, 2006 [website]. http://www.cdc.gov/injury/wisqars. Accessed March 25, 2010.)

condition, including loss of subcutaneous fat, muscle wasting, presence of edema, or ascites.

Box 18-6 presents possible clinical manifestations of nutritional deficiencies that can occur in older adults. The PT should remember that before ascribing any physical findings elicited during physical examination to nutritional problems, he or she should consider whether the findings are consistent with normal aging or with an underlying disease state.

Clinical Features of Dehydration

Dehydration, a decrease in total body water, is the most common fluid and electrolyte disturbance in older adults.[64] In many cases, cognitive or physical disabilities reduce the ability to recognize thirst, express thirst, or obtain access to water.[53] In addition, healthy older individuals seem to have reduced thirst in response to fluid deprivation.[24] Older adults also produce less concentrated urine after fluid deprivation. Because older subjects have higher vasopressin levels in response to dehydration, the reduced capacity to concentrate the urine is most likely the result of renal changes that occur with normal aging.[24]

Among older patients, hypernatremia (dehydration with elevated sodium levels in the serum) is most common in those who do not drink sufficient water to satisfy their thirst or in those whose thirst sensation is reduced by impaired CNS functioning. A net deficit of water is associated with vomiting, diarrhea, and hyperpyrexia (excessive sweating). In general, older patients appear to be predisposed to the development of hypernatremia. They have an increased sensitivity to dehydration as a result of physiologic changes, including an increase in fat and

a decrease in lean body mass, which corresponds with reduced total body water.

Surgery, febrile illnesses, infirmity, and diabetes mellitus account for most of these incidences.[42] Diuretic fluids, such as coffee and soft drinks, can aggravate hypernatremia, and some pharmacologic agents can lead to dehydration. Dehydration often is iatrogenic, resulting from low-salt diets and volume-depleting drugs, which include most cardiovascular medications (particularly diuretics), many psychotropic and gastrointestinal medications, and many commonly used pain-relieving drugs prescribed or purchased over the counter. Drug-related changes with age involve the kidneys' reduced ability to conserve water and concentrate urine, increased secretion of antidiuretic hormone, and impaired renal sodium conservation.

The PT should consider dehydration as part of the medical screening process when examining an older adult. Physical, rather than biochemical, parameters are indicators of dehydration.[89] PTs should encourage hydration when physical signs are observed. The following examination findings common to dehydration should alert the primary care therapist to further assess an older person for this condition:

- Weight loss
- Agitation or lethargy
- Lightheadedness
- Confusion or altered mental status
- Syncope
- Orthostatic hypotension
- Weakness
- Tongue dryness
- Sternal skin turgor

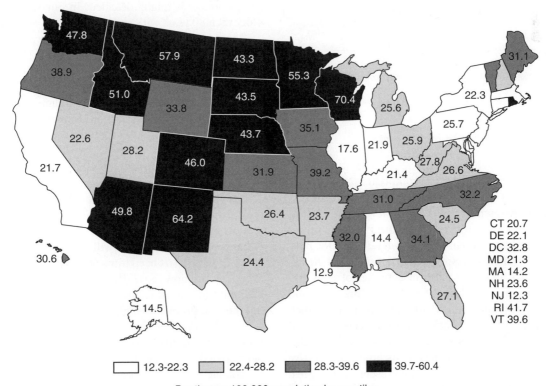

CT 20.7
DE 22.1
DC 32.8
MD 21.3
MA 14.2
NH 23.6
NJ 12.3
RI 41.7
VT 39.6

| | 12.3-22.3 | | 22.4-28.2 | | 28.3-39.6 | | 39.7-60.4 |

Deaths per 100,000 population by quartiles

FIGURE 18-2 Age-adjusted fatal fall injury rates among women aged 65 years and older, United States, 2000-2003. (From Centers for Disease Control Prevention: *Injury prevention & control: data & statistics [WISQARS]*, 2006 [website]. http://www.cdc.gov/injury/wisqars. Accessed March 25, 2010.)

Physical Manifestations of Malnutrition

Nutrient Deficiency	Physical Manifestation
Protein	Edema, hypoalbuminemia, enlarged liver, diarrhea
Protein, energy	Muscle wasting; sparse, thin, dry, brittle hair; dry, inelastic skin; muscle weakness
Vitamin A	Poor visual accommodation to dark, dryness of the eyes, hair loss, impaired taste, gooseflesh
Vitamin D	Bowed legs, beading of ribs, other skeletal deformities (rickets)
Vitamin K	Bleeding (poor coagulation of blood)
Thiamin (vitamin B$_1$)	Cardiac enlargement; mental confusion; irritability; calf muscle tenderness and foot drop; hyporeflexia; hyperesthesia; paresthesia
Riboflavin (vitamin B$_2$)	Fissures around mouth; reddened, scaly, greasy skin around nose and mouth; magenta-colored tongue
Niacin (vitamin B$_3$)	Bright red, swollen, painful tongue; depression; insomnia; headaches; dizziness; dementia; diarrhea
Pyridoxine (vitamin B$_6$)	Neuropathies; glossitis; nasolabial seborrhea
Folic acid	Red, painful, shiny, smooth tongue; skin hyperpigmentation
Vitamin B$_{12}$	Mild dementia; sensory losses in hands and feet; red, smooth, shiny, painful tongue; mild jaundice; optic neuritis; anorexia; diarrhea
Vitamin C	Joint tenderness and swelling; hemorrhages under the skin; spongy gums that bleed easily; poor wound healing; petechiae
Essential fatty acids	Sparse hair growth; dry, flaky skin; depression and psychosis; dementia
Calcium	Poor reflexes; poor cardiovascular accommodation to activity; slow mental processing; depression; dementia
Magnesium	Lethargy and weakness; anorexia and vomiting; tremor; convulsions
Iodine	Goiter
Iron	Pallor; pale, atrophic tongue; pale conjunctivae
Zinc	Sluggish muscle contraction; poor wound healing; diminished taste and appetite; dermatitis; hair loss; diarrhea

From Bottomley JM: Exploring nutritional needs in the elderly. In Bottomley JM, Lewis CB: *Geriatric rehabilitation: a clinical approach*, 3rd ed, Upper Saddleback, NJ, 2008, Prentice Hall, p 111.

Comprehensive Components of Geriatric Assessment

The four essential components of a comprehensive geriatric assessment are physical health, functional health, mental health, and social health. Assessment of a geriatric patient's physical health typically includes a geriatric medical history; physical examination; and assessment such as for gait, risk for falls, mobility, and incontinence. Assessment of functional health includes the patient's ability to perform activities of daily living (ADLs), such as feeding himself or herself, dressing, and bathing, as well as instrumental activities of daily living, which include light housework, yard work, money management, and transportation. A comprehensive geriatric assessment also addresses an older patient's mental health, including a cognitive assessment to determine whether dementia or delirium is present and an affect assessment to determine whether such mental disorders as depression are involved. Finally, the comprehensive assessment examines the patient's social health, including

economic condition, presence or absence of caregivers and their ability to give care, whether the patient has a durable power of attorney for health care, and whether the patient has completed estate planning.

Medical Diagnostic Challenges

For many disease states in older adults, the atypical presentation of illness cannot be overemphasized. The classic signs and symptoms of disease may be absent in older adults, or diseases may have unusual presentations, with clinical symptoms and signs that can be confusing. Congestive heart failure, for example, may have the presenting problem of urinary incontinence. Older adults may not experience angina; rather, cardiac blockage often presents itself as shortness of breath. Hyperthyroidism may present as lethargy and intellectual blunting. Hypothyroidism may lack symptoms of fatigue, skin findings, and constipation and may produce confusion alone.[45] It is not uncommon to find clinically important congestive heart failure without the presence of rales. The clinical signs of pulmonary consolidation occur much later in older adults in the presence of pneumonia. At other times, disease may present nonspecifically as failure to thrive, loss of appetite, and altered alertness or, to the caregiver, as simply a change.[41]

Infections in older adults are especially challenging to identify. Delay in diagnosis and lack of treatment contribute substantially to mortality from infection in older adults.[89] An older individual's core temperature is often lower than normal because of inactivity, a decrease in metabolic rate, and reduced neuroendocrine activity (see Chapter 9). The result is that fevers go undetected and older adults may be in the advanced stages of infection when the pathology is finally detected. In one study, 48% of persons older than 80 years with an infection were afebrile.[89]

Because of the often complex and atypical presentation of medical conditions in older adults, the PT must be an astute observer. The old axiom, "When you hear hoofbeats under your window, you should think of horses before you think of zebras,"[75] does not always hold true in older patients. Uncommon presentations of common medical conditions are a frequent occurrence in this population.[41] As PTs move toward establishing functional and physical therapy diagnoses, it is imperative that they look beyond the obvious when assessing and diagnosing symptoms in this population.

The symptoms of illness may not adhere to typical differential diagnostic algorithms. One of the most common symptoms in an outpatient setting is a loss in cognitive ability, or confusion. Patients or family members will often say, "I can't seem to think clearly," "Dad hasn't been himself lately," or "Mom used to do this every day and now can't." These symptoms usually result from an alteration in mental status—a sentinel event for many underlying medical problems in older adults. Although a common fear is that the older adult has suffered a stroke, other conditions are more often the underlying cause of a change in cognition or behavior. The change should not automatically be considered neurologic in origin. A sudden increase in restlessness, confusion, apathy, agitation, or lethargy can indicate an array of diagnoses. Changes in sleeping patterns or decreased appetite also can signal underlying acute medical problems. These are only a few examples of a long list of nonspecific and atypical presentations in the older adult.

The Three Ds: Delirium, Depression, and Dementia

Delirium

When a change in mental status occurs, one must differentiate dementia from delirium or depression. Delirium has an acute onset, most often related to a physical cause. Acute illness, medication toxicity, or other adverse drug interactions are often contributors to sudden confusion. If the accompanying physical condition is adequately treated, symptoms of delirium will disappear. In contrast, dementia has a slower, progressively worsening onset. However, nutritional or neuroendocrine disorders such as a vitamin B_{12} deficiency or hypothyroidism can cause symptoms that mimic those of dementia but are reversible. These should be ruled out in a differential diagnosis. Conversely, Alzheimer's disease, the most common type of dementia, has been linked to physical symptoms such as urinary incontinence and gait apraxia.[73] Dementias are characterized by a slow onset of increasing intellectual impairment, including disorientation, memory loss, reduced ability to reason and make sound judgments, loss of social skills, and development of regressed or antisocial behavior.[46] Depression may be superimposed on dementia as a reaction to the perceived loss of intellectual skills and leads to further cognitive impairment.[94]

Depression

Depression has been coined the common cold of older adults.[7,81] According to the Agency on Aging, in 2004 11% of noninstitutionalized men and 17% of noninstitutionalized women older than 65 years had clinically relevant depressive symptoms.[83] Nevertheless, studies have shown that it is not aging per se that is related to depression, but added variables such as cognitive impairment, incontinence, chronic conditions, and disabilities, as well as significant personal and emotional losses.[23]

Depression is usually associated with cognitive symptoms such as poor concentration and indecisiveness, in addition to low self-esteem, feelings of guilt, and hopelessness. At its extreme, depression is manifested by suicidal ideations.[81] Somatic symptoms often accompany depression in older adults, and an atypical symptomatic description of symptoms should alert the therapist to explore for the presence of depression. In addition, somewhat unique to this population are manifestations of memory loss, disorientation, and distractibility. Box 18-7 lists symptoms that patients often report when they have depression. It is important for the primary care PT to recognize depressive symptoms (see Chapters 5 and 8) and appreciate that older adults in particular may see depression as a character flaw and will not admit to being depressed.

Depression may occur because of the older person's adjustment to new family roles, new body image, or increased dependency. Physical and functional losses have a significant effect on emotional well-being. Research indicates that a relationship between depressive symptoms and functional change is present but complex, and not necessarily linear. Therefore, a decline in function will vary by the task assessed.[36]

The primary care therapist should understand some of the themes that emerge when working with the depressed older

---

BOX 18-7

Manifestations of Depression

- Fatigue
- Altered sleep patterns
- Weight gain or loss
- Tearfulness
- Agitation
- Heart palpitations
- Sadness
- Nonspecific generalized weakness
- Anxiety
- Irritability
- Fear
- Anger
- Depersonalization
- Feeling of isolation

Adapted from Jefferson M: *Handbook of medical psychiatry,* 2nd ed, St. Louis, 2004, Mosby.

---

patient, and determining the presence of depression may greatly affect subsequent treatment outcomes. The depressed older person often will be unmotivated and noncompliant with treatment recommendations, because he or she fails to find value in being and consequently sees little need for exercise, activity, or even attending physical therapy sessions. See Chapter 5 for a description of communication strategies when working with a patient who is depressed and for information about recognizing patients who may be considering suicide.

Dementia

Recognition and documentation of dementia in the primary care setting have been found to be inconsistent, and such cognitive deficits often go undiagnosed in the early stages.[85] However, the diagnosis of mild cognitive impairment (MCI) is becoming more prevalent. Mild cognitive difficulties can be noted for years before the person meets the complete criteria of being diagnosed with dementia.[63] A person with MCI experiences memory problems more than the normal expected with aging but does not show symptoms of dementia, such as impaired judgment or reasoning, and has the ability to perform ADLs.

However, early symptoms of dementia can affect the most complex ADLs, with the most noticeable deficit being memory loss.[47,62,69,82] Memory loss often shows up as difficulty remembering recently learned facts and decreased ability to acquire new information. There continues to be debate as to whether MCI is a preclinical stage of Alzheimer's disease or whether it is a different diagnostic entity.[59,77] Cognitive impairment in older primary care patients has been found to have an effect on morbidity and mortality after controlling for the confounding effects of demographic and comorbid chronic conditions.[79] The mortality rate increases steeply with the degree of severity of dementia. The remaining life expectancy of the older adult with dementia is affected by the severity of the dementia, the patient's age, and his or her general physical health.[51]

Alzheimer's disease and multi-infarct dementia are the two most common forms of dementia. Each has a fairly characteristic pattern of onset and findings. Alzheimer's disease, involving multiple areas of cognition and function, begins gradually and is slowly progressive.[48] It is not associated with focal neurologic deficits or abrupt changes in severity. Patients typically begin with short-term memory deficits and progress to severely regressed behavior, an inability to learn or remember new tasks, and loss of ability to perform ADLs.[62] Early diagnosis is key, because it can initiate the process of patients and family adapting to and managing disease symptoms.[48] Moreover, certain pharmacologic interventions can impede symptom progression and significantly improve quality of life.

Many cognitive, behavioral, and psychological instruments are used in primary care settings to screen for dementia.[45] However, preexisting impairments in speech, vision, or hearing can complicate the therapist's assessment of cognitive changes. Such instruments also may help rule out depression as a cause for a change in mental status. In acute situations, using a few questions from the Mini-Mental State Examination, such as asking the patient to identify the place and date, or asking who is the current and immediate past president of the United States, can provide a brief assessment of cognition[26a]. A baseline evaluation and subsequent use of the entire scale are necessary to assist in determining progression of dementia. Other tests, such as the clock drawing test and categorical naming, have been shown to aid in differentiating between normal cognition and the presence of dementia secondary to Alzheimer's disease.[52]

Multi-infarct dementia, which has as its pathophysiologic basis irreversible brain damage resulting from repetitive ischemic injury caused by emboli or bleeding, is usually of more rapid onset and progresses in a stepwise fashion, with abrupt worsening and subsequent plateaus of function.[1] The patient often has focal neurologic deficits, such as paresis and paresthesias.[19] Examples of sudden onset of symptoms include confusion, wandering in familiar places, and laughing or crying inappropriately. It is important to distinguish between Alzheimer's and multi-infarct dementias. The prevention of recurrent cerebral infarction may arrest the progression of multi-infarct dementia. Normalization of blood pressure, controlling diabetes and cholesterol, and managing heart disease are effective interventions known to decrease the risk of infarcts.[47,69]

Reversible dementia, such as that resulting from hypothyroidism, vitamin B_{12} deficiency, and normal pressure hydrocephalus, can become fixed and unresponsive to treatment unless identified and treated at an early stage. Normal-pressure hydrocephalus can be differentiated from other dementias in that there is a triad of symptoms. These include gait disturbances, cognitive dysfunction, and urinary incontinence.[95] Gait disturbances are usually the earliest symptoms in normal-pressure hydrocephalus and are described as apraxia, with patients having difficulties in turning, starting, and stopping when ambulating. Superimposed illnesses can cause a rapid decline in mental status, which may resolve as the underlying illness is treated.

Regardless of the cause of dementia, when reversible causes have been ruled out, the main tasks of a clinical team include addressing the patient's emotional needs, such as grieving for lost function; altering the environment so that the patient's remaining skills can be maximized to accomplish ADLs; and educating the family. It is beneficial for the primary care PT to recognize signs and clusters of the varying cognitive impairments and understand when to treat and when to consult with others.

Elder Abuse

Because the practice of rehabilitation typically involves the development of an ongoing relationship with the patient and may include frequent contact with the patient's families, PTs must know how to identify and effectively intervene in situations of suspected abuse. Types of elder maltreatment include caregiver neglect and self-neglect, emotional and psychological abuse, fiduciary exploitation, and physical abuse. The abuser profile may include the following:

- Often lives with the victim
- Is a relative and primary caregiver
- Has little or no caregiver experience
- May have a history of chemical dependency or other mental disorders

Abusive behavior by family toward people with dementia is common, with a third reporting important levels of abuse and half some abusive behavior.[16] Elder abuse occurs most often in the home rather than institutional settings, and victims most likely know their perpetrator.[39,49] Both depression and dementia have been identified as particularly strong risk factors associated with abuse of older adults.[4,22] Other risk factors for mistreatment of older people include advanced age, low income, functional or cognitive impairment, a history of violence, and recent stressful events.[36]

Assessment consists of a comprehensive history and physical examination, including scrutiny of the musculoskeletal system, neurologic and cognitive testing, and a detailed social history.[33] See Chapter 8 for additional information about screening for abuse. Clinical findings listed in Box 18-8 that cannot be explained medically, or are accompanied by implausible stories, may signal elder abuse.

To intervene properly, clinicians need to be familiar with state laws governing reporting procedures and patient privacy.

Common Medical Conditions in Older Adults

As age advances, there is a significant increase in the diseases highlighted in Box 18-9. Some of these medical conditions are explored elsewhere in this text, and others are discussed in the following sections.

BOX 18-8

Manifestations of Potential Elder Abuse

BEHAVIORAL
- Agitation, anger
- Fear
- Confusion
- Anxiety
- Withdrawal

PHYSICAL
- Burns, bruises, lacerations, rashes
- Diarrhea, fecal impaction
- Incontinence
- Poor hygiene

Musculoskeletal Pathologies

SARCOPENIA. Sarcopenia is an age-associated loss in lean muscle mass and results in a significant decrease in muscle power.[48] This process starts earlier in the life cycle and is accelerated with inactivity. Although the condition itself is not considered pathologic, it can progress to the point that it affects functional capabilities such as standing, transfers, and ambulation, and it increases the likelihood of falls.[46] Clinically, the surface muscles appear atrophied, and manual muscle tests reveal a decrease in maximal force produced. Patients often complain of poor endurance in activities such as walking and tasks that require repeated muscle activity.

OSTEOPOROSIS. Osteoporosis is primarily a disease of older adults. Of the 10 million Americans estimated to have osteoporosis, 8 million are women and 2 million are men.[80] Presenting features of this disease are a decrease in height; postural changes; including a forward head; kyphosis in the thoracic spine; a decrease in lordosis of the lumbar spine; and accommodative hip and knee flexion[34] (Figure 18-3).

The most common fracture sites include the vertebral column (thoracic and lumbar), femoral neck, and radius.[72] Figure 18-4 depicts age-specific incidence rates for common fractures in the aged, with the vertebral column (thoracic and lumbar), femur,

BOX 18-9
Common Medical Conditions of Older Adults

- Hypertension
- Atherosclerosis
- Myocardial degeneration
- Osteoarthritis
- Osteoporosis
- Cerebrovascular accidents
- Cancer

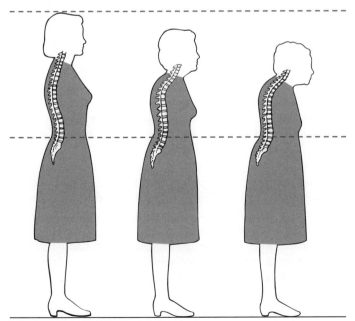

FIGURE 18-3 Postural changes associated with osteoporosis. (From Touhy T: *Ebersole and Hess' gerontological nursing & healthy aging,* 3rd ed, St. Louis, 2009, Mosby.)

and radius being the most common sites. Osteoporosis often is asymptomatic until a fracture occurs and a seemingly benign activity, such as leaning over to tie one's shoe, sitting upright in bed, or a cough or sneeze, may be the precipitating event; note that all include some element of trunk flexion. Symptoms of pain and muscle splinting are often noted immediately over the site of fracture. In addition, increased pain with trunk flexion and an increased kyphotic spinal curve suggests vertebral body compression fracture. For femoral head or neck fractures, increased pain with hip internal rotation, a position of comfort with the leg in external rotation and abduction, both possibly accompanied by a shortened leg, may be noted.

Osteoporosis may not be a presenting diagnosis for the patient. Recognizing risk factors for osteoporosis, the primary care PT can initiate a patient referral to the patient's primary care physician. Box 18-10 outlines risk factors for older adults who may have undiagnosed osteoporosis.

PAGET'S DISEASE. Paget's disease of bone[55] is a chronic affliction of the adult skeleton featuring one or more areas of aggressive osteoclast-mediated bone resorption preceding imperfect osteoblast-mediated bone repair. Paget's disease is rarely diagnosed before the age of 40, and men are more commonly affected than women. The prevalence of Paget's disease includes 1% of the population, depending on age and country of residence. It typically manifests in middle or advanced age.

Paget's disease typically involves one bone or a few bones, primarily the skull or pelvis, or a vertebra, femur, or tibia. Although often asymptomatic and identified only by abnormal findings on plain films, symptomatic patients present with bone pain, pathologic fractures, and deformities in the long bones, clavicles, and skull. The long bones, such as the tibia or femur, may be bowed. Another classic sign of Paget's disease is hypervascularity of the skin covering the involved bones.

Paget's disease may also lead to other medical conditions, such as osteoarthritis (OA) caused by bone changes, loss of hearing if the skull and bones of the inner ear are affected, and cardiovascular disease if there is more than 15% of skeletal involvement. The heart then needs to work harder to pump blood to the affected bones and may result in left ventricular hypertrophy.

OSTEOARTHRITIS. From 2005 to 2006, 46% of men and 54% of women older than 65 years self-reported arthritis as a leading chronic health condition.[12] In general, joint destruction occurs gradually and progresses slowly, but the symptoms of OA can occur insidiously or acutely. Pain is described as a deep ache, can occur at rest, and may awaken the individual at night. Stiffness of the involved joint(s) occurs after periods of inactivity and usually is resolved after a relatively short period of movement. Loss of flexibility is associated with soft tissue contractures, intraarticular loose bodies, osteophytes, and loss of joint surface congruity.[70] This condition is important to differentiate from joint rheumatic disorders, which can cause rapid joint destruction (see Chapter 7).

RHEUMATOID ARTHRITIS. The initial manifestations of rheumatoid arthritis (RA) typically occur at younger ages, but with aging, the potential multisystem complications associated with this autoimmune systemic illness can affect quality of life. Onset of the disease usually occurs between 30 and 50 years of age; 70% of those affected are women.[12] RA is a systemic disease; therefore,

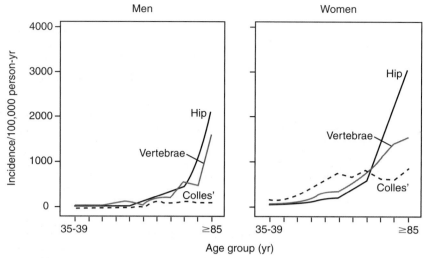

FIGURE 18-4 Age-specific incidence rates for hip, vertebral, and Colles' fractures in Rochester, Minnesota. (From Cooper C, Melton LJ 3rd: Epidemiology of osteoporosis. *Trends Endocrinol Metab* 3:224-229, 1992.)

BOX 18-10

Factors Associated with Osteoporosis

- Female gender
- Older age
- Family history
- Small skeletal frame
- Lean muscle mass
- History of fractures
- Decreased sex hormones—low estrogen levels in women, including menopause, amenorrhea; low levels of testosterone and estrogen in men
- Inactive lifestyle
- Diet—low calcium intake; low vitamin D intake; excessive intake of protein, sodium, caffeine
- Smoking
- Alcohol abuse
- Steroid medications
- Anorexia nervosa
- Rheumatoid arthritis
- Gastrointestinal absorption disorders

Adapted from National Osteoporosis Foundation: *Fast facts on osteoporosis* (website). http://www.nof.org/osteoporosis/diseasefacts.htm#riskfactors. Accessed January 30, 2010.

BOX 18-11

Body Areas Commonly Affected by Initial Attack of Gout

- First metatarsal phalangeal joint
- Midfoot
- Ankle
- Knee
- Wrist
- Fingers
- Elbow

Adapted from Centers for Disease Control and Prevention: *Injury prevention & control: data & statistics (WISQARS), 2006* (website). http://www.cdc.gov/injury/wisqars. Accessed March 25, 2010.

---

extra-articular signs and symptoms are often present, including fever, fatigue, malaise, poor appetite, weight loss, nutritional deficiencies, weakness, anemia, enlarged spleen, and lymphadenopathy. RA typically is characterized by the abrupt onset of symmetric joint swelling, erythema, and pain. Inflammation of the synovial membrane results in the release of proteolytic enzymes that perpetuate inflammation and joint damage.[70]

Symptoms usually are insidious and progress slowly as the disease progresses. Inflammation and musculoskeletal symptoms are localized to the specific joint, although multiple joints are usually involved. Morning stiffness is more pronounced and of longer duration than in OA. Intense pain can occur after periods of rest. Involved joints tend to be the small joints of the hands and feet, wrists, shoulders, elbows, hips, knees, and ankles; but essentially every joint can be involved. Eventually, deformities occur, affecting mobility and basic ADLs (see Chapter 7).

GOUT. Needle-like crystals of uric acid (monosodium urate crystals) are deposited in joints, tendons, and bursae that incite a rapidly progressive inflammatory reaction. When crystals other than monosodium urate crystals are found, such as calcium pyrophosphate dihydrate crystals, the condition is called *pseudogout.* The result is the abrupt onset of severe pain and development of an acutely tender and inflamed joint that can rapidly incapacitate the individual. Although up to 50% of first bouts of gout occur in the hallux, the metatarsal phalangeal joint or other joints may be the site of involvement. Commonly affected joints are listed in Box 18-11 .

In middle age, gout is episodic, but in later years it tends to occur with greater frequency and in more joints.[48] Certain diuretics used to treat congestive heart failure or hypertension may contribute to gout, because they interfere with the secretion of uric acid from the kidney, thereby causing an elevated level of uric acid. Other causes of gout include rapid tissue turnover, such as seen in lymphoma, leukemia, psoriasis, and pernicious anemia, and acidosis of any cause, including diabetes, alcohol abuse, or renal failure, can also precipitate gout.

It is appropriate to refer a patient to an urgent care clinic or emergency room if he or she presents with an acute onset of an isolated inflamed joint associated with intense pain, edema, erythema, and warmth (see Chapter 7). The most common treatments for an acute attack of gout are high doses of nonsteroidal anti-inflammatory drugs or corticosteroids, which are taken orally or injected into the affected joint. Patients often begin to improve within a few hours of treatment, and the attack usually is resolved within approximately 1 week.

TEMPORAL ARTERITIS AND POLYMYALGIA RHEUMATICA. Inflammation of small and medium-sized arteries derived from the aortic arch gives rise to giant cell arteritis. This condition is associated with a spectrum of disorders that include polymyalgia rheumatica (PMR), which is seen in those older than 50 years.[46] Neck, shoulder, and pelvic girdle stiffness and pain; an elevated erythrocyte sedimentation rate; low-grade anemia; fever; weight loss; elevated globulin levels; and rapid response to steroids are the characteristics of PMR. Of clinical significance is the high incidence of sudden monocular blindness, which can result from obliteration of the ophthalmic artery by temporal arteritis (TA).[8] The visual changes may be preceded by a sudden onset of a unilateral temporal headache and scalp sensitivity. This potential outcome necessitates urgent evaluation and treatment (prednisone if diagnosed) by a physician of anyone suspected of having PMR or TA. The diagnosis is established by biopsy of the temporal artery, looking for evidence of arteritis (see Chapter 7).[44]

SPINAL STENOSIS. Men and women older than 50 years are most likely to have spinal stenosis.[12] Many people can have narrowing of the spinal canal without symptoms or restrictions in their activities. However, older adults who present with symptoms of spinal stenosis will experience less pain with flexion and increased pain with extension. Box 18-12 depicts common inherited and acquired causes of spinal stenosis.

The significance of this condition is the risk for progressive neurologic loss, including cauda equina syndrome. Any patient with lower limb complaints that suggest claudication should be questioned regarding weakness and abnormal sensation, bowel and bladder function, and saddle paresthesia or anesthesia. Patients with neurogenic claudication stemming from spinal stenosis often describe a previous history of back pain only and then a transition toward increasingly severe leg symptoms (see Chapter 20).

Cardiovascular Pathologies

ISCHEMIC HEART DISEASE. Myocardial ischemia occurs when the demand for oxygen by cardiac muscle outweighs the available supply of oxygen.[20] Factors affecting oxygen demands can include exercise, anxiety disorders, or spontaneous fluctuations in heart rate and blood pressure. A decrease in available blood flow may be a result of decreased aortic driving pressure or increased coronary vascular resistance.[50]

A person may experience stable angina with exercise that is often described as pressure, heaviness, or tightness in the middle of the chest, over the heart, or in the shoulder or arm. Especially in older adults, ischemic angina often lasts for several minutes and is alleviated by rest and/or nitroglycerin. Unstable angina is characterized by a change in an anginal pattern or pain experienced at rest. Unstable angina may occur with less exertion than stable angina, may last longer, or may become less responsive to medicine.

MYOCARDIAL INFARCTION. Myocardial infarction (MI) results from prolonged ischemia and is precipitated in most cases by an occlusive coronary thrombus at the site of a preexisting atherosclerotic plaque. It may also result from a prolonged

---

BOX 18-12
Causes of Spinal Stenosis

Inherited Causes	Acquired Causes
Narrow spinal canal	Degenerative aging process
Scoliosis	Osteoarthritis
Achondroplasia	Herniated disk
	Spondylolisthesis
	Rheumatoid arthritis

---

vasospasm resulting in inadequate blood flow to the heart or excessive metabolic demand. This causes a complete interruption of blood flow, most often to the left ventricle and rarely to the right ventricle. An inflammatory response occurs within 18 to 24 hours after the infarction, and the formation of fibrous scar tissue is complete within 6 to 8 weeks.[20]

A symptom difference between an MI and ischemia is the quality and duration of the pain. Pain presentation with an MI is usually more severe and prolonged and is unrelieved with rest. Patients with prescribed nitroglycerin are instructed to go to an emergency department.[30] if their pain does not subside after three doses because of the possibility of an evolving MI.[20] Of importance for therapists working with older adults is knowledge that a silent MI is much more likely in this age group.[33] Of all MIs, 20% to 23% present without chest pain, but women and those older than 75 years are considerably more likely to experience a silent MI.[33] Symptoms of shortness of breath and possibly confusion can indicate an MI in older adults.

CARDIOMYOPATHIES. Cardiomyopathies consist of multiple conditions in which there is a primary disorder of the myocardial cells, with resultant myocardial dysfunction. Congestive heart failure is one example; the heart is not contracting strongly enough to meet the body's peripheral vascular needs. The hypertrophied heart is stiff and does not easily fill with blood. As a result, the heart contracts vigorously, but there is little forward circulation to show for the effort, and the body's energy and oxygen needs are not met. As a result, fluid builds up in the pulmonary circulation, causing pulmonary edema, difficulty breathing, low blood oxygen, and further difficulty in meeting the metabolic needs of the contracting cardiac muscle. Manifestations of cardiomyopathy generally include dyspnea, orthopnea, tachycardia, palpitations, peripheral edema, and distended jugular vein.[29]

CONDUCTION SYSTEM DISEASES. Conduction system diseases are those that affect the rate and rhythm of the heart's contractions.[29] The electrical wave that results in the coordinated contraction of the heart muscle is propagated in the two pacemaker sites in the heart and carried along specialized pathways that spread the wave throughout the heart, also known as the *conduction system*. These pacemakers and pathways can be damaged by many different agents, including those that result in cardiomyopathies and myocardial infarction. Table 18-1 provides a brief overview of the various types of dysrhythmias.[29]

VALVE DYSFUNCTION. Age-related pathology of an otherwise normal valve results from the gradual buildup of scar tissue and calcium on the valve leaflets. Valvular disease of are of two types, stenosis or narrowing of the valve, which restricts blood flow, and insufficiency or regurgitation, which results in the backward flow of blood. Both conditions increase the workload on

TABLE 18-1

Common Dysrhythmias

	SYMPTOMS	
Dysrhythmia	In Healthy Individuals with No Underlying Cardiovascular Disease	In Individuals with Underlying Cardiovascular Disease
Tachycardias		
Supraventricular tachycardia	No symptoms; abrupt-onset palpitations, lightheadedness, nausea, fatigue	May precipitate congestive heart failure (CHF), acute coronary insufficiency, myocardial infarction (MI), pulmonary edema
Sinus tachycardia	Awareness of the heart rate on exertion or with anxiety	Secondary to some precipitating factor (e.g., fever, anemia, MI)
Paroxysmal atrial tachycardia (PAT)	Sudden onset; precipitated by coffee, smoking, exhaustion	Supraventricular tachycardia; spontaneous onset of regular palpitations that can last for hours; may be obscured by myocardial insufficiency and CHF in older patients; increased anxiety and fatigue
Bradycardia		
sinus bradycardia	Physiologic in very fit young adults	In older patients, may suggest sinus nodal and conduction system pathology; can produce syncope or CHF

Adapted from Frownfelter D, Dean E: *Cardiovascular and pulmonary physical therapy, evidence and practice,* 4th ed, St. Louis, 2006, Mosby.

the heart and greatly reduce its efficiency.[76] The aortic valve is involved more often in older adults, with aortic stenosis usually being asymptomatic until middle or old age. Stenosis of the aortic valve results in a progressive increase in resistance to the flow of blood out of the heart and, as a result, the heart pumps blood against increasingly greater afterload.

Patients can experience angina without coronary artery disease, because even normal coronary arteries are unable to deliver sufficient blood to meet the metabolic demands of the overtaxed heart muscle. As the stenosis increases, transient decreases in cardiac output caused by arrhythmias or ischemia result in syncope.[76] Finally, when the heart is no longer able to compensate by hypertrophy for the increasing resistance to flow, congestive heart failure supervenes. See Chapter 11 for a description of auscultation as a clinical tool that may detect aortic valve dysfunction before any symptoms are noted.

Rheumatic valve disease, caused by a history of rheumatic fever, is the most common cause of mitral stenosis and insufficiency in the older adult.[71] Congestive heart failure, arrhythmias, and embolization of blood clots from the heart to the brain and other organs are the most common complications associated with mitral valve disease. Patients with these disorders require medical management, including the use of anticoagulants to prevent emboli, diuretics to control congestive heart failure, and medications to control the heart rate.[76] Nutritional support often is required to ensure compliance with a low-sodium diet. Protective intervention should focus on maintenance of maximal functional capabilities, with close monitoring of the older person's vital signs (see Chapter 11) and subjective responses of perceived tolerance to increasing activity levels.

HYPERTENSION. Hypertension is another common condition affecting the cardiovascular system. Older adults with systolic blood pressures greater than 160 mm Hg and diastolic pressures greater than 95 mm Hg clearly are at increased risk for stroke, congestive heart failure, and renal failure. Isolated systolic hypertension carries a similar risk. See Chapter 11 for a detailed discussion of hypertension and the assessment of blood pressure and other related vascular measures.

Orthostatic hypotension is defined as a 20–mm Hg drop in systolic and/or a 10–mm Hg drop in diastolic blood pressure

within 3 minutes of standing.[51] Orthostatic hypotension has a low prevalence (6%) in healthy older adults but is common in older adults with disease and who are taking medications.[51,89] At-risk individuals exhibit orthostatic hypotension readings, a finding that is not expected in healthy older adults.[89]

HEART FAILURE. Heart failure is the general decline of cardiac performance with age and with inactivity; it affects older adults' ability to function at their maximum. Chronic heart failure is multifactorial, but some literature suggests that the failing heart is an engine out of fuel.[57] According to the American Heart Association, symptoms include shortness of breath, increased heart rate, and fatigue. These symptoms often reflect problems with getting enough oxygen to the working muscle through a failing circulatory system.[2]

Individuals with a seriously reduced cardiac reserve report a significant need for rest after even mild physical activity.[46] ADLs are notably difficult for these older adults, and lying down to rest can induce a sharp recurrence or increase of dyspnea. Sleeping in a recliner versus in a bed is common to maintain a posture that optimizes pulmonary function.

The primary care PT can assist patients in ensuring that they are receiving adequate medical care. Care for these patients should include prescription by a physician for medications such as beta blockers, angiotensin-converting enzyme (ACE) inhibitors, or angiotensin II blockers to manage the heart failure.[2] The therapist can educate the patient in energy conservation techniques and assist the patient in obtaining and using equipment to conserve oxygen demand while completing ADLs. It is critical to provide instruction in exercise and activities to maintain strength, flexibility, balance, and endurance for patients with limited cardiac function.

Respiratory Pathologies

PNEUMONIA. Pneumonia is the most common infectious cause of death in older adults and the most common infection requiring hospitalization.[57] The increased incidence of pneumonia with aging is caused in part by weakening of the local pulmonary defenses, including reduced cough reflex, relative immobility, and decreased ciliary action. However, the high mortality of pneumonia is largely a result of its more subtle and atypical presentation in older adults. Typical symptoms such as a productive cough, fever, and pleuritic chest pain often are absent, but subtler symptoms, such as mild confusion, alteration of sleep-wake cycles, increased congestive heart failure, and loss of appetite, are more common. Noting any of the aforementioned manifestations should prompt the therapist to auscultate the chest wall (see Chapter 11) and refer the patient to his or her physician if abnormal sounds are detected.

OBSTRUCTIVE AND RESISTIVE LUNG DISEASE. Conditions that cause obstruction to air flow in the lungs are called *obstructive airway diseases*. Chronic obstructive pulmonary disease (COPD) is a mixture of small airway disease and parenchymal destruction emphysema[65] and is never completely reversible. In the older adult, structural damage to the lungs often results from cigarette smoking, infections, toxic exposures, or any combination of these. Asthma is an obstructive pulmonary disease that causes reversible airway restriction. Many older adults have been managing asthma most of their lives or asthma may manifest itself later in life, commonly precipitated by influenza.[9] *Emphysema* is a term used to describe the permanent destruction of alveoli, with the resulting expansion of the remaining alveoli. A consequence of emphysema is a reduction in the area in which gas exchange can occur. This causes a perfusion-ventilation mismatch and hypoxia. Emphysema is associated with increased airway resistance resulting from collapse of small airways.

Chronic bronchitis is a different disease process in which there is chronic inflammation of the small airways, with resulting increased mucus, airway plugging, and destruction of small airways.[29] As a consequence, air flow is reduced because of permanent narrowing of the small airways. There is often a reversible component of the airway obstruction superimposed on the chronic changes. Cigarette smoking is the leading cause of chronic bronchitis and multiplies the deleterious effects of other environmental agents, such as asbestos, silica, coal dust, and fibers. Emphysema and chronic bronchitis often coexist.

Patients with obstructive airway diseases usually manifest disabilities that result from hypoxia, hypercapnia (elevated carbon dioxide), and/or dyspnea. Both hypoxia and hypercapnia can cause confusion, fatigue, and worsening heart failure. Dyspnea is usually the most limiting symptom of COPD. Functional impairment caused by COPD can be severe, and COPD often is fatal. See Chapter 9 for a detailed discussion of symptoms associated with pulmonary disorders and Chapter 11 for a discussion of auscultation for pulmonary disorders.

Restrictive lung diseases are characterized by reduced total lung capacity (TLC), vital capacity, and/or resting lung volume. Accompanying characteristics are preserved air flow and normal airway resistance, which are measured as the functional residual capacity (FRC).[74] There are three main categories of restrictive lung diseases:

- Intrinsic lung diseases involving the collagen-vascular systems include scleroderma, polymyositis, dermatomyositis, systemic lupus erythematosus, RA, and ankylosing spondylitis.
- Idiopathic fibrotic disorders may include acute interstitial pneumonia and idiopathic pulmonary fibrosis (IPF).
- Extrinsic disorders include nonmuscular diseases of the chest wall, which may involve kyphosis and contribute to restrictive lung disease. Neuromuscular diseases manifest as respiratory muscle weakness and include myopathy or myositis, quadriplegia, and phrenic neuropathy.

Interventions for the primary care PT include patient education on the relationship between activity and pulmonary function and energy conservation techniques, in addition to monitoring exercise tolerance and modifying the exercise as needed. A consult with a respiratory therapist may be appropriate to determine airway flow and maximal exercise tolerance. The use of medications is also a major component of managing patients with obstructive and restrictive pulmonary disease. Therefore, numerous team members have a role in the patient's care.

Neurologic and Neurosensory Pathologies

PARKINSON'S DISEASE. Parkinson's disease (PD) is the most common type of parkinsonism, a clinical syndrome caused by lesions in the basal ganglia, predominantly in the substantia nigra, that produce deficits in motor behavior.[91] There is a characteristic tetrad of symptoms associated with PD, including resting tremor, cogwheel rigidity, bradykinesia or akinesia, and impairment of postural reflexes. Of this tetrad, only resting tremor is truly suggestive of PD, an early symptom that may remain prominent even late in the disorder.[88] In contrast to PD, parkinsonism is a clinical rather than a causative entity because it is associated with several pathologic processes that damage the extrapyramidal system.[90] With PTs having expertise in movement and movement dysfunction, the PT in primary care settings may be the first professional to recognize parkinsonism symptoms in older adults.

CERVICAL SPONDYLOSIS. Cervical spondylosis, another pathology often seen in older adults, is caused by impingement on the cervical spinal cord by bony spurs resulting from severe degenerative arthritis.[68] Because patients may develop a gait ataxia with spasticity, incontinence, and reduced sensation in the lower extremities, this condition can be overlooked while other neurologic disorders are considered first in the diagnostic process. Also causing confusion is that the patient may have few if any direct cervical spine symptoms other than a slightly decreased range of motion. Cervical computed tomography scanning, myelography, and magnetic resonance imaging can often establish the location and extent of spinal cord impingement (see Chapter 20).[68]

PERIPHERAL NERVOUS SYSTEM DISORDERS. Peripheral nervous system disorders often are diagnosed in older adults. With aging, the number and size of peripheral nerve fibers diminish, with a concomitant decrease in conduction velocity.[76] The peripheral nerves are also easily affected by nutritional deficiencies, toxins, and endocrine disorders. The resulting neuropathies can cause significant loss of position sense, resulting in instability, falls, or chronic pain[43] and dysesthesia (unpleasant sensation often induced by a gentle touch).

A common example of a peripheral nervous disorder is diabetic neuropathy, which can take several forms. Distal sensory polyneuropathy affects the hands and feet, with diminished sensation and burning pain, and motor neuropathy, resulting in distal muscle wasting and weakness. Diffuse autonomic neuropathy (not a peripheral neuropathy) results in orthostatic hypotension, neurogenic bladder, and bowel immotility.[30] For a patient with diabetes and lower extremity sensory neuropathy, a comprehensive foot examination can prevent pressure ulceration and the serious complications of skin breakdown.

VESTIBULAR DISORDERS. Vestibular symptoms have been reported in more than 50% of older adults.[46] The central mechanisms involved in the control of balance do not appear to change excessively with age but are more likely to be affected by degenerative neurologic diseases such as Alzheimer's disease or PD. However, age-related changes in the peripheral vestibular system occur and affect balance. Hair cell receptors decrease in number, there is a loss of the vestibular receptor ganglion cells, and the myelinated nerve cells of the vestibular system decrease by as much as 40%.[5,46] Partial loss of vestibular function in older adults can lead to symptoms of dizziness, with less ability of the nervous system to accommodate to positional changes. Coupled with vestibular losses, there may be concomitant losses in vision and somatosensation, which severely affect sensory input used in the maintenance of balance.

Various pathologic conditions can affect the peripheral vestibular system, producing vertigo or disequilibrium. Benign paroxysmal positional vertigo (BPPV) is a common form of vertigo in older adults. In general, BPPV is associated with the deposition of otoliths (otoconial material) in the cupula of the posterior semicircular canal. The otoliths adhere to the cupula and can retard its return to a resting position after head rotation. In addition, otoliths can obstruct the flow of endolymph, producing symptoms in the affected posterior semicircular canal by impeding or stopping stimulation to the vestibular nerve. These conditions can be unilateral or bilateral. When patients present with acute or chronic intermittent dizziness, BPPV needs to be considered. BPPV is readily treated by PTs by performing the Epley maneuver (see Chapter 7).

Acute vestibular neuritis, also known as *labyrinthitis,* is the second most common cause of vertigo in older adults. It is associated with a viral infection that causes inflammatory changes of branches of the vestibular nerve. In older adults, the onset usually is preceded by upper respiratory or gastrointestinal infections. The chief symptom is the acute onset of prolonged severe rotational vertigo that is exacerbated by movement of the head. Symptoms include spontaneous horizontal rotatory nystagmus, postural imbalance, and nausea. Habituation exercises help resolve symptoms after the infection clears.[24]

Ménière's disease is a disorder of the inner ear that can cause hearing problems and vestibular symptoms in older adults. The patient complains of a sensation of fullness of the ear, a reduced ability to hear, and tinnitus. These symptoms are accompanied by rotational vertigo, postural imbalance, nystagmus, and nausea and vomiting.[61]

Bilateral vestibular disorders may occur secondary to other diseases or can be drug-induced in older adults. Conditions that may lead to bilateral vestibular problems include meningitis, labyrinthine infections, otosclerosis, Paget's disease, polyneuropathy, bilateral tumors (acoustic neuromas in neurofibromatosis), ototoxic drugs, inner ear autoimmune disease, and congenital malformations of the inner ear. Autoimmune conditions such as RA, psoriasis, ulcerative colitis, and Cogan's syndrome (iritis accompanied by vertigo and sensorineural hearing loss) can lead to a progressive bilateral sensorineural hearing loss, often accompanied by bilateral loss in vestibular function. In addition, the toxic effects of alcohol may cause an acute vertigo because the dehydration created by alcohol may change the specific gravity of the endolymph. Other agents that may cause vertigo include organic compounds of heavy metals.

Endocrine Pathologies

DIABETES MELLITUS. Diabetes mellitus is a chronic endocrine disease that affects a significant number of older people in the United States.[43] The complex nature of diabetes creates a broad spectrum of physical complications and reactions that can make the condition extremely dangerous. It is the leading cause of blindness and retinopathy and is detected in 40% of diabetic patients.[89] Older adults with diabetes have higher rates of premature death and disability, hypertension, stroke, and coronary artery disease. Often adding to the medical complexity in older adults with diabetes is the presence of polypharmacy, depression, cognitive impairment, urinary incontinence, injurious falls, and pain. Symptoms of diabetes include increased urination, thirst, hunger, fatigue and lethargy, weight loss, and numbness or tingling in the feet and hands. Although there is no cure, the disease can be controlled by achieving and maintaining normal levels of blood glucose.[30] This requires a careful balance of four critical components—diet, exercise, education for self-monitoring, and drug therapy.

Therapists must be vigilant for signs of hyperglycemia and hypoglycemia. Hyperglycemia may be caused by a missed insulin dose, overeating, failure to follow the diabetic diet, or infection. The signs include excessive thirst and urination, dry mouth, drowsiness, flushed dry skin, fruitlike breath odor, nausea, vomiting, and difficulty breathing. Signs of hypoglycemia may be caused by excessive insulin, skipping of a snack or meal, illness, excessive exercise, or drinking alcohol. Symptoms include anxiety, chills, cold sweats, cool pale skin, confusion, drowsiness, excessive hunger, headache, nausea, anxiety shakiness, vision changes, and unusual fatigue. It may be difficult to differentiate the symptoms of hyperglycemia from those of hypoglycemia. If possible, determine when the individual last ate and when he or she last took insulin. The consumption of a sugar-containing food (e.g., orange juice or honey) will reverse symptoms of hypoglycemia. Extreme hypoglycemia needs to be treated as a medical emergency by calling 911 or having the person transported to the emergency department.

THYROID DISEASE. Diseases of the thyroid gland, although often diagnosed at younger ages, are more common in the older population. Significant morbidity and even death can result from excessive or insufficient thyroid hormone. In hyperthyroidism and hypothyroidism, presentation of the syndrome can be very different in the older adult from that in younger patients. As is the rule in most illnesses in older adults, the initial manifestation may be more subtle, and symptoms and signs less specific, including change in mentation.[54]

Hypothyroidism results from failure of the thyroid gland to produce and secrete sufficient thyroid hormone, despite maximal stimulation of the gland by thyroid-stimulating hormone (TSH).[66] Slight vague symptoms may be present, such as dry skin, chronic myalgias and arthralgias, lethargy, confusion, weight gain, edema, depression, apathy, sensitivity to sedatives, and cold intolerance (see Chapter 7).

Patients with severe hypothyroidism develop hypothermia and cognitive dysfunction resembling delirium. This hypofunction is seen most often in hospitalized older patients who experience the stress of surgery or other acute illness.

For older adults, hyperthyroidism typically results from an excess of thyroid hormone released from a multinodular enlarged thyroid gland (goiter). Although many symptoms of hyperthyroidism in older adults are similar to those in the younger patient, as with hypothyroidism, they usually are more subtle. Common manifestations include muscle weakness, weight loss, fatigue, exophthalmos, diarrhea, and agitation.

Summary

If the unprecedented increase in life expectancy has a down side, it is the increased incidence of chronic age-related disorders. As PTs work to foster healthy aging, we must seek ways to prevent the disabling disorders that prevent many older people from enjoying their longevity. Under a primary care model of geriatric intervention, successful patient management must extend beyond diagnosis and disease treatment and include promotion of function and prevention of decline. Achieving this goal requires a seamless continuum of management and interdisciplinary care. We also must focus on improving our understanding of the science of aging so that preventive approaches can be used to decrease the development of chronic illness and disability in older adults.

REFERENCES

1. Alzheimer's Disease Education and Referral Center: Symptoms (website). http://www.nia.nih.gov/Alzheimers/AlzheimersInformation/Symptoms. Accessed March 19, 2010.
2. American Heart Association: Signs of symptoms of heart failure, 2009 (website). http://www.americanheart.org/presenter.jhtml?identifier=339. Accessed January 24, 2010.
3. American Physical Therapy Association. The guide to physical therapist practice. 2nd ed. Alexandria, VA: American Physical Therapy Association; 2001.
4. Anetzberger GJ, Palmisano BR, Sanders M, et al. A model intervention for elder abuse and dementia. Gerontologist 2000;40:492–7.
5. Baloh RH, Honrubia V. Clinical neurophysiology of the vestibular system. 3rd ed. New York: Oxford University Press; 2001.
6. Bell AJ, Talbot-Stern JK, Hennessy A: Characteristics and outcomes of older patients presenting to the emergency department after a fall: a retrospective analysis. Med J Austral 2000;173:176–7.
7. Bettes S. Depression: the "common-cold" of the elderly, Western Gerontological Society Generations, Spring 1979, 15–16.
8. Boyer CG. Vision problems. In: Camevali EPC, editor. Nursing management for the elderly. Philadelphia: JB Lippincott; 1989.
9. Bramann SS, Kaemmerlen JT, Davis SM. Asthma in the elderly. A comparison between patients with recently acquired and long-standing disease. Am Rev Respir Dis 1992;143:336–40.
10. Buchner DM, Wagner EH. Preventing frail health. Clin Geriatr Med 1992;8:1–7.
11. Cassel K. Successful aging. How increased life expectancy and medical advances are changing geriatric care. Geriatrics 2001;56:35–9.
12. Centers for Disease Control and Prevention: Injury prevention & control: data & statistics (WISQARS), 2010 (website). http://www.cdc.gov/injury/wisqars/index.html. Accessed March 19, 2010.
13. Centers for Medicare and Medicaid Services: Medicare and you, 2010 (website). http://www.medicare.gov/Publications/Pubs/pdf/10050.pdf. Accessed March 19, 2009.
14. Cohen HJ, Feussner JR, Weinberger M, et al. A controlled trial of inpatient and outpatient geriatric evaluation and management. N Engl J Med 2002;346:905–12.
15. Committee on the Future of Health Care Workforce for Older Americans: Retooling for an aging America: building the health care workforce, 2008 (website). http://www.iom.edu/Reports/2008/Retooling-for-an-Aging-America-Building-the-Health-Care-Workforce.aspx. Accessed March 19, 2010.
16. Cooper C, Selwood A, Blanchard M, et al. Abuse of people with dementia by family carers: representative cross sectional survey. BMJ 2009;338:155.
17. Coronado VG, Thomas. KE, Sattin RW, Johnson RL. The CDC traumatic brain injury surveillance system: characteristics of persons aged 65 years and older hospitalized with a TBI. J Head Trauma Rehabil 2005;20:215–28.
18. Counsell SR, Callahan CM, Buttar AB, et al. Geriatric Resources for Assessment and Care of Elders (GRACE): a new model of primary care for low-income seniors. J Am Geriatr Soc 2006;54:1136–41.
19. Cummings JL, Miller B, Hill MA, Neshkes R. Neuropsychiatric aspects of multi-infarct dementia and dementia of the Alzheimer type. Arch Neurol 1987;44:389–93.
20. De Turk WF, Cahalin LP. Cardiovascular and pulmonary physical therapy. New York: McGraw Hill; 2004.
21. Duerksen DR, Yeo TA, Siemens JL, O'Connor MP. The validity and reproducibility of clinical assessment of nutritional status in the elderly. Nutrition 2000;16:740–4.
22. Dyer CB, Pavlik VN, Murphy KP, Hyman DJ. The high prevalence of depression and dementia in elder abuse or neglect. J Am Geriatr Soc 2000;48:205–8.
23. Ferrucci LI, Guralnik J. Aging and prevalance of depression. Gerontologist 1990;30(314A).
24. Fetter M. Vestibular system disorders. In: Herman SJ, editor. Vestibular rehabilitation. Philadelphia: FA Davis; 1994. p. 80–9.
25. Fillet HM, Gutterman R, Orland BI, et al. Polypharmacy management in Medicare managed care: changes in prescribing by primary care physicians resulting from a program promoting medication reviews. Am J Managed Care 1999;5:587–94.
26. Fineberg HV. Retooling for an aging America. Medscape J Med 2008;10:188.
26a. Folstein MF, Folstein SE, McHugh PR. "Mini-mental state". A practical method for grading the cognitive state of patients for the clinician. J Psychiatr Res 1975;12:189–98.
27. Fried LP, Guralnik JM. Disability in older adults: evidence regarding significance, etiology, and risk. J Am Geriatr Soc 1997;45:92–100.
28. Fried TR, Mor V. Frailty and hospitalization of long-term stay nursing home residents. J Am Geriatr Soc 1997;45:265–9.
29. Frownfelter D, Dean E. Cardiovascular and pulmonary physical therapy: evidence and practice. 4th ed. St. Louis: Mosby; 2006.
30. Gambert SR. Diabetes in the elderly: a practical guide. New York: Raven Press; 1990.
31. Gambert SR, Guansing AR. Protein-calorie malnutrition in the elderly. J Am Geriatr Soc 1980;28:272–5.
32. Ganto JG, Goldberg RJ, Hand MM, et al. Symptom presentation of women with acute coronary syndromes: myth vs reality. Arch Intern Med 2007;167:2405–13.
33. Gray-Vickery P. Recognizing elder abuse. Nursing 1999;29:52–3; 1999.
34. Ham R, Sloane P, Warshaw G, Bernard M, Flaherty E. Primary care geriatrics: a case-based approach. 5th ed. St. Louis: Mosby; 2006.
35. Herrman H, Saxena S, Moodie R, editors: Promoting mental health: concepts, emerging evidence, practice, 2004 (website). http://www.who.int/mental_health/evidence/ en/promoting_mhh.pdf. Accessed March 25, 2010.
36. Hybels CF, Pieper CF, Blazer DG. The complex relationship between depressive symptoms and functional limitations in community-dwelling older adults: the impact of subthreshold depression. Psychol Med 2009;39:1677–88.
37. Jager TE, Weiss H, Coben JH, Pepe PE. Traumatic brain injuries evaluated in U.S. emergency departments, 1992-1994. Acad Emerg Med 2000;359:134–40.
38. Jefferson M. Handbook of medical psychiatry. 2nd ed. St. Louis: Mosby; 2004.
39. Jogerst GJ, Dawson JD, Hartz AJ, et al. Community characteristics associated with elder abuse. J Am Geriatr Soc 2000;48:513–8.
40. Johnson HA. In: Johnson HA, editor. Relations between normal aging and disease. Is aging physiological or pathological? vol. 28. New York: Raven Press; 1985. p. 239–47.
41. Keen P: Atypical presentation of medical conditions in the elderly. American Academy of Nurse Practitioners 16th Annual National Conference, Austin, TX, 2001.
42. Lavizzo-Mourey R, Johnson J, Stolley P. Risk factors for dehydration among elderly nursing home residents. J Am Geriatr Soc 1988;36:213–8.
43. Leland JY. Chronic pain: primary care treatment of the older patient. Geriatrics 1999;54:3–28.
44. Levine SM, Hellman DB. Giant cell arteritis. Curr Opin Rheumatol 2002;14:3–10.
45. Lewis CB. Assessment instruments. In Geriatric rehabilitation: a clinical approach. Upper Saddle River, NJ: Prentice Hall; 2003. p. 152–90.
46. Lewis CB, Bottomley JM. Geriatric rehabilitation. 3rd ed. Upper Saddle River, NJ: Prentice Hall; 2008.
47. Linn RW, Wolf PA, Bachman DL, et al. The "preclinical phase" of probable Alzheimer's disease. A 13-year prospective study of Framingham cohort. Arch Neurol 1995;52:485–90.
48. Marin DB, Sewell MC, Schlechter A. Alzheimer's disease. Accurate and early diagnosis in the primary care setting. Geriatrics 2002;57:36–40.

49. Marshall CE, Benton D, Brazier JM. Elder abuse. Using clinical tools to identify clues of mistreatment. Geriatrics 2000;55:42–4.

50. Mattson P. Pathophysiology concepts of altered health states. 3rd ed. Philadelphia: JB Lippincott; 1990.

51. Medow M, Stewart JM, Sanyal S, et al. Pathophysiology, diagnosis, and treatment of orthostatic hypotension and vasovagal syncope. Cardiol Rev 2008;16:4–20.

52. Mendez MA, Ala T, Underwood KL. Development of scoring criteria for the clock drawing task in Alzheimer's disease. J Am Geriatri Soc 1992;40:1095–9.

53. Miller PD, Krebs RA, Neal BJ, McIntyre DO. Hypodipsia in geriatric patients. Am J Med 1982;73:354–6.

54. Morely JE. The aging endocrine system. Postgrad Med 1983;73:107–20.

55. Whyte MP. Clinical practice. Paget's disease of bone. N Engl J Med 2006;355:593–600.

56. Mukamel DB, Peterson DR, Temkin-Greener H, et al. Program characteristics and enrollees' outcomes in the Program of All-Inclusive Care for the Elderly (PACE). Milbank Q 2007;85:499–531.

57. Neubauer S. The failing heart—an engine out of fuel. N Engl J Med 2007;356:1140–51.

58. World Health Organization. Constitution of the World Health Organization, 1946 (website). http://apps.who.int/gb/bd/PDF/bd47/EN/constitution-en.pdf. Accessed March 25, 2010.

59. Palmer KB, Berger AK, Monastero R, et al. Predictors of progression from mild impairment to Alzheimer disease. Neurology 2007;68:1596–602.

60. Pearlman DN, Branch LG, Ozminkowski RJ, et al. Transitions in health care use and expenditures among frail older adults by payor/provider type. J Am Geriatr Soc 1997;45:550–7.

61. Perez-Garriques H, et al. Time course of episodes of definitive vertigo in Meniere's disease. Arch Otolaryngol Head Neck Surg 2008;134:1149–54.

62. Pernecsky R, Pohl C, Sorg C, et al. Complex activities of daily living in mild cognitive impairment: conceptual and diagnostic issues. Age Ageing 2006;35:240–5.

63. Petersen RS, Stevens JC, Gangulii M, et al. Practice parameter: early detection of dementia: mild cognitive impairment (an evidence-based review). Neurology 2001;56:1133–42.

64. Phillips PA, Rolls BJ, Ledingham JG, et al. Reduced thirst after water deprivation in healthy elderly men. N Engl J Med 1984;311(12):753–9.

65. Rabe KF, Hurd S, Anzueto A, et al. Global strategy for the diagnosis, management, and prevention of chronic pulmonary disease. Am J Respir Crit Care Med 2007;176:532–55.

66. Robuschi G, Safran M, Braverman LE, et al. Hypothyroidism in the elderly. Endocrinol Rev 1987;8:142–53.

67. Roglieri JL, Futterman R, McDonough KL, et al. Disease management interventions to improve outcomes in congestive heart failure. Am J Managed Care 1997;3:1831–9.

68. Roh JT, Teng A, Yoo JU, et al. Degenerative disorders of the lumbar and cervical spine. Orthop Clin North Am 2005;36:255–62.

69. Saxton JL, Lopez OL, Ratcliff G. Preclinical Alzheimer's disease: neuropsychological test performance 1.5 to 8 years prior to onset. Neurology 2004;63:2341–7.

70. Schiller AL. Bones and joints. In: Rubin E, Farber JL, editor. Pathology. 2nd ed. Philadephia: JB Lippincott; 1994. p. 1273–347.

71. Schneider EL, Reed JD. Modulations of aging processes. In: Finch CE, Schenider EL, editors. Handbook of biology of aging. New York: Academic Press; 1985.

72. Scott J. Osteoporosis and hip fractures. Rheum Dis Clin North Am 1990;16:717–40.

73. Sevush S, Minagar A, Peruyera G. Ventricular dilation on magnetic resonance imaging predicts early onset of urinary incontinence in patients with probable Alzheimer's disease. Program and abstracts of the 125th Annual Meeting of the American Neurological Association; October 15-18, 2000; Boston. Poster 43.

74. Kanaparthi LK, Lessnan KD, Sharma S. Restrictive lung disease, 2008 (website). http://emedicine.medscape.com/article/301760-overview. Accessed March 25, 2010.

75. Shem S. The house of God. New York: Bantam Doubleday; 1979.

76. Shepard RJ. Physical activity and aging. 2nd ed. Gaithersburg, MD: Aspen Publishers; 1987.

77. Small BG, Robinson B. Early identification of cognitive deficits: preclinical Alzheimer's and mild cognitive impairment. Geriatrics 2007;62:19–23.

78. Stevens JA, Corso PS, Finkelstein EA, Miller TR. The costs of fatal and non-fatal falls among older adults. Inj Prev 2006;12:290–5.

79. Stump TE, Callahan CM, Hendrie HC. Cognitive impairment and mortality in older primary care patients. J Am Geriatr Soc 2001;49:934–40.

80. Taxel P. Osteoporosis: detection, prevention, and treatment in primary care. Geriatrics 1998;53:22–3.

81. Travis, LA, Lyness JM. Minor depression. Diagnosis and management in primary care. Geriatrics 2002;57:65–6.

82. Twamley ER, Ropacki SA, Bondi MA. Neuropsychological and neuroimaging changes in preclinical Alzheimer's disease. J Int Neuropsychol Soc 2006;12:707–35.

83. U.S. Department of Health and Human Services: Agency for Healthcare Research and Quality; 2008. Adapted from Health and Retirement Study: A Longitudinal Study of Health, Retirement, and Aging. Sponsored by the NIA; 2010. http://hrsonline.isr.umich.edu/index.php?p=dbook Accessed 4 April 13, 2010.

84. U.S. Department of Health and Human Services. Medicare & you, 2010 (website). http://www.medicare.gov/publications/pubs/pdf/10050.pdf. Accessed April 14, 2010.

85. Valcour VG, Masaki KH, Curb JD, Blanchette PL. The detection of dementia in the primary care setting. Arch Intern Med 2000;160:2964–8.

86. Vellas BJ, Wayne SJ, Romero, et al. Fear of falling and restriction of mobility in elderly fallers. Age Ageing 1997;26:189–93.

87. Vellas B, Guigoz Y, Garry PJ, et al. The Mini Nutritional Assessment (MNA) and its use in grading the nutritional state of elderly patients. Nutrition 1999;15:116–22.

88. Victor A, Ropper AH. Adams and Victor's principle of neurology. 9th ed. New York: McGraw-Hill; 2009.

89. Wasserman M, Levinstein M, Keller E, et al. Utility of fever, white blood cells, and differential count in predicting bacterial infections in older adults. J Am Geriatr Soc 1989;37:537–43.

90. Waters CH. Diagnosis & management of Parkinson's disease. 6th ed. Caddo, OK: Professional Communications, Inc; 2008.

91. Winograd CH, Lindenberger EC, Chavez CM, et al. Identifying hospitalized older patients at varying risk for physical performance decline: a new approach. J Am Geriatr Soc 1997;45:604–9.

92. Woolf SH, Kamerow DB, Lawrence RS, et al. The periodic health examination of older adults: the recommendations of the U.S. Preventive Services Task Force. Part I. Counseling, immunizations, and chemoprophylaxis. J Am Geriatr Soc 1990;38:817–23.

93. Woolf SH, Kamerow DB, Lawrence RS, et al. The periodic health examination of older adults: the recommendations of the U.S. Preventive Services Task Force. Part II. Screening tests. J Am Geriatr Soc 1990;38:933–42.

94. Wright SP. Distinguishing between depression and dementia in older persons:neuropsychological and neuropathological correlates. J Geriatr Psychiatry Neurol 2007;20:189–98.

95. Zarrouf F, Griffith J, Jesse J. Cognitive dysfunction in normal pressure hydrocephalus (NPH): a case report and review of the literature. W V Med J 2009;105(22):24–6.

A Health and Wellness Perspective in Primary Care   19

Janet R. Bezner, PT, PhD

Objectives

After reading this chapter, the reader will be able to:

1. Understand and differentiate between the terms health and wellness.
2. Describe the relationship between health behaviors and health.
3. Demonstrate the ability to screen clients for health behaviors.
4. Integrate the results from an Health Risk Assessment (HRA) or general health and wellness screening tool into intervention planning for a client.
5. Apply the transtheoretical model by assessing and addressing stages of change, decisional balance, and the processes of change with a client adopting a habit of regular physical activity.
6. Apply the construct of self-efficacy in designing a physical activity intervention with a client.
7. Identify clients who might benefit from motivational interviewing and apply the skills with a client who desires to become more physically active.

As the subject of this text, the role of the physical therapist (PT) in primary care has been established. The American Academy of Family Physicians states that primary care practices include the provision of "health promotion, disease prevention, health maintenance, counseling, and patient education"[2] among other things and that nonphysician primary care providers work in collaborative teams to provide some of these services. The American Physical Therapy Association (APTA) has established the role of the PT in health promotion and wellness through its policies, educational offerings, description of PT practice in *The Guide to Physical Therapist Practice*,[3a] and other initiatives. In the context of primary care, how does the PT provide health and wellness services and to whom are these services provided? In this chapter, the various terms used in the context of health and wellness will be defined and described, and the need for health promotion and wellness services will be discussed. Furthermore, health and wellness screening tools and behavior change interventions will be presented to enable the PT to provide health promotion and wellness services to clients.

Definitions of Health and Wellness Terms

The term *health* is commonly thought of as the absence of disease. The World Health Organization (WHO) has defined health as "a state of complete physical, mental and social well-being and not merely the absence of disease and infirmity."[40] This definition implies that there is more to health than our physical state and, indeed, including mental and social dimensions of health in a general health definition suggests that health is a broad concept and multiple factors affect health.

At the first International Conference on Health Promotion in Ottawa, Canada in 1986, health promotion was defined as the process of enabling people to increase control over, and to improve, their health.[39] Recognizing the multiple factors affecting health from the previous definition of health, health status is affected by genetic predisposition, the behaviors and actions taken or not taken, and numerous social and environmental factors. The action of promoting health, then, involves empowering individuals to make choices and making changes in the environment that positively affect health. An ecologic approach to health promotion, touted by health promoters, the Institute of Medicine, and other professional groups, maintains that improvement of the health status and quality of life of a group of individuals requires that attention be given to the ecosystem in which people reside and work and its subsystems, such as family, organizations, community, culture, and physical environment.[6,14,18] An illustration of an ecologic model is shown in Figure 19-1, with the multiple subsystems in the model occupying the concentric circles around the individual at the center. The provision of health promotion in a primary care model requires the PT to recognize the influences on the health of the individual and to engage in efforts to influence not just the individual level, but the other levels as well. This approach is consistent with the notion of social responsibility as described in the professionalism core values document of the APTA.[4] Social responsibility is the promotion of a mutual trust between the profession and the larger public that necessitates responding to societal needs for health and wellness.

Wellness is a term that has been the subject of much interest over the past decade. Numerous definitions exist, with the first offered by Dunn in 1961: "an integrated method of functioning which is oriented to maximizing the potential of which an individual is capable, within the environment where he is functioning."[11] WHO has defined wellness as "the optimal state of health of individuals and groups. There are two focal concerns, the realization of the fullest potential of an individual physically, psychologically, socially, spiritually and economically, and the fulfillment of one's role expectations in the family, community, place of worship, workplace and other settings."[34] Common to these definitions is the notion that wellness is multidimensional and goes beyond physical well-being; that wellness is salutogenic, or health-causing; and that wellness is consistent with a systems view or an ecologic model, as noted earlier.

For many people, including the public, the term *wellness* is interchangeable with physical health or physical well-being, which commonly consists of physical activity, efforts to eat nutritiously, and getting adequate sleep. Research has indicated that when the public is asked to rate their general health, they narrowly focus on their physical health status, choosing not to

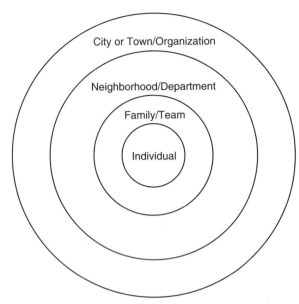

FIGURE 19-1 Ecologic model.

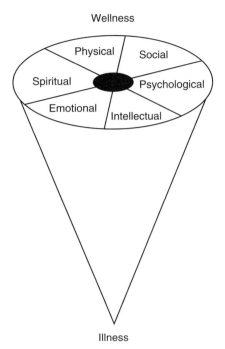

FIGURE 19-2 Wellness model.

consider their emotional, social, or spiritual health.[27] Referring back to the definitions of wellness from Dunn and WHO, and consistent with numerous other theorists, it is noteworthy that wellness, as it is defined, includes more than just physical parameters. Among the dimensions included in various wellness models are physical, spiritual, intellectual, psychological, social, emotional, occupational, and community or environmental.[1]

The second characteristic of wellness is that it has a salutogenic or health-causing focus[5] in contrast to a pathogenic focus in an illness model. Emphasizing that which causes health (e.g., is salutogenic) supports Dunn's original definition that implied wellness involves "maximizing the potential of which the individual is capable." In other words, wellness is not just preventing illness or injury or maintaining the status quo; rather, it involves choices and behaviors that emphasize optimal health and well-being beyond the status quo.

Third, wellness is consistent with a systems or ecologic perspective. In an ecologic model, each element of the system is independent and contains its own subelements, in addition to being a subelement of a larger system.[19,24,33] Furthermore, the elements in a system are reciprocally interrelated, indicating that a disruption of homeostasis at any level of the system affects the entire system and all its subelements.[19,33] Therefore, overall wellness is a reflection of the state of being within each dimension and a result of the interaction among and between the dimensions of wellness. Figure 19-2 illustrates a model of wellness reflecting this concept. Vertical movement in the model occurs between the wellness and illness poles as the magnitude of wellness in each dimension changes. The top of the model represents wellness because it is expanded maximally, whereas the bottom of the model represents illness. Bidirectional horizontal movement occurs within each dimension along the lines extending from the inner circle. As per systems theory, movement in every dimension influences and is influenced by movement in the other dimensions.[1] As an example, an individual who experiences a knee injury and undergoes surgery to repair the anterior cruciate ligament will probably experience at least a

short-term decreased physical wellness. Applying systems theory and according to the model, this individual may also experience a decrease in other dimensions—for example, emotional and/or social wellness in the postoperative period. The overall effect of the changes in these dimensions will be a decrease in overall wellness, which anecdotally is known to occur when an individual experiences an illness or injury. Being aware of the influence of health on wellness can provide the PT with additional information that might be useful in the creation of intervention programs that not only restore health but also address wellness.

Health and Wellness Behaviors

Numerous articles in the print and other media remind us of the state of Americans' health. Of the leading causes of death, many are preventable with positive lifestyle choices. In 2004, Mokdad and colleagues[23] determined that the top three actual causes of death in the United States in the year 2000 were, in order, tobacco, poor diet and physical inactivity, and alcohol consumption. They concluded that at least half of premature deaths in the United States are attributable to behavior or lifestyle causes.[23] Therefore, interventions that promote healthy behaviors, such as smoking cessation, selecting healthy food choices, and physical activity, are sorely needed and could have a significant effect on overall health and wellness. Because health behaviors are deeply rooted in lifestyle, defined as a pattern of behavior developed over time as a result of cultural, social, and economic conditions, usually without a specific purpose but with health consequences,[14] they are difficult to change. Anyone who has attempted to diet or be regularly physically active understands the challenge of changing a lifestyle behavior. Adopting healthy behaviors and stopping unhealthy behaviors require knowledge of the predisposing, enabling, and reinforcing factors related to the adoption of healthy behaviors, along with knowledge of the science of behavior change.[13] Before the PT reviews the science of behavior change, it is appropriate to identify the ways in which clients who would benefit from behavior change can be identified in a physical therapy practice.

Approaches to Screening Clients for Health and Wellness Interventions

As discussed in Chapter 8, the performance of a comprehensive examination includes the collection of health history information and questions about health habits. Current health habits such as smoking, drinking alcohol, use of recreational drugs, diet, and physical activity provide valuable information that can serve as a starting point for a conversation about behavior change and the adoption of positive health habits. Regardless of whether a patient is seeing the PT for a specific diagnosis related to an injury or disease or presents directly to the PT for guidance with a physical activity program, routine collection and review of health habit information provide an opportunity to address health and wellness needs with all clients. This approach is consistent with the role of the PT as a primary care provider in which the health and well-being of all clients served is addressed.

In addition to screening questions about health habits presented in Chapter 8, specific questions can be asked about health behaviors in a number of ways. The Documentation Template for Physical Therapist Patient/Client Management in *The Guide to Physical Therapist Practice*[3a] includes several questions that can serve to screen patients for healthy behaviors. The general health status questions on the inpatient form, as an example, include the following:

22. GENERAL HEALTH STATUS
    a. Patient/client rates health as: Excellent, Good, Fair, Poor
    b. Major life changes during the past year?
       (1) Yes
       (2) No
23. SOCIAL/HEALTH HABITS (Past and Current)
    a. Alcohol
    b. Smoking
       (1) Currently smokes tobacco?
          (a) Yes
             1. Cigarettes: # packs per day _____
             2. Cigars/pipes: # per day _____
       (2) Smoked in past?
          (a) Yes, Year quit: _____
          (b) No
    c. Exercise
       (1) Exercises beyond normal daily activities and chores?
          (a) Yes, Describe the exercise: _____
             1. On average, how many days per week does patient/client exercise or do physical activity? _____
             2. For how many minutes, on an average day? _____
          (b) No

A commonly used screening tool for health habits is a health risk assessment (HRA). The purpose of an HRA is to assess an individual's risk for contracting disease based on a combination of behaviors (e.g., smoking, physical activity, diet) and biomedical markers (e.g., blood pressure, weight, cholesterol). HRAs are available for purchase from various vendors and can also be accessed free on some vendor websites. Table 19-1 includes a list of HRA resources. There are other general screening tools that can be used to assess a patient's or client's overall perception of his or her well-being or functional status. Two of these tools are reviewed subsequently.

Perceived Wellness Survey

The Perceived Wellness Survey (PWS) was created by Adams and associates[1] to fill a void in the wellness assessment arena. The PWS is based on the definition and characteristics of wellness discussed earlier. It is a 36-item self-assessment scale that measures perceived wellness in six dimensions—physical, social, psychological, emotional, spiritual, and intellectual. The scale is available for use in practice and research and is easily scored by the clinician (Appendix 19-1). The PWS results can be used during intervention planning as another source of information about the client. For example, scoring the PWS results from the client in Appendix 19-2 yields subscale scores between 1 and 6 for each of the six dimensions of the PWS. In this case, the scores are as follows:

Physical, 5.0
Social, 5.5
Psychological, 3.6
Emotional, 3.8
Spiritual, 2.8
Intellectual, 5.3

TABLE 19-1

Health Risk Assessment (HRA) Options

Company	HRA Website	Details About Services
InfoTech	*Wellness Checkpoint* http://www.wellness checkpoint.com	Integrated suite of web-based health risk assessment and information management services; includes comprehensive reports and follow-up
HPN Worldwide	*Health Power Profile* http://www.hpn.com/hra.htm	Can purchase paper or online access; includes comprehensive reports and follow-up
WellSource	*Personal Wellness Profile* http://www.wellsource.com/health-risk-assessments.html	Can purchase paper or online access to several different versions of assessment forms; includes comprehensive reports and follow-up
WellSteps	*WellSteps* http://www.wellsteps.com/index.php	Free, requires one-time registration; includes comprehensive report and follow-up interventions and planning
Real Age	*What's Your Real Age?* http://www.realage.com	Free, requires one-time registration; includes report and frequent e-mail reminders based on health risks

The dimensions in which the client scores highest can be considered strengths, or assets. In this case, the client's strengths are the social, intellectual, and physical dimensions. In other words, this client perceives a strong social network, has a good perception of his or her physical self, and perceives that intellectual stimulation is important. Keeping these strengths in mind while planning the intervention will result in an intervention program that is better suited to the client. For example, the client might respond well to an intervention program involving group exercise or exercise with another person. Furthermore, the client might respond well to additional information about her or his condition or conversation about the condition and healing process (intellectual dimension). Although there are no good or bad or right or wrong answers or scores on the PWS, the information assessed provides insight into the beliefs and perceptions of the client and therefore can be useful.

Medical Outcomes Study Short Form 36

The Medical Outcomes Study Short Form 36 (MOS SF-36) is also a self-report questionnaire consisting of 36 questions that has been used in thousands of studies.[36] It provides an eight-scale profile of physical and mental health and well-being. There are two summary measures—physical health and mental health—and eight scales—four in each of the two summary measures. The physical health measure includes physical functioning (PF), role—physical (RP), bodily pain (BP), and general health (GH). The mental health measure includes the subscales vitality (VT), social functioning (SF), role—emotional (RE), and mental health (MH). The clinician can obtain the instrument online (www.sf-36.org) and administer the tool in a paper or electronic format. Assistance with scoring is also available.

Short of using a specific HRA or general assessment tool such as the PWS or MOS SF-36 with your clients, specific questions can be incorporated into the health history and habits screening form to assess key behaviors, as demonstrated previously with the examples from *The Guide to Physical Therapist Practice*[3a] documentation templates. Common questions include the following:

- Do you perform physical activity 3 days or more per week for at least 30 minutes a day? Yes/No
- Compared with others your age, would you say your health is excellent, good, fair, poor?
- Do you eat 3 to 5 fruits and/or vegetables per day? Yes/No

The answers to these questions provide the basis for a conversation with clients about health habits. The ability to approach these topics with clients is a skill worth developing. As a result of the plethora of health information available in the media, on the Internet, and from health care providers, most clients are aware of what they should be doing, and the last thing they want or need is a lecture from someone else about what they should be doing. Approaching these sensitive issues carefully and skillfully will result in a better outcome.

Designing Interventions for Health Behavior Change

Clients who express an interest in adopting a healthy behavior such as physical activity are typically ready to engage in the intervention. These clients are not unlike typical clients treated by PTs who are motivated to get better by their functional limitations, which are interrupting gainful participation in life. However, not all clients who could benefit from adopting a healthy habit identified by the PT will be ready to engage, either physically or psychologically. Healthy habits, such as regular physical activity and eating a balanced diet, are complex behaviors influenced by myriad cultural, environmental, and genetic factors. Therefore, the PT will benefit from additional tools to help identify someone who is ready to engage and to counsel those clients who are not ready. A number of cognitive-behavioral theories have been created to assist with understanding the knowledge, attitude, belief, efficacy, intention, and behavior that underlie the adoption and maintenance of health behaviors.[13] Review of all of these theories is beyond the scope of this chapter. Key theories and tools are included here that will enable the clinician to plan more effective interventions for clients.

Assessment of Physical Readiness

Before the initiation of a physical activity program, individuals should be assessed to ensure safety and minimize risks.[3] Screening can be performed using a self-report questionnaire, such as the Physical Activity Readiness Questionnaire (PAR-Q; Appendix 19-3). Based on the answers to the seven questions on the PAR-Q, individuals between the ages of 15 and 69 years can be appropriately cleared to increase their level of physical activity or be referred for further evaluation. Clients who answer no to all the questions can participate safely in up to moderate physical activity. Clients who want to participate in vigorous activities should have a more thorough examination.[3]

Assessment of Psychological Readiness

Prochaska and Velicer[26] have identified a phenomenon about behavior change that has been applied to numerous health behaviors to determine the intervention that is most appropriate for a client at a specific point in time. Prochaska posited that clients exist and move along a continuum, from not being aware that a change is necessary to maintaining a new behavior for longer than 6 months. In other words, the stage dimension in the transtheoretical model (TTM) describes behavior change as more of a process rather than an event (e.g., the medical decision to get a flu shot). Medical decisions that require a behavior change process are the target of TTM research and theory.[25] The TTM, also called *stages of change,* contains five stages (Table 19-2). Identifying the stage in which a client falls at a specific point in time enables a more tailored intervention to be developed and implemented. For example, if a client wishes to develop a regular physical activity habit, yet is in the preparation stage, providing an exercise prescription would be inappropriate and unlikely to be followed because the client is not yet ready to engage in regular physical activity. Appropriate and tailored interventions for clients in the preparation stage include identifying and assisting in problem solving to remove obstacles to the behavior, helping the client identify social support, verifying that the client has the underlying skills for behavior change, encouraging small initial steps, developing a plan and telling others about the change, focusing on costs and benefits, setting short- and long-term goals, establishing rewards, and developing time management skills.

TABLE 19-2

Transtheoretical Model Stages of Change

Stage	Description
Precontemplation	Not intending to take action in the foreseeable future (next 6 months) Uninformed or underinformed of consequences and risks May have tried and failed, may feel demoralized and/or defensive Tends to avoid reading, talking, or thinking about the high-risk behavior Labeled as "unmotivated" or "hard to reach"
Contemplation	Plans to change in the next 6 months Aware of the pros and cons of changing but is ambivalent about them Rule of thumb is "when in doubt, don't act" May be stuck here for years as a "chronic contemplator"
Preparation	Intends to take action in next month or so May have started to take some significant action in the past year Generally has a plan of action An unstable phase Appropriate recruit for an action-oriented intervention program
Action	Has made specific, overt changes in his or her behavior in past 6 months Must attain a level of action that is sufficient to reduce risks (e.g., recommended levels of physical activity, total abstinence from alcohol or cigarettes, 25% of calories from fat) High risk for relapse because benefits may not be readily apparent
Maintenance	Has stuck with the behavior for at least 6 months but fewer than 5 years Working to prevent relapse, yet is increasingly confident that he or she can sustain the changes made

Data from Prochaska JO: Decision making in the transtheoretical model of behavior change, *Med Decis Making* 28:845-849, 2008.

TABLE 19-3

Stage of Change for Physical Activity Questionnaire

Stage	Question*
Precontemplation	I presently do not exercise and do not plan to start exercising in the next 6 months.
Contemplation	I presently do not exercise, but I have been thinking about starting to exercise within the next 6 months.
Preparation	I presently get some exercise, but not regularly.
Action	I presently exercise on a regular basis, but I have begun doing so only within the past 6 months.
Maintenance	I presently exercise on a regular basis and have been doing so for longer than 6 months.

*Client instructions: Select the statement that best describes you in relation to your exercise habits.
Modified from Cardinal JB: Construct validity of stages of change for exercise behavior, *Am J Health Promot* 12:68-74, 1997.

Table 19-3 shows an example of an assessment tool that can be used to identify what stage a client is in for the behavior of physical activity. This tool can be easily added to an intake questionnaire so that the stage of change can be routinely assessed. Scales measuring stage of change are behavior-specific because stage of change is behavior-specific, meaning that a client could, for example, be in the precontemplation stage for one health behavior and in the action stage for another health behavior.

In addition to the stages of change, there are other constructs in the TTM that are useful to understand and apply to enhance the efficacy of the intervention, including decisional balance and processes of change. Decisional balance is a construct in which an individual weighs the pros and cons of changing. Researchers who have studied decisional balance across a wide range of studies and behaviors indicate that from precontemplation to action, the pros of changing a behavior, such as becoming physically active regularly, must increase twice as much as the cons of changing must decrease.[16,25] As a result, moving from precontemplation to action requires primary focus on increasing the pros or benefits of change. As clients progress to contemplation and preparation, progress can be further enhanced by the addition of interventions focusing on removing or diminishing the cons of change.[16] A tool to assess decisional balance can be found in Appendix 19-4.

Moving decisional balance from a negative balance (more cons) to a positive balance (more pros) is necessary but not sufficient for successful long-term behavior change.[25] The processes of change, the third construct in the TTM, are helpful at each stage to reinforce positive behaviors and to move clients toward action and maintenance. The processes of change are the strategies and techniques used by clients to modify their thoughts, feelings, behavior, and/or environment.[20] Whereas the stages of change explain when people change, the processes of change describe how people change.[20] Research by Marcus and associates[20,21] has indicated that for the adoption of a physical activity behavior, all 10 of the processes of change are important at all the stages of change, using some processes more at specific stages. The processes are categorized into cognitive and behavioral strategies, as follows (with application for physical activity in parentheses):

- *Cognitive strategies:* Increasing knowledge (reading and thinking about physical activity), being aware of risks (being inactive is unhealthy), caring about consequences to others (the effect of inactivity on family and friends), comprehending benefits (of being physically active), and increasing awareness of healthy (physically active) opportunities
- *Behavioral strategies:* Substituting alternatives (encourage client to be physically active at times that are not typical, such as when tired or stressed), enlisting social support (find a partner to provide support for being physically active, rewarding yourself for being physically active), committing yourself (making promises, plans, and commitments to be active), and reminding yourself (establish reminders to be active)[20]

In research performed with employees of retail and industrial manufacturer worksites, Marcus and coworkers[21] discovered that those in the preparation stage for physical activity tended to use the behavioral processes more often than the contemplators, and the use of the cognitive processes did not differ between the two stages. Employees in the action stage used the cognitive and behavioral processes more often than those in the preparation stage. Compared with those in the action stage, those in maintenance used fewer cognitive strategies, whereas the use of behavioral strategies was the same in both stages.[21] Applying this information in practice, a clinician should consider applying primarily the cognitive strategies in early stages (precontemplation and contemplation) and incorporating behavioral strategies in earnest when the client reaches the preparation stage. The processes of change provide additional information to enable the development of a more tailored and more successful intervention plan. The clinician can use the stages of change, decisional balance, and processes of change within the TTM to identify the stage the client is in, set a realistic goal for the client based on stage, assess and address the pros and cons of changing to move the client toward action, and apply the processes of change to enhance movement through the stages, resulting in an intervention plan that is specifically tailored for the client and that will lead to long-term behavior change.

Self-Efficacy

As noted by Glanz and coworkers,[13] social cognitive theory (SCT) was developed by Bandura to explain the multiple influences on behavior change created by the interactions of factors specific to the person, attributes of the behavior, and the environment. A primary construct in SCT is self-efficacy, or the confidence that a person feels about performing a particular activity.[13] Clients who perceive that they can perform a behavior successfully will be more likely to engage in that behavior. Like the TTM, self-efficacy is behavior-specific, such that self-efficacy to perform one behavior is likely to be independent of self-efficacy to perform another behavior. Self-efficacy has been shown to be related to a number of health behaviors and to be specifically related to physical activity—clients with greater self-efficacy for physical activity are more physically active.

Self-efficacy can be enhanced in a number of ways.[22] Most simply, successful accomplishment of the desired behavior will improve self-efficacy. In terms of physical activity, it is important to set achievable, small goals when beginning a physical activity habit so that the client is successful, which will improve self-efficacy. Ongoing greater mastery of the physical movement will continue to enhance self-efficacy. Observational learning, or vicarious learning, is the reinforcement that a client receives from watching or observing another person like him or her engaging successfully in the desired behavior. This method of improving self-efficacy is especially useful for sedentary and older individuals. Social persuasion can also enhance self-efficacy, especially when it comes from an individual whom the client respects and believes. Finally, ensuring that the client appropriately interprets physical experiences with physical activity can result in improving self-efficacy. For example, when a sedentary client begins a physical activity habit, it is likely that he or she will experience physiologic symptoms such as muscle soreness or fatigue. To prevent the client from interpreting these states as negative consequences of the physical activity, the clinician can prepare the client to anticipate these symptoms and teach the client to monitor change in the feelings as a sign of progress.[22] Efforts to improve self-efficacy have been shown to positively influence the attainment of a regular habit of physical activity.[9,15,32,38]

Motivational Interviewing

Clients in the contemplation stage of the TTM are ambivalent about behavior change. They recognize the pros and cons of adopting the behavior, but the pros do not yet outweigh the cons. The client who is ambivalent would benefit from counseling to push him or her off the fence, so to speak, and move him or her to the preparation phase, where action planning toward the behavior can begin. Motivational interviewing (MI), originally described by Miller in 1983[22a] as an intervention for problem drinking, in which motivation is a common obstacle to change, is useful for clients who are in the contemplation phase for a health-related behavior. MI is a client-centered counseling style useful for eliciting the client's own motivations for changing a behavior in the interest of his or her own health. Because the client steers the conversation, it involves guiding more than directing and is also known as a collaborative approach that honors the client's autonomy.[31]

There are four guiding principles of MI: (1) to resist the righting reflex, (2) to understand and explore the client's own motivations, (3) to listen with empathy, and (4) to empower the client while encouraging hope and optimism.[31]

RESIST THE RIGHTING REFLEX. Consider what happens when a client is making a choice that the clinician knows is not beneficial for health (e.g., not being physically active regularly), the client is aware of the best choice (to be physically active), the clinician knows well what the better choice is, and the clinician has a strong desire to help the client. This combination of factors usually creates a situation in which the clinician strongly argues for the best choice and, because the client is ambivalent, the client naturally argues for his or her choice, the choice that is not beneficial for health. This scenario is played out numerous times and, as a result, clients do not change and health status suffers. The way in which a clinician talks with a client about the client health can significantly influence the client's motivation for behavior change and, when the clinician is in the role of arguing for change, it is likely that the client will resist because nobody wants to admit that they are wrong or unmotivated. A better approach is for the clinician to resist the temptation to tell the client what to do but rather to get the client to verbalize the arguments for changing behavior. This role for the clinician is based heavily on the notion that people tend to believe what they hear themselves say.[31] Techniques to increase change talk, or statements made by the client that are favorable toward changing behavior (e.g., recognizing disadvantages of current behavior, stating advantages of changing behavior, expressing optimism for change, expressing intention to change), include focusing specifically on listening reflectively during conversations, emphasizing client autonomy, and avoiding giving advice without permission.[8]

UNDERSTAND YOUR CLIENT'S MOTIVATIONS. Although the clinician may have had success adopting the same behavior that he or she is trying to help the client adopt, the motivations for doing so may differ. A better approach is to discover the client's own concerns, values, and motivations for changing the behavior.

Linking behavior change to a client's values produces powerful results and often reveals a discrepancy in the client's current behavior and most important goals and values, a discrepancy of which the client was not aware and that can commonly push him or her off the fence of ambivalence.[31]

LISTEN WITH EMPATHY. Empathy is a skill familiar to PTs and is central to using MI successfully. Clinicians who apply MI generally listen more than talk and use open-ended questions, letting the client state the reasons for changing behavior and the obstacles that must be overcome.[31] See Chapter 5 for additional strategies to enhance patient-therapist rapport and empathy. Davis has written a text that is another excellent resource.[10]

EMPOWER THE CLIENT. The fourth principle is based on the belief that clients who take an active role in their own health care will achieve better outcomes. An important goal is to empower a client to adopt a health behavior, such as physical activity, in a way that works best for the client, considering the client's unique life and lifestyle. The clinician's role is to support the client to find the best way to adopt the behavior, provide hope and optimism that the client can be successful, build self-efficacy in the client, and help the client solve problems to overcome barriers and setbacks. In other words, the clinician's role is to determine the client's expertise in how best to adopt the new behavior successfully.[31]

The following process can be used to apply the principles of MI with a client.

IDENTIFY THE TARGET BEHAVIOR. MI is best applied when a specific behavior has been identified that the client has selected. In a situation in which there are multiple behaviors that a client could change (e.g., smoking, physical activity, eating), an Agenda-Setting Chart (Appendix 19-5) can be used to facilitate the client's selection of the most appropriate behavior to focus on first. The clinician presents the chart and tells the client that the chart contains areas that are commonly related to disease or illness and asks the client to select the area that he or she is most interested in talking about. The blank areas can be used to add additional areas that the client thinks are more important "right now." Providing the opportunity for the client to select the behavior on which to focus honors the principles of MI described and empowers the client to determine the priority right now.

EXPLORE THE CLIENT'S VALUES AND PRIORITIES. To identify a discrepancy that may exist between the client's current behavior and important goals and values, it is important for the clinician to understand the values that the client considers most important. This information may surface in the course of building a relationship with the client or can be directly solicited. An easy way to identify the client's most important values is to ask the client to identify his or her top three values from a list of common values, such as considerate, disciplined, family, friendship, independence, inner peace, health, helpfulness, honesty, responsible, and spirituality. When presenting a generic list of values for the client to consider, provide an opportunity for the client to add additional values that are not on the list. It is important for the clinician not to judge the values selected but to ask the client to indicate the three or four most important and set the list aside. If the opportunity arises in the course of the conversation about the health behavior to point out a discrepancy between the client's current behavior and the values that he or she selected, the clinician can use this information in context.[30]

IDENTIFY IMPORTANCE AND CONFIDENCE ABOUT THE BEHAVIOR. The importance of changing the behavior and the confidence that the client has to make this change are helpful pieces of information that enable the clinician to understand more about the behavior and to elicit change talk from the client. These questions are illustrated in Figure 19-3. After the client indicates how important it is to change the behavior, the clinician asks "Why did you select a score of ___ and not a 1?" This question produces change talk from the client, who discusses why the behavior is important to him or her.[31] As a result of this question and the following discussion, the clinician knows how important it is to the client to change the behavior, and why it is important. The confidence question is similarly processed. After the client selects a number indicating his or her level of confidence to change right now, the clinician asks "Why did you give yourself a ___ and not a 1?"[31] The discussion that follows provides insight into self-efficacy and any barriers that may exist.

ASSESS DECISIONAL BALANCE. The next step is to identify the pros and cons of changing behavior. A decisional balance tool can be used such as the one shown in Appendix 19-4, or the clinician can ask a series of questions that will enable the exploration of ambivalence. If the behavior being discussed is physical inactivity, the following questions are relevant:

1. What do you like about being physically inactive?
2. What are the not so good things about being physically inactive?

The clinician must ensure that he or she listens without judgment or disapproval, but with honest interest and curiosity about how the client feels about the behavior. After the client answers the two questions, the clinician can summarize his or her understanding of the pros and cons of the behavior and ask the client, "Where does this leave you now?" This question provides an opportunity for the client to go the next step in exploring how to create the desired change.[31]

When engaged in the process outlined, the clinician looks for opportunities to build self-efficacy, express hope and optimism that the client can be successful, and point out any discrepancies between the client's priority values or goals and current behavior(s) and resists the temptation to tell the client how to change—until or unless the client asks directly. As noted earlier, the goal of MI is to resolve ambivalence, not to create an action

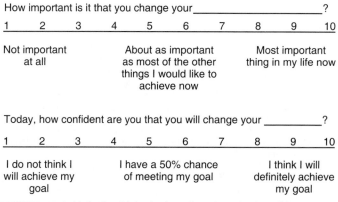

FIGURE 19-3 Motivational interviewing—importance and confidence questions. (Adapted from Rhode R: Motivational Interviewing, from the *American Journal of Health Promotion Conference*, Las Vegas, March 20-23, 2006.)

plan for performing the desired behavior. Executing the process outlined will often result in enhanced client understanding about the ambivalence and the discrepancy between the behavior and his or her values. The clinician can end the conversation with an offer to talk further with the client about the behavior when the client is ready, again empowering the client to take the next step.

Limitations of MI include that it is not easy to learn or apply, especially for health care providers who are used to a more prescriptive, expert-driven approach than the facilitative, client-centered approach of MI.[29] MI requires practice to apply, as well as feedback from another clinician. The literature is unclear on what parts of MI work or why it works, although more research on the use of MI with health behaviors such as physical activity and eating behaviors is emerging.[7,17,28,35,37]

Summary

There is a clear need for all health care providers to address the overall health status of members of society, because lifestyle diseases account for most morbidity and mortality.[23] PTs are in a unique position to support clients in adopting a habit of regular physical activity, a health habit that prevents numerous diseases and improves quality and quantity of life for those with disease.[12] Assessing and addressing overall health habits is an important part of a primary care approach to practice as well and, with a set of tools and an approach based on evidence, PTs can successfully partner with clients to promote health and enhance quality and quantity of life.

REFERENCES

1. Adams T, Bezner J, Steinhardt M. The conceptualization and measurement of perceived wellness: integrating balance across and within dimensions. Am J Health Promotion 1997;11:208–18.
2. American Academy of Family Physicians: Primary care (website). http://www.aafp.org/online/en/home/policy/policies/p/primarycare.html. Accessed August 16, 2009.
3. American College of Sports Medicine. The ACSM's guidelines for exercise testing and prescription. 7th ed. Philadelphia: Lippincott Williams & Wilkins; 2006.
3a. American Physical Therapy Association. Guide to physical therapist practice. 2nd ed. Phys Ther 2001;81:9–746.
4. American Physical Therapy Association. Professionalism in physical therapy: core values (website). http://www.apta.org/AM/Template.cfm?Section=Professionalism1&Template=/TaggedPage/TaggedPageDisplay.cfm&TPLID=97&ContentID=21263. Accessed December 1, 2009.
5. Antonovsky A. Unraveling the mystery of health—how people manage stress and stay well. San Francisco: Jossey-Bass Publishers; 1987.
6. Best A, Stokols D, Green LW, et al. An integrative framework for community partnering to translate theory into effective health promotion strategy. Am J Health Promot 2003;18:168–76.
7. Carels RA, Darby L, Cacciapaglia HM, et al. Using motivational interviewing as a supplement to obesity treatment: a stepped-care approach. Health Psychol 2007;26:369–74.
8. Catley D, Harris KJ, Mayo MS, et al. Adherence to principles of motivational interviewing and client within-session behavior. Behav Cognit Psychother 2006;34:43–56.
9. Dallow CB, Anderson J. Using self-efficacy and a transtheoretical model to develop a physical activity intervention for obese women. Am J Health Promot 2003;17:373–81.
10. Davis CM. Patient-practitioner interaction: an experiential manual for developing the art of health care. Thorofare, NJ: Slack; 2006.
11. Dunn HL. High level wellness. Arlington, VA: RW Beatty; 1961.
12. Exercise is Medicine: Health and fitness professionals (website). http://www.exerciseismedicine.org/fitpros.htm. Accessed October 18, 2009.
13. Glanz K, Rimer BK, Viswanath K. Health behavior and health education: theory, research, and practice. San Francisco: Jossey-Bass; 2008.
14. Green LW, Kreuter MW. Health program planning: an educational and ecological approach with PowerWeb bind-in card. 4th ed. New York: McGraw Hill; 2005. p 413.
15. Griffin-Blake CS, DeJoy DM. Evaluation of social-cognitive versus stage-matched, self-help physical activity interventions at the workplace. Am J Health Promot 2006;20:200–9.
16. Hall KL, Rossi JS. Meta-analytic examination of the strong and weak principles across 48 health behaviors. Prev Med 2008;46:266–74.
17. Harland J, White M, Drinkwater C, et al. The Newcastle exercise project: a randomised controlled trial of methods to promote physical activity in primary care. BMJ 1999;319:828–32.
18. Institute of Medicine of the National Academies: Who will keep the public healthy? Workshop Summary, Washington DC, May 22, 2003 (website). http://www.iom.edu/Reports/2003/Who-Will-Keep-the-Public-Healthy-Workshop-Summary.aspx. Accessed March 26, 2010.
19. Jasnoski ML, Schwartz GE. A synchronous systems model for health. Am Behav Scientist 1985;28:468–85.
20. Marcus BH, Forsyth LH. Motivating people to be physically active. Champagne, IL: Human Kinetics; 2003.
21. Marcus BH, Rossi JS, Selby VC, et al. The stages and processes of exercise adoption and maintenance in a worksite sample. Health Psychol 1992;11:386–95.
22. McAuley E, Courneya KS. Adherence to exercise and physical activity as health-promoting behaviors: attitudinal and self-efficacy influences. Appl Prev Psychol 1993;2:65–77.
22a. Miller WR. Motivational interviewing with problem drinkers. Behav Psychother 1983;11:147–72.
23. Mokdad AH, Marks JS, Stroup DF, Gerberding JL. Actual causes of death in the United States, 2000. JAMA 2004;291:1238–45.
24. Nicholas DR, Gobble DC, Crose RG, Frank B. A systems view of health, wellness and gender: implications for mental health counseling. J Mental Health Counsel 1992;14:8–19.
25. Prochaska JO. Decision making in the transtheoretical model of behavior change. Med Decis Making 2008;28:845–9.
26. Prochaska JO, Velicer WF. The transtheoretical model of health behavior change. Am J Health Promot 1997;12:38–48.
27. Ratner PA, Johnson JL, Jeffery B. Examining emotional, physical, social and spiritual health as determinants of self-rated health status. Am J Health Promot 1998;12:275–82.
28. Resnicow K, Jackson A, Wang T, et al. A motivational interviewing intervention to increase fruit and vegetable intake through black churches: results of the Eat for Life Trial. Am J Publ Health 2001;91:1686–93.
29. Resnicow K, Kilorio C, Soet JE, et al. Motivational interviewing in health promotion: it sounds like something is changing. Health Psychol 2002;21:444–51.
30. Rhode R. Motivational Interviewing, from the American Journal of Health Promotion Conference, Las Vegas; March 20-23, 2006.
31. Rollnick S, Miller WR, Butler CC. Motivational interviewing in health care. New York: Guilford Press; 2008.
32. Rovniak LS, Hovell MF, Wojcik JR, et al. Enhancing theoretical fidelity: an e-mail-based walking program demonstration. Am J Health Promot 2005;20:85–95.
33. Seeman J. Toward a model of positive health. Am Psychol 1989;44:1099–109.
34. Smith BJ, Tang KC, Nutbeam D. WHO health promotion glossary: new terms. Health Promot Int 2006;21:340–5.
35. VanWormer JJ, Boucher JL. Motivational interviewing and diet modification: a review of the evidence. Diabet Educator 2004;30:404–16.
36. Ware JE: SF-36 health survey update (website). http://www.sf-36.org/tools/sf36.shtml. Accessed December 1, 2009.
37. West DS, DiLillo V, Bursac Z, et al. Motivational interviewing improves weight loss in women with type 2 diabetes. Diabetes Care 2007;30:1081–7.
38. Williams BR, Bezner J, Chesbro SB, Leavitt R. The relationship between achievement of walking goals and exercise self-efficacy in postmenopausal African American women. Topics Geriatr Rehabil 2008;24:305–14.
39. World Health Organization: The Ottawa Charter for health promotion (website). http://www.who.int/healthpromotion/conferences/previous/ottawa/en/. Accessed December 1, 2009.
40. World Health Organization. Preamble to the Constitution of the World Health Organization. Geneva: World Health Organization; 1948.

Appendix **19-1** **Perceived Wellness Survey (PWS)**[1]

The following statements are designed to provide information about your wellness perceptions. Please carefully and thoughtfully consider each statement, then select the *one* response option with which you *most* agree.

	Very Strongly Disagree					Very Strongly Agree
1. I am always optimistic about my future.	1	2	3	4	5	6
2. There have been times when I felt inferior to most of the people I knew.	1	2	3	4	5	6
3. Members of my family come to me for support.	1	2	3	4	5	6
4. My physical health has restricted me in the past.	1	2	3	4	5	6
5. I believe there is a real purpose for my life.	1	2	3	4	5	6
6. I will always seek out activities that challenge me to think and reason.	1	2	3	4	5	6
7. I rarely count on good things happening to me.	1	2	3	4	5	6
8. In general, I feel confident about my abilities.	1	2	3	4	5	6
9. Sometimes I wonder if my family will really be there for me when I am in need.	1	2	3	4	5	6
10. My body seems to resist physical illness very well.	1	2	3	4	5	6
11. Life does not hold much future promise for me.	1	2	3	4	5	6
12. I avoid activities that require me to concentrate.	1	2	3	4	5	6
13. I always look on the bright side of things.	1	2	3	4	5	6
14. I sometimes think I am a worthless individual.	1	2	3	4	5	6
15. My friends know they can always confide in me and ask me for advice.	1	2	3	4	5	6
16. My physical health is excellent.	1	2	3	4	5	6
17. Sometimes I don't understand what life is all about.	1	2	3	4	5	6
18. In general, I feel pleased with the amount of intellectual stimulation I receive in my daily life.	1	2	3	4	5	6
19. In the past, I have expected the best.	1	2	3	4	5	6
20. I am uncertain about my ability to do things well in the future.	1	2	3	4	5	6
21. My family has been available to support me in the past.	1	2	3	4	5	6
22. Compared with people I know, my past physical health has been excellent.	1	2	3	4	5	6
23. I feel a sense of mission about my future.	1	2	3	4	5	6
24. The amount of information that I process in a typical day is just about right for me (i.e., not too much and not too little).	1	2	3	4	5	6
25. In the past, I hardly ever expected things to go my way.	1	2	3	4	5	6
26. I will always be secure with who I am.	1	2	3	4	5	6
27. In the past, I have not always had friends with whom I could share my joys and sorrows.	1	2	3	4	5	6
28. I expect to always be physically healthy.	1	2	3	4	5	6
29. I have felt in the past that my life was meaningless.	1	2	3	4	5	6
30. In the past, I have generally found intellectual challenges to be vital to my overall well-being.	1	2	3	4	5	6
31. Things will not work out the way I want them to in the future.	1	2	3	4	5	6
32. In the past, I have felt sure of myself among strangers.	1	2	3	4	5	6
33. My friends will be there for me when I need help.	1	2	3	4	5	6
34. I expect my physical health to get worse.	1	2	3	4	5	6
35. It seems that my life has always had purpose.	1	2	3	4	5	6
36. My life has often seemed void of positive mental stimulation.	1	2	3	4	5	6

Appendix **19-2** PWS Scoring Sheet[1]

SCORING SHEET

Instructions: Record your score from the PWS instrument for each numbered item below. Note the * items indicating reverse scoring. Add the numbers in each column and divide by 6 to determine each subscale score.
*Reverse score (e.g., 1 = 6, 2 = 5, 3 = 4, 4 = 3, 5 = 2, and 6 = 1).

PSYCHOLOGICAL

Item Number	Score
1.	3
*7.	3=4
13.	4
19.	4
*25.	4=3
*31.	3=4
Total = 22	
Divided by 6 = 3.6	

PHYSICAL

Item Number	Score
*4.	2=5
10.	6
16.	5
22.	4
28.	5
*34.	2=5
Total = 30	
Divided by 6 = 5.0	

EMOTIONAL

Item Number	Score
*2.	4=3
8.	5
*14.	3=4
*20.	3=4
26.	3
32.	4
Total = 23	
Divided by 6 = 3.8	

SPIRITUAL

Item Number	Score
5.	2
*11.	3=4
*17.	4=3
23.	2
*29.	4=3
35.	3
Total = 17	
Divided by 6 = 2.8	

SOCIAL

Item Number	Score
3.	5
*9.	2=5
15.	6
21.	6
*27.	2=5
33.	6
Total = 33	
Divided by 6 = 5.5	

INTELLECTUAL

Item Number	Score
6.	5
*12.	1=6
18.	5
24.	5
30.	5
*36.	1=6
Total = 32	
Divided by 6 = 5.3	

Appendix **19-3** Physical Activity Readiness-Questionnaire

Physical Activity Readiness
Questionnaire - PAR-Q
(revised 2002)

PAR-Q & YOU

(A Questionnaire for People Aged 15 to 69)

Regular physical activity is fun and healthy, and increasingly more people are starting to become more active every day. Being more active is very safe for most people. However, some people should check with their doctor before they start becoming much more physically active.

If you are planning to become much more physically active than you are now, start by answering the seven questions in the box below. If you are between the ages of 15 and 69, the PAR-Q will tell you if you should check with your doctor before you start. If you are over 69 years of age, and you are not used to being very active, check with your doctor.

Common sense is your best guide when you answer these questions. Please read the questions carefully and answer each one honestly: check YES or NO.

YES	NO		
☐	☐	**1.**	**Has your doctor ever said that you have a heart condition <u>and</u> that you should only do physical activity recommended by a doctor?**
☐	☐	**2.**	**Do you feel pain in your chest when you do physical activity?**
☐	☐	**3.**	**In the past month, have you had chest pain when you were not doing physical activity?**
☐	☐	**4.**	**Do you lose your balance because of dizziness or do you ever lose consciousness?**
☐	☐	**5.**	**Do you have a bone or joint problem (for example, back, knee or hip) that could be made worse by a change in your physical activity?**
☐	☐	**6.**	**Is your doctor currently prescribing drugs (for example, water pills) for your blood pressure or heart condition?**
☐	☐	**7.**	**Do you know of <u>any other reason</u> why you should not do physical activity?**

If

you

answered

YES to one or more questions

Talk with your doctor by phone or in person BEFORE you start becoming much more physically active or BEFORE you have a fitness appraisal. Tell your doctor about the PAR-Q and which questions you answered YES.

- You may be able to do any activity you want — as long as you start slowly and build up gradually. Or, you may need to restrict your activities to those which are safe for you. Talk with your doctor about the kinds of activities you wish to participate in and follow his/her advice.
- Find out which community programs are safe and helpful for you.

NO to all questions

If you answered NO honestly to <u>all</u> PAR-Q questions, you can be reasonably sure that you can:

- start becoming much more physically active — begin slowly and build up gradually. This is the safest and easiest way to go.
- take part in a fitness appraisal — this is an excellent way to determine your basic fitness so that you can plan the best way for you to live actively. It is also highly recommended that you have your blood pressure evaluated. If your reading is over 144/94, talk with your doctor before you start becoming much more physically active.

DELAY BECOMING MUCH MORE ACTIVE:

- if you are not feeling well because of a temporary illness such as a cold or a fever — wait until you feel better; or
- if you are or may be pregnant — talk to your doctor before you start becoming more active.

PLEASE NOTE: If your health changes so that you then answer YES to any of the above questions, tell your fitness or health professional. Ask whether you should change your physical activity plan.

<u>Informed Use of the PAR-Q</u>: The Canadian Society for Exercise Physiology, Health Canada, and their agents assume no liability for persons who undertake physical activity, and if in doubt after completing this questionnaire, consult your doctor prior to physical activity.

No changes permitted. You are encouraged to photocopy the PAR-Q but only if you use the entire form.

NOTE: If the PAR-Q is being given to a person before he or she participates in a physical activity program or a fitness appraisal, this section may be used for legal or administrative purposes.

"I have read, understood and completed this questionnaire. Any questions I had were answered to my full satisfaction."

NAME _____

SIGNATURE _____ DATE_____

SIGNATURE OF PARENT _____ WITNESS _____
or GUARDIAN (for participants under the age of majority)

Note: This physical activity clearance is valid for a maximum of 12 months from the date it is completed and becomes invalid if your condition changes so that you would answer YES to any of the seven questions.

 © Canadian Society for Exercise Physiology   Supported by: Health Canada   Santé Canada

continued on other side...

Continued

...continued from other side

PAR-Q & YOU

Physical Activity Readiness
Questionnaire - PAR-Q
(revised 2002)

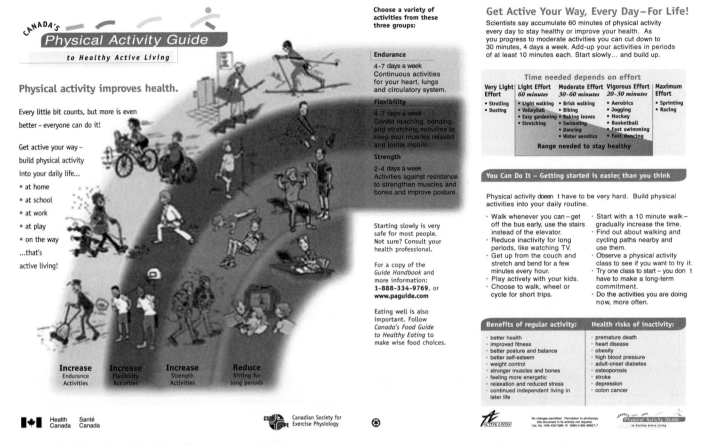

CANADA'S Physical Activity Guide
to Healthy Active Living

Physical activity improves health.

Every little bit counts, but more is even better – everyone can do it!

Get active your way – build physical activity into your daily life...

- at home
- at school
- at work
- at play
- on the way

...that's active living!

Increase Endurance Activities

Increase Flexibility Activities

Increase Strength Activities

Reduce Sitting for long periods

Choose a variety of activities from these three groups:

Endurance
4-7 days a week
Continuous activities for your heart, lungs and circulatory system.

Flexibility
4-7 days a week
Gentle reaching, bending and stretching activities to keep your muscles relaxed and joints mobile.

Strength
2-4 days a week
Activities against resistance to strengthen muscles and bones and improve posture.

Starting slowly is very safe for most people. Not sure? Consult your health professional.

For a copy of the *Guide Handbook* and more information:
1-888-334-9769, or **www.paguide.com**

Eating well is also important. Follow *Canada's Food Guide to Healthy Eating* to make wise food choices.

Get Active Your Way, Every Day–For Life!

Scientists say accumulate 60 minutes of physical activity every day to stay healthy or improve your health. As you progress to moderate activities you can cut down to 30 minutes, 4 days a week. Add-up your activities in periods of at least 10 minutes each. Start slowly... and build up.

Time needed depends on effort

Very Light Effort	Light Effort 60 minutes	Moderate Effort 30-60 minutes	Vigorous Effort 20-30 minutes	Maximum Effort
• Strolling • Dusting	• Light walking • Volleyball • Easy gardening • Stretching	• Brisk walking • Biking • Raking leaves • Swimming • Dancing • Water aerobics	• Aerobics • Jogging • Hockey • Basketball • Fast swimming • Fast dancing	• Sprinting • Racing
		Range needed to stay healthy		

You Can Do It – Getting started is easier than you think

Physical activity doesn't have to be very hard. Build physical activities into your daily routine.

- Walk whenever you can – get off the bus early, use the stairs instead of the elevator.
- Reduce inactivity for long periods, like watching TV.
- Get up from the couch and stretch and bend for a few minutes every hour.
- Play actively with your kids.
- Choose to walk, wheel or cycle for short trips.

- Start with a 10 minute walk – gradually increase the time.
- Find out about walking and cycling paths nearby and use them.
- Observe a physical activity class to see if you want to try it.
- Try one class to start – you don't have to make a long-term commitment.
- Do the activities you are doing now, more often.

Benefits of regular activity:	Health risks of inactivity:
· better health · improved fitness · better posture and balance · better self-esteem · weight control · stronger muscles and bones · feeling more energetic · relaxation and reduced stress · continued independent living in later life	· premature death · heart disease · obesity · high blood pressure · adult-onset diabetes · osteoporosis · stroke · depression · colon cancer

Health Canada   Santé Canada

CSEP SCPE   Canadian Society for Exercise Physiology

ACTIVE LIVING

No changes permitted. Permission to photocopy this document in its entirety not required. Cat. No. H39-429/1998-1E ISBN 0-662-86627-7

Physical Activity Guide to Healthy Active Living

Source: Canada's Physical Activity Guide to Healthy Active Living, Health Canada, 1998 http://www.hc-sc.gc.ca/hppb/paguide/pdf/guideEng.pdf
© Reproduced with permission from the Minister of Public Works and Government Services Canada, 2002.

FITNESS AND HEALTH PROFESSIONALS MAY BE INTERESTED IN THE INFORMATION BELOW:

The following companion forms are available for doctors' use by contacting the Canadian Society for Exercise Physiology (address below):

The **Physical Activity Readiness Medical Examination (PARmed-X)** – to be used by doctors with people who answer YES to one or more questions on the PAR-Q.

The **Physical Activity Readiness Medical Examination for Pregnancy (PARmed-X for Pregnancy)** – to be used by doctors with pregnant patients who wish to become more active.

References:

Arraix, G.A., Wigle, D.T., Mao, Y. (1992). Risk Assessment of Physical Activity and Physical Fitness in the Canada Health Survey Follow-Up Study. **J. Clin. Epidemiol.** 45:4 419-428.

Mottola, M., Wolfe, L.A. (1994). Active Living and Pregnancy, In: A. Quinney, L. Gauvin, T. Wall (eds.), **Toward Active Living: Proceedings of the International Conference on Physical Activity, Fitness and Health**. Champaign, IL: Human Kinetics.

PAR-Q Validation Report, British Columbia Ministry of Health, 1978.

Thomas, S., Reading, J., Shephard, R.J. (1992). Revision of the Physical Activity Readiness Questionnaire (PAR-Q). **Can. J. Spt. Sci.** 17:4 338-345.

For more information, please contact the:

Canadian Society for Exercise Physiology
202-185 Somerset Street West
Ottawa, ON K2P 0J2
Tel. 1-877-651-3755 • FAX (613) 234-3565
Online: www.csep.ca

The original PAR-Q was developed by the British Columbia Ministry of Health. It has been revised by an Expert Advisory Committee of the Canadian Society for Exercise Physiology chaired by Dr. N. Gledhill (2002).

Disponible en français sous le titre «Questionnaire sur l'aptitude à l'activité physique - Q-AAP (revisé 2002)».

 CSEP SCPE © Canadian Society for Exercise Physiology   Supported by: 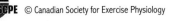 Health Canada   Santé Canada

Appendix **19-4** **Decisional Balance**[20]

SCALE

1 = Not at all important
2 = Slightly important
3 = Moderately important
4 = Very important
5 = Extremely important

1. I would have more energy for my family and friends if I were regularly physically active.	1	2	3	4	5
2. Regular physical activity would help me relieve tension.	1	2	3	4	5
3. I think I would be too tired to do my daily work after being physically active.	1	2	3	4	5
4. I would feel more confident if I were regularly physically active.	1	2	3	4	5
5. I would sleep more soundly if I were regularly physically active.	1	2	3	4	5
6. I would feel good about myself if I kept my commitment to be regularly physically active.	1	2	3	4	5
7. I would find it difficult to find a physical activity that I enjoy and that is not affected by bad weather.	1	2	3	4	5
8. I would like my body better if I were regularly physically active.	1	2	3	4	5
9. It would be easier for me to perform routine physical tasks if I were regularly physically active.	1	2	3	4	5
10. I would feel less stressed if I were regularly physically active.	1	2	3	4	5
11. I feel uncomfortable when I am physically active because I get out of breath and my heart beats very fast.	1	2	3	4	5
12. I would feel more comfortable with my body if I were regularly physically active.	1	2	3	4	5
13. Regular physical activity would take too much of my time.	1	2	3	4	5
14. Regular physical activity would help me have a more positive outlook on life.	1	2	3	4	5
15. I would have less time for my family and friends if I were regularly physically active.	1	2	3	4	5
16. At the end of the day, I am too exhausted to be physically active.	1	2	3	4	5

DECISIONAL BALANCE SCORING

Compute the averages of the 10 pro items and the 6 con items:
Pros = items 1, 2, 4, 5, 6, 8, 9, 10, 12, 14
Cons = items 3, 7, 11, 13, 15, 16
Decisional balance = pros minus cons

Decisional balance score greater than 0 shows more pros than cons. A score less than 0 indicates more cons than pros.

Appendix **19-5** **Agenda-Setting Chart**

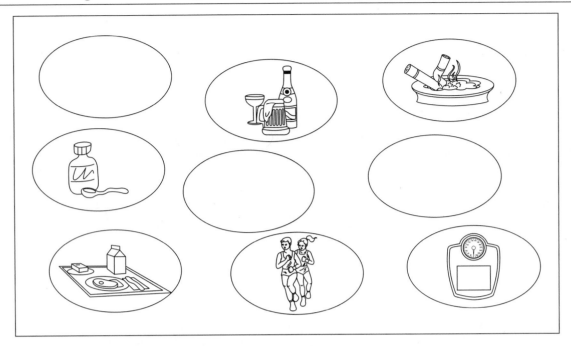

"Do Not Want To Miss List" of Nine Conditions

20

William G. Boissonnault, PT, DPT, DHSc, FAAOMPT

Objectives

After reading this chapter, the reader will be able to:

1. Have increased awareness of the diagnostic challenges associated with each disorder.
2. Understand appropriate medical screening history red flags, tests and measures, and published clinical guidelines.
3. Have an awareness of the current medical diagnostic tests for each condition.

The numerous published case reports and series in the *Physical Therapy Journal* and *Journal of Orthopaedic and Sports Physical Therapy* have demonstrated that screening by physical therapists (PTs) has led to a wide variety of diagnoses being made (ultimately by physicians). The conditions diagnosed include acute injuries, chronic pain conditions, and diseases of almost all body systems, with therapist referrals sometimes being of an urgent nature. The general goal of this chapter is to highlight nine medical conditions that carry great significance in terms of incidence; heath care costs in morbidity, mortality, dollars, and resources; and diagnostic challenges for clinicians. Some conditions, such as myocardial infarct, are among the most common disorders in the United States, whereas others, such as cauda equina and cervical myelopathy, are rare in the general population but involve potentially urgent surgical referrals in common outpatient populations (e.g., patients with low back or neck pain). Considering the detailed examination that PTs carry out, and the usually excellent rapport that therapists develop with patients and family, PTs are in an excellent position to detect clinical red flags and make timely referrals.

Box 20-1 lists the nine disorders discussed in this chapter.

BOX 20-1

"Do Not Want To Miss List" of Nine Conditions

Major depression
Suicide risk
Femoral head and neck fractures
Cauda equina syndrome
Cervical myelopathy
Abdominal aortic aneurysm
Deep venous thrombosis
Pulmonary embolism
Atypical myocardial infarction

Major Depression

Depression is common in the United States—in the general population and in patients in rehabilitation—with major depression carrying significance related to morbidity, mortality (approximately 15% of these patients will commit suicide), and health care costs. Early recognition and referral are critical for appropriate treatment to be implemented. Chapters 5, 17 (depression associated with pregnancy and postpartum), and 18 (geriatric population) include additional information on depression. Estimates are that the lifetime risk for major depression is 10% to 25% for women and 5% to 12% for men[2]; in primary care settings, the prevalence ranges from 5% to 13% for adults.[42] Although more than 50% will experience remission in their condition, the estimates are that approximately half of these individuals will relapse in the subsequent year.[42]

Risk Factors

See Box 20-2 for a list of important risk factors related to major depressive disorder.[2,42,47]

Clinical Manifestations

For the general population, a two-question initial screening is recommended, with a positive response leading to a more detailed assessment. This screening tool asks the following questions: "Over the past 2 weeks have you felt (1) down, depressed or hopeless, and/or (2) little interest or pleasure in doing things?" A positive response carries a sensitivity of 96% (95% CI, 90% to 99%) and a specificity of 57% (95% CI, 53% to 62%).[46] Figure 20-1 illustrates a decision-making flow chart for clinicians.

Awareness of and application of these screening tools should facilitate PTs' willingness to screen for this condition. One of the obstacles leading to delayed diagnosis is reluctance on the part of clinicians to broach this topic with patients. Haggman and colleagues[23] have noted some clinics' unwillingness to participate in their study based on the therapists' thinking that the topic of depression is too invasive and could potentially upset or deter new patients.

Suicide Risk

Although suicide risk is not exclusively tied to a history of major depression and chemical dependency, they are considered key risk factors. See the earlier discussion of depression (and Chapters 5, 17, and 18) and Chapter 8 for chemical dependency screening details. Suicide was the 11th leading cause of death in the United States in 2001, with approximately 500,000 individuals seeking care in emergency departments related to suicide

---

BOX 20-2

Risk Factors Related to Major Depressive Disorder

- Current or previous history of major depression
- Women, especially during pregnancy or postpartum
- History of diabetes, myocardial infarction, cancer, stroke, chemical dependency
- Suffering from significant loss, including change in social status
- Positive family history (first-degree relative)

---

attempts. In persons aged 15 to 24 years, suicide is the third leading cause of death. Estimates are that 2% to 3% of patients seen in primary care settings have had suicide ideation within the last 4 weeks. In addition, 50% to 67% of individuals committing suicide will have seen a physician within 4 weeks of the act.[20]

Risk Factors

Box 20-3 lists suicide risk factors. Men aged 65 years or older are the highest risk group for completed suicides. Race is also a factor, with approximately 75% of completed suicides involving white men. Estimates are that approximately 90% of those committing suicide have a history of psychiatric illness, with most having major depression (odds ratio [OR], 33.1; 95% CI, 10.9% to 99.6%) and/or alcohol abuse (OR, 16.7; 95% CI, 3.9% to 71.4%). The sense of hopelessness is a factor that could be associated with patients commonly seen by physical therapists, especially those with chronic progressive disorders or chronic unrelenting conditions.[8,20]

Clinical Manifestations

A sense of hopelessness and the sense of giving up can be expressed in a number of ways:

- "I don't know how much longer I can take this."
- Stopping therapy, with potential for continued progress
- Stopping other forms of treatment (e.g., medications)

Patients expressing thoughts of death (100% sensitivity, 81% specificity, 5.9% positive predictive value) and wishing they were dead (92% sensitivity, 93% specificity, 14% positive predictive value) are also relevant to screening patients for suicidal ideation.[20] However, it is important to understand that many individuals with suicidal ideation will not volunteer their plan so, when concerned, asking patients whether they are having thoughts of attempting to harm themselves is critical.

If a patient responds "yes" to the question of having thoughts of attempting to harm himself or herself, the clinician should initiate the facility's protocol related to this scenario. This should include important follow-up questions regarding whether the patient has a plan in place, whether resources related to the patient's plan are readily available (e.g., patient own a gun, has filled a medication prescription), and who should then be contacted.

Femoral Head and Neck Fractures

A timely referral for diagnostic imaging can prevent a nondisplaced fracture from progressing to a displaced fracture. In the case of femoral head and neck injuries, surgical intervention will subsequently follow. The relevance of femoral head and neck fractures is that once the injury occurs, significant morbidity, mortality, and health care issues arise.[6,7]

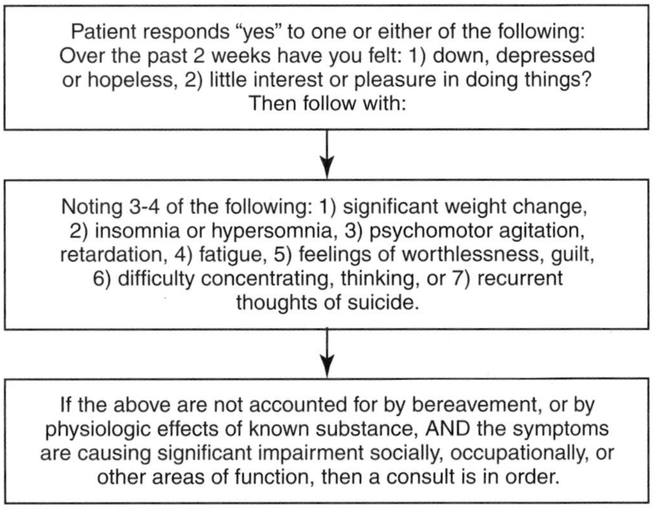

FIGURE 20-1 Flow chart for PTs showing sequence of screening questions. Because of the high sensitivity value associated with the initial two questions, a "no" response to both, especially in an individual without a history of depression in the past year, makes it very unlikely a major depressive episode is present. Because of the low specificity value, a "yes" response is not diagnostic but requires that additional patient information be collected.

BOX 20-3

Common Risk Factors Associated with Suicide Risk

- Gender
  - Males (higher rate of suicide completion)
  - Females (higher rate of suicide attempts)
- Widowed, divorced, living alone
- History of psychiatric illness
  - Primarily major depression and/or alcohol abuse
- Previous suicide attempt
- History of chronic progressive illnesses
- Recent significant loss (e.g., death of loved one, loss of job)
- Unemployed
- Sense of hopelessness
- Family history of suicide completion or attempts

Fractures have been described as being the second most frequently noted musculoskeletal injury in the general population (22%), exceeded only by sprains and strains (38%).[41] Osteoporosis-related fractures most commonly involve the femur and lumbar vertebrae and, compared with all stress fracture sites, the location most likely to progress to a displaced fracture is the head and neck of the femur.[41] An estimated 30% of those suffering a hip fracture die within 1 year, and the estimated direct cost following hip fracture in the United States is $40,000 during the first year and up to $5000 in subsequent years.[7] Braithwaite and associates[6] have described a lifetime cost of hip fracture to be more than $80,000 per injury. DeFranco and coworkers[14] have estimated that 11% of stress fractures in athletes involve the femoral neck, and File and colleagues[15] have estimated that the incidence of delayed diagnosis of hip fracture ranges from 2% to 9%. In athletes and military servicemen and women, once the femoral fracture occurs, return to normally high levels of activity is significantly compromised.[5]

The classic manifestations of fractures include the following:
- Pain and local tenderness
- Deformity
- Edema
- Ecchymosis
- Loss of general function and mobility

With displaced femoral head and neck fractures, the primary loss of function and mobility relate to compromised weight-bearing status, and the onset of pain is related to major trauma, typically a fall. There may or may not be ecchymosis or edema, and palpatory tenderness is questionable for these lesions; often, palpation may lead to a patient response of "that is the painful area but you are not deep enough." The common deformity includes a shortened lower limb, with a position of comfort being external rotation and abduction. Any clinician seeing such a patient will take the appropriate action. Conversely, a nondisplaced femoral head or neck fracture can have a more confusing and much less severe presentation, resulting in a delay in diagnosis, placing the individual at high risk for progression to a displaced fracture.

Nondisplaced femoral fractures can be categorized as insufficiency or fatigue fractures. Insufficiency fractures involve bone that is deficient in mineral density or elastic resistance, whereas fatigue fractures are associated with bone of normal density and elasticity. Both types of fractures, with the associated pain onset, are typically not marked by major trauma or mechanism of injury. A patient with compromised bone density may sustain a fracture as a result of relatively minor trauma, such as a slip versus a fall, sneezing, lifting a gallon of milk out of a car, or trying to open a window that is stuck. These patients often do not come into the clinic with a diagnosis of osteoporosis, but other items in their medical history should raise suspicion of compromised bone density.

Risk Factors

Risk factors are different for insufficiency and fatigue fractures. Box 20-4 lists a variety of disorders, medications, and substances that may compromise bone density[21,22] (see Chapters 17 and 18 for additional information related to osteoporosis). These risk factors are in addition to those such as gender (female), age (older than 50 years, and then further risk in those older than 70 years), and ectomorphic body build.[21] The PT should assume that patients with these factors in their medical history have reduced bone density, and thus should have heightened vigilance for insufficiency fractures. The therapist should use a different definition of trauma that could result in fracture compared with patients who do not have this type of medical history.

Fatigue fractures (called stress fractures, or osseous stress reaction injuries; see Chapter 14) are typically associated with those involved in repetitive activity (e.g., athletes, military personnel, dancers). See Box 20-5 for a list of risk factors associated with fatigue fractures.

Clinical Manifestations

Bony lesions of the femoral head and neck regions typically present with pain noted in the groin, greater trochanteric, and/or buttock regions. Referred pain into the anteromedial thigh and knee could be the chief presenting complaint, potentially causing diagnostic confusion. The pain will be provoked with increased weight bearing and relieved with reduced weight bearing but,

---

BOX 20-4

Disorders, Medications, and Substances Associated With Compromised Bone Density

DISORDER
- Chronic renal failure
- GI malabsorption syndrome
- Rheumatoid arthritis
- Ankylosing spondylitis
- Hyperparathyroidism
- Hyperthroidism
- Hypogonadism
- Type 2 diabetes
- Multiple sclerosis
- Chronic alcohol dependency
- Cushing's syndrome

MEDICATION OR SUBSTANCE USE OR ABUSE
- Aluminum
- Anticonvulsants
- Corticosteroids
- Cytotoxic drugs
- Excessive thyroxine
- Heparin, warfarin (Coumadin)
- Methotrexate
- Caffeine (>three cups daily of caffeinated coffee)
- Tobacco
- Soft drinks

BOX 20-5

Factors Associated With Increased Risk of Developing Fatigue Fractures

- Female gender; hormonal, menstrual irregularities
- Involvement in running, jumping, marching activities
- Change in training program or routine (e.g., new activity, increased activity intensity, change in footwear and training surface)
- Nutritional deficiencies
- Leg length discrepancy
- Diminished muscle strength

---

over time, the individual will tolerate less weight bearing and get less relief when the limb is unloaded. Johansson and associates[27] have reported an average delay of 14 weeks in diagnosing femoral neck stress fractures in athletes, and Johnson and coworkers[28] have reported a 4- to 12- week delay in diagnosis in military recruits. The delay has been attributed to various factors: the insidious onset of pain (pain can be initially mild—many will not present with an antalgic gait); hip range-of-motion (ROM) testing often reveals minor if any pain provocation (many will present with normal ROM and strength)[10]; and/or plain films are often negative (plain film radiographs can be negative for 2 to 3 months after the onset of stress fracture–related pain[19,31]).[11,27]

A useful test to include when suspicion of a nondisplaced femoral fracture is high is the patellar-pubic percussion test.[15,40] Figure 20-2 illustrates the examination technique.

AUSCULTATORY PERCUSSION ASSESSMENT OF BONY INTEGRITY. There is a difference in pitch when comparing the uninvolved leg with the painful limb. The involved limb produces a sound that is duller and diminished in quality, which is indicative of bony abnormality. Tiru and associates[40] have used this test on

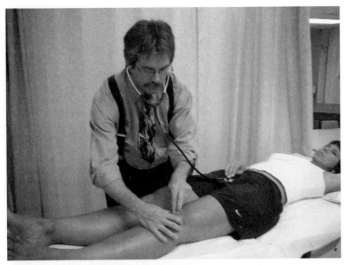

FIGURE 20-2 Patellar-pubic percussion test. The patient is comfortably positioned supine **(1)**; the legs are placed in a symmetric position **(2)**; the head of the stethoscope is positioned in the midline, on the pubic symphysis **(3)**; and the therapist holds the patella in place **(4)** and percusses sharply on the patella **(5)**.

290 patients with suspected occult femoral neck fracture; their analyses revealed a sensitivity of 0.96 (95% CI, 0.87 to 0.99), specificity of 0.86 (95% CI, 0.49 to 0.98), positive predictive value of 0.98, and negative predictive value of 0.75; the likelihood ratios for a positive test were 6.73 and for a negative test, 0.75. A positive test would warrant strong consideration of advanced imaging (magnetic resonance imaging [MRI] or bone scan).

FULCRUM TEST. Johnson and colleagues[28] have described another special test for femoral shaft stress fractures, the fulcrum test. The patient is sitting, with the therapist placing his or her forearm under the patient's thigh (in the area of pain). The therapist then applies gentle downward pressure on the dorsum of the knee, with a positive response being pain provocation. Weishaar and associates[43] have described this technique in the context of two patients presenting with thigh pain secondary to stress fractures.

Cauda Equina Syndrome

Although relatively uncommon, cauda equina carries risk of significant irreversible neurologic compromise, often requiring urgent surgical intervention. Loss of bladder, bowel, and sexual function are potentially associated serious morbidities.[18] The estimates of cauda equina incidence range from 1% to 16% of those with disk herniation and 1% to 3% of those undergoing disk surgery.[18,26] In addition to lumbar disk herniation, tumor, infections, spinal stenosis, and hematoma have been linked with cauda equina.[29]

Risk Factors

Various conditions carry an increased risk of cauda equina compromise, including the following:

- Low back injury, central disk herniation
- Congenital or acquired spinal stenosis (degenerative disk or facet joint disease, degenerative spondylolisthesis)
- Spinal fracture
- Ankylosing spondylitis
- Tuberculosis, Pott's disease

Clinical Manifestations

Cauda equina is rare in patients with low back pain only, with an estimate of 4 in 10,000.[26] Although limb and perhaps back pain can be present, the classic presentation is marked by neurologic compromise—motor and sensory deficits, urinary and bowel dysfunction, and sexual dysfunction (Box 20-6).

The PT's initial concern regarding the presence of cauda equina may be the observation of gait ataxia and/or balance problems. Patients' complaints of legs feeling heavy and weak or difficulty in navigating stairs or ramps should be warning signs to perform a detailed neurologic screening (see Chapters 12 and 13) and ask detailed questions regarding bladder, bowel, and sexual function. The latter can be challenging because many patients are embarrassed talking about these activities. Questions regarding these functions must be very specific (see Chapter 9) considering that many patients may interpret "no pain" with urination or defecation as "having no problems". Typically, pain during these functions is not associated with cauda equina syndrome and, if the patient is asked only about incontinence, he or she may not indicate that urinary retention is present. Chou and coworkers[9] have described urinary retention as being the most frequently noted cauda equina manifestation (90% sensitivity); without urinary retention, the probability of cauda equina is estimated to be 1 in 10,000.

The onset of these symptoms may be abrupt and subsequently more alarming to patients, or they may be slow and gradual.[18,29] In summary, a recent literature review on cauda equina syndrome has found significant inconsistencies regarding definitions of cause and clinical presentation; the authors recommended careful and detailed examination of patients with low back and leg symptoms.[18]

Cervical Myelopathy

There are parallels between the diagnostic challenges for cauda equina and cervical myelopathy. Coronado and coworkers[12] have described the discord between MRI findings of cervical spine stenosis and spinal cord compromise and classic symptoms (e.g., neck pain, paresthesia, progressive hand clumsiness) associated with these findings. Clinical manifestations associated with both conditions can be highly variable in terms of symptomatic presentation, including progression of the disorder. This diagnostic challenge is of concern, considering the potentially serious ramifications associated with cervical spinal cord compromise. Combining patient data from a detailed history and physical examination, leading to radiographic and/or electrodiagnostic assessment, provides the best opportunity for a timely referral to a physician.[3]

Risk Factors

Cervical myelopathy is typically associated with cervical spine spondylotic changes. Cervical spondylosis is very common in older adults and is the most common cause of nontraumatic spastic paraparesis and quadriparesis. Although Matz and colleagues[32] have reported wide variation in the natural history of cervical spondylotic myelopathy, neurologic symptoms associated with spinal degeneration generally start in individuals in their mid-50s to 60s. The incidence increases with each subsequent decade. Spinal degeneration can occur in younger populations with a history of significant neck trauma (e.g., motor vehicle accident, sports injury). Cervical myelopathy can also occur at younger ages in individuals with rheumatoid arthritis. The associated cervical instability can lead to spinal cord compromise.[3,21]

Clinical Manifestations

As with cauda equina, the primary symptoms of cervical myelopathy tend to be neurologic in nature opposed to severe pain complaints. The symptoms are often marked by a slow stepwise progression, but long periods of symptomatic stability can occur.[32] Box 20-7 provides an overview of potential examination findings.

As noted for cauda equina syndrome, questioning regarding urinary function needs to be very specific and exact; there should be no misunderstanding on the patient's part of what he or she is being asked (see Chapter 9). Hand impairment may be manifested by poor handwriting, difficulty with buttoning clothing, and other activities that require hand dexterity. The patient may note difficulty navigating stairs or sidewalk curbs, and/or the therapist may note a slow, stiff gait and possibly a wide base of support as the patient walks to the examination room.[3] Close observation of patients during the entire encounter may reveal subtle signs of potential neurologic involvement, leading to a detailed screening of the nervous system (see Chapters 12 and 13). Coronado and associates[12] have concluded that based on current evidence, a high index of suspicion is often key to the diagnosis of this condition. Identifying patients at increased risk for cervical myelopathy and observing subtle signs of neurologic compromise, leading to a detailed neurologic assessment, can result in a timely referral.

Abdominal Aortic Aneurysm

Visceral causes of back pain are relatively uncommon, constituting up to an estimated 2% of all back pain episodes.[26] When specific age groups are considered, however, the probability of certain disorders occurring increases significantly. For example, most abdominal aortic aneurysms (AAAs) occur in individuals aged 60 years and older, and most AAA-related deaths occur in those 65 years and older. AAA rupture is the 10th leading cause of death in men aged 65 years and older, and ranks 13th in women aged 75 years and older.[13,17]

By definition, an AAA is an abdominal aortic (distal to the renal arteries) vessel diameter of 3 cm or more. Relative risk for abdominal aorta rupture increases as the diameter approaches 5 to 6 cm. The surgery itself carries significant risks, with a

---

BOX 20-7

Potential Examination Findings of Cervical Myelopathy

HISTORY
- Impaired hand dexterity (clumsiness)
- Gait, balance difficulties (legs weak, stiff)
- Numbness, paresthesia—extremities (upper and possibly lower)
- Neck stiffness
- Urinary dysfunction (retention, and possible urgency and frequency)

PHYSICAL EXAMINATION
- Hand—intrinsic atrophy
- Muscle weakness, often of triceps; hand intrinsic
- Muscle weakness of lower extremities (proximal muscles)
- Upper motor neuron signs (hyperactive deep tendon reflexes, clonus, positive Babinski's and Hoffman's signs)

BOX 20-8

Abdominal Aortic Aneurysm (AAA) Risk Factors

- Age
- Male gender
- History of smoking
- History of hypercholesterol and coronary heart disease
- Family history of AAA

---

mortality rate of up to 4.2% and a complication rate of 32%.[17] If the AAA is generating pain, typically the complaint will be back pain, common in those seeking PT services. Therapists must consider the visceral origins of back pain, especially in those in high-risk groups.

Risk Factors

Most AAAs are primarily associated with atherosclerotic vessel changes, with an inflammatory variant deemed secondarily responsible for approximately 5% to 10% of all aneurysms.[24] Considering the association between atherosclerosis and AAAs, some of the risk factors are similar to those associated with coronary heart disease. Box 20-8 lists risk factors for an AAA.

Age and male gender are important risk factors, because the prevalence of AAA is five to six times greater in men than women, and the odds ratios of diagnosing an AAA of 4 cm or larger increases by 1.71 (95% CI, 1.61 to 1.82) for every 7-year interval of age.[17] The prevalence in women increases on average 10 years later in men, with most ruptures occurring in women aged 80 years or older. A history of smoking carries a three to five times greater risk for developing an AAA. The effect of smoking plus age consideration was demonstrated by a study inviting men aged 65 to 74 years of age with a lifetime consumption of smoking more than 100 cigarettes into an AAA screening; it was estimated that this would result in an 89% reduction in AAA-related deaths in this age group.[17] Those with an inflammatory AAA can present at younger ages.[33]

Clinical Manifestations

Unfortunately, in most individuals, the AAA is asymptomatic but, as noted, if pain is a symptom, it will most likely be back pain. In addition to back pain, abdominal, hip, groin, or buttock pain is possible. The pain will have nonmechanical qualities, with possibly an increase in pain intensity noted with general activity, but typically is unchanging with specific spinal movements and postures. At some point, the pain may wake an individual from sleep, and simply changing positions in bed does not provide relief. The pain will be of insidious onset and may progress slowly or quickly. Individuals may also note early satiety, weight loss, and nausea.[21,22]

Considering that an AAA is often described as a palpable abdominal mass, abdominal palpation should be a valuable screening tool. However, the overall accuracy of detecting an AAA with abdominal palpation is 68% sensitivity (95% CI, 60% to 76%) and 75% specificity (95% CI, 68% to 82%). However, if individual girth (>100 cm) and size (diameter ≥5 cm) of the aneurysm are considered, the sensitivity is 100%.[16] Not surprisingly, the smaller the individual's girth, the more likely one will palpate the pulse of a normal aorta (false-positive finding). In fact, I have often observed an abdominal pulse when thin patients are lying supine.

To help with this dilemma, clinicians can use auscultation for a bruit to accompany the palpation findings. Auscultation for an AAA-related bruit carries very low sensitivity (17%), but higher specificity (95%).[30] So, for relatively thin patients with a prominent abdominal pulse, the clinician can auscultate along the course of the aorta; if no bruit is noted, one can be relatively certain that there is no aneurysm of 5 cm diameter or more. Figure 20-3 illustrates abdominal palpation over the abdominal aorta.

Abdominal auscultation over the aorta should occur approximately along the midline and 2 inches cephalad to the umbilicus; hearing a pulse would be considered abnormal at that point in the examination. A short videoclip can be found on the *Journal of Orthopaedic and Sports Physical Therapy* website; an icon will be found with the videoclip describing abdominal palpation and

auscultation related to screening for an AAA.[33a] Also note the study by Mechelli and colleagues.[33]

Finally, in the discussion of screening for AAA, the presence of vessel dissection should be determined. For some individuals, once the vessel begins to leak, death follows quickly, but not for all. If an individual describes back or abdominal pain as hot, searing, ripping, tearing pain that stops all activity until it begins to pass, vascular dissection must be considered as the cause. Depending on the time relationship between the dissection event and next clinic visit, the hot horrible pain could have resolved days prior to the visit. Asking patients about their symptom status since the last visit may reveal a pain pattern unusual for the patient and concerning to the therapist.

Deep Venous Thrombosis

Deep venous thrombosis (DVT) affects approximately 2 million individuals in the United States annually, making it the third most common cardiovascular disease.[1] Considering the risk factors associated with DVT, it is not surprising that it is a relatively common condition in patients seeking physical therapy services. DVT carries significant risk for the development of pulmonary embolism, postphlebitic syndrome, and chronic thromboembolic pulmonary hypertension.[38] Approximately 70% to 80% of lower extremity DVTs develop in the proximal veins (popliteal and superficial femoral veins in particular), and the remainder develop in the calf (anterior tibial, peroneal, and posterior tibial veins).[38,45] A sobering estimation is that approximately 50% of those with a DVT are asymptomatic in the early stages.[21] Clinicians are challenged to identify patients at greater risk for this condition in lieu of the obvious calf pain, swelling, and redness.

Risk Factors

Multiple risk factors exist for developing DVT, providing clinicians with a sense of when to be more vigilant for the condition. The presence of any single item listed[21,22] in Box 20-9 does not mean that the patient has or will develop DVT. However, some of the risk factors, combined with symptoms and signs, can provide the clinician with a useful clinical decision-making rule. Immobility must be interpreted in different ways, including bed rest for longer than 3 days, a long car ride or plane trip, and/or

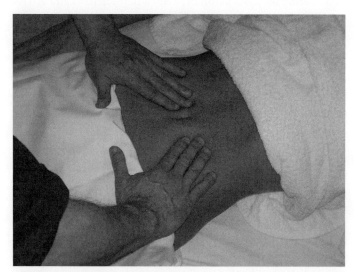

FIGURE 20-3 Abdominal palpation over the aorta. Once a pulse has been detected with midabdominal palpation, the PT places fingertips with deep and gentle pressure along the sides of the pulse, noting the presence of a laterally expansive pulsation. Such a finding would further warrant abdominal auscultation for a bruit.

BOX 20-9

Risk Factors Associated With Development of Deep Venous Thrombosis (DVT)

- Previous history of DVT
- History of cancer
- History of congestive heart failure
- History of systemic lupus erythematosus
- Receiving chemotherapy
- Major surgery
- Major trauma
- Immobility
- Limb paralysis
- Women during pregnancy
- Women taking oral contraceptives, hormone replacement therapy
- Age >60 yr

secondary to a neurologic disorder (e.g., traumatic brain injury, stroke, spinal cord injury).

Clinical Manifestations

As noted, approximately 50% of individuals with DVT are asymptomatic in the early disease phase. Box 20-10 lists potential clinical manifestations of DVT.

The pain and discomfort typically are worsened with walking and relieved with rest and elevation. However, as the condition worsens, the patient will experience comparatively less relief of symptoms with rest.[21,22]

Clinical Decision Rule

No specific symptoms or signs are diagnostic for DVT, but a specific cluster of risk factors and clinical manifestations can be used to establish probability of the condition, thus aiding the clinician in recognizing when a referral should be made. Table 20-1 presents the clinical decision rule for DVT and probability.

A recent study has described a slight modification allowing for determining the presence of DVT as being likely or unlikely. Scarvelis and Wells[38] have described adding another clinical

---

BOX 20-10
Clinical Manifestations Associated with Deep Venous Thrombosis

- Ache, tightness, tenderness
- General edema
- Pitting edema
- Prominent superficial venous plexus
- Increased local skin temperature

TABLE 20-1
Clinical Decision Rule for Deep Venous Thrombosis (DVT)

Clinical Characteristic	Score*
Active cancer (treatment ongoing, within previous 6 mo, or palliative)	1
Paralysis, paresis, or recent plaster immobilization of lower extremities	1
Recently bedridden >3 days, or major surgery in past 12 wk requiring general or regional anesthesia	1
Localized tenderness along distribution of deep venous system	1
Swelling of entire leg	1
Calf swelling > 3cm, more than asymptomatic side (measured 10 cm below tibial tuberosity)	1
Pitting edema confined to symptomatic leg	1
Collateral superficial veins (nonvaricose veins)	1
Alternative diagnosis is as or more likely than DVT	−2

*Key: The score is determined as follows:
−2 to zero = low probability of DVT (5%; 95% CI, 4.0%-8.0%)
1-2 = moderate probability of DVT (17%; 95% CI, 13%-23%)
≥3 = high probability of DVT (53%; 95% CI, 44%-61%)
From Wells PS, Anderson DR, Bormanis J, et al: Value of assessment of pretest probability of deep-vein thrombosis in clinical management, *Lancet* 350:1795-1798, 1997; and Wells PS, Owen C, Doucette S, et al: Does this patient have deep venous thrombosis? *JAMA* 295:199-207, 2006.

---

characteristic to the original clinical decision rule—previously diagnosed DVT = +1, a score of 2 or more indicates that DVT is likely, and a score lower than 2 indicates that DVT is unlikely. Although originally written for physicians, the provided clinical decision rule is relevant for PTs. Each of the 10 criteria represents patient information that would be routinely collected by a PT. Use of a tool such as the clinical decision rule not only assists therapists in recognizing the high probability of DVT but also provides concise information that can be easily expressed to the patient's physician during the referral and/or consultation process.

Pulmonary Embolism

Pulmonary embolism (PE) is associated with high morbidity and mortality, highlighting the critical nature of timely detection. Hull[25] has described PE as one of the "great masqueraders" of medicine because of the often nonspecific presenting symptoms and signs, and Wells and coworkers[44] have estimated that 50% of PEs go undiagnosed. In addition, Scarvelis and colleagues[37] have estimated that more than 50% of PE-related deaths are potentially preventable, in part if an earlier diagnosis had been made. The PE is most frequently associated with a blood clot (DVT), air, fat, or bone marrow; it has been estimated that proximal lower limb DVTs are the most common cause of these episodes (approximately 70%), but the clot origin can also be the upper limb.[48] The estimates of PE-related mortality range from 5% to 20%.[34] PTs provide services to high-risk populations, such as patients who have undergone operative hip, knee, or shoulder procedures. Commonly reported risk factors and clinical manifestations are presented in the next sections but, as with DVT, single factors rarely provide the needed guidance for clinical decision making and diagnosis. Research clustering using a combination of risk factors, symptoms, and signs can provide clinicians with a useful screening tool.

Risk Factors

Box 20-11 lists commonly reported risk factors associated with PE. Age also is a factor—the incidence of PE increases with age (especially in those older than 60 years)—and women have a higher incidence than men older than 50 years.[35] Considered to be minor risk factors are congenital heart disease, congestive heart failure, indwelling catheter, chronic obstructive pulmonary disease, oral contraceptives, and hormone replacement therapy.[21]

BOX 20-11
Risk Factors Associated With Development of Pulmonary Embolism (PE)

- Previous history of PE
- History of DVT
- Immobility
- History of abdominal, pelvic surgery
- Total hip, knee replacement
- Late-stage pregnancy
- Lower limb fractures
- Malignancy of pelvis or abdomen

Clinical Manifestations

As with DVT, individuals with PE can be asymptomatic, depending on the size and location of the clot. Box 20-12 lists common symptoms and signs potentially related to PE.[21,48]

Chapters 9 and 11 provide descriptions and definitions of these manifestations. Young and Flynn have analyzed the most common manifestations of PE: dyspnea, tachypnea, and pleurtic chest pain.[48] They concluded that for patients having no chest pain or dyspnea, there is a moderate to strong chance that PE is not present (Table 20-2).

Clinical Decision Rule

Wells and colleagues[44] have provided clinicians with a clinical decision rule for determining the probability of PE (Table 20-3). As with the DVT clinical decision rule, the established criteria include patient information routinely collected by PTs. A maximum point score would be 12.5 points. This tool provides therapists with a mechanism to identify individuals at risk for PE, resulting in a physician referral, and with specific criteria supporting the therapist's concerns.

Atypical Myocardial Infarction

Chapter 6 provides descriptions of pain associated with myocardial infarction (MI), including the classic pattern of angina—left-sided chest tightness, pressure, and pain with possible referral into the left upper extremity. All PTs, and most of the public, will be alarmed by this presentation, thinking that the heart could be involved. Unfortunately, not everyone suffering an MI presents in this classic pattern; it is less typical for women than men,

leading to delayed diagnosis and potentially poorer outcomes. Death rates associated with cardiovascular disease for women have exceeded those for men since the mid-1980s, and cardiac death is the leading cause of death in women of all ages.[39,49] One reason for the potentially delayed diagnosis and treatment in women is that only approximately 50% of women with an MI have chest pain.[49] Knowledge of other possible clinical manifestations of MI in women is critical for more timely recognition and referral.

Risk Factors

The primary risk factors for MI are similar to those associated with coronary artery disease and can be categorized into modifiable and nonmodifiable risk factors. Box 20-13 lists frequently noted risk factors; their presence should raise the clinician's concern about the possibility of occult heart disease.[21,22]

Clinical Manifestations

As noted, approximately 50% of women experience the expected chest pain (with or without left upper extremity pain) with their ischemic heart disease. Other potential pain locations include

---

BOX 20-12

Clinical Manifestations Associated With Pulmonary Embolism

- Dyspnea
- Tachypnea
- Pleuritic chest pain, intensified with deep respiration and cough
- Persistent cough
- Apprehension, anxiety
- Tachycardia
- Palpitations

TABLE 20-2

Sensitivity, Specificity, and Likelihood Ratios of the Most Common Symptoms of Pulmonary Embolism

Parameter	Dyspnea with Chest Pain
Sensitivity	0.97
Specificity	0.10
Likelihood ratio	
Positive	1.08
Negative	0.30

Adapted from Young BA, Flynn TW: Pulmonary emboli: the differential diagnosis dilemma, *J Orthop Sports Phys Ther* 35:637-644, 2005.

TABLE 20-3

Wells Criteria for Determining Probability of Pulmonary Embolism (PE)*

Criterion	Value (points)
Clinical signs of DVT	3.0
Heart rate >100 beats/min	1.5
Immobilization for 3 days or longer, or surgery in previous 4 wk	1.5
Previous diagnosis of PE or DVT	1.5
Hemoptysis	1.0
Patients with cancer receiving treatment, treatment stopped in past 6 mo, or receiving palliative care	1.0
Alternative diagnosis less likely than PE	3.0

*Pretest probability of PE is low with a score <2 points, moderate with a score of 2-6 points, and high with a score >6 points.

Adapted from Wells PS, Anderson DR, Rodger M, et al: Derivation of a simple clinical model to categorize patients probability of polmonary embolism: increasing the models utility with the Simpli RED d-dimer, *Thromb Haemost* 2000; Mar 83(3): 416-20.

BOX 20-13

Risk Factors Associated With Myocardial Infarction

MODIFIABLE RISK FACTORS
- Cigarette smoking
- High cholesterol levels (low-density lipoprotein and total serum cholesterol levels)
- Hypertension
- Diabetes
- Obesity
- Sedentary lifestyle
- Excessive alcohol consumption

NONMODIFIABLE RISK FACTORS
- Age: >55 yr for women; >45 yr for men
- Family history
- Ethnicity (highest in African Americans)

upper abdominal and epigastric; neck, jaw, and tooth; interscapular and mid to lower thoracic; and right arm pain (possibly isolated at the biceps region). The pain may or may not be associated with exertion.[4,39,49] The upper abdominal discomfort may be interpreted by the individual as being indigestion or heartburn. In fact, the woman may be taking antacids to treat the indigestion, but without relief. In addition to pain, Box 20-14 lists other manifestations associated with women and MI.

The shortness of breath may occur at night, and the fatigue can be extreme. See Chapters 9 and 11 for further descriptions of manifestations of cardiac disease. The manifestations noted, as related to MI and women, may also be present for some men. Not all men have the classic substernal left-sided chest wall pain and pressure. The findings noted would lead the therapist to assess heart rate, blood pressure, and respiratory rate (see Chapter 11).

Older Adults

Older adults are more likely to experience a silent attack (infarction without pain). It is estimated that 21% to 68% of older adults experience the expected, classic exertional angina pain pattern.[36] Those that do experience pain may have a presentation different from that seen in younger populations. Rittger and associates[36] have noted that pain perception in older adults is not only significantly less severe, but also delayed. The cause of this phenomenon is postulated to be multifactorial, including impaired autonomic nerve responsiveness and central pain mechanisms. The literature has described dyspnea as being the most common manifestation in older adults.

Summary

This chapter has presented a screening overview of nine serious medical conditions for which patients with common complaints such as back pain, neck pain, or limb symptoms (e.g., pain, tingling, numbness) may present to PTs, or the condition may present as a secondary health issue (e.g., major depression) associated with chronic back pain. The therapist's concern regarding the presence of these conditions should warrant immediate contact with the patient's primary care physician. The tools presented are screening and not diagnostic tools, but the associated disease probability provides therapists with guidance about the level of their concern. This can then be communicated, not just to the physician, but also to the patient, encouraging the patient to follow through with the PT's consult recommendation. As noted at the beginning of this chapter, these conditions are not the only serious conditions that PTs may encounter clinically. Therapists can work closely with primary care physicians in a particular setting and identify other conditions more commonly seen at those clinics that would carry the same degree of significance and concern.

REFERENCES

1. Anand SS, Wells PS, Hunt D, et al. Does this patient have deep venous thrombosis? JAMA 1998;279:1094–9.
2. American Psychiatric Association. Diagnostic and statistical manual of mental disorders. 4th ed. Washington DC: American Psychiatric Association; 2000.
3. Baron EM, Young WF. Cervical spondylotic myelopathy: a brief review of its pathophysiology, clinical course, and diagnosis. Neurosurgery 2007;60:S35–41.
4. Berg J, Bjorck L, Dudas K, et al. Symptoms of a first acute myocardial infarction in women and men. Gender Med 2009;6:454–62.
5. Boden BP, Osbahr DC. High-risk stress fractures: evaluation and treatment. J Am Acad Orthop Surg 2000;8:344–53.
6. Braithwaite RS, Col NF, Wong JB. Estimating hip fracture morbidity, mortality and costs. J Am Geriatr Soc 2003;51:364–70.
7. Brauer CA, Coca-Perraillon M, Cutler DM, Rosen AB. Incidence and mortality of hip fractures in the United States. JAMA 2009;302:1573–9.
8. Brown GK, Beck AT, Steer R, Grisham JR. Risk factors for suicide in psychiatric outpatients: a 20-year prospective study. J Consult Clin Psychol 2000;68:371–7.
9. Chou R, Qaseem A, Snow V, et al. Diagnosis and treatment of low back pain: a joint clinical practice guideline from the American College of Physicians and the American Pain Society. Ann Intern Med 2007;147:478–91.
10. Clement DB, Ammamm W, Taunton JE, et al. Exercise-induced stress fractures to the femur. Int J Sports Med 1993;14:348–53.
11. Clough TM. Femoral neck stress fracture: the importance of a clinical suspicion and early review. Br J Sports Med 2002;36:308–9.
12. Coronado R, Hudson B, Sheets C, et al. Correlation of magnetic resonance imaging findings and reported symptoms in patients with chronic cervical dysfunction. J Man Manip Ther 2009;17:148–53.
13. National Center for Health Statistics. National Vital Statistics Report: Deaths, percent of total deaths, and death rates for the 15 leading causes of death in 5 year age groups, by race and sex: United States, 2001-2006; (website). http://www.cdc.gov/nchs/data/dvs/LCWKI_2001.pdf. Accessed December 15, 2009.
14. DeFranco MJ, Recht M, Schils J, et al. Stress fractures of the femur in athletes. Clin Sports Med 2006;25:89–103.
15. File P, Wood JP, Kreplick LW. Diagnosis of hip fracture by the auscultatory percussion technique. Am J Emerg Med 1996;16:173–6.
16. Fink HA, Lederle FA, Roth CS, et al. The accuracy of physical examination to detect abdominal aortic aneurysm. Arch Intern Med 2000;160:833–6.
17. Fleming C, Whitlock EP, Beil TL, Lederle FA. Screening for abdominal aortic aneurysm: a best-evidence systematic review of the U.S. Preventive Services Task Force. Ann Intern Med 2005;142:203–11.
18. Fraser S, Roberts L, Murphy E. Cauda equina syndrome: a literature review of its definition and clinical presentation. Arch Phys Med Rehabil 2009;90:1964–8.
19. Fredericson M, Jennings F, Beaulieu C, Matheson GO. Stress fractures in athletes. Topics Magn Reson Imaging 2006;17:309–25.
20. Gaynes BN, West SL, Ford CA, et al. Screening for suicide risk in adults: a summary of the evidence for the U.S. Preventive Services Task Force. Ann Intern Med 2004;140:822–35.
21. Goodman CC, Fuller KS, editors. Pathology: implications for the physical therapist. 3rd ed. St. Louis: Saunders Elsevier; 2009.
22. Gorroll AH, Mulley AG, editors. Primary care medicine. 5th ed. Philadelphia: Lippincott Williams & Wilkins; 2006.
23. Haggman S, Maher CG, Refshauge KM. Screening for symptoms of depression by physical therapists managing low back pain. Phys Ther 2004;84:157–166.
24. Hellmann DB, Grand DJ, Freischlag JA. Inflammatory abdominal aortic aneurysm. JAMA 2007;2297:395–400.
25. Hull RD. Diagnosing pulmonary embolism with improved certainty and simplicity. JAMA 2006;295:213–5.
26. Jarvik JG, Deyo RA. Diagnostic evaluation of low back pain with emphasis on imaging. Ann Intern Med 2002;137:586–97.
27. Johansson C, Ekenman I, Tornkvist H, et al. Stress fractures of the femoral neck in athletes. Am J Sports Med 1990;18:524–8.

BOX 20-14

Clinical Manifestations Associated With Myocardial Infarction in Women

- Shortness of breath
- Fatigue
- Sleep disturbance
- Nausea (with or without vomiting)
- Palpitations
- Dizziness
- Diaphoresis
- Anxiety

28. Johnson AW, Weiss CB, Wheeler DL. Stress fractures of the femoral shaft in athletes—more common than expected. A new clinical test. Am J Sports Med 1994;22:248–56.

29. Lavy C, James A, Wilson-MacDonald J, Fairbank J. Cauda equina syndrome. BMJ 2009;338:881–8.

30. Lederle FA, Walker JM, Reinke DB. Selective screening for abdominal aortic aneurysms with physical examination and ultrasound. Arch Intern Med 1988;148:1753–8.

31. Matheson GO, Clement DB, McKenzie DC, et al. Stress fractures in athletes. Am J Sports Med 1987;15:46–58.

32. Matz PG, Anderson PA, Holly LT, et al. The natural history of cervical spondylotic myelopathy. J Neurosurg Spine 2009;1:104–11.

33. Mechelli F, Proboski Z, Boissonnault W. Differential diagnosis of a patient referred to physical therapy with low back pain: abdominal aortic aneurysm. J Orthop Sports Ther 2008;38:551–7.

33a. Mechelli F, Proboski Z, Boissonnault W. Differential diagnosis of a patient referred to physical therapy with low back pain: abdominal aortic aneurysm. J Orthop Sports Ther 2008;38:551–7 (website). http://www.jospt.org/issues/articleID.14249 type.2/article_detail.asp#relatedVideo.

34. Reidel M. Acute pulmonary embolism 1: pathophysiology, clinical presentation and diagnosis. Heart 2001;85:229–40.

35. Stein PD, Huang H, Afzal A, Noor HA. Incidence of acute pulmonary embolism in a general hospital: relation to age, sex, and race. Chest 1999;116:909–13.

36. Rittger H, Reiber J, Breithardt OA, et al. Influence of age on pain perception in acute myocardial ischemia: a possible cause for delayed treatment in elderly patients. Int J Cardiol January 4, 2010 (Epub).

37. Scarvelis D, Anderson J, Davis L, et al. Hospital morality due to pulmonary embolism and an evaluation of the usefulness of preventive interventions. Thromb Res 2010;125(2):166–70.

38. Scarvelis D, Wells PS. Diagnosis and treatment of deep-vein thrombosis. CMAJ 2006;175:1087–92.

39. Shaw LJ, Bugiardini R, Merz NB. Women and ischemic heart disease. J Am Coll Cardiol 2009;54:1561–75.

40. Tiru M, Goh SH, Low BY. Use of percussion as a screening tool in the diagnosis of occult hip fracture. Singapore Med J 2002;43:467–9.

41. American Academy of Orthopaedic Surgeons. The burden of musculoskeletal diseases in the United States. Rosemont, IL: American Academy of Orthopaedic Surgeons; 2008.

42. U.S. Preventive Services Task Force. Screening for depression in adults: U.S. Preventative Services Task Force recommendation statement. Ann Intern Med 2009;151:784–92.

43. Weishaar MD, McMillian DM, Moore JH. Identification and management of 2 femoral shaft stress injuries. J Orthop Sports Phys Ther 2005;35:665–73.

44. Wells PS, Anderson DR, Rodger M, et al. Excluding pulmonary embolism at the bedside without diagnostic imaging: management of patients with suspected pulmonary embolism presenting to the emergency department by using clinical model and d-dimer. Ann Intern Med 2001;135:98–107.

45. Wells PS, Owen C, Doucette S, et al. Does this patient have deep venous thrombosis? JAMA 2006;295:199–207.

46. Whooley MA, Avins AL, Miranda J, Browner WS. Case-finding instruments for depression: two questions are as good as many. J Gen Intern Med 1997;12:439–45.

47. Wisner KL, Parry BL, Piontek CM. Postpartum depression. N Engl J Med 2002;347:194–9.

48. Young BA, Flynn TW. Pulmonary emboli: the differential diagnosis dilemma. J Orthop Sports Phys Ther 2005;35:637–44.

49. Zbierajewski-Eischeid SJ, Loeb SJ. Myocardial infarction in women: promoting early diagnosis and risk management. Dimens Crit Care Nurs 2009;28:1–6.

Page numbers followed by f, t or b indicate figures, tables, or boxes, respectively.

401